FIELD GUIDE TO WILDERNESS MEDICINE

FIELD GUIDE TO WILDERNESS MEDICINE

THIRD EDITION

Paul S. Auerbach, MD, MS, FACEP, FAWM
Clinical Professor of Surgery
Division of Emergency Medicine
Stanford University School of Medicine
Stanford, California

Howard J. Donner, MD
Wilderness Medicine Consultant, Educator, Guide
Mountain Medical Seminars
Ashland, Oregon

Eric A. Weiss, MD, FACEP
Associate Professor of Surgery
Division of Emergency Medicine
Stanford University School of Medicine
Stanford, California

MOSBY

ELSEVIER

MOSBY
ELSEVIER

1600 John F. Kennedy Blvd.
Suite 1800
Philadelphia, PA 19103-2899

FIELD GUIDE TO WILDERNESS MEDICINE   ISBN: 978-1-4160-4698-1
Third Edition

Notice

Knowledge and best practice in this field are constantly changing. As new research and experience broaden our knowledge, changes in practice, treatment, and drug therapy may become necessary or appropriate. Readers are advised to check the most current information provided (i) on procedures featured or (ii) by the manufacturer of each product to be administered, to verify the recommended dose or formula, the method and duration of administration, and contraindications. It is the responsibility of the practitioner, relying on their own experience and knowledge of the patient, to make diagnoses, to determine dosages and the best treatment for each individual patient, and to take all appropriate safety precautions. To the fullest extent of the law, neither the Publisher nor the Authors assume any liability for any injury and/or damage to persons or property arising out of or related to any use of the material contained in this book.

The Publisher

Library of Congress Cataloging-in-Publication Data

Auerbach, Paul S.
Field guide to wilderness medicine/Paul S. Auerbach, Howard J. Donner, Eric A. Weiss.—3rd ed.
    p. ; cm.
        Includes bibliographical references and index.
        ISBN 978-1-4160-4698-1
        1. Outdoor medical emergencies—Handbooks, manuals, etc. I. Donner, Howard J. II. Weiss, Eric A., M.D. III. Title.
        [DNLM: 1. Emergencies—Handbooks. 2. Emergency Treatment—Handbooks. 3. Wounds and Injuries—therapy—Handbooks. WB 39 A917f 2008]
RC88.9.O95A938 2008
616.02'5—dc22   2007046673

Acquisitions Editor: Dolores Meloni
Developmental Editor: Julie Mirra
Publishing Services Manager: Frank Polizzano
Senior Project Manager: Robin E. Hayward
Designer: Steven Stave

Printed in Canada.

Last digit is the print number: 9 8 7 6 5 4 3 2 1

Working together to grow
libraries in developing countries

www.elsevier.com | www.bookaid.org | www.sabre.org

ELSEVIER   BOOK AID International   Sabre Foundation

This book is dedicated to our future wilderness medicine experts: Brian, Lauren and Dan (the "Mammal") Auerbach; Danny Weiss; and Evan Donner.

Preface

Accompanying the Fifth Edition of the textbook *Wilderness Medicine,* this Third Edition of *Field Guide to Wilderness Medicine* is modified and expanded to reflect what we have learned and observed since the Second Edition. We continue to direct our efforts to presenting clinical and therapeutic information that is appropriate for a trained health care provider to practice medicine in the field. To the best extent possible, we have streamlined our recommendations so that this guide does not take up more than its fair share of space in a pack or duffel.

As always, the guide relies upon the collected wisdom from contributors to the textbook. They are tireless and wise, and I am grateful for their remarkable skills, enthusiasm, and generosity. Based on their comments and those of countless readers, each edition improves upon its predecessor, and creates a practical and accessible book to assist the practitioners of wilderness medicine.

The Wilderness Medical Society is joined by many energetic training, education, and experiential organizations, such as the National Outdoor Leadership School, Outward Bound, Stonehearth Open Learning Opportunities, Wilderness Medical Associates, Divers Alert Network, and Advanced Wilderness Life Support; academic medical centers; university outdoor programs; the military; and independent experts who advance and promote the specialty of wilderness medicine. This book is dedicated to everyone who has advanced or is advancing sound medical practice in the outdoors.

Be cautious, be safe, and seek every opportunity to help your fellow man. I hope this field guide makes you more confident and effective as you do your best to practice the art of wilderness medicine. I also hope that you take the time to better understand the challenges faced by our planet. To preserve the wilderness, we must fulfill our responsibilities to understand global environmental science and be proactive in preserving the landscape.

—*Paul S. Auerbach*

Acknowledgments

The wilderness medicine community includes many extraordinary individuals. For the creation of this book, I thank Drs. Howard Donner and Eric Weiss; the special support and friendship of Drs. Luanne Freer, Robert Norris, Brownie Schoene, Eric Johnson, Peter Hackett, and Jay Lemery; and the editorial team at Elsevier. —*Paul S. Auerbach*

I am pleased to acknowledge the following for their kind assistance: Craig Sturbenz; Debra Wheeler, MD; Valeska Armisen, MD; Lance Ferguson, MD; Howard Backer, MD; Steve Lyons; and Catherine Soutter. —*Howard J. Donner*

Although this book "is dedicated to our future wilderness medicine experts," it is with gratitude and appreciation that I acknowledge and thank my colleagues and friends who have shared my passion for wilderness medicine in the past. Their experience, wisdom and devotion to wilderness medicine are reflected in many parts of the book. In particular I would like to extend my gratitude to Paul Auerbach, Howard Donner, Peter Hackett, Findlay Russell, Robert Norris, Joseph Serra, Lanny Johnson, Tim Erickson, Henry Herrmann, Jim Bagian, Brownie Schoene, Gene Allred, and Gary Kibbee. Most of all, I am grateful to my father, Gerald Weiss, who taught me to love and to respect the wilderness, and who inspired me to pursue a life of learning and teaching. —*Eric A. Weiss*

Cover photos courtesy of the following:
Crystal Crag from Mammoth Crest, photo by Mathias Schar, MD; Black and White or Not, photo by Gordon Giesbrecht, PhD; Truk Lagoon, Federated States of Micronesia, photo by Ian Jones, MD; Galapagos Sally Lightfoot Crab, and Machu Picchu, photos by Paul S. Auerbach, MD; Death Canyon, Grand Teton National Park, photo by Tim Floyd, MD.

Contents

Color plates follow page xvi

FIELD GUIDE TO WILDERNESS MEDICINE

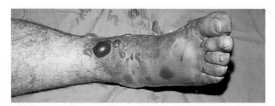

Plate 1. Edema and blister formation 24 hours after frostbite injury occurring in an area covered by a tightly fitted boot. (Courtesy Cameron Bangs, MD.)

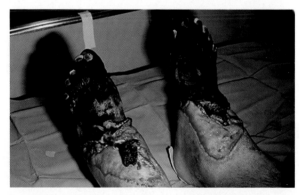

Plate 2. Gangrenous necrosis 6 weeks after frostbite injury shown in Plate 1. (Courtesy Cameron Bangs, MD.)

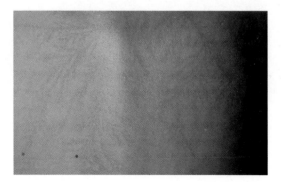

Plate 3. Feathering burns from lightning injury. (Courtesy Mary Ann Cooper, MD.)

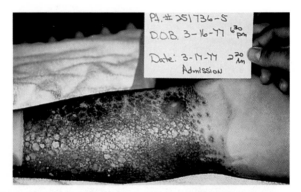

Plate 4. Punctate burns from lightning injury. (Courtesy Arthur Kahn, MD.)

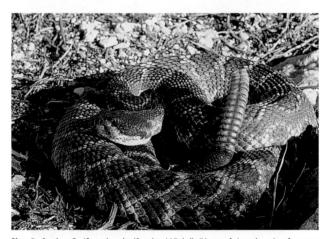

Plate 5. Southern Pacific rattlesnake *(Crotalus viridis helleri)* is one of nine subspecies of western rattlesnakes (*C. viridis* spp.) (Courtesy Michael Cardwell/Extreme Wildlife Photography.)

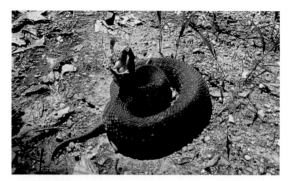

Plate 6. Cottonmouth water moccasin *(Agkistrodon piscivoris)*. The open-mouthed threat gesture is characteristic of this semiaquatic pit viper. (Courtesy Sherman Minton, MD.)

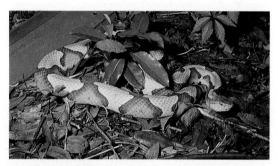

Plate 7. Southern copperhead *(Agkistrodon contortrix contortrix)* has markings that make it almost invisible when lying in leaf litter. (Courtesy Michael Cardwell and Carl Barden Venom Laboratory.)

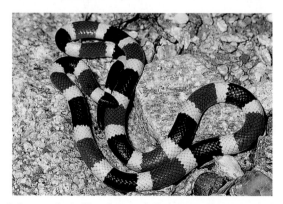

Plate 8. Senoran coral snake. *(Micruroides curyxanthus)* is also known as the Arizona coral snake. No documented fatality has followed a bite by this species. (Courtesy Michael Cardwell and Jude McNally.)

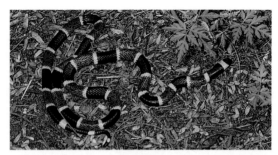

Plate 9. Texas coral snake. *(Micrurus fulvius tenere)* has a highly potent venom but is secretive, and bites are uncommon. (Courtesy Michael Cardwell and the Gladys Porter Zoo.)

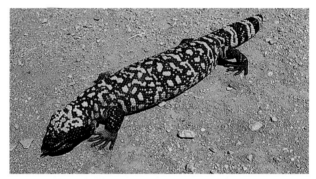

Plate 10. Gila monster *(Heloderma suspectum)* is one of only two known venomous lizards and the only species found in the United States. (Courtesy Michael Cardwell/Extreme Wildlife Photography.)

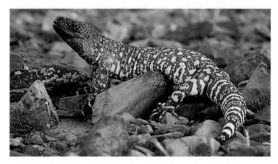

Plate 11. Mexican beaded lizard *(Heloderma horridum)* is located south of the Gila monster's range in Mexico. (Courtesy Michael Cardwell/Extreme Wildlife Photography.)

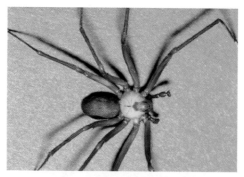

Plate 12. Brown recluse spider *(Loxosceles recluse)*. (Courtesy Indiana University Medical Center.)

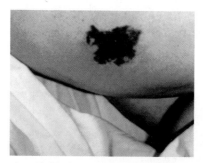

Plate 13. Brown recluse spider bite after 24 hours, with central ischemia and rapidly advancing cellulitis. (Courtesy Paul S. Auerbach, MD.)

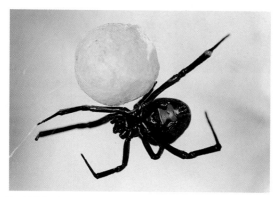

Plate 14. Adult female. *Latrodectus mactans* with fresh egg case. (Courtesy Michael Cardwell & Associates.)

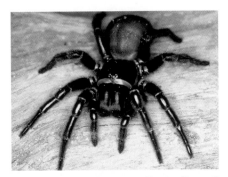

Plate 15. Funnel-web spider (*Atrax* species) wearing a wedding ring. (Courtesy Sherman Minton, MD.)

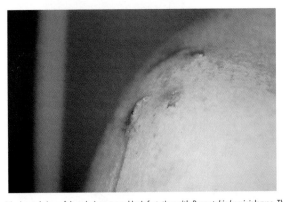

Plate 16. Lateral view of three lesions caused by infestation with *Dermatobia hominis* larvae. The nodules were initially assumed to be furunculosis. A central breathing aperture is present in each nodule. Serosanguineous fluid is draining from two of the nodules. Larval spiracles are visible emerging from the uppermost nodule. (From Brewer TF, Wilson ME, Gonzalez E, Felsenstein D: Bacon therapy and furuncular myiasis. JAMA 270:2087, 1993.)

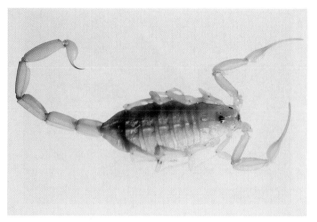

Plate 17. *Centruroides exilicauda* (*Centruroides sculpturatus*), the bark scorpion of Arizona.

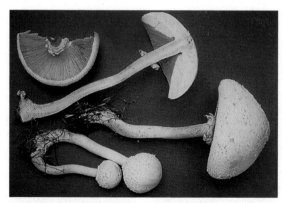

Plate 18. *Chlorophyllum molybdites.* A gastrointestinal irritant. (Courtesy Roger Phillips, rogersmushrooms.com.)

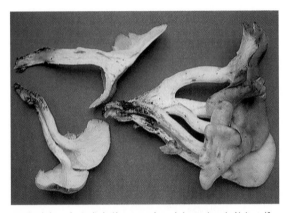

Plate 19. *Omphalotus olearius* (jack o' lantern mushroom). A gastrointestinal irritant. (Courtesy Roger Phillips, rogersmushrooms.com.)

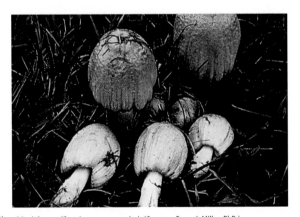

Plate 20. Inky cap *(Corprinus atramentarius)*. (Courtesy Orson J. Miller, PhD.)

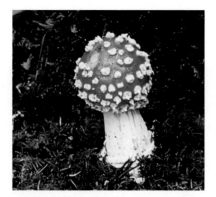

Plate 21. *Amanita muscaria.*

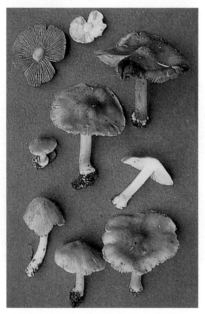

Plate 22. *Inocybe cookei.* Contains muscarinic toxins. (Courtesy Roger Phillips, rogersmushrooms.com.)

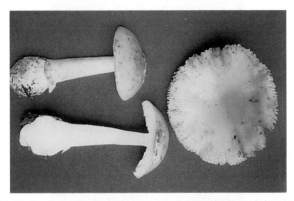

Plate 23. *Amanita pantherina.* Contains the neurotoxins ibotenic acid and isoxazole derivatives. (Courtesy Roger Phillips, rogersmushrooms.com.)

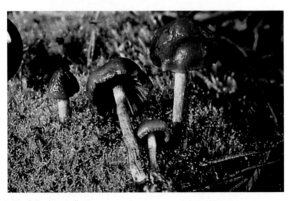

Plate 24. *Psilocybe caerulipes.*

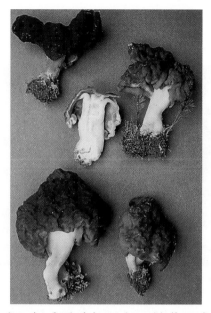

Plate 25. *Gyromitra esculenta*. Contains the hepatotoxin gyromitrin. (Courtesy Roger Phillips, rogersmushrooms.com.)

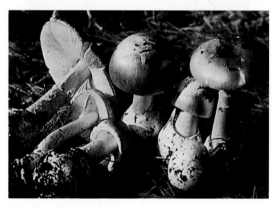

Plate 26. Death cap. *(Amanita phalloides)*.

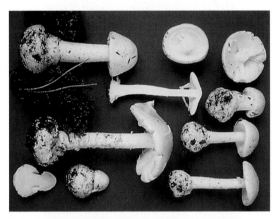

Plate 27. *Amanita virosa.* Causes delayed hepatotoxicity. (Courtesy Roger Phillips, rogersmushrooms.com.)

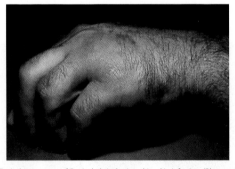

Plate 28. Typical appearance of *Erysipelothrix rhusiopathiae* skin infection. (Photograph by Paul S. Auerbach, MD.)

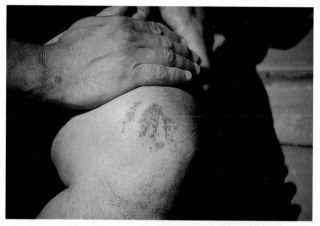

Plate 29. Fernlike hydroid "print" on the knee of a diver. (Photograph by Paul S. Auerbach, MD.)

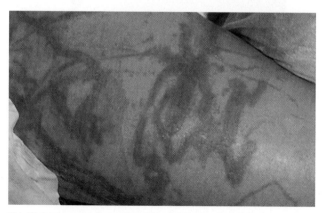

Plate 30. Intense necrosis (here at 48 hours) is typical of a severe box-jelly fish *(Chironex fleckeri)* sting. Skin darkening can be rapid with cellular death. (Courtesy John Williamson, MD.)

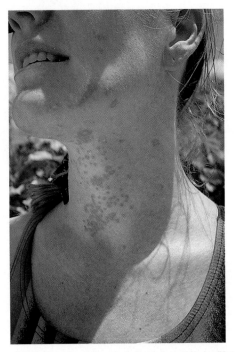

Plate 31. Seabather's eruption on the neck of a diver in Cozumel, Mexico. (Photograph by Paul S. Auerbach, MD.)

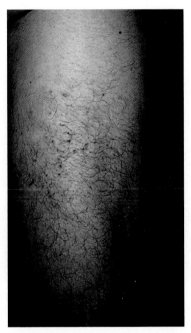

Plate 32. Thigh of the author demonstrating multiple sea urchin punctures from black sea urchins *(Diadema)*. Within 24 hours, the black markings were absent, indicative of spine dye without residual spines. (Photograph by Ken Kizer, MD.)

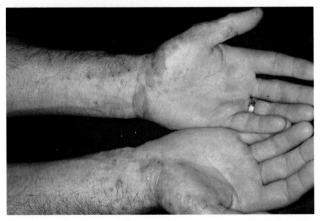

Plate 33. Sea moss dermatitis. Dermatitis of palms and forearms from a moving sea moss entangled in nets. (Courtesy of Edgar Maeyens, Jr., MD.)

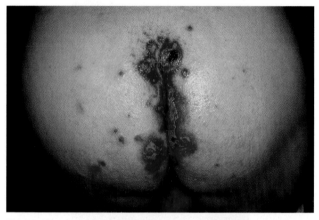

Plate 34. *Microcoleus lyngbyaceus.* Rare and extreme example of superficial necrosis and inflammation secondary to dermonecrotic toxins. (Courtesy of Edgar Maeyens, Jr., MD.)

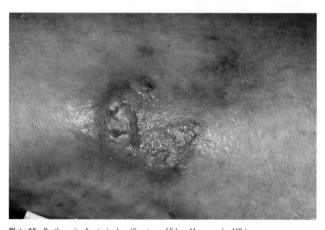

Plate 35. Prothecosis of anterior leg. (Courtesy of Edgar Maeyens, Jr., MD.)

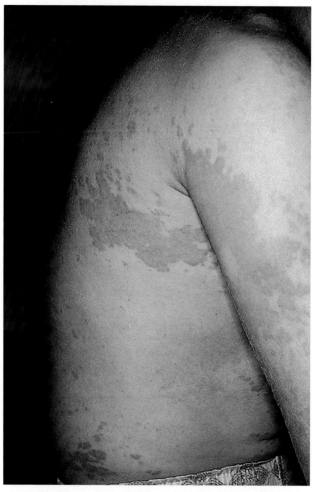

Plate 36. Aquagenetic urticaria. Pruritic punctate and perifollicular wheals characteristic of the rash of aquagenic urticaria. (Courtesy of Edgar Maeyens, Jr., MD.)

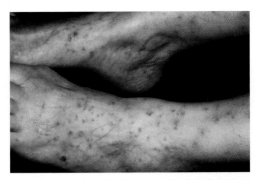

Plate 37. Schistosome cercarial dermatitis of the feet and ankles. (Courtesy of Edgar Maeyens, Jr., MD.)

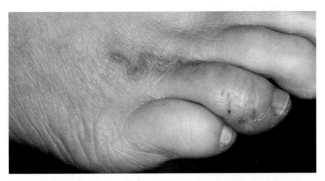

Plate 38. Cutaneous larva migrans. (Courtesy of Edgar Maeyens, Jr., MD.)

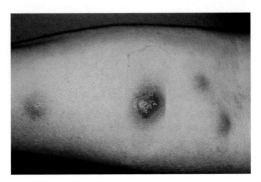

Plate 39. Nodular lymphangitis from *Mycobacterium marinum*. (Courtesy of Edgar Maeyens, Jr., MD.)

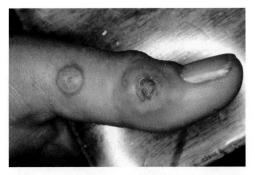

Plate 40. Seal finger secondary to *Mycoplasma*. (Courtesy of Edgar Maeyens, Jr., MD.)

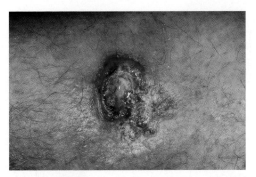

Plate 41. *Aeromonas hydrophila.* Trauma-induced necrotic ulcer of the anterior leg of a fisherman. (Courtesy of Edgar Maeyens, Jr., MD.)

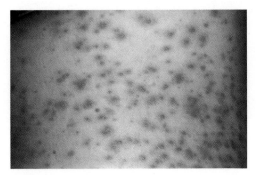

Plate 42. Hot tub folliculitis. (Courtesy of Edgar Maeyens, Jr., MD.)

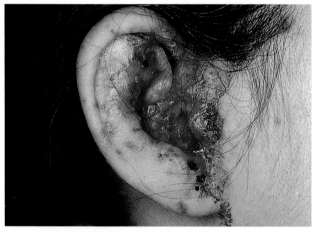

Plate 43. Malignant otitis externa. (Courtesy Edgar Maeyens, MD.)

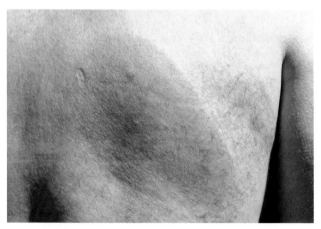

Plate 44. Rash of erythema migrans. (Courtesy of Paul Auerbach, MD.)

High-Altitude Medicine

1

▶ DEFINITIONS

High altitude occurs between 1500 to 3500 m (4950 to 11,500 ft). This altitude is marked by decreased exercise performance and increased ventilation at rest. Altitude illness is common with rapid ascent above 2500 m (8200 ft).

Very high altitude ranges from 3500 to 5500 m (11,500 to 18,050 ft). Arterial partial pressure of oxygen (PaO_2) falls below 60 mm Hg, and maximal arterial oxygen saturation (SaO_2) drops below 90%. Extreme hypoxia may occur during exercise or sleep and with altitude sickness. Severe altitude illness (e.g., high-altitude pulmonary edema [HAPE] and high-altitude cerebral edema [HACE]) occurs most commonly in this group.

Extreme altitude exists above 5500 m (roughly 18,000 ft). Marked hypoxemia and hypocapnia occur, and successful acclimatization is impossible. Abrupt ascent to this altitude without supplemental oxygen is extremely dangerous.

▶ HIGH-ALTITUDE ILLNESS

High-Altitude Headache

Signs and Symptoms
1. Often the first symptom of altitude exposure
2. May be the only symptom following altitude exposure
3. May or may not portend the development of acute mountain sickness (AMS, see later)

Treatment
1. Oxygen is very effective if available.
2. Nonsteroidal antiinflammatory drugs (NSAIDs) or acetaminophen, or both, are generally effective.
3. AMS treatment agents such as acetazolamide and dexamethasone (see later) may be used to prevent or treat high-altitude headache.

Acute Mountain Sickness

Signs and Symptoms (Primary)
1. Headache, usually throbbing, bitemporal or occipital, worse at night and with Valsalva's maneuver or stooping over
2. Anorexia
3. Nausea
4. Vomiting
5. Frequent awakening during sleep

6. Dizziness or lightheadedness
7. Fatigue, lassitude
8. Feels like a "hangover"

Other Signs and Symptoms
1. Periodic breathing and sensation of suffocation, not necessarily associated with AMS
2. Sensation of inner chill
3. Facial pallor
4. Dyspnea on exertion
5. Irritability
6. Funduscopic venous tortuosity and dilation
7. Absence of normal-altitude diuresis

Natural Course
1. Highly variable
2. Symptoms may start within 2 hours after arrival at altitude.
3. Symptoms rarely start after 36 hours at a given altitude.
4. Most patients resolve within 3 days.
5. Some patients progress despite remaining at a fixed altitude.

Treatment
1. Do not proceed to a higher sleeping altitude.
2. Monitor the victim for progression of illness (to pulmonary or cerebral edema).
3. If symptoms worsen despite an additional 24 hours of acclimatization, descend. Often a descent of 500 to 1000 m (1650 to 3300 ft) is sufficient.
4. Immediately descend if victim has ataxia, altered consciousness, or pulmonary edema.
5. For mild AMS, halt the ascent and wait for acclimatization to occur (12 hours to 4 days). Administer acetazolamide, 125 to 250 mg PO bid, for 2 days while at altitude or until symptoms have diminished.
6. Ginkgo biloba, 100 mg bid, may prevent and reduce symptoms of AMS.
7. Administer aspirin, 650 mg; acetaminophen, 650 to 1000 mg; or ibuprofen, 400 to 600 mg, for headache.
8. Administer prochlorperazine, 5 mg PO or IV, for nausea and vomiting.
9. Avoid sedative-hypnotics.
10. Minimize exertion.
11. Consider descending 500 to 1000 m.
12. Consider administering oxygen, 0.5 to 1.5 L/minute, by nasal cannula or simple (open type) facemask during sleep. This is particularly effective for headache.
13. Consider administering dexamethasone, 4 mg PO or IM q6h, in conjunction with descent, for progressive

neurologic symptoms or ataxia, or if the patient cannot tolerate acetazolamide.

14. Consider undertaking a 2- to 6-hour treatment in a portable hyperbaric bag (i.e., Gamow Bag) inflated to 2 psi. Maintaining 2 psi inside the bag is equivalent to a descent of 1000 to 3000 m (3281 to 9900 ft) depending on the starting altitude. The hyperbaric bag can be used with or without supplemental oxygen. The Gamow Bag requires constant pumping, so recruit additional rescuers or friends for relief (Box 1-1).

Box 1-1. Field Treatment of High-Altitude Illness

HIGH-ALTITUDE HEADACHE AND MILD ACUTE MOUNTAIN SICKNESS
Stop ascent, rest, and acclimatize at same altitude
Acetazolamide, 125 to 250 mg bid, to speed acclimatization
Symptomatic treatment as needed with analgesics and antiemetics
OR descend 500 m or more

MODERATE TO SEVERE ACUTE MOUNTAIN SICKNESS
Low-flow oxygen, if available
Acetazolamide, 125 to 250 mg bid, with or without dexamethasone, 4 mg PO, IM, or IV q6h
Hyperbaric therapy
OR immediate descent

HIGH-ALTITUDE CEREBRAL EDEMA
Immediate descent or evacuation
Oxygen, 2 to 4 L/minute
Dexamethasone, 4 mg PO, IM, or IV q6h
Hyperbaric therapy

HIGH-ALTITUDE PULMONARY EDEMA
Minimize exertion and keep warm
Oxygen, 4 to 6 L/minute until improving, then 2 to 4 L/minute
If oxygen is not available:
Nifedipine, 10 mg PO q4h by titration to response, or 10 mg PO once, followed by 30 mg extended release q12 to 24h
Inhaled beta-agonist
Consider sildenafil 50 mg every 8 hours
Hyperbaric therapy
OR immediate descent

PERIODIC BREATHING
Acetazolamide, 62.5 to 125 mg at bedtime as needed

High-Altitude Cerebral Edema

Signs and Symptoms
1. Ataxic gait is the hallmark of diagnosis. Ataxia in the face of recent ascent to very high altitude is HACE until proven otherwise.
2. Altered consciousness (confusion, drowsiness, stupor, coma)
3. Severe lassitude
4. Headache
5. Nausea and vomiting
6. Hallucinations (rare)
7. Cyanosis or pallor
8. Hypoxemia associated with concomitant pulmonary edema
9. Seizures (rare)
10. Cranial nerve palsy (rare)

Treatment
1. Immediately descend at least 500 to 1000 m, or more as needed.
2. Administer dexamethasone, 4 to 8 mg IV, IM, or PO, followed by 4 mg q6h.
3. Administer oxygen, 2 to 4 L/minute by nasal cannula or simple (open type) facemask, to maintain SaO_2 greater than 90%. Higher O_2 concentrations and a non-rebreather mask may be required.
4. If the victim is comatose, manage the airway and drain the bladder.
5. Consider giving furosemide, 20 mg, or bumetanide, 1 mg PO, IM, or IV, if intravascular volume is thought to be adequate (monitor blood pressure).
6. Consider undertaking a 2- to 6-hour treatment in a portable hyperbaric bag (e.g., Gamow Bag) inflated to 2 psi. Maintaining 2 psi inside the bag is equivalent to a descent of 1000 to 3000 m (3281 to 9900 ft) depending on the starting altitude. The hyperbaric bag can be used with or without supplemental oxygen.
7. If neurologic symptoms persist despite treatment with oxygen, steroids, and descent, a cerebrovascular accident (CVA or stroke) may be present. Carefully evaluate the situation.

High-Altitude Pulmonary Edema

Signs and Symptoms
1. Decreased exercise performance and increased recovery time
2. Dyspnea on exertion
3. Cough (dry or productive)

4. Tachycardia and tachypnea at rest
5. Fatigue, weakness, lassitude
6. Low-grade fever
7. Headache
8. Anorexia
9. Cyanotic nail beds and lips
10. Audible chest rales
11. Orthopnea is uncommon with mild to moderate disease
12. Pink or blood-tinged sputum (late finding)
13. Mental changes, ataxia, decreased level of consciousness, coma
14. Hypoxemia on pulse oximetry or arterial blood gas (ABG) analysis (Table 1-1)

Treatment
1. Immediately descend at least 500 to 1000 m.
2. Administer oxygen, 2 to 4 L/minute, by nasal cannula or simple (open type) facemask to maintain SaO_2 greater than 90%. Higher O_2 concentrations and a non-rebreather mask may be required.

TABLE 1-1. Severity Classification of High-Altitude Pulmonary Edema

GRADE	SYMPTOMS	SIGNS	CHEST FILM
1 Mild	Dyspnea on exertion, dry cough, fatigue while moving uphill (if any)	HR (rest) <90-100; RR (rest) <20; dusky nail beds; localized rales	Minor infiltrate involving <25% of one lung field
2 Moderate	Dyspnea, weakness, fatigue on level walking; raspy cough; headache; anorexia	HR 90-100; RR 16-30; cyanotic nail beds; rales present; ataxia may be present	Some infiltrates involving 50% of one lung or smaller area of both lungs
3 Severe	Dyspnea at rest, productive cough, orthopnea, extreme weakness	Bilateral rales; HR >110; RR >30; facial and nail-bed cyanosis; ataxia; stupor; coma; blood-tinged sputum	Bilateral infiltrates >50% of each lung

HR, heart rate; RR, respiratory rate.
Modified from Hultgren HN: In Staub NC (ed): New York, Dekker, 1978, pp 437-469.

3. If supplemental oxygen is not available, consider giving nifedipine, 20 to 30 mg sustained-release capsule q12h or 10 mg sublingually (PO), the latter dose repeated as needed to reduce pulmonary arterial pressure without causing persistent hypotension.
4. Use an inhaled beta-agonist (albuterol MDI, 2 puffs q4h, or salmeterol, 2 puffs q8–12h).
5. Keep the victim warm.
6. Consider using pursed-lip breathing or a continuous positive airway pressure (CPAP) mask.
7. Consider undertaking a 2- to 6-hour treatment in a portable hyperbaric bag (i.e., Gamow Bag) inflated to 2 psi. Maintaining 2 psi inside the bag is equivalent to a descent of 1000 to 3000 m (3281 to 9900 feet) depending on the starting altitude. The hyperbaric bag can be used with or without supplemental oxygen.
8. Consider a PDE-5 inhibitor such as sildenafil or tadalafil (not yet well studied for treatment but effective for prevention, discussed next).

Prevention
Agents that block hypoxic pulmonary hypertension will block the onset of HAPE. Anecdotal evidence suggests that acetazolamide, 125 to 250 mg PO bid or 500-mg sustained-release capsule q24h, prevents HAPE in persons with a history of recurrent episodes. Nifedipine, 20-mg sustained-release capsule q8h, may also accomplish this. Studies suggest that the inhaled beta-agonist salmeterol MDI, 2 puffs q8–12h, may prevent HAPE. Recent studies suggest that the PDE-5 inhibitors sildenafil and tadalafil may effectively prevent HAPE. Optimum dosage recommendations have not been established. Regimens for sildenafil have varied from a single dose of 50 to 100 mg just prior to exposure to 40 mg three times per day. Study regimens for tadalafil included 10 mg every 12 to 24 hours. Recently, dexamethasone has been shown to prevent HAPE in susceptible subjects. The dose used was 8 mg every 12 hours starting 2 days prior to exposure.

▶ OTHER ALTITUDE DISORDERS

Sleep Disturbances
Sleep disturbances are common at high altitude and are believed to result from cerebral hypoxia.

Signs and Symptoms
1. Increased wakefulness
2. Periodic breathing

3. Frequent arousal
4. Decreased rapid eye movement (REM) sleep

Periodic Breathing

Signs and Symptoms
Nocturnal hyperpnea followed by apnea, reflecting alternating periods of respiratory alkalosis (hyperpnea)

Treatment of Sleep Disturbances and Periodic Breathing
1. Give acetazolamide, 62.5 mg to 125 mg PO, in the evening.
2. Use hypnotics cautiously (especially in patients with altitude sickness) because of the potential for respiratory depression.
3. If the disturbed sleep is thought to be unrelated to altitude and a sleep agent is elected, use triazolam, 0.125 to 0.25 mg, temazepam, 15 mg, or zolpidem, 10 mg.

Peripheral Edema

Signs and Symptoms
Edema of the hands, face, and ankles

Treatment
1. Examine the victim for signs of AMS, HAPE, or HACE.
2. In the absence of AMS, administer a diuretic (furosemide, 10 to 20 mg PO) or acetazolamide, 125 to 250 mg.
3. Maintain adequate intravascular hydration.
4. Consider limiting ascent until resolved.

High-Altitude Pharyngitis and Bronchitis

Signs and Symptoms
1. Sore throat
2. Chronic cough (dry or productive)
3. Dry or cracking nasal passages

Treatment
1. Maintain adequate hydration.
2. Give lozenges or hard candies.
3. Use an antitussive agent (codeine, 30 mg PO q8-12h).
4. Administer steam inhalation.
5. Give antibiotics if sputum becomes purulent (relatively ineffective).
6. Give nasal saline spray prn.
7. Apply topical nasal ointment (mupirocin, bacitracin, or petroleum jelly [Vaseline]).

High-Altitude Retinal Hemorrhages
Common in trekkers and climbers above 15,000 feet

Signs and Symptoms
1. Usually asymptomatic
2. Requires an ophthalmoscope for definitive diagnosis
3. If bleeding is premacular, field deficits may occur.

Treatment
1. No specific treatment
2. Descent is recommended if hemorrhages are extensive or symptomatic (field deficit) to prevent progression.
3. Supplemental oxygen may hasten resolution.

Focal Neurologic Conditions without Cerebral Edema

Various localizing neurologic signs occur that are usually transient and do not necessarily occur in the setting of AMS. Syndromes include the following:
1. Migraine
2. Cerebral vascular spasm
3. Transient ischemic attack (TIA)
4. Stroke with permanent focal neurologic dysfunction

Factors contributing to stroke at altitude may include polycythemia, dehydration, increased intracranial pressure, cerebrovascular spasm, and coagulation abnormalities.

Signs and Symptoms
1. Transient hemiplegia
2. Hemiparesis
3. Transient global amnesia
4. Unilateral paresthesias
5. Aphasia
6. Scotoma
7. Cortical blindness

Treatment
1. Supportive measures
2. Oxygen
3. Descent
4. Steroids may be worthwhile for the underlying treatment of AMS or HACE.
5. When supplemental oxygen is not available, CO_2 rebreathing may be of benefit (increases cerebral blood flow). Add ventilatory "deadspace" by having the victim breathe through a 6-inch piece of respiratory tubing (or similar device).
6. Victims with signs and symptoms of TIA at high altitude should be started on aspirin.

High-Altitude Flatus Expulsion (HAFE)

Signs and Symptoms
Excessive flatulence of colonic gas

Treatment
1. Administer oral simethicone, 80 mg PO prn.
2. Encourage a carbohydrate diet.
3. Apologize to tentmates.

High-Altitude Deterioration

Signs and Symptoms
1. Acclimatization impossible, with victim's condition deteriorating and marked by weight loss, lethargy, weakness, headache, and poor-quality sleep.
2. Very common at extreme altitude in the so-called "death zone," 7500 m (≈25,000 ft) and above
3. More common in persons with chronic diseases, particularly those associated with hypoxemia

Treatment
The only definitive treatment is descent to a lower altitude.

Chronic Mountain Polycythemia (a Problem of Long-Term High-Altitude Dwellers)

Signs and Symptoms
1. Headache
2. Insomnia
3. Lethargy
4. Plethoric appearance
5. Polycythemia (hemoglobin >20 g/dL of blood; hematocrit >60%)

Treatment
1. Descend to a lower altitude.
2. Administer supplemental oxygen during sleep.
3. Perform a phlebotomy.
4. Give medroxyprogesterone acetate, 20 to 60 mg/day, as a respiratory stimulant.
5. Give acetazolamide, 125 to 250 mg PO bid, as a respiratory stimulant.

Ultraviolet Keratitis ("Snowblindness")

Signs and Symptoms
1. Eye pain
2. Sensation of grittiness in the eyes
3. Sensitivity to light
4. Tearing
5. Conjunctival erythema
6. Chemosis
7. Eyelid swelling

Treatment
1. Remove contact lenses.
2. Give a topical anesthetic for evaluation but not repetitively (inhibits corneal re-epithelialization).
3. Administer aspirin or ibuprofen orally.
4. Use external cool compresses.
5. Instill a mydriatic-cycloplegic agent to reduce ciliary spasm and dilate the pupil, the latter to prevent synechiae.
6. Consider a topical nonsteroidal antiinflammatory agent (i.e., ketorolac ophthalmic solution, 1 drop qid).
7. Avoid topical corticosteroids.
8. Patch the affected eye(s) for 24 hours; then reexamine. Do not patch the eye if there is a purulent discharge, facial rash consistent with herpes zoster, or any suggestion of corneal ulcer.
9. If the victim has both eyes affected and must use one eye, patch the more severely affected eye.
10. Encourage the victim to rest.

Acclimatization

Acclimatization is the key to successful habitation at high altitude. Beginning at an altitude of 1500 m (4950 ft), the following physiologic changes are noted:
1. Increased ventilation, which decreases alveolar carbon dioxide and increases alveolar oxygen. This is mediated in part by the hypoxic ventilatory response (carotid body), which can be affected positively by respiratory stimulants (progesterone, almitrine) and negatively by alcohol, sedative-hypnotics, and fragmented sleep. Acetazolamide is a respiratory stimulant that acts on the central respiratory center.
2. Renal bicarbonate excretion in response to increased ventilation, hypocapnia, and the resulting respiratory alkalosis. Without this correction in pH, the alkalosis would inhibit the central respiratory center and limit ventilation. Ventilation reaches a maximum after 4 to 7 days at the same altitude. Acetazolamide facilitates this process.
3. Hypoxic pulmonary vasoconstriction leads to increased pulmonary artery pressure. This is not completely ameliorated by the administration of oxygen at altitude.
4. Red blood cell mass increases over a period of weeks to months. This may lead to polycythemia. Long-term acclimatization leads to increased plasma volume as well.

How to Acclimatize to Altitude

1. Avoid abrupt ascent to sleeping altitudes above 3000 m (9850 ft).
2. Spend 2 or 3 nights at 2500 to 3000 m (8200 to 9850 ft) before further ascent.
3. Add an extra night of acclimatization for every 600 to 900 m (1980 to 2970 ft) of ascent.
4. Make day trips to a higher altitude with a return to lower altitude for sleep.
5. Avoid alcohol and sedative-hypnotics for the first two nights at altitude.
6. Be aware that mild exercise may be beneficial and extreme exercise deleterious.
7. Administer acetazolamide, 125 mg PO bid or 5 mg/kg/day divided bid, starting 24 hours before ascent. An alternative dose is one 500-mg sustained-release capsule q24h.
   a. Continue the drug during the ascent and until acclimatization has occurred (generally for 48 hours at maximum altitude).
   b. Do not use in the presence of allergy to sulfa derivatives.
   c. Side effects include peripheral paresthesias, polyuria, nausea, drowsiness, impotence, myopia, and altered (bitter) taste of carbonated beverages.
   d. Dexamethasone, 4 mg PO q4h, can be used if acetazolamide is contraindicated. It is best reserved for treatment, rather than prophylaxis, of AMS.
   e. Studies with Ginkgo biloba have had inconsistent results. Some studies show that ginkgo (nonprescription), 100 mg bid, taken 3 to 5 days before ascent, and continued, may be effective for preventing symptoms. Potency and quality vary. Consumer Labs at www.consumerlabs.com compares available preparations. Acetazolamide is probably the superior agent.

▶ **COMMON MEDICAL CONDITIONS AND HIGH ALTITUDE**

Persons with certain preexisting illnesses might be at risk for adverse effects on ascent to high altitude, either because of exacerbation of their illnesses or because these illnesses might affect acclimatization and susceptibility to altitude illness. Certain populations, such as pregnant women and the elderly, also require special consideration (Box 1-2).

Based on available research, it seems prudent to recommend that only women with normal, low-risk pregnancy

---

Box 1-2. Advisability of Exposure to High and Very High Altitude for Common Conditions (without Supplemental Oxygen)

PROBABLY NO EXTRA RISK
Young and old
Fit and unfit
Obesity
Diabetes
After coronary artery bypass grafting (without angina)
Mild chronic obstructive pulmonary disease (COPD)
Asthma
Low-risk pregnancy
Controlled hypertension
Controlled seizure disorder
Psychiatric disorders
Neoplastic diseases
Inflammatory conditions

CAUTION
Moderate COPD
Compensated congestive heart failure (CHF)
Sleep apnea syndromes
Troublesome arrhythmias
Stable angina/coronary artery disease
High-risk pregnancy
Sickle cell trait
Cerebrovascular diseases
Any cause for restricted pulmonary circulation
Seizure disorder (not on medication)
Radial keratotomy

CONTRAINDICATED
Sickle cell anemia (with history of crises)
Severe COPD
Pulmonary hypertension
Uncompensated CHF

---

undertake a sojourn to altitude. For these women, exposure to an altitude at which Sao_2 will remain above 85% most of the time (up to 3000 m [9843 ft] altitude) appears to pose no risk of harm, but further study is necessary to place these recommendations on a more solid scientific footing.

Avalanche Safety and Rescue

2

The factors that contribute to avalanche release are terrain, weather, and snow pack. Terrain factors are fixed; however, the state of the weather and snow pack change daily, even hourly. Precipitation, wind, temperature, snow depth, snow surface, weak layers, and settlement are all factors that contribute to avalanche potential. A comprehensive review of snow pack evaluation and route finding is beyond the scope of this field guide. Anyone venturing into avalanche terrain must be familiar with avalanche hazard evaluation and appropriate route selection. This chapter focuses on aspects of personal safety and rescue.

▶ SAFETY EQUIPMENT

Proper equipment is essential for maintaining safety. This safety equipment should include the following:

Snow Shovel
The snow shovel is an essential piece of equipment for anyone traveling in avalanche country. All personnel should carry one.
1. It can be used to dig snow pits for stability evaluation and snow caves for overnight shelter.
2. A shovel is necessary for digging in avalanche debris because such snow is far too hard for digging with hands or skis.
3. The shovel should be sturdy and strong enough, yet light and small enough to fit into a pack. Shovels are made of aluminum or high-strength plastic and can be collapsible.

Collapsible Probe Pole or Ski Pole Probe
1. This may be used to assist in pinpointing a victim following a transceiver (rescue beacon) search and is essential if the victim is without a transceiver.
2. Organized rescue teams keep rigid poles in 10- or 12-foot lengths as part of their rescue caches.
3. The recreationist can buy probe poles of tubular aluminum or carbon fiber that come in 2-foot sections that fit together to make a full-length probe.
4. Ski poles with removable grips and baskets can be screwed together to make an avalanche probe. These are largely inferior to dedicated commercial probes.
5. Although entirely suboptimal, a tent pole, the tail of a ski, or a ski pole with the basket removed can substitute for this piece of equipment in an absolute emergency.

Avalanche Rescue Beacons (Rescue Transceivers)

1. Avalanche rescue beacons are now the most frequently used personal rescue devices worldwide.
2. Transceivers emit an electromagnetic signal on a frequency of 457 kHz.*
3. A buried victim's transceiver emits the signal, and the rescuer's unit can be set to receive the signal.
4. The signal carries 20 to 30 m (60 to 100 ft) and, when used properly, can guide searchers to the victim.
5. It is essential to confirm that all members of the party have their transceivers set to "transmit" before travel.
6. Merely possessing a beacon does not ensure its lifesaving capability. Frequent practice is required to master a beacon-guided search.
7. Skilled practitioners can find a buried unit in less than 5 minutes once they pick up the signal. Because speed is of the essence in avalanche rescue, beacons are lifesavers.
8. Beacons should be strapped close to the body under a layer of clothing.
9. Always check batteries before trips and carry extras. Use high-quality batteries.
10. Never use rechargeable batteries in an avalanche rescue transceivers. The transceiver could lose power without warning or prior indication of low power.
11. Check every party member's beacon periodically throughout the trip.
12. Keep beacons dry and free from battery corrosion.
13. Beacon technology is evolving rapidly and has improved radically over the past decade.
14. Modern beacons generally employ a computer chip to process the signal, displaying a digital readout of the distance and general direction to the buried unit.
15. Avalanche rescue beacon searches have become highly specialized, and search technique depends largely on the specific model and type. It is essential to learn the specifics of any model used prior to an avalanche burial.
16. Box 2-1 provides a generic overview of a search, but these instructions should not take the place of the unit's type-specific instructions.

---

*In 1986 the International Commission for Avalanche Alpine Rescue (ICAR) adopted a new standard for an avalanche beacon frequency of 457 kHz. This new frequency has a much greater range and effectiveness than any other single- or dual-frequency beacon. The sale and use of 2.275-kHz beacons ceased on December 1, 1995. Be certain that all beacons are single-frequency 457 kHz. A single-frequency 2.275 kHz beacon is incompatible with 457-kHz beacons and now obsolete.

Box 2-1. Avalanche Transceiver Search

INITIAL SEARCH

1. Have everyone switch their transceivers to "receive" and turn the volume to "high."
2. If enough people are available, post a lookout to warn others of further slides.
3. Should a second slide occur, have rescuers immediately switch their transceivers to "transmit."
4. Have rescuers space themselves no more than 30 m (100 ft) apart and walk abreast along the slope.
5. For a single rescuer searching within a wide path, zigzag across the rescue zone. Limit the distance between crossings to 30 m (100 ft).
6. For multiple victims, when a signal is picked up, have one or two rescuers continue to focus on that victim while the remainder of the group carries out the search for additional victims.
7. For a single victim, when a signal is picked up, have one or two rescuers continue to locate the victim while the remainder of the group prepares shovels, probes, and medical supplies for the rescue.

Avalanche Airbag System (ABS) (Fig. 2-1)

The ABS is a new avalanche rescue device designed in Germany and introduced in Europe.

1. Although it was originally designed for guides and ski patrollers, it can be used by anyone venturing into avalanche terrain.
2. The airbag is based on the principle of "inverse segregation," which causes larger particles to rise to the surface. A person is already a large particle. The airbag makes the user an even larger particle.
3. The airbag is integrated into a special backpack, and the user deploys it by pulling a ripcord-like handle.
4. Empiric data suggest that the ABS system significantly reduces fatality in avalanche burial.
5. This device should never be used to justify taking additional risks.

AvaLung (Fig. 2-2)

1. The AvaLung is an emergency breathing device designed to extract air from the snow surrounding a buried avalanche victim.
2. It is worn as a vest or independent device over the outer layer of clothing.

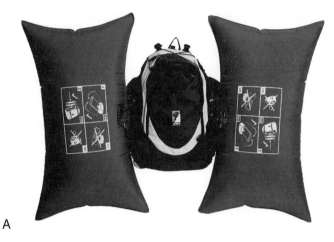

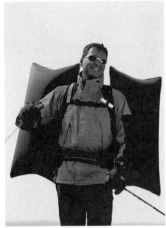

Figure 2-1. **A,** A small-size Avalanche ABS backpack with deployed airbags. The airbags are stowed in outside pockets of the backpack. **B,** Integrated into a backpack, the Avalanche ABS is deployed by pulling the white "T" handle. (Courtesy Peter Aschauer, GmbH.)

3. If buried, the victim can breathe through a mouthpiece and flex-tube connected to the vest.
4. The victim inhales oxygenated air coming from the surrounding snow, which passes through a membrane in the vest.
5. The exhaled air, rich in carbon dioxide, passes through a one-way valve and into another area of the snow posterior

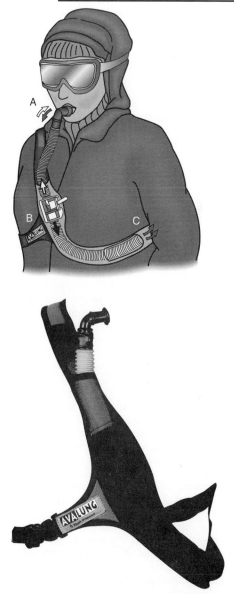

Figure 2-2. The AvaLung 2 (Black Diamond Equipment, Ltd., Salt Lake City, UT) is a breathing device intended to prolong survival during avalanche burial by diverting expired air away from inspired air drawn from the snow pack.

to the victim to greatly reduce the effects of carbon dioxide contaminating the air space.

6. The AvaLung has worked well in simulated burials, allowing the victim to breathe for 1 hour in tightly packed snow. It has already been effective in actual avalanche burials.

7. Like the ABS system (described earlier), this device should never be used to justify taking additional risks.

▶ CROSSING AN AVALANCHE SLOPE

Travel through avalanche terrain always involves risk. Before crossing a potential avalanche slope, take the following precautions:

1. Never ski alone in dangerous conditions.

2. Tighten up clothing; fasten zippers; and wear hat, gloves, and goggles.

3. If wearing a heavy mountaineering pack, loosen it before crossing so that it can be jettisoned if necessary. A heavy pack may increase potential for traumatic injury.

4. Conversely, a lighter pack or "day pack" is probably best left on to protect the spine.

5. Remove ski pole straps and ski runaway straps because attached poles and skis will add to potential for trauma. In avalanche terrain, always use releasable bindings on snowboards and mountaineering skis (including telemark skis).

6. Check transceiver batteries, and be sure that all rescue transceivers are set to "transmit."

7. Cross slopes at a high point, and stay on ridges. The person highest on a slope runs the least risk of being buried should the slope slide.

8. If crossing below the slope, remember that avalanches can be triggered from the flats below. This is generally a safe route if far enough from the slope. However, avalanches have been triggered in valleys up to 0.5 mile from the slope.

9. Cross potential avalanche slopes as quickly as possible. Never stop moving in the middle of an avalanche slope.

10. When climbing or descending an avalanche path, stay close to the sides. This makes it easier to escape to the side should the slope begin to slide.

11. Only allow one member of the group to cross at a time. This exposes one person at a time to danger, and it puts less weight on the snow. Watch this person carefully as he or she crosses.

12. Try to move toward natural islands of safety such as large rock outcroppings or dense trees.

13. Anticipate an avalanche. Plan your escape route ahead of time.

▶ **VICTIM SURVIVAL**

1. Escape to the side. The moment the snow begins to move, try to escape by skiing or moving quickly to the side of the avalanche, similar to the method a swimmer uses to ferry to the side of a river. Turning skis or a snow machine downhill in an effort to outrun the avalanche invariably fails because the avalanche will overtake you.

2. Shout, and then close your mouth. Shouting alerts companions, and closing the mouth may help prevent snow inhalation.

3. If knocked off your feet, kick off your skis and toss away ski poles. A lightweight mountaineering pack is probably protective. If you are wearing a heavy multiday mountaineering pack, jettison it because it will drag you down rather than allow you to stay near the surface.

4. Try to grab on to some fixed object (hanging on allows more snow to go past, reducing odds of burial).

5. Once knocked off your feet you should get your hands up to your face. Halsted Morris (former long-time education coordinator for the Colorado Avalanche Information Center) recommends reaching across the face and grabbing a jacket collar or the pack strap where it crosses the shoulder. This may not position your hands directly in front of your face, but you can use the crook of your elbow to create an air pocket.

6. Attempting to place your hands immediately in front of your face will increase the probability of maintaining an airspace in a tumbling ride. It also leaves your hands in a position to create a breathing space around your mouth and nose after the avalanche stops.

7. Once the avalanche stops it is nearly impossible to move the hands to the face to create an air pocket. Without an air pocket the consequences of a burial are usually fatal, unless the victim is uncovered in minutes.

▶ **RESCUE**

Although it is usually safe to move onto the bed surface of an avalanche that has just completed its run, beware when the fracture has occurred at mid slope, leaving a large mass of snow hanging above the fracture.

1. If enough rescuers are available and conditions remain unstable, post one person in a safe place and have him or her shout a warning should a second avalanche slide begin. This allows rescuers to switch their transceivers back to "transmit."

2. Mark the victim's last-seen location with a piece of equipment, clothing, or anything that can be seen from a distance down the slope.
3. Without a transceiver: Search the fall line below the victim's last-seen location for clues. If the victim is without a transceiver, make shallow probes at likely burial spots with an avalanche probe, ski pole, or tree limb. Likely burial spots are the uphill sides of trees and rocks and benches or bends in the slope where snow avalanche debris is concentrated. The "toe" of the debris is also a place where many victims come to rest.
4. Using transceivers: If the group was using transceivers, have all survivors immediately switch their units to "receive." With skilled rescuers, when a signal is received, the search can be quickly narrowed and the victim pinpointed within a few minutes.
5. Surface and "scuff" search: Even when using transceivers, visually check the avalanche path for any equipment or body parts that may be sticking out of the snow.
6. If the accident occurs in a ski area and several rescuers are available, send one person immediately to notify the ski patrol. If only one rescuer is present, yell for help and stay on scene to initiate rescue. Always search the surface for clues before leaving to notify the ski patrol. Remember that the odds of an organized search finding a live victim are very small. If the avalanche occurs in backcountry terrain, rapid recovery is so essential to the victim's survival that all rescuers should search for the victim. By the time organized rescue personnel return to search, it is unlikely that buried persons will be alive.
7. Keep all rescue gear with you or organized and in a safe location. Do not contaminate the scene.
8. For specific transceiver search technique, refer to the manual that came with your unit and practice often (minimally once at the start of each ski season) (see Box 2-1).

Probe Search (Only Applicable in the Initial Search if Victim Is without Transceiver)

1. Spot probe (e.g., look for areas likely to contain the victim).
   a. The fall line below last-seen area
   b. Around the victim's equipment on the surface
   c. Places where snow is piled up against trees or boulders
   d. Where the slope decreases
   e. Benches or bends in the slope
   f. At the "toe" of the avalanche
   g. Areas of deceleration, or anywhere the avalanche deposition is built up

 h. Do not "jam" the probe into the ground; rather, push the probe steadily downward.

 i. Studies show that avalanche victims infrequently survive below 6 ft (1.5 m).

 j. A live recovery is more probable if you probe additional areas rather than probing deeper.

2. Three-hole-per-step probe

 a. By this time, the objective is usually to recover the body.

 b. Probers stand with arms out, wrist to wrist.

 c. Probers first probe between their feet and then probe 50 cm to the right and then 50 cm to the left (Fig. 2-3).

 d. At a command from the leader, the line advances 50 cm (one step).

 e. This method gives an 88% chance of finding the victim on the first pass.

Shoveling

1. Victim depth and precise position should be rapidly pinpointed by final probe placement (remember, it is faster to probe than dig).

2. Although speed is essential when digging out the victim, try to:

 a. Avoid standing on top of the victim, which may collapse the victim's air space.

 b. Begin digging starter hole approximately 1.5 times the burial depth of the victim below the victim (i.e., downhill from the probe).

 c. Starter hole should be 6 ft (2 m) or one "wingspan" wide.

 d. Initially dig on knees, throwing snow to side.

 e. When waist deep, throw snow downhill.

 f. Instruct rescuers to take care not to injure the victim with their shovels.

 g. Provide airway measures immediately on encountering patient.

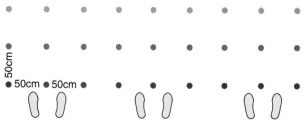

Figure 2-3. Fine avalanche probing (three-hole-per-step method).

▶ AVALANCHE VICTIM

Avalanches kill in two ways:

1. Asphyxiation secondary to airway occlusion by snow, increased carbon dioxide levels, pressure of snow on the thorax, and formation of an ice mask around the nose and mouth after burial
2. Trauma secondary to the wrenching action of snow in motion and the potential for impact with trees, rocks, loose equipment, and cliffs

Prognostic features for low survival potential include the following:

1. Complete burial of victim. Survival probabilities greatly diminish with increasing burial depth. No avalanche victim in the United States has survived a burial deeper than 2 m (6.5 ft) without protection by a structure.
2. Prolonged burial time. In the first 15 minutes after the avalanche, more persons are found alive than dead. Within 15 to 30 minutes, an equal number of people are found dead and alive. After 30 minutes, more people are found dead than alive, and the survival rate rapidly diminishes thereafter. Trained search dogs can locate buried victims very quickly, but they are typically brought to the scene after victims have been buried for an extended period. Consequently, very few live rescues have been done using search dogs.
3. Another factor that affects survival is the position of the victim's head (i.e., whether the victim was buried face up or face down). The most favorable position is face up. Data from a limited number of burials show the victim is twice as likely to survive if buried face up rather than face down. If buried face up, an airspace forms around the face as the back of the head melts into the snow; if buried face down, an airspace cannot form as the face melts into the snow (Table 2-1).

TABLE 2-1. Injuries in Survivors of Avalanche Burial (Partial and Total)

	UTAH	EUROPE
TOTAL INJURIES	*9 (TOTAL, 91 AVALANCHE ACCIDENTS)*	*351 (TOTAL, 1447 AVALANCHE ACCIDENTS)*
Major orthopedic	3 (33%)	95 (27%)
Hypothermia requiring treatment at hospital arrival	2 (22%)	74 (21%)
Skin/soft tissue	1 (11%)	84 (25%)
Craniofacial	—	83 (24%)
Chest	3 (33%)	7 (2%)
Abdominal	—	4 (1%)

From Grossman MD, Saffle JR, Thomas F, Tremper B: J Trauma 29:1705-1709, 1989.

Care of the Victim (Fig. 2-4)

Treatment
1. Manage the ABCs (airway, breathing, and circulation).
2. Immobilize the spine as needed.
3. Stabilize any fractures or other injuries.
4. Provide thermal stabilization (see Chapter 3). Handle the victim gently in anticipation of hypothermia.
5. Provide for evacuation.

References

1. Brugger H, Durrer B: On-site treatment of avalanche victims: ICAR-MEDCOM-Recommendation. High Alt Med Biol 3:421-425, 2002.
2. Brugger H, Durrer B, Adler-Kastner L: On-site triage of avalanche victims with asystole by the emergency doctor. Resuscitation 31:11-16, 1996.

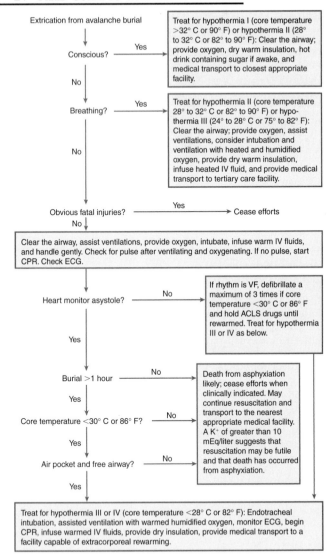

Figure 2-4. Assessment and medical care of extricated avalanche burial victim.

Hypothermia

3

▶ **DEFINITION**

Accidental hypothermia is the unintentional decline of at least approximately 2° C (3.6° F) in the normal human core temperature of 37.2° C to 37.7° C (99° F to 99.8° F) that occurs in the absence of any causation originating in the preoptic and anterior hypothalamic nuclei. It is both a symptom and a clinical disease entity. Hypothermia occurs in mild, moderate, or severe forms (Table 3-1).

▶ **GENERAL TREATMENT**

1. Consider rescue scene safety factors including unstable snow, ice, and rock fall.
2. Handle all victims of moderate or severe hypothermia carefully to avoid unnecessary jostling or sudden impact. Rough handling can cause ventricular fibrillation.
3. The rescuer should stabilize injuries, protect the spine, splint fractures, and cover open wounds.
4. Prevent further heat loss; insulate the victim from above and below.
5. Anticipate an irritable myocardium, hypovolemia, and a large temperature gradient between the periphery and the core.
6. Assume problematic intravenous access on hypodynamic, volume-depleted, and vasoconstricted hypothermic patients. Consider intraosseous ("IO") infusion systems. Many civilian and military rescue groups now carry IO needles and adapters.
7. Treat hypothermia before treating frostbite.

▶ **DISORDERS**

Mild Hypothermia
Mild hypothermia is diagnosed when the body temperature is between 37° C (98.6° F) and 33° C (91.4° F).

Signs and Symptoms
1. Shivering
2. Dysarthria
3. Poor judgment, perseveration, or neurosis
4. Amnesia
5. Apathy or moodiness
6. Ataxia

TABLE 3-1. Characteristics of the Four Zones of Hypothermia

CORE TEMPERATURE		CHARACTERISTICS
°C	°F	
Mild		
37.6	99.6 ± 1	Normal rectal temperature
37.0	98.6 ± 1	Normal oral temperature
36.0	96.8	Increase in metabolic rate and blood pressure and preshivering muscle tone
35.0	95.0	Urine temperature 34.8° C; maximum shivering thermogenesis
34.0	93.2	Amnesia, dysarthria, and poor judgment develop; maladaptive behavior; normal blood pressure; maximum respiratory stimulation; tachycardia, then progressive bradycardia
33.0	91.4	Ataxia and apathy develop; linear depression of cerebral metabolism; tachypnea, then progressive decrease in respiratory minute volume; cold diuresis
Moderate		
32.0	89.6	Stupor; 25% decrease in oxygen consumption
31.0	87.8	Extinguished shivering thermogenesis
30.0	86.0	Atrial fibrillation and other arrhythmias develop; poikilothermy; pupils and cardiac output two thirds of normal; insulin ineffective
29.0	85.2	Progressive decrease in level of consciousness, pulse, and respiration; pupils dilated; paradoxical undressing
Severe		
28.0	82.4	Decreased ventricular fibrillation threshold; 50% decrease in oxygen consumption and pulse; hypoventilation
27.0	80.6	Loss of reflexes and voluntary motion
26.0	78.8	Major acid-base disturbances; no reflexes or response to pain
25.0	77.0	Cerebral blood flow one third of normal; loss of cerebrovascular autoregulation; cardiac output 45% of normal; pulmonary edema may develop
24.0	75.2	Significant hypotension and bradycardia
23.0	73.4	No corneal or oculocephalic reflexes; areflexia
22.0	71.6	Maximum risk of ventricular fibrillation; 75% decrease in oxygen consumption

TABLE 3-1. Characteristics of the Four Zones of Hypothermia—cont'd

CORE TEMPERATURE		CHARACTERISTICS
Profound		
20.0	68.0	Lowest resumption of cardiac electromechanical activity; pulse 20% of normal
19.0	66.2	Electroencephalographic silencing
18.0	64.4	Asystole
13.7	56.8	Lowest adult accidental hypothermia survival
15.0	59.2	Lowest infant accidental hypothermia survival
10.0	50.0	92% decrease in oxygen consumption
9.0	48.2	Lowest therapeutic hypothermia survival

7. Initial hyperreflexia, tachypnea, tachycardia, elevated systemic blood pressure
8. Hunger, nausea, fatigue, dizziness

Treatment
If the victim is awake:
1. Gently remove all wet clothing and replace it with dry clothing.
2. Insulate the victim with sleeping bags, cloth pads, bubble wrap, blankets, or other suitable material.
3. Always insulate the victim from the ground up. Use adequate insulation underneath the victim.
4. If the victim is capable of purposeful swallowing (will not aspirate), encourage drinking of warm and sweet drinks, warm gelatin (Jell-O), reconstituted fruit beverages, juice, or decaffeinated tea or cocoa. Avoid heavily caffeinated drinks.
5. If a mildly hypothermic victim is well hydrated and insulated from further cooling, he or she can often walk out to safety.

Moderate Hypothermia
Moderate hypothermia is diagnosed when the body temperature is between 32° C (89.6° F) and 27° C (80.6° F).

Signs and Symptoms
1. Stupor progressing to unconsciousness
2. Loss of shivering reflex

3. Atrial fibrillation and other arrhythmias, bradycardia
4. Poikilothermy
5. Mild to moderate hypotension
6. Diminished respiratory rate and effort, bronchorrhea
7. Dilated pupils
8. Diminished neurologic reflexes and voluntary motion
9. Decreased ventricular fibrillation threshold
10. Prolonged PR, QR, and QTc intervals; J (Osborne) wave
11. Paradoxical undressing

Treatment
If the victim is confused, stuporous, or unconscious and shows obvious signs of life:
1. Handle gently and immobilize the victim (reduces the potential for ventricular fibrillation).
2. Consider helicopter evacuation to prevent jostling.
3. Maintain the victim in a horizontal position to avoid orthostatic hypotension.
4. Do not encourage ingestion of oral fluids. The small contribution to hydration and rewarming is outweighed by the risk of aspiration.
5. Do not massage or vigorously manipulate the victim's extremities.
6. Provide oxygenation commensurate with the victim's clinical condition.
   a. Options include simple administration of oxygen by nasal cannula or facemask, bag-valve-mask ventilation, or endotracheal intubation.
   b. If endotracheal intubation is performed, avoid overinflation of the tube cuff with frigid air, which will expand and kink the tube as the air within the cuff warms.
7. If intravenous (IV) capability exists, initiate an IV line and administer 250 to 500 mL of heated (37° C to 41° C [98.6° F to 105.8° F]) 5% dextrose in normal saline (NS) solution. If NS solution is unavailable, use any crystalloid, preferably with dextrose. Avoid lactated Ringer's solution because a cold liver poorly metabolizes lactate. The fluid can be infused rapidly and warmed by any of the following techniques:
   a. Place the IV bag underneath the victim's back, shoulder, or buttocks.
   b. Tape heat-producing packets to the IV bag.
   c. Use an IV fluid-compressor inflatable cuff.
   d. If heated fluids are unavailable, administer fluid heated to the rescuer's skin temperature (i.e., >86° F [30° C]). This can be accomplished by carrying plastic IV bags next to the skin during rescue.

8. Consider treatment of hypoglycemia, specifically, therapy with 50% dextrose, 25 g IV.
9. Consider treatment of opiate effects, specifically, therapy with naloxone, 0.8 to 1.6 mg IV.
10. Consider treatment for benzodiazepine ingestion, specifically, therapy with flumazenil, 0.2 mg IV.
11. Stabilize the victim's body temperature.
    a. Remove wet clothing and replace it with dry clothing; insulate the victim from above and below.
    b. Be cautious with immersion warming in the field because this may cause core temperature "after drop."
    c. Place hot water bottles or padded heat packs in the axillae and groin area and around the neck. Wrap hot water bottles with insulation (e.g., fleece) to prevent thermal burns.
    d. Initiate external warming using blankets, sleeping bags, or shelter. In the field, the patient should be wrapped. The wrap starts with a large plastic sheet on which is placed an insulated sleeping pad. A layer of blankets, sleeping bag, or bubble wrap insulating material is laid over the sleeping bag. The victim is placed on the insulation, the heating bottles are put in place along with IVs, and the entire package is wrapped layer over layer. The plastic is the final closure. The face should be partially covered, but a tunnel should be created to allow access for breathing and monitoring of the victim.
    e. A warmed-air-circulating heater pack may be used as an adjunct.
    f. Consider inhalation rewarming if available and personnel are well trained in its use (with active humidification if possible).

Severe Hypothermia

Severe hypothermia is diagnosed when the body temperature falls below 26° C (78.8° F).

Signs and Symptoms
1. Absent neurologic reflexes (deep tendon, corneal, oculocephalic)
2. Absent response to pain
3. Pulmonary edema
4. Acid-base abnormalities
5. Coagulopathy, thrombocytopenia
6. Significant hypotension
7. Significant risk for ventricular fibrillation

8. Flat electroencephalogram
9. Asystole

Treatment

When the victim is confused, stuporous, or unconscious and shows obvious signs of life, follow the treatment guidelines for moderate hypothermia. When no immediate signs of life are present, do the following:

1. Determine if the victim is breathing.
   a. Because chest rise may be difficult to discern, listen and feel carefully around the nose and mouth. A "vapor trail" is usually absent. If a stethoscope is available, auscultate for breath sounds in the absence of discernible ventilation.
   b. If the victim is not breathing, assist with oxygenation and ventilation by endotracheal intubation or the next best method available.
2. Feel for a pulse (best done at the carotid or femoral arteries). Do this for at least 1 minute. If a stethoscope is available, auscultate for heart sounds in the absence of a palpable pulse.
3. Unnecessary chest compressions of cardiopulmonary resuscitation (CPR) may initiate ventricular fibrillation and thus may be catastrophic.
4. Most wilderness rescue environments will preclude the use of a cardiac monitor or defibrillator. If a cardiac monitor is available, use it.
   a. If ventricular fibrillation or apparent asystole is determined, defibrillate one time with 2 watt-sec/kg up to 200 watt-sec. Use benzoin to affix nonadherent electrodes. Do not defibrillate if electrical complexes are seen on a cardiac monitor. Defibrillation rarely succeeds below a core temperature of 30° C (86° F). If the victim is in asystole or ventricular fibrillation, begin CPR.
   b. If electrical complexes are seen on a cardiac monitor, assess for a central pulse to determine if true electromechanical dissociation exists. This is a difficult judgment call. The victim may have a low blood pressure that cannot be appreciated by the rescuer, in which case the chest compressions of CPR might initiate ventricular fibrillation.
4. If resuscitation is not successful in the field, continue warming and CPR until the victim arrives at a hospital or you cannot continue because of fatigue or danger to yourself.
5. If the resuscitation is successful, follow the preceding protocol for moderate or severe hypothermia.
6. Use pneumatic military antishock trousers (MAST) only for temporary stabilization of a major pelvic fracture (Box 3-1).

> ### Box 3-1. Preparing Hypothermic Patients for Transport
>
> 1. The patient must be dry. Gently remove or cut off wet clothing and replace it with dry clothing or a dry insulation system. Keep the patient horizontal, and do not allow exertion or massage of the extremities.
> 2. Stabilize injuries (i.e., the spine; place fractures in the correct anatomic position). Open wounds should be covered before packaging.
> 3. Initiate intravenous infusions (IVs) if feasible; bags can be placed under the patient's buttocks or in a compressor system. Administer a fluid challenge.
> 4. Active rewarming should be limited to heated inhalation and truncal heat. Insulate hot water bottles in stockings or mittens and then place them in the patient's axillae and groin.
> 5. The patient should be wrapped. Begin building the wrap by placing a large plastic sheet on the available surface (floor, ground), and on it place an insulated sleeping pad. A layer of blankets, a sleeping bag, or bubble wrap insulating material is laid over the sleeping pad. The patient is then placed on the insulation. Heating bottles are put in place along with IVs, and the entire package is wrapped layer over layer, with the plastic as the final closure. The patient's face should be partially covered, but a tunnel should be created to allow access for breathing and monitoring.

Rewarming Options

Passive External Rewarming in the Field
1. Cover the victim with dry insulating materials in a warm environment.
2. Block the wind.
3. Keep the victim dry.
4. Insulate the patient from the ground (e.g., foam pad).
5. Use a windproof tarp, tent fly, or an aluminized (reflective) body cover such as a "space blanket."
6. Rescue groups typically carry specialized casualty evacuation bags. These are often windproof, waterproof, and well insulated. Many offer specialized zippers and openings for patient access.

Active External Rewarming in the Field
1. Apply hot water bottles, chemical heat packs, or warmed rocks to areas of high circulation such as around the neck, in the axillae, and in the groin. Take care to avoid thermal burns by insulating the heated objects adequately.
2. Use skin-to-skin contact by putting a normothermic rescuer in contact with the victim inside a sleeping bag. This

method may suppress shivering and reduce rewarming rates in mildly hypothermic persons. It may, however, be one of few options in remote locations or with severely hypothermic, nonshivering victims, especially when evacuation will be delayed.

3. Use a forced-air warming system within a sleeping bag.
4. Immerse the victim in a warm (40° C [104° F]) water bath. Be cautious with immersion warming in the field because this may increase core temperature "after drop."
5. Place the hands and feet in warm (40° C [104° F]) water.
6. Do not rub or massage cold extremities in an attempt to rewarm them.

Core Rewarming in the Field (note that the impact of these modalities on the rate of rewarming in the field may not be significant)

1. Use heated (40° C to 45° C [104° F to 113° F]), humidified oxygen inhalation.
2. Administer heated (40° C to 42° C [104° F to 107.6° F]) IV solutions.

▶ CARDIOPULMONARY RESUSCITATION

Handle all victims gently to avoid creating a situation of ventricular fibrillation in the nonarrested heart.

1. Carefully determine the victim's cardiopulmonary status.
   a. Feel for a carotid or femoral pulse.
   b. Watch the chest for motion (breathing) for at least 30 seconds.
   c. Listen with the ear close to the victim's nose for breathing for at least 30 seconds.
2. If a hypothermic victim has any sign of life, do not begin the chest compressions of CPR, even if a peripheral pulse cannot be appreciated.
3. Manage the airway.
   a. If the victim is breathing at a suboptimal rate, assist with mouth-to-mouth or mouth-to-mask technique.
   b. If endotracheal intubation is available, perform it for standard indications (oxygenation, ventilation, and protection of the airway).
4. If the victim is without any sign of life, begin standard CPR.
   a. A single rescuer who is fatigued may continue at slower rates of compression and artificial breathing with some expectation that these may be adequate because of the protective effects of hypothermia.
   b. Continue CPR until the victim is brought to a hospital, the rescuer is fatigued, or the rescuer is endangered.

5. Do not begin CPR if the victim has suffered obviously fatal injuries.
   a. A serum potassium (K^+) level greater than 10 mEq/L in the presence of hypothermia is a strong prognostic marker for death.
   b. Remember that a victim who appears dead may recover from hypothermia, so if in doubt, begin the resuscitation.

4 Frostbite and Trench Foot

FROSTBITE

▶ DEFINITIONS

In mild frostbite there is no tissue loss, whereas in severe frostbite, tissue loss occurs. In another classification, severity of frostbite is divided into first, second, third, and fourth degrees.

▶ DISORDERS

First-Degree Frostbite

Signs and Symptoms
1. Numbness
2. Erythema
3. White or yellowish plaque
4. Edema
5. Occasional blue mottling
6. Skin insensate and firm with normal or diminished pliability

Second-Degree Frostbite

Signs and Symptoms
1. Superficial blisters with clear or milky fluid
2. Erythema and edema surrounding blisters (see Plate 1)

Third-Degree Frostbite

Deeper blisters characterized by hemorrhagic fluid

Fourth-Degree Frostbite

Signs and Symptoms
1. Injury that extends through the skin into muscle and beyond
2. Leads to mummification and bone involvement (see Plate 2)

Proposed Classification

A newer proposed classification (Table 4-1) is based on the risk of amputation of the affected part for the hand and foot. This classification may have greater clinical relevance by attempting to guide treatment considerations and planning. The classification relies on early bone scanning but includes useful clinical considerations as well (Tables 4-2 and 4-3).

TABLE 4-1. Proposed Classification for Severity of Frostbite Injuries of the Extremities

	GRADE 1	GRADE 2	GRADE 3	GRADE 4
Extent of initial lesion at day 0 after rapid re-warming	Absence of initial lesion	Initial lesion on distal phalanx	Initial lesion on middle (or) prox-imal pha-lanx	Initial lesion on carpal/tarsal
Bone scanning at day 2	Useless	Hypofixa-tion of radio-tracer uptake area	Absence of radio-tracer	Absence of radio-tracer uptake area on the car-pal/tarsal
Blisters at day 2	Absence of blis-ters	Clear blis-ters	Hemor-rhagic blisters on the digit	Hemor-rhagic blisters over car-pal/tarsal
Prognosis at day 2	No ampu-tation	Tissue am-putation	Bone ampu-tation of digit	Bone ampu-tation of the limb ± sys-temic in-volvement ± sepsis
Sequelae	No sequelae	Fingernail sequelae	Functional sequelae	Functional sequelae

From Cauchy E, Chetaille E, Marchand V, Marsigny B: Retrospective study of 70 cases of severe frostbite lesions: A proposed new classification scheme. Wilderness Environ Med 12:248-255, 2001.

▶ **PROGNOSIS**

Favorable Prognostic Signs (after Rewarming)
1. Sensation to pinprick
2. Normal color
3. Warmth
4. Large clear blebs that appear early and extend to tips of the digits

Unfavorable Prognostic Signs (after Rewarming)
1. Small dark blebs that appear late and do not extend to the tips of the digits

TABLE 4-2. Management of Frostbite Injuries of the Extremities

On day 0, treatment consists of rapid rewarming for 2 hours in 38° C water bath, with intravenous infusion of 400 mg chlorohydrate of bluflomedil (vasodilator) and 250 mg aspirin. Subsequent treatment depends on the extent of the initial lesion, as follows:

GRADE 1: ABSENCE OF INITIAL LESION	GRADE 2: INITIAL LESION OVER DISTAL PHALANX	GRADE 3: INITIAL LESION OVER MIDDLE (OR) PROXIMAL PHALANX	GRADE 4: INITIAL LESION OVER CARPAL/ TARSAL
No hospitalization	Hospitalization 2 days	Hospitalization 8 days	Hospitalization intensive care unit
Oral treatment for 1 wk (aspirin, vasodilator)	Possibly a bone scan at day 2	Bone scan at day 2	Bone scan at day 2
Recovery	Oral treatment for 3 wk (aspirin, vasodilators), dressing	IV administration for 8 days (aspirin, vasodilators), dressing	IV administration for 8 days (aspirin, vasodilators), dressing
	Recovery with moderate sequelae	Bone scan near day 8	Possibly antibiotics
		Bone amputation near day 30	Early bone amputation near day 3 if sepsis
		Bone amputation of the digit with functional sequelae	Bone amputation of the limbs with systemic involvement

From Cauchy E, Chetaille E, Marchand V, Marsigny B: Retrospective study of 70 cases of severe frostbite lesions: A proposed new classification scheme. Wilderness Environ Med 12:248-255, 2001.

2. Absence of edema
3. Cyanosis that does not blanch with pressure

TABLE 4-3. Probability of Amputation Based on the Extent of the Initial Lesion

	EXTENT (LEVEL OF INVOLVEMENT)	PROBABILITY OF BONE AMPUTATION (95% CI)
Hand	5 (carpal/tarsal)	100
	4 (metacarpal/metatarsal)	100
	3 (proximal phalanx)	83
	2 (intermediate phalanx)	39
	1 (distal phalanx)	1
Foot	5 (carpal/tarsal)	100
	4 (metacarpal/metatarsal)	98
	3 (proximal phalanx)	60
	2 (intermediate phalanx)	23
	1 (distal phalanx)	0
Hand and foot	5 (carpal/tarsal)	100
	4 (metacarpal/metatarsal)	98
	3 (proximal phalanx)	67
	2 (intermediate phalanx)	31
	1 (distal phalanx)	1

Adapted from Cauchy E, Chetaille E, Marchand V, Marsigny B: Retrospective study of 70 cases of severe frostbite lesions: A proposed new classification scheme. Wilderness Environ Med 12:248-255, 2001.

Note
1. No prognostic technique is absolutely accurate in the immediate post-thaw period.
2. Radioisotope scanning or other diagnostic modalities may be used to aid prognosis at 2 to 3 weeks following injury. Earlier scans (at day 2) have been used recently to provide earlier insight into prognosis (see Table 4-1).

▶ TREATMENT

Treatment of All Degrees of Frostbite
The preferred field treatment is rapid rewarming if the affected tissue can be kept warm enough after the thaw to avoid refreezing, which might be disastrous.
1. Protect the victim from the environment and provide appropriate shelter.
2. Transfer or evacuation arrangements must protect the victim from cold exposure.
3. Replace constricting and wet clothing with dry, loose wraps or garments.
4. Do not attempt rewarming during transport unless it will be "rapid" (see next section). Do not attempt partial or slow rewarming.

5. Do not attempt rewarming using the radiant warmth from a campfire or the exhaust from a car heater or tailpipe.
6. Do not attempt rewarming if the victim is severely hypothermic, unless done in conjunction with systemic rewarming.
7. Do not attempt rewarming if part or all the victim's foot is involved, and he or she will need to put the boot back on and continue to walk or climb. Rewarm only when the boot can remain off. NOTE: This does not necessarily apply for frostbite of the toes only.
8. As stated earlier, do not attempt rewarming if there is any chance of refreezing.
9. If field conditions make it impossible to rewarm in the field or if contraindications exist, transport the victim. If transport will precede rewarming (victim can be brought to definitive medical attention within 2 hours), pad all affected parts as best possible. During transport do the following:
   a. Keep the victim well hydrated (PO or IV).
   b. Keep the victim warm.
   c. Administer oxygen.
   d. Elevate the injured extremity.
   e. Protect from further trauma.
   f. Place sterile gauze fluffs between fingers and toes to prevent maceration.
   g. Use fluffy sterile dressings to maintain hands and feet in position of function.
   h. Keep sleeping bag, blankets, and other pressure-generating objects off toes by improvising a foot cradle.
   i. Prohibit tobacco use.
   j. Consider antiprostaglandin therapy (i.e., ibuprofen, 400 mg PO q12h).

Rapid Rewarming Techniques—"Field Rewarming"

1. Always treat hypothermia before or along with rewarming frostbitten extremities.
2. Immerse affected tissues in gently circulating water warmed to 40° C to 42° C (104° F to 108° F).
3. Rewarm until the skin is pliable and erythematous at the most distal parts of the frostbitten extremities.
4. Allow active motion, but do not massage injured parts.
5. Manage pain with analgesics (may require intravenous narcotics).
6. After thawing is complete, keep the victim and tissues warm. Do not allow refreezing.

Extended Field Care

1. Evacuate as soon as practical.
2. Keep the victim well hydrated (PO or IV).

3. Apply padded and sterile (or as clean as possible) dressings to all blistered areas. Place sterile gauze fluffs between fingers and toes to prevent maceration.
4. Do not rupture blisters.
5. If blisters rupture spontaneously, apply topical aloe vera or antiseptic (e.g., mupirocin) ointment.
6. Pad with sterile cotton gauze or soft cloth between fingers and toes.
7. Pad all splints.
8. Elevate the affected parts.
9. Keep sleeping bag, blankets, and other pressure-generating objects off toes by improvising a foot cradle.
10. If injury is deep, change dressings daily. If blisters are present, perform daily irrigation with disinfected lukewarm water, encourage active range of motion, and air dry or gently blot dry with sterile gauze.
11. Encourage active movement of extremities, but not passive motion (i.e., do not manipulate).
12. Administer antiprostaglandin therapy (ibuprofen, 400 mg PO q12h).
13. Observe daily for development of new areas of blistering or infection.
14. If the injury is extensive or blisters are ruptured, administer an oral antibiotic in a dose appropriate for age.
15. Prohibit tobacco use.
16. If indicated and available, administer antitetanus prophylaxis.
17. The use of adjunctive therapies such as dextran, heparin, pentoxifylline, and other agents is controversial and usually reserved for the hospital environment.

▶ PREVENTION

1. Maintain adequate systemic hydration.
2. Wear properly fitted, nonconstricting clothing, particularly footgear.
   a. Avoid wrinkles in socks.
   b. Keep mittens, gloves, and footgear dry.
   c. Wear mittens in preference to gloves.
   d. Keep fingernails and toenails properly trimmed.
   e. Carry extra garments.
3. Do not handle cold liquids or metals. (NOTE: Fuel and metal cameras are common culprits.)
4. Maintain an adequate diet in the cold.
5. Avoid fatigue and sleep loss.
6. Maintain oxygenation, using supplemental oxygen at altitude.
7. Maintain a dry, warm environment.

8. Do not overwash skin; allow natural oils to accumulate.
9. Wind and high altitude greatly increase risk.
10. Avoid ingested alcohol and inhaled tobacco.
11. Persons with preexisting Raynaud's phenomenon or prior cold injury should exercise special caution.
12. Tetanus immunity should be current.

TRENCH FOOT (IMMERSION FOOT)

Trench foot follows exposure to nonfreezing cold and wet conditions over a number of days, leading to neurovascular damage without ice crystal formation.

▶ OVERVIEW

1. Injury occurs when tissue is exposed to cold and wet conditions at temperatures ranging from 0° C to 15° C (32° F to 59° F).
2. Injury may extend proximally and involve the knees, thighs, and buttocks.
3. Usually insidious in onset.

Signs and Symptoms
1. Red skin that becomes pale and extremely edematous
2. Early numbness, painful paresthesias
3. Leg cramps
4. During the first few hours to days: limb hyperemia with swelling, then diffuse discoloration, mottling, and numbness
5. Delayed capillary refill or petechial hemorrhages possible
6. After 2 to 7 days: hyperemia predominant, with regional skin temperature variation, edema, blisters, and ulceration
7. After 7 days, nature of the pain changes to "shooting or stabbing"
8. Sensory deficits may diminish, but paresthesias continue; anesthesia may remain extensive
9. Anhidrosis often present

Treatment
1. Keep the affected area dry and warm.
2. Initial treatment is similar to that for frostbite, with the exception that rapid rewarming (thawing) is not necessary.
3. As with frostbite, elevate the affected extremity.
4. Recovery during the "posthyperemic" phase may be hastened by physiotherapy.

Prevention
1. Maintain body core temperature.
2. Remain active; encourage blood flow to the feet.
3. Make certain footwear fits properly and does not constrict.
4. Keep feet dry, continually changing socks (up to two to three times per day in some situations).
5. Limit sweat accumulation.
6. Take special care if wearing "vapor barrier boots."
7. Recent studies have shown effectiveness of silicone foot preparations.

5 Heat Illness

▶ DEFINITIONS

The term *heat illness* encompasses a spectrum of syndromes ranging from muscle cramps to heatstroke, which is a life-threatening emergency. Predisposing factors include the following:

1. Environmental temperature exceeding 35° C (95° F) with humidity level greater than 80%
2. Dehydration, as indicated by dark yellow–colored urine
3. Obesity
4. Cardiovascular disease
5. Fever
6. Hyperactivity
   a. Seizures
   b. Psychosis
   c. Cocaine or amphetamine intoxication
7. Muscular exertion
   a. Hard labor
   b. Strenuous exercise
8. Burns (including sunburn)
9. Drugs
   a. Anticholinergic agents (antihistamines, phenothiazines, antispasmodics)
   b. Beta-adrenergic blockers, angiotensin-converting enzyme (ACE) inhibitors, diuretics
10. Extremes of age, either very young or old
11. Fatigue or lack of sleep

Heat stress can be predicted by evaluation of the wet-bulb globe temperature (WBGT) index. Whereas a regular thermometer measures the dry-air temperature, a wet-bulb thermometer (WBT) measures the effect of humidity on temperature. The globe thermometer measures the effect of radiant heat. Because the WBGT is complex and 70% of the value is derived from the WBT, a simple alternative in the field is to use a sling psychrometer. This instrument has a thermometer with a wick surrounding the bulb attached to an aluminum frame with a hinged handle. After the wick is moistened, the psychrometer is slung over the head for approximately 2 minutes. Air passing over the wetted thermometer bulb cools the bulb in inverse proportion to the humidity. The WBGT can be used as a guide for recommended activity levels (Table 5-1).

TABLE 5-1. Wet Bulb Globe Temperature and Recommended Activity Levels

°C	°F	RECOMMENDATIONS
15.5	60	No precautions necessary
16.2-21	61-70	No precautions if adequate hydration maintained
22-24	71-75	Unacclimatized: curtail exercise
		Acclimatized: exercise with caution; rest periods and water breaks every 20 to 30 minutes
24.5-26.6	76-80	Unacclimatized: avoid hiking or sports or sun exposure
		Acclimatized: heavy to moderate work with caution
27-30	81-85	Limited brief activity for acclimatized, fit persons only
31	88	Avoid activity and sun exposure

▶ **DISORDERS**

Heat Edema

Signs and Symptoms
Peripheral edema develops during the first few days in a hot environment.

Treatment
Be aware that the edema is usually self-limited and does not require medical therapy.

"Prickly Heat" (Miliaria Rubra)

Signs and Symptoms
1. Erythematous, papular, pruritic rash developing on actively sweating skin
2. In dry climates, rash confined to skin sufficiently occluded by clothing to produce local high humidity
3. Skin that does not sweat effectively, predisposing to heat exhaustion and heatstroke

Treatment
1. Cool and dry affected skin.
2. Administer antihistamines (diphenhydramine, 25 to 50 mg q4-6h) to relieve itching.
3. Desquamation of the affected epidermis and recovery of sweat gland function occurs in 7 to 10 days.

Heat Syncope

Signs and Symptoms
Syncope occurs after prolonged standing in a hot environment.

Treatment
1. Perform a secondary assessment after a primary survey to assess for any trauma that may have occurred because of a fall.
2. Place the victim in the Trendelenburg position.
3. Cool the victim and administer oral fluids (at least 1 L over 1 hour) when he or she is awake and alert. A carbohydrate-containing beverage can be absorbed by the body up to 30% faster than plain water. To disinfected water, add a powdered sports drink mix; a 6% or 7% carbohydrate concentration such as diluted Gatorade (one third to one half strength) is ideal. Higher carbohydrate concentrations should be avoided because they can produce stomach cramps and delay absorption.
4. Note that colder fluids are more easily absorbed from the stomach.
5. Unacclimatized individuals working in the heat for 8 hours a day can develop a salt deficit and electrolyte imbalance unless a small amount of salt is added to their drinking water. The ideal concentration is a 0.1% salt solution, which can be prepared by dissolving two 10-grain salt tablets or ¼ tsp of table salt in a quart of water. Crush the salt tablets before attempting to dissolve them. Salt tablets should not be eaten by themselves. They irritate the stomach, produce vomiting, and do not treat the dehydration that is also present.

Heat Cramps

Signs and Symptoms
1. Painful, spasmodic muscle cramps that usually occur in heavily exercised muscles
2. Recurrent cramps that may be precipitated by manipulation of the muscle
3. Onset during exercise or after the work effort

Treatment
1. Administer an oral rehydration solution containing 3.5 g sodium chloride (¼ tsp salt) and 1.5 g potassium chloride in 1 L drinking water. Many sport drinks such as Gatorade will do just as well. Due to the high osmolality, dilute Gatorade half strength with water.
2. Allow the victim to rest in a cool environment.

Heat Exhaustion

Signs and Symptoms
1. Flu-like symptoms (malaise, headache, weakness, nausea, anorexia)
2. Vomiting
3. Orthostatic hypotension
4. Tachycardia
5. Core body temperature usually less than 38° C to 39° C (100.4° F to 102.2° F) and often normal
6. Sweating
7. Normal mental status and normal findings on neurologic examination

Treatment
1. Stop all exertion and move the victim to a cool and shaded environment.
2. Remove restrictive clothing.
3. Administer an oral rehydration solution (see earlier).
4. Place ice or cold packs on the neck, chest wall, axillae, and groin. (Do not place ice directly against skin.) Fanning the victim, while spraying with tepid water and soaking the victim in cool water, is also an effective cooling method.

Heatstroke

Heatstroke is a true medical emergency; if not promptly and effectively treated, the mortality approaches 80%. Environmental heatstroke can be thought of as the end stage of heat exhaustion, when compensatory mechanisms for dissipating heat fail. The transition from heat exhaustion to heatstroke is often noted when a victim shows abnormal mental status and neurologic function.

Signs and Symptoms
1. Elevated core body temperature, usually above 40.5° C (105° F)
2. Altered neurologic state (confusion, disorientation, bizarre behavior, ataxia, seizures, coma). Loss of coordination is one of the earliest manifestations.
3. Tachycardia
4. Hypotension
5. Tachypnea
6. Sweating present or absent

Treatment
1. Provide rapid cooling. The prognosis is a function of the magnitude and duration of hyperthermia. The faster cooling is accomplished, the lower the morbidity and mortality.

   a. Place ice or cold packs on the neck, axillae, chest wall, and groin.

   b. Wet with tepid water, then fan rapidly to facilitate evaporative cooling.

   c. Immerse in cool water if available.

2. Protect the airway, and do not give anything by mouth because of the risk of vomiting and aspiration.
3. Administer fluid intravenously (1 to 2 L normal saline solution).
4. Treat for shock; specifically, administer oxygen if available.
5. Treat seizures and combative behavior with a benzodiazepine (diazepam, 2 to 5 mg IV adult dose) or a barbiturate.
6. Suppress shivering by administering a benzodiazepine or chlorpromazine (25 to 50 mg IM or IV).
7. Evacuate the victim immediately to the nearest medical facility. Continue to cool the victim during transport until his or her core body temperature has fallen to 38° C to 39° C (100.4° F to 102.2° F).
8. Recheck the temperature at least every 30 minutes.

Hyponatremia

Symptomatic hyponatremia is diagnosed when serum sodium is less than 130 mEq/L and is generally caused by drinking large volumes of water or markedly hypo-osmotic fluids. It may be difficult to differentiate between hyponatremia from water intoxication and heat exhaustion/heatstroke in the field because of considerable overlap of symptoms. A major difference is that in heat illnesses, core body temperature is generally greater than 39° C (102.2° F), whereas in hyponatremia, core temperature is usually normal or close to normal.

Signs and Symptoms
1. Weakness
2. Anorexia
3. Vomiting
4. Muscle cramps
5. Altered neurologic state (lethargy, apathy, confusion, disorientation, agitation, psychosis, seizures, coma)

Treatment
1. Fluid restriction in stable asymptomatic patient. If the victim is mentating and capable of safely consuming oral liquids, have him or her drink a full-strength (not diluted) sports beverage such as Gatorade.
2. If available, administer intravenous normal saline at 250 to 500 mL per hour until the victim is well hydrated.

3. If hyponatremia is severe (<120 mEq/L) and develops rapidly (within 24 hours) with central nervous system manifestations, administer 3% saline solution at 25 to 100 mL/hr.

▶ **ACCLIMATIZATION**

Physiologic acclimatization to a hot environment is an important adaptive response. It usually requires 8 to 11 days to reach maximum benefit and mandates some amount of daily exercise (1 to 2 hours/day). With acclimatization, sweating is initiated at lower body temperatures and the sweat rate may more than double (up to 1 to 3 L/hour or up to 15 L/day). Sodium is conserved in both urine and sweat, in contrast to the unacclimatized state.

Work in the heat mandates constant fluid replenishment. Because net water absorption in the gut is about 20 mL/minute or 1200 mL/hour, compensation for high sweat rates requires rest periods with reduced sweat rates and time for hydration. Thirst is a poor indicator of adequate hydration because it is not stimulated until plasma osmolarity rises 1% to 2% above normal.

6

Wildland Fires

▶ SENSIBLE LAND DEVELOPMENT PRACTICES

1. Create access to adequate water sources.
2. Do not stack firewood next to houses.
3. Do not pile slash (e.g., branches, stumps, logs, and other vegetative residues) on home sites or along access roads.
4. Do not build structures on slopes with unenclosed stilt foundations.
5. Remove trees and shrubs growing next to structures, under eaves, and among stilt foundations.
6. Do not create roads that are steep, narrow, winding, unmapped, unsigned, unnamed, and bordered by slash or dense vegetation because these are prone to be difficult, if not impossible, for fire suppression vehicles to negotiate.
7. Do not place a dwelling or group of dwellings in an area without at least two or more access roads for simultaneous ingress and egress.
8. Do not create roads and bridges without the grade, design, and width to permit simultaneous evacuation by residents and access by firefighters and emergency medical personnel and their equipment.
9. Do not place dwellings and other structures on excessive slopes, within continuous or heavy fuel situations, or in box canyons.
10. Place constructed firebreaks and fuel breaks around home sites and within clusters of dwellings.
11. Be certain to prune, thin, landscape, or otherwise reduce living fuels, vegetation, and litter that readily contribute to spot fire development and fire intensity.
12. Do not construct homes with flammable building materials such as wooden shake shingles.
13. Do not expose propane tanks to the external environment.
14. Create a system that will allow delivery of water effectively before and during passage of a fire front in and around the structure.

▶ **EARLY WARNING SIGNALS OR INDICATORS ASSOCIATED WITH EXTREME FIRE BEHAVIOR**

Fuel

1. Continuous fine fuels, especially fully cured (dead) grasses
2. Large quantities of medium and heavy fuels (e.g., deep duff layers, dead-down logs)

3. Abundance of bridge or ladder fuels in forest stands (e.g., branches, lichens, suspending needles, flaky or shaggy bark, small conifer trees, tall shrubs extending from the ground surface upward)
4. Tight tree crown spacing in conifer forests
5. Presence of numerous snags
6. Significant amounts of dead material in elevated, shrubland fuel complexes
7. Seasonal changes in vegetation (e.g., frost kill)
8. Fire, meterorologic, or insect and disease impacts (e.g., preheated canopy or crown scorch, snow-, wind-, or ice-damaged stands, drought-stressed vegetation, or mountain pine beetle–killed stands)

Weather
1. Extended dry spell
2. Drought conditions
3. High air temperatures
4. Low relative humidity
5. Moderately strong, sustained winds
6. Unstable atmosphere (visual indicators include gusty winds, dust devils, good visibility, and smoke rising straight up)
7. Towering cumulus clouds
8. High, fast-moving clouds
9. Battling or shifting winds
10. Sudden calm
11. Virga (a veil of rain beneath a cloud that does not reach the ground)

Topography
1. Steep slopes
2. South- and southwest-facing slopes in northern hemisphere
3. North- and northeast-facing slopes in southern hemisphere
4. Gaps or saddles
5. Chutes, chimneys, and narrow or box canyons

Fire Behavior
1. Many fires that start simultaneously
2. Fire that smolders over a large area
3. Rolling and burning pine cones, agaves, logs, hot rocks, and other debris igniting fuel downslope
4. Frequent spot fires developing and coalescing
5. Spot fires occurring out ahead of the main fire early on

6. Individual trees readily candling or torching out
7. Fire whirls that cause spot fires and contribute to erratic burning
8. Vigorous surface burning with flame lengths starting to exceed 1 to 2 m (3 to 6 ft)
9. Sizable areas of trees or shrubs that begin to readily burn as a "wall of flame"
10. Black or dark, massive smoke columns with rolling, boiling vertical development
11. Lateral movement of fire near the base of a steep slope

▶ CONDITIONS THAT PRODUCE A CROWN FIRE

1. Dry fuel
2. Low humidity and high temperatures
3. Heavy accumulations of dead and downed fuels
4. Small trees in the understory, or "ladder fuels"
5. Steep slope
6. Strong winds
7. Unstable atmosphere
8. Continuous crown layer

▶ TEN STANDARD FIREFIGHTING ORDERS

1. Keep informed of fire weather conditions, changes, and forecasts and how they may affect the area where you are located.
2. Know what the fire is doing at all times through personal observations, communication systems, or scouts.
3. Base all actions on current and expected behavior of the fire.
4. Determine escape routes and plans for everyone at risk and make certain that everyone understands routes and plans.
5. Post lookouts to watch the fire if you think there is any danger of being trapped, of increased fire activity, or of erratic fire behavior.
6. Be alert, keep calm, think clearly, and act decisively to avoid panic reactions.
7. Maintain prompt and clear communication with your group, firefighting forces, and command and communication centers.
8. Give clear, concise instructions and be sure that they are understood.
9. Maintain control of the people in your group at all times.
10. Fight the fire aggressively, but provide for safety first.

▶ **EIGHTEEN "WATCH OUT!" SITUATIONS IN THE WILDLAND FIRE ENVIRONMENT**

1. You are moving downhill toward a fire but must be aware that fire can move swiftly and suddenly uphill. Constantly observe fire behavior, fuels, and escape routes, assessing the fire's potential to run uphill.
2. You are on a hillside where rolling, burning material can ignite fuel from below. When below a fire, watch for burning materials, especially cones and logs, that can roll downhill and ignite a fire beneath you, trapping you between two coalescing fires.
3. Wind begins to blow, increase, or change direction. Wind strongly influences fire behavior, so be prepared to respond to sudden changes.
4. The weather becomes hotter and drier. Fire activity increases, and its behavior changes more rapidly as ambient temperature rises and relative humidity decreases.
5. Dense vegetation with unburned fuel is between you and the fire. The danger in this situation is that unburned fuels can ignite. If the fire is moving away from you, be alert for wind changes or spot fires that may ignite fuels near you. Do not be overconfident if the area has burned once because it can reignite if sufficient fuel remains.
6. You are in an unburned area near the fire where terrain and cover make travel difficult. The combination of fuel and difficult escape makes this dangerous.
7. Travel or work in an area you have not seen in daylight. Darkness and unfamiliarity create a dangerous combination.
8. You are unfamiliar with local factors influencing fire behavior. When possible, seek information on what to expect from knowledgeable people, especially those from the area.
9. By necessity, you have to make a frontal assault on a fire with tankers. Any encounter with an active line of fire is dangerous because of proximity to intense heat, smoke, and flames, along with limited escape opportunities.
10. Spot fires occur frequently across the fireline. Generally, increased spotting indicates increased fire activity and intensity. The danger is that of entrapment between coalescing fires.
11. The main fire cannot be seen, and you are not in communication with anyone who can see it. If you do not know the location, size, and behavior of the main fire, planning becomes guesswork, which is an unfavorable response.

12. An unclear assignment or confusing instructions have been received. Make sure that all assignments and instructions are fully understood.
13. You are drowsy and feel like resting or sleeping near the fireline in unburned fuel. This may lead to fire entrapment. No one should sleep near a wildland fire. If resting is absolutely necessary, choose a burned area that is safe from rolling material, smoke, reburn, and other dangers or seek a wide area of bare ground or rock.
14. Fire has not been scouted and sized up.
15. Safety zones and escape routes have not been identified.
16. You are uninformed on strategy, tactics, and hazards.
17. No communication link with crew members or supervisor has been established.
18. A line has been constructed without a safe anchor point.

▶ WILDLAND-URBAN "WATCH OUT!" SITUATIONS

1. Access is poor (e.g., narrow roads, twisting and single-lane routes).
2. Local bridges are narrow and/or have light or unknown load limits.
3. Winds are strong, and erratic fire behavior is occurring.
4. The area contains garages with closed, locked doors.
5. The water supply is inadequate to attack the fire.
6. Structure windows are black or smoked over.
7. There are septic tanks and leach lines.
8. A structure is burning with puffing rather than steady smoke.
9. Construction of structures includes wood, with shake shingle roofs.
10. Natural fuels occur within 9 m (30 ft) of the structures.
11. Known or suspected panicked individuals are in the vicinity.
12. Structure windows are bulging, and the roof has not been vented.
13. Additional fuels can be found in open crawl spaces beneath the structures.
14. Firefighting is taking place in or near chimney or canyon situations.
15. Elevated fuel or propane tanks are present.

▶ VEHICLE BEHAVIOR IN A FIRE SITUATION

1. The engine may stall and not restart.
2. The vehicle may be rocked by convection currents.
3. Smoke and sparks may enter the cab.
4. The interior, engine, or tires may ignite.

5. Temperatures increase inside the cab because heat is radiated through the windows.
6. Metal gas tanks and containers rarely explode.
7. If it is necessary to leave the cab after the fire has passed, keep the vehicle between you and the fire.
8. If smoke obstructs visibility, turn on the headlights and drive to the side of the road away from the leading edge of the fire. Try to select an area of sparse vegetation offering the least combustible material.
9. Attempt to shield your body from radiant heat energy by rolling up the windows and covering up with floor mats or hiding beneath the dashboard. Cover as much skin as possible.
10. Stay in the vehicle as long as possible. Unruptured gas tanks rarely explode, and vehicles usually take several minutes to ignite.
11. Grass fires create about 30 seconds (maximum) of flame exposure, and chances for survival in a vehicle are good. Forest fires create higher-intensity flames lasting 3 to 4 minutes (maximum) and lowering changes for survival. Staying in a vehicle improves chances for surviving a forest fire. Remain calm.
12. A strong, acrid smell usually results from burning paint and plastic materials, caused by small quantities of hydrogen chloride released from breakdown of polyvinyl chloride. Hydrogen chloride is water soluble, and discomfort can be relieved by breathing through a damp cloth. Urine is mostly water and can be used in emergencies.

The decision to evacuate a building or remain and defend is not an easy one. Several principles should guide the evaluation decision:

1. A fire within sight or smell is a fire that endangers you.
2. More unattended houses burn down.
3. Evacuation when fire is close is too late; evacuation must be done well before danger is apparent.
4. More people are injured and killed in the open than in houses.
5. Learn beforehand about community refuges.
6. Evacuate only to a known safe refuge.

Before fire approaches a dwelling, take the following precautions:

1. If you plan to stay, evacuate your pets and livestock and all family members not essential to protecting the home well in advance of the fire's arrival.
2. Be properly dressed to survive the fire. Wear long pants and boots, and carry for protection a long-sleeved shirt or jacket made of cotton fabrics or wool. Synthetics should not be worn because they can ignite and melt. Wear a hat

that can offer protection against radiation to the face, ears, and neck areas. Wear leather or natural fiber gloves and have a handkerchief handy to shield the face, water to wet it, and safety goggles.

3. Remove combustible items from around the house, including lawn and poolside furniture, umbrellas, and tarp coverings. If they catch fire, the added heat could ignite the house.

4. Ensure that anything that might be tossed around by strong fire-induced winds is secured.

5. Ensure that the areas around any external propane tanks are fuel free for a considerable distance.

6. Close outside attic, eave, and basement vents to eliminate the possibility of sparks blowing into hidden areas within the house. Close window shutters.

7. Place large plastic trash cans or buckets around the outside of the house and fill them with water. Soak burlap sacks, small rungs, and large rags to use in beating out burning embers or small fires. Inside the house, fill bathtubs, sinks, and other containers with water. Toilet tanks and water heaters are important water reservoirs.

8. Place garden hoses so that they will reach any place on the house. Use the spray gun type of nozzle, adjusted to spray.

9. If you have portable gasoline-powered pumps to take water from a swimming pool or tank, make sure they are operating and in place.

10. Place a ladder against the roof of the house opposite the side of the approaching fire. If you have a combustible roof, wet it down or turn on any roof sprinklers. Turn on any special fire sprinklers installed to add protection. Do not waste water. Waste can drain the entire water system quickly.

11. Back your car into the garage and roll up the car windows. Disconnect the automatic garage door opener (otherwise, in case of power failure, you cannot remove the car). Close all garage doors.

12. Place valuable papers and mementos inside the car in the garage for quick departure, if necessary. In addition, place all pets in the car.

13. Close windows and doors to the house to prevent sparks from blowing inside. Close all doors inside the house to prevent drafts. Open the damper on any fireplace to help stabilize outside-inside pressure, but close the fireplace screen so that sparks will not ignite the room. Turn on a light in each room to make the house more visible in heavy smoke.

14. Turn off pilot lights.

15. If you have time, take down drapes and curtains. Close all Venetian blinds or noncombustible window coverings to reduce the amount of heat radiating into the house. This provides added safety in case the windows give way because of heat or wind.
16. As the fire approaches, go inside the house. Stay calm; you are in control of the situation.
17. After the fire passes, check the roof immediately. Extinguish any sparks or embers. Then check the attic for hidden burning sparks. If you have a fire, enlist your neighbors to help fight it. For several hours after the fire, recheck for smoke and sparks throughout the house.

▶ IF YOU CANNOT ESCAPE AN APPROACHING WILDFIRE

1. Select an area that will not burn—the bigger the better or, failing that, an area with the least amount of combustible material, and one that offers the best microclimate (e.g., depression in the ground).
2. Use every means possible to protect yourself from radiant and convective heat emitted by the flames (e.g., boulders, rock outcrops, large downed logs, trees, snags).
3. Protect your airway from heat at all costs and try to minimize smoke exposure.
4. Try to remain as calm as possible.
5. If you are caught out in the open and are likely to be entrapped or burned over by a wildfire and not able to take refuge in a vehicle, building, or fire shelter:
   a. Retreat from the fire and reach a safe haven.
   b. Burn out a safety area.
   c. Hunker in place.
   d. Pass through the fire edge into the burned-out area.

▶ SURVIVING A WILDLAND FIRE ENTRAPMENT OR BURNOVER

When entrapment or burnover by a wildland fire appears imminent, injuries or death may be avoided by following these basic emergency survival principles and procedures:
1. Acknowledge the stress you are feeling. Most people are afraid when trapped by fire. Accept this fear as natural so that clear thinking and intelligent decisions are possible. If fear overwhelms you, judgment is seriously impaired and survival becomes more a matter of chance than good decision making.
2. Protect yourself against radiation at all costs. Many victims of forest fires die before the flames reach them. Radiated

heat quickly causes heatstroke. Find shielding to reduce heat rays quickly in an area that will not burn, such as a shallow trench, crevice, large rock, running stream, large pond, vehicle, building, or the shore water of a lake. Do not seek refuge in an elevated water tank. Avoid wells and caves because oxygen may be used up quickly in these restricted places; consider them a last resort. To protect against radiation, cover the head and other exposed skin with clothing or dirt.

3. Regulate your breathing. Avoid inhaling dense smoke (which can impair both your judgment and eyesight). Keep your face near the ground, where there is usually less smoke. Hold a dampened handkerchief over the nose. Match your breathing with the availability of relatively fresh air. If there is a possibility of breathing superheated air, place a dry, not moist, cloth over the mouth. The lungs can withstand dry heat better than moist heat.

4. Do not run blindly or needlessly. Unless a clear path of escape is indicated, do not run. Move downhill and away from the flank of the fire at a 45-degree angle where possible. Conserve your strength. If you become exhausted, you are much more prone to heatstroke and may easily overlook a place of safe refuge.

5. Burn out fuels to create a safety zone if possible. If you are in dead grass or low shrub fuels and the approaching flames are too high to run through, burn out as large an area as possible between you and the fire edge. Step into the burned area and cover as much of your exposed skin as possible. This requires time for fuels to be consumed and may not be effective as a last-ditch effort, nor does this work well in an intense forest fire.

6. Lie prone on the ground. In a critical situation, lie face-down in an area that will not burn. Your chance of survival if the fire overtakes you is greater in this position than standing upright or kneeling.

7. Enter the burned area whenever and wherever possible. Particularly in grass, low shrubs, or other low fuels, do not delay if escape means passing through the flame front into the burned area. Move aggressively and parallel to the advancing fire front. Choose a place on the fire's edge where the flames are less than 1 m (3 ft) deep and can be seen through clearly, and where the fuel supply behind the fire has been mostly consumed. Cover exposed skin and take several breaths, then move through the flame front as quickly as possible. If necessary, drop to the ground under the smoke for improved visibility and to obtain fresh air.

▶ **PERSONAL GEAR FOR A RESCUE MISSION
ON A WILDLAND FIRE INCIDENT**

1. Boots (leather, high-top, lace-up, nonslip soles, extra leather laces)
2. Socks (cotton or wool, at least two pairs)
3. Pants (natural fiber, flameproof, loose fitting, hems lower than boot tops)
4. Belt or suspenders
5. Shirt (natural fiber, flameproof, loose fitting, long sleeves)
6. Gloves (natural fiber or leather, extra pair)
7. Hat (hard hat and possibly a bandana, stocking cap, or felt hat)
8. Jacket
9. Handkerchiefs or scarves
10. Goggles
11. Sleeping bag and ground cover
12. Map
13. Protective fire shelter
14. Food
15. Canteen
16. Radio (AM radio will receive better in rough terrain; FM is more line-of-sight; emergency personnel should have a two-way radio)
17. Bolt cutters (carried in vehicles to get through locked gates during escape from flare-ups or in the rescue of trapped people)
18. Miscellaneous items (mess kit, compass, flashlight, extra batteries, toilet paper, pencil, notepaper, flagging tape, flares, matches (windproof), can opener, wash cloth, toiletries, insect repellent, plastic bags, knife, first aid kit, and lip balm)

▶ **HOW TO REPORT A WILDLAND FIRE TO LOCAL
AUTHORITIES**

A caller should be prepared to provide the following information when reporting a fire:
1. Name of person giving the report
2. Where the person can be reached immediately
3. Where the person was at the time the fire was discovered
4. Location of the fire; orient the fire to prominent landmarks such as rods, creeks, and mileposts on the highways.
5. Description of the fire: color and volume of the smoke, estimated size, and flame characteristics if visible
6. Whether anyone is fighting the fire at the time of the call

▶ PORTABLE FIRE EXTINGUISHERS

Extinguishers are chosen based on the three major classes of fires:

Class A fires: fueled by ordinary combustible materials such as wood, paper, cloth, upholstery, and many plastics—use water, dry chemical, or liquefied gas extinguishers

Class B fires: fueled by flammable liquids and gases such as kitchen greases, paints, oil, and gasoline—use carbon dioxide or dry chemical extinguishers

Class C fires: fueled by live electrical wires or equipment such as motors, power tools, and appliances—use dry chemical or liquefied gas extinguishers

Burns and Smoke Inhalation

7

The severity of a burn injury is related to the cause of the burn, size and depth of the burn, and the part of the body that is burned. Treatment plans including first aid and the necessity for evacuation are based on the overall burn size in proportion to the victim's total body surface area (TBSA) (Fig. 7-1). Scalds are a common cause of burns. Water at 60° C (140° F) creates a deep partial-thickness or full-thickness burn in 3 seconds. At 68.9° C (156° F), the same burn occurs in 1 second. When hot liquids soak clothing, the heat is retained and applied for a longer time period to the skin. Common causes of flame burns in an outdoor setting are misadventures from using cooking stoves fueled by white gasoline, taking lanterns into tents, smoking in sleeping bags, and starting or improving campfires with gasoline or kerosene. Cooking oil and grease, when hot enough to use for cooking, may be in the range of 204.4° C (400° F). Contact burns may occur from handling hot rocks or stepping on hot embers buried in sand.

▶ GENERAL TREATMENT

1. Remove all burned clothing from the victim.
2. Assess the airway and perform a primary and secondary survey.
3. Administer 100% oxygen if smoke inhalation is suspected.
4. Treat smaller burns by applying cool water compresses or immersion. Take care to avoid inducing hypothermia. Do not use ice packs except on small burns, and limit application to no longer than 10 minutes.
5. Remove any jewelry from burned or distal parts.
6. For a chemical burn, flush the site with a copious amount of water.

▶ DISPOSITION

1. A burn less than 5% total body surface area (TBSA), excluding a deep burn of the face, hand, foot, perineum, or circumferential extremity, can be treated successfully in a wilderness setting if adequate first-aid supplies are available and wound care is performed diligently.
2. A minor burn that involves less than 15% TBSA in the 10- to 50-year-old age group or less than 10% in a child younger than age 10 years or an adult older than age 50 years can usually be treated in an outpatient setting. If a burn covers

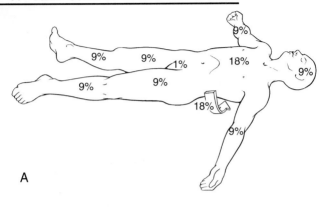

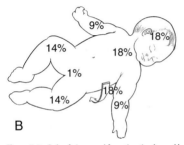

Figure 7-1. Rule of nines used for estimating burned body surface. **A,** Adult. **B,** Infant.

more than 50% of a hand or foot, it should be evaluated by a physician as soon as possible.

3. A major burn victim should be evacuated immediately to a burn center. A major burn is defined as any of the following:
   a. Partial-thickness burn greater than 25% TBSA in the 10- to 50-year-old age group or greater than 20% in a child younger than age 10 years or an adult older than age 50 years
   b. Full-thickness burn greater than 10% TBSA in anyone
   c. Serious burn involving the hand, face, foot, or perineum
   d. Burn complicated by inhalation injury
   e. Electrical burn
   f. Burn in an immunocompromised patient, infant, or elderly person

▶ **DISORDERS**

First-Degree Burn

Signs and Symptoms
1. Only involves the epidermis
2. Erythema (dermal vasodilation) and pain without blisters
3. Prototype: mild sunburn
4. When over a large surface area: fever, weakness, chills, vomiting

Treatment
1. Cool the burn with wet compresses. (Do not use ice directly on skin.) When the burn is acquired suddenly, immediately apply very cold water to limit the extent of tissue damage.
2. Apply aloe vera gel or lotion topically to the burn.
3. Administer ibuprofen, aspirin, or another nonsteroidal antiinflammatory drug (NSAID). An adult dose is ibuprofen, 800 mg q8h.
4. For severe sunburn without blistering, administer oral prednisone in a rapid taper (80 mg on the first day, 60 mg on the second, 40 mg on the third, 20 mg on the fourth, and 10 mg on the fifth).
5. Be aware that topical corticosteroid creams or ointments have no benefit and anesthetic sprays with benzocaine may cause sensitivity reactions.
6. Erythema and pain should subside over 2 to 3 days.

Superficial Partial-Thickness Burn
(Formerly Second-Degree Burn)

Signs and Symptoms
1. Involves the upper layer of dermis and creates clear, filled blisters.
2. Blisters may not appear until several hours after injury.
3. When blisters are removed, the skin is moist and erythematous, blanches with pressure, and is hypersensitive to touch.
4. If infection is prevented, the burn heals spontaneously within 3 weeks without functional impairment.

Deep Partial-Thickness Burn
(Formerly Second-Degree Burn)

Signs and Symptoms
1. Possible damage to hair follicles and sweat glands
2. Usually blister formation
3. Wound surface mottled pink and white immediately after injury, or may be dry, with a cherry red appearance

4. Wound possibly less sensitive to touch than surrounding normal skin. The victim complains of discomfort rather than pain.
5. When pressure is applied to the burn, capillary refill returns slowly or is absent.
6. If infection is prevented, the burn heals in 3 to 9 weeks with scar formation.

Treatment
1. Remove the victim from the source of the burn.
   a. If clothing is on fire, roll victim on the ground or wrap in a blanket to extinguish the flames.
   b. If the burn is chemical, use large amounts of water (minimum 10 minutes of active rinsing) to wash the agent(s) off. Do not apply a specific neutralizing agent, which may generate heat and worsen the injury.
   c. If the eyes are involved, copiously irrigate them.
   d. Because phosphorus ignites on contact with air, keep any phosphorus still in contact with the victim's skin covered with water.
2. Evaluate the airway for smoke inhalation. If present, administer oxygen by facemask, 5 to 10 L/minute, and transport the victim to a medical facility (see "Smoke Inhalation and Thermal Airway Injury" later). Be alert for vomiting into the facemask.
3. If the victim shows signs of shock, elevate the victim's legs 30 cm (12 inches) off the ground and administer humidified oxygen.
4. Irrigate gently with cool water or saline solution to remove all loose dirt and skin. Wash the burn gently with plain soap and water and dry with a clean towel. Wash water should be suitable for drinking (e.g., disinfected) but does not absolutely need to be sterile or bottled.
5. Peel off or trim any necrotic skin with sharp débridement.
6. Drain large (>2.5 cm [1 inch]), thin, fluid-filled blisters and trim the dead skin if a sterile dressing can be applied.
7. Leave small, thick blisters intact.
8. Apply aloe vera gel or an antibacterial ointment to the burn.
9. Cover the burn with a dressing, and change the dressing at least once a day. Maintain mobility of the wound area and avoid dependent positioning, particularly during rest and sleep.
   a. Use cool, moist dressings (not ice) if the area is small (<10% TBSA).
   b. Use dry, nonadherent dressings if the surface area is large to avoid overcooling the victim.

10. Give oral balanced salt solutions to achieve rehydration if the transport time will be more than 30 minutes, the thermal injuries involve more than 20% TBSA, or there is evidence of shock.
    a. Prompt the victim to drink or sip enough fluid to keep the urine clear and copious. Encourage drinking of liquids with electrolytes such as sports beverages rather than water or soda pop.
    b. If this is not possible, administer lactated Ringer's or normal saline solution without glucose through a large-bore percutaneous catheter, preferably inserted through unburned skin. The arm is the preferred site. Administer 4 mL/kg/% TBSA/24 hour. Half the calculated 24-hour fluid total is given over the first 8 hours from the time the burn occurred (not the time the intravenous line was established). The second half is infused over the remaining 16 hours. The rate should be adjusted to support the victim's vital signs and maintain a urine output of 1 mL/kg/hour.
    c. Note that fluid resuscitation at the scene may be difficult for children because of the difficulties achieving cannulation of small veins.
11. Avoid chilling the victim by placing a clean sheet under the person and then covering with another clean sheet, followed by clean blankets.
12. Note that antibiotics are only used if the burn becomes infected.
    a. If infection is present, pus, foul odor, cloudy blisters, increased redness and swelling in the normal skin around the burn, and fever greater than 38.3° C (101° F) will be noted.
    b. If an antibiotic is necessary, give dicloxacillin, cephalexin, or erythromycin. Be sure to change all dressings daily.

Full-Thickness Burn (Formerly Third-Degree Burn)

Signs and Symptoms
1. Involves all layers of the dermis and can heal only by wound contracture, epithelialization from the wound margin, or skin grafting
2. Leathery, firm, depressed when compared with adjoining normal skin, and insensitive to light touch or pinprick
3. Rarely blanches with pressure; may have a dry, white ("waxy") appearance with or without small clotted blood vessels that appear as purple or maroon lines under the surface. An immersion scald may have a red appearance, but it does not blanch with pressure.

4. Can be difficult to differentiate from a deep partial-thickness burn
5. Develops classic burn eschar that separates from underlying viable tissue

Fourth-Degree Burn

Signs and Symptoms
1. Involves all layers of skin plus subcutaneous fat and deeper structures
2. Almost always has a charred appearance

Treatment
1. Follow the same instructions as for second-degree burn.
2. Be aware that immediate evacuation to a burn center is recommended.
3. Field considerations for fourth-degree burns are the same as for full-thickness burns.
4. Escharotomy. If an extremity burn is circumferential and the burn eschar is dry and leathery, performance of escharotomy is justified, even in a wilderness setting when monitoring equipment is not available. Escharotomy does not require an anesthetic. The burned extremity should be rinsed well and cleansed with soap and water. A scalpel is used to perform an incision through the eschar into the subcutaneous tissue. Ideally, only the eschar is incised because subcutaneous fat is often viable and can cause bleeding. A "give" is felt as the scalpel passes through the eschar and into the fat. After the long initial incision is made, a short, push-type maneuver is performed by laying the belly of the scalpel blade along the entire length of the incision to ensure that all constricting tissue has been freed. A popping open of the incision occurs as the scalpel moves from one end of the incision to the other. The first incision is made along the lateral aspect of the extremity. The extremity should soften and any signs or symptoms of ischemia should resolve within a few minutes. If this does not occur, a second incision should be made along the medial aspect of the extremity. On completion of the procedure, a moist dressing such as antibiotic/antiseptic cream or ointment should be applied. A compression wrap and elevation of the extremity after the procedure will assist in maintaining hemostasis.

Carbon Monoxide Poisoning

Signs and Symptoms
1. If resulting from a fire: dyspnea, burns of the mouth and nose, singed nasal hairs, sooty sputum, brassy cough
2. Headache, nausea, vomiting, tachypnea, dizziness, loss of manual dexterity

3. Sometimes subtle perception and memory abnormalities or frank confusion and lethargy
4. Abnormal skin and nail bed color, with "chocolate cyanosis" or a cherry-red color
5. Bullae
6. Unconsciousness leading to coma
7. Possible cardiac arrest
8. Late complications (after first 48 hours): personality disorders, chronic headaches, seizures, Parkinson's disease (generally after 2 to 40 days)

Treatment
1. Administer 100% oxygen by a non-rebreathing mask.
2. Consider initiating evacuation to a hyperbaric chamber for any victim who displays abnormal neurologic signs or symptoms or who is pregnant.

Smoke Inhalation and Thermal Airway Injury

Signs and Symptoms
1. Facial burns
2. Intraoral or pharyngeal burns
3. Singed nasal hairs
4. Soot in the mouth or nose, carbonaceous sputum
5. Hoarseness, inspiratory stridor with a barking sound that seems to originate in the neck, or expiratory wheezing
6. Shortness of breath and coughing that produces carbonaceous black sputum
7. Muffled voice, drooling, difficulty swallowing
8. Swollen tongue
9. Agitation

Treatment
1. Once the injury has occurred, no measures can be taken to limit its progress, so evacuate the victim immediately.
2. Administer humidified oxygen at 5 to 10 L/minute by facemask.
3. Consider initiating intubation and ventilation if stridor or dyspnea is present. Note that progressive edema can produce complete airway obstruction.
4. Administer a bronchodilator (albuterol, 200 to 400 μg [2 to 8 full inhalations, depending on preparation] by metered-dose inhaler with a spacer q15–20 minutes prn).

Solar Radiation and Photoprotection

8

Erythemogenic doses of ultraviolet (UV) energy are defined as multiples of the minimal erythema dose (MED)—the lowest dose to elicit perceptible erythema. In a day's time, a person can receive 15 MEDs of ultraviolet B (UVB) but only 2 to 4 MEDs of ultraviolet A (UVA). So, although humans are exposed to 10-fold to 100-fold more UVA than UVB, more than 90% of sunlight-induced erythema is attributable to UVB. However, UVA exposure contributes significantly to development of skin cancer. Almost all ultraviolet C (UVC) is absorbed by the earth's ozone layer.

▶ ACUTE SUNBURN

Sunburn represents a local cutaneous inflammatory and vascular-mediated reaction. UVB erythema has its onset 2 to 6 hours after exposure, peaks at 12 to 36 hours, and fades over 72 to 120 hours. UVA erythema has an onset within 4 to 6 hours, peaks in 8 to 12 hours, and fades in 24 to 48 hours.

Signs and Symptoms
1. Painful erythema of skin, commonly viewed as "first degree" in burn description
2. Blistering, low-grade fever, chills, nausea, vomiting, diarrhea in severe cases

Treatment (Box 8-1)
Sunburn is self-limited, and its treatment is largely symptomatic.
1. Cool water soaks or compresses may provide immediate relief. Moisturizers are sometimes helpful.
2. Topical anesthetics are sometimes useful. It is generally preferable to use the nonsensitizing anesthetics containing menthol, camphor, and pramoxine rather than potentially sensitizing anesthetics containing benzocaine and diphenhydramine. Refrigerating topical anesthetics before application provides added relief.
3. Anecdotal remedies (controlled studies are lacking) include aloe, baking soda, and oatmeal (Aveeno).
4. Topical steroids may blanch reddened skin but should not be used on blistered skin.
5. Systemic steroids (e.g., 3- to 5-day prednisone taper) enjoy anecdotal support.
6. Diclofenac gel, a topical nonsteroidal antiinflammatory drug (NSAID), alleviates pain, erythema, and edema for up to 48 hours when applied after exposure.

Box 8-1. Sunburn Treatments

PAIN CONTROL
Acetylsalicylic acid
Nonsteroidal antiinflammatory drugs

SKIN CARE
Cool soaks, compresses
Nonmedicated moisturizers
Topical anesthetics
- Prax lotion (pramoxine)
- Sarna anti-itch lotion (menthol plus camphor)
- Aveeno anti-itch concentrated lotion (pramoxine plus camphor plus calamine)
- Neutrogena Norwegian Formula soothing relief moisturizer (lidocaine plus camphor)

STEROIDS
Topical
Systemic

---

7. Oral NSAIDs including aspirin provide analgesia and may reduce sunburn erythema.

▶ PHOTOPROTECTION

The essential element in avoiding UV radiation (UVR)–induced injury is a comprehensive approach to protection.

Sunscreens
Sun Protection Factor (SPF)

1. The ability of a sunscreen to protect the skin from UVR-induced erythema is measured by the sun protection factor (SPF).
2. The SPF is defined as a ratio, in which the numerator is the UVR required to produce minimal erythema (1 MED) in sunscreen-protected skin and the denominator is the UVR required to produce minimal erythema in unprotected skin.
3. SPF 15 sunscreen or clothing blocks 93% of UVB. Histologically an SPF 30 sunscreen provides better protection against sunburn cell formation than does an SPF 15 sunscreen (Table 8-1).
4. Although UVB is primarily responsible for the burning effects from the sun, both UVB and UVA radiation can cause skin cancer. Additionally, UVA rays penetrate more deeply into the skin and are largely responsible for premature wrinkles, aged skin, and photosensitivity. Although standards do not yet exist, "broad-spectrum" sunscreens that include UVA and UVB protection are recommended (see later).

TABLE 8-1. Skin Protection Factor (SPF) and
Ultraviolet B (UVB) Absorption

SPF	UVB ABSORPTION (%)
2	50.0
4	75.0
8	87.5
15	93.3
30	96.7
50	98.0

Sunscreen Vehicles
1. Sunscreen vehicles affect efficacy.
2. The ideal vehicle spreads easily; maximizes skin adherence; minimizes interaction with the active sunscreening agent; and is noncomedogenic, nonstinging, nonstaining, and inexpensive.
3. Sunscreens are a leading cause of photoallergic contact dermatitis. Oxybenzone is the most commonly implicated.
4. PABA (para-aminobenzoic acid) sensitizes approximately 4% of exposed subjects.
5. Creams and lotions (emulsions): spread easily, penetrate well.
6. Oils: spread easily, but thinly; certain oils are comedogenic.
7. Ointments and waxes: may be preferable for extreme conditions; resist chapping and frostbite.
8. Gels: nongreasy but wash or sweat off easily; alcoholic gels may cause stinging.
9. Sticks: waxes are impractical for large surface area.
10. Aerosols: wasteful and may form an uneven layer.
11. Sunscreens are increasingly being incorporated into cosmetics.

Sunscreen Application
1. Adequate coverage of just the face, ears, and dorsal hands requires 2 to 3 g, which requires an 8-oz bottle of sunscreen every 80 to 120 days.
2. Apply liberally and frequently. Apply 15 to 30 minutes before water exposure. Reapply after every exit from the water.
3. Cover all exposed areas.
4. Take care to avoid having the sunscreen run into the eyes.

5. The concomitant use of sunscreen and insect repellent containing deet can lower the effective SPF by 34%.
6. Safe Sea jellyfish safe sunblock, available in SPF 15 or 30, contains chemical agents that inhibit stings by jellyfish and other nematocyst-bearing stinging creatures.

UVA Protection
Recently, more efficient UVA blocking agents have become available.
1. Common UVA blocking agents include avobenzone, ecamsule, and micronized TiO_2 and ZnO.
2. No accepted standard for UVA protectiveness exists.
3. Sunscreens with a labeling claim of UVA protection allow transmission of 6% to 52% of UVA.

Substantivity
1. The ability of a sunscreen to resist water wash-off is referred to as *substantivity*. "Water-resistant" sunscreens retain their SPF after 40 minutes of immersion, and "very water-resistant" sunscreens after 80 minutes.
2. By applying sunscreen 15 to 30 minutes before water exposure, substantivity can be increased.
3. Reapplication after swimming or sweating helps ensure protection.
4. Cold churning water, sand abrasion, and toweling may add to sunscreen loss, hence the development of so-called "surfshop" sunscreens.

Stability
1. Keep sunscreens out of glove compartments and similar locations where they are exposed to extreme temperatures for prolonged periods.
2. Shelf life is presumed to be at least 1 year for most commercially available sunscreens; however, data are lacking (Table 8-2).

Clothing Protection
1. Clothing varies considerably in its ability to block UV.
2. Standardized testing of clothing has produced the ultraviolet protection factor (UPF), analogous to SPF in sunscreens.
3. The single most important factor in determining SPF is the tightness of the weave, followed by the actual fabric. For instance, Lycra blocks nearly 100% of UVR when lax and only 2% when maximally stretched. Other determinants include wetness and color. Dry, dark fabrics have a higher SPF than do otherwise identical wet, white fabrics.

TABLE 8-2. Select Sunscreen Products

PRODUCT	SPF	ACTIVE INGREDIENTS
High-SPF Waterproof Broad-Spectrum Creams/Lotions		
Bain de Soleil Oil-Free Protecteur Sunscreen Lotion	35	A, B, OC, S
Banana Boat Sport 50	30	B, C, OC, S
Blue Lizard Australian Sunscreen Lotion	30+	B, C, OC, ZO
Bullfrog SuperBlock Lotion	45	B, C, MA, OC, S, TI
Coppertone Sport Ultra Sweatproof	30	B, C, S
Dermatone Sunscreen Lotion	36	C, PBSA, ZO
Durascreen Lotion	30	B, C, PBSA, S, TI
Hawaiian Tropic Ozone Sunblock	70	B, C, PB, S, TI
Kiss My Face Sunblock Lotion	30	C, TI
Neutrogena Ultra Sheer Dry-Touch Sunblock	55	A, B, OC, S
Ocean Potion Anti-Aging Sunblock	50	A, B, C, S
Ombrelle Sunscreen Lotion Extreme	40	A, B, OC, S
Panama Jack Sunscreen Lotion	45	B, C, OC, S
Sea & Ski Sport	50	B, C, S, ZO
Solbar PF Cream	50	B, C, OC, S
TI Screen Moisturizing Sunscreen Lotion	30	A, B, C, OC, S
Water Babies Sunblock Lotion	45	B, C, S
High-SPF Gels		
Bullfrog Quik Gel	36	B, C, OC, S
Coppertone Sport Sunblock Gel	30	A, B, OC, S
Pre-Sun Ultra Gel	30	A, B, C, S
TI-Screen Sports Gel	20	B, C, S
High-SPF Sprays		
Banana Boat Sport Quik Block Sunblock Spray	48	A, B, C, OC, S
Bullfrog Fast Blast Spray Sunblock	36	B, C, OC, S
Coppertone Sport Sunblock Spray	30	B, C, S
Neutrogena Healthy Defense Oil-Free Spray	30	A, C, S
TI-Screen Sunscreen Spray	23	B, C, MA, OC
High-SPF Sticks		
Banana Boat Sport Sunscreen Stick	30	B, C, OC, S
Bullfrog Quik Stick	36	B, C, OC, S
Hawaiian Tropic Ozone Oil-free Sunblock Stick	50+	A, B, OC, S
Neutrogena Healthy Defense Sunblock Stick	30	A, C, S
Ocean Potion Sport Stick	60	A, B, S
Shade Sunblock Stick	30	B, C, S

Continued

TABLE 8-2. Select Sunscreen Products—cont'd

PRODUCT	SPF	ACTIVE INGREDIENTS
Specialty Sunscreens		
AloeGator Super Waterproof Gel	40+	B, C, OC, S
Bullfrog Surfer Formula Gel	36	B, C, OC
Dermatone Skin Protector Pomade	23	B, C, PB
SolRx ProSport	44	B, C, OC, S
Lip Screens		
Banana Boat Aloe Vera Lip Balm	30	B, C, PB, S
Coppertone Sport Lip Guard	15	B, C
Dermatone Medicated Lip Balm	23	B, PB
Hawaiian Tropic Aloe Vera Sunblock Lip Balm	45+	C, OC, S
Neutrogena Lip Moisturizer	15	B, C
TI-Screen Lip Protectant	15	B, C
"Physical" Sunscreens		
Neutrogena Sensitive Skin Sunblock Lotion	30	TI
Pre-Sun Sensitive Skin Sunblock	28	TI
Vanicream Sunscreen	15	TI, ZO
Moisturizers Containing Higher SPF Sunscreen		
Antihelios SX Daily Moisturizing Cream	15	A, E, OC
Aveeno Positively Radiant Daily Moisturizer	15	A, C, S
Eucerin Extra Protective Moisture Lotion	30	C, OC, PBSA, TI, ZO
Lubriderm Daily Moisture Lotion	15	B, C, S
Neutrogena Healthy Defense Daily Moisturizer	30	C, OC, PBSA, ZO
Oil of Olay Complete Defense Daily UV Moisturizer	30	C, OC, S, ZO
Purpose Dual Treatment Moisture Lotion	15	C, MA, TI

A, avobenzone; B, benzophenones; C, cinnamates; E, ecamsule; MA, methyl anthranilate (meradimate); OC, octocrylene; PB, PABA, or PABA ester; PBSA, phenylbenzimidazole sulfonic acid (ensulizole); S, salicylates; TI, titanium dioxide; ZO, zinc oxide.

A typical dry, white cotton T-shirt has an SPF of 5 to 9. Ladies' hosiery generally has an SPF of less than 3.

4. In the United States, sun-protective clothing is regulated as a medical device. For example, one approved product, Solumbra, is made of tightly woven nylon with an SPF of 30+.

5. A hat with a brim wide enough to protect the nose, cheeks, and chin is highly protective.

Sunglasses

1. Glasses, contact lenses, and sunglasses protect the corneas from most UVB and variable amounts of UVA.
2. Acute exposure to high levels of UVR may result in acute UV photokeratitis.
3. UV is now implicated in a myriad of ocular disorders including cataracts, macular degeneration, and retinitis pigmentosa.
4. Standard sunglasses transmit 15% to 25% of visible light; mountaineering sunglasses transmit 5% to 10%, which is necessary to reduce luminance to a comfortable range.
5. Side-shields or deeply wrapped lens designs should be used in mountaineering environments. Table 8-3 provides desirable characteristics in selecting sunglasses for environments with high levels of luminance and UVR.

Sun Avoidance

1. Avoid excessive midday sun, from 10 AM to 3 PM.
2. Seek shade whenever possible. Overhead shade cloths provide more protection than clothing of the same fabrics.
3. Automobile windshields typically block UVB and some UVA, whereas side windows block only UVB. Transparent plastic films can be applied to block more than 99% of UVR.
4. Apply sunscreens liberally and begin their use early in life.

TABLE 8-3. Sunglasses Selection Criteria for Mountaineering

SUBJECT	CHARACTERISTICS
UV absorption	99% to 100%
Visible light transmittance	5% to 10%*
Lens material	Polycarbonate or CR-39†
Optical quality	Clear image without distortion‡
Frame design features	Large lenses; side shields or "wraparound" design; fit close to face; good stability on face during movement; lightweight; durable

*Glasses with less than 8% transmittance of visible light should not be worn while driving. Sunglasses or any tinted lenses with a visible light transmittance of less than 80% should not be worn while driving at night.
†Glass lenses typically have very good optical clarity and scratch resistance but are heavier and more expensive.
‡Hold the sunglasses at arm's length and move them back and forth. If the objects are distorted or move erratically, the optical quality is probably less than desirable. Also, compare the image quality between several different pairs of sunglasses to get a basis for comparison.

9

Lightning Injury

Although the chances of being struck by lightning are minimal, 200 to 400 persons are victims of lightning strikes in the United States each year, resulting in an average of 67 deaths per year. Worldwide estimates are up to 240,000 annual injuries with up to 24,000 deaths. Lightning is the electrical discharge associated with thunderstorms, and an initial stroke can show a potential difference between the tip and the earth that ranges from 10 to 200 (average 30) million volts. Up to 30 strokes that comprise a single lightning flash give lightning its flickering quality. The main stroke usually measures 2 to 3 cm in diameter, and its temperature at the hottest has been estimated to range from 8000° C to 50,000° C (14,432° F to 90,032° F), or four times as hot as the surface of the sun. Thunder results from the shock waves generated by the nearly explosive expansion of the heated and ionized air. Thunder is seldom heard over distances greater than 10 miles (16 km).

Lightning can cause injury by (1) direct hit, (2) splash as the bolt first hits an object and then jumps to the victim, (3) contact with a conductive material that is hit or splashed by lightning, (4) step voltage where the bolt hits the ground or a nearby object and then flows like a wave in a pond to the victim, (5) ground current, (6) surface arcing, (7) upward streamer current, or (8) blunt trauma from the explosive force of the positive and negative pressure waves (thunder) it produces. The "flashover phenomenon" describes the situation wherein the electrical current of lightning travels appreciably over the body's surface, rather than through it. This likely accounts for vaporized moisture on the skin and unique skin burn patterns.

▶ DISORDERS

Box 9-1 lists the types of immediate injuries that can occur with any of the effects of lightning, which is best described as a unidirectional massive current impulse.

Signs and Symptoms
1. Generally, a history of a lightning strike or near strike
2. Disarray of clothing and belongings
3. Feathering burns (see Plate 3)
4. Linear or punctate (see Plate 4) burns with tympanic membrane rupture and confusion in an outdoor setting
5. Confusion, amnesia, or lack of consciousness in a person found indoors after or during a thunderstorm

Box 9-1. Types of Immediate Injuries Attributable to Lightning

1. Cardiopulmonary arrest
   a. Immediate cardiac arrest that may be brief because of inherent automaticity
   b. Respiratory arrest, caused by paralysis of the medullary respiratory center, that lasts longer and leads to secondary cardiac arrest from hypoxia
2. Neurologic injury
   a. Seizures
   b. Deafness
   c. Confusion or amnesia
   d. Blindness
   e. Dizziness
   f. Extremity paralysis
   g. Headache, nausea, and postconcussion syndrome
3. Contusions and fractures
4. Chest pain and muscle aches
5. Tympanic membrane rupture
6. Superficial punctate and feathering burns (see Plates 3 and 4)
7. Partial-thickness burns

6. Muscle aches and body tingling
7. In more severe cases, skin mottled, extremities paralyzed, pulse difficult to ascertain at the wrist because muscles of the radial artery are in spasm

Treatment
Note that lightning victims are not "charged" and thus pose no hazard to rescuers.

1. Assess and treat first those victims who appear dead because they may ultimately recover if properly resuscitated.
   a. Assess airway, breathing, and circulation.
   b. Perform CPR if indicated. If no pulse is obtained within 30 minutes of starting resuscitation, it is reasonable to stop CPR. However, be aware that dilated pupils should not be taken as the sole sign of brain death in the lightning victim.
   c. If you successfully obtain a pulse with CPR, continue ventilation until spontaneous adequate respirations resume, the victim is pronounced dead, continued resuscitation is deemed not feasible, or you are in danger.
2. Stabilize and splint any fractures.

3. Be aware that the victim may have been thrown a considerable distance by the strike. Initiate and maintain spinal precautions if indicated.
4. Administer oxygen and intravenous fluids if available. Apply a cardiac monitor if available.
5. Prepare for transport to a medical facility.

Prevention

To calculate the approximate distance in miles that you are from a flash of lightning, count in seconds the time from when you see the flash until when you hear the thunder, and divide that number by five. If you see lightning and hear thunder before you can count to 30 seconds, you should be seeking shelter. Activities should not be resumed for at least 30 minutes after the last lightning is seen and the last thunder heard.

1. When a thunderstorm threatens (lightning may travel nearly horizontally as far as 10 miles [16 km] or more in front of a thunderstorm), seek shelter in a substantial building or inside a metal-topped vehicle (not a tent or a convertible automobile). If you are in a car, stay in it. If it is a convertible and there is no other shelter, huddle on the ground at least 45 m (50 yards) away from the vehicle.
2. If you are in a tent, stay as far away from the poles and wet cloth as possible.
3. Do not count on rubber-soled shoes or raincoats to provide protection. Similarly, the rubber tires on a car do not provide any protection—electrical energy travels along the outside of the car body and dissipates into the ground.
4. Do not stand under a tall tree in an open area or on a ridge or hilltop.
5. Move away from open water, and do not stand near a metal boat. If you are swimming, get out of the water.
6. Move away from tractors and other metal farm equipment. Avoid tall objects, such as ski lifts, boat masts, flagpoles, and power lines.
7. Get off motorcycles, bicycles, and golf carts. Put down golf clubs, umbrellas, and fishing poles.
8. Stay away from wire fences, clotheslines, metal pipes, and other metallic paths that could carry lightning to you from some distance.
9. Avoid standing in small, isolated sheds or other small structures in open areas.
10. Once you are indoors, avoid being near windows, open doors, fireplaces, or large metal fixtures. Be aware that a cellular telephone can transmit loud static that can cause acoustic damage.

11. In a forest, seek shelter in a low area under a thick growth of saplings or small trees. Avoid the tallest trees, staying a distance from the tree at least equal to the tree's height. Avoid the entrances to caves.

12. In an open area, go to a low place such as a ravine or alley.

13. If you are totally in the open:
    a. Stay far away from single trees to avoid lightning splashes.
    b. Drop to your knees and bend forward, putting your hands on your knees.
    c. If it is available, place insulating material (e.g., sleeping pad, life jacket, rope) between you and the ground. Do not lie flat on the ground.

14. If your hair stands on end, you hear high-pitched or crackling noises, or you see a blue halo around objects, there is electrical activity around you that typically precedes a lightning strike. If you can, leave the area immediately. If you are unable to do this, crouch down on the balls of your feet and tuck your head down. Do not touch the ground with your hands.

15. When a thunderstorm is about to pass, maintain a cautious approach because this continues to be a dangerous time.

10 Emergency Airway Management

Emergencies involving the airway are among the most urgent conditions necessitating medical intervention. Airway management in the field is a combination of careful physical and scene assessment, recognition of risk, optimization of airway mechanics, and communication to bring the victim to definitive care.

The conscious or semiconscious person with an airway emergency instinctively seeks an optimal posture for air exchange. The unconscious person, unless deeply anesthetized, paralyzed, or profoundly hypoxic, continues effort to breathe until death is very near. If a victim shouts or cries out, the airway is intact and the lungs are filling. If a victim is breathing but obstructed, determination should be made as to why. If a victim is making no respiratory effort at all, a choice must be made about whether to initiate CPR.

▶ RECOGNITION OF AIRWAY OBSTRUCTION

Cyanosis can be present without airway compromise, and significant airway compromise can be present without cyanosis.

Signs and Symptoms
The two most important aspects of respiratory assessment are as follows:
1. The presence or absence of attempts to breathe (assesses the integrity of the central nervous system).
2. If attempts to breathe are being made, ascertain the degree of labor and posture adjustment required to support air exchange. This assesses the patency of airway corridors in combination with elasticity of the lungs and strength of the chest wall.

Additional Signs and Symptoms
1. Labored respirations are typified by a rate that is forcefully rapid, irregular, or gasping.
2. Unusual sounds or noisy respirations could be present.
3. Accessory muscles of the chest wall, shoulders, neck, and abdomen strain with the effort. If respiratory effort causes chest wall retractions, there may be an airway emergency in evolution.
4. In the obstructed airway, expiration tends to be prolonged.
5. Partial obstruction can be recognized by:
   a. Decreased volume exchange (decreased air entry by auscultation or decreased chest rise by inspection)
   b. Increased transit time during inhalation or exhalation

6. No pause between breaths is an ominous sign. This suggests that there is a significant airway obstruction.

Head and Tongue Positioning

The most common causes of upper airway obstruction are the following:

1. A floppy tongue and lax pharyngeal muscles from decreased muscle tone of the genioglossus muscle, which contracts to move the tongue forward during inspiration and dilate the pharynx.
2. Soft tissue enlargement from infection, edema, or hypertrophy.
3. Teeth. These play an important role in preserving the size and patency of the oropharynx. Edentulous persons (the young, elderly, poorly dentitioned, and recently traumatized) are vulnerable to upper airway obstruction.

Treatment of Airway Obstruction

Upper airway obstruction is almost always improved by optimal head positioning, mouth opening, clearing of nasal passages, and/or tongue manipulation.

1. Open the mouth of an unconscious person.
2. Note the position of the tongue and the presence of vomitus, foreign debris, or pooled secretions.
3. Listen to the quality and consistency of respiratory noises.
4. In the obtunded infant or small child, the site of upper airway obstruction is usually between the tip of the tongue and the hard palate in the front of the mouth.
5. In an obtunded adult, the site of upper airway obstruction is usually between the base of the tongue and the posterior oropharynx (back of the throat) (Fig. 10-1).
6. When the tongue is retrodisplaced, it causes the epiglottis to fold over and close off the tracheal introitus, which results in a secondary site of upper airway obstruction.
7. Relief of both of these sources of obstruction can be obtained by lifting the jaw upward (Fig. 10-2), by "dislocating" the jaw hinge to simultaneously keep the mouth open and the jaw lifted, or by traction on the tongue.
8. The optimal head position for airway alignment and patency varies with age. However, no matter the person's age, the most desirable posture is maintaining a "neutral" (not flexion, not hyperextension) head position with the chin "proudly" jutted forward: nose in the "sniffing" position, mouth open, tongue resting on the floor of the mouth, and angle of the mandible perpendicular to the ground.

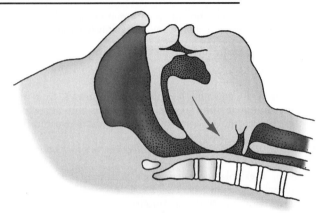

Figure 10-1. Tongue position in the unconscious adult. Note airway obstruction by the base of the tongue against the posterior pharyngeal wall with closure of the epiglottis over the trachea.

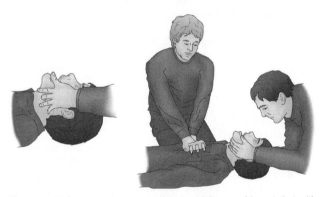

Figure 10-2. Triple maneuver airway support: Maintain axial alignment of the cervical spine, lift up on the angle of the mandible, and hold open the mouth. Located midway between the chin and the angle of the mandible, the facial artery pulse may be monitored at the same time.

9. The least desirable head position in any age group is with the neck flexed and chin pointed toward the chest. Flexion also increases unfavorable stresses on a potentially unstable cervical spine.
10. Extreme hyperextension of the head in any age group stresses ligaments and angulates the airway and is to be avoided.

11. Because of prominence of the cranial occiput in an infant, an infant's airway is best supported with a shoulder roll or built-up surface for the back.
12. The child does best without a pillow or with a built-up cushion for the back and only a small pad for the occiput.
13. The adult's airway is best supported in the sniffing position with a small pillow under the head, the chin pointed in the air, and preserved natural lordosis of the cervical spine. Improvisationally, the sniffing position can be achieved with a soda can behind the neck and a folded T-shirt under the head.
14. If the mechanism of injury or physical examination suggests a possible cervical spine injury, efforts to stabilize the neck and head should be undertaken. The victim should be spared neck flexion, hyperextension, or lateral rotation. Fortunately, the best head position for the airway is also good for the cervical spine. If a cervical spine immobilization method is employed, the airway should be evaluated for obstruction both before and after application.

Body Positioning

The supine position may be neither desirable nor achievable. Because of gravity, some airways are better maintained in a side-lying or prone position. Nontraditional positioning for stabilization and transport may be necessary because of burns, vomiting, management of secretions, or location of impaled objects. Principles of transport for patients in nonsupine positions relate to preservation of good perfusion and mechanical alignment in all body parts under pressure, maintaining neck straightness, and assuring the ability of the rescuer to monitor airway patency. In a nonsupine position, the same airway posture is sought: minimal torsion of the cervical spine, neck in a sniffing position, mouth open, and tongue on the floor of the mouth (Fig. 10-3).

▶ NONINVASIVE AIRWAY MANEUVERS

If the upper airway is obstructed, there are four basic noninvasive airway-opening maneuvers. All noninvasive airway maneuvers except tongue traction and the internal jaw lift can be conjoined with rescue breathing or bag-valve-mask assisted ventilation.
1. The most simple is the head tilt, chin lift. The heel of one of the rescuer's hands is pressed down on the victim's forehead, and the fingers of the other hand are placed under the chin to lift it up. The intended result is the sniffing position.

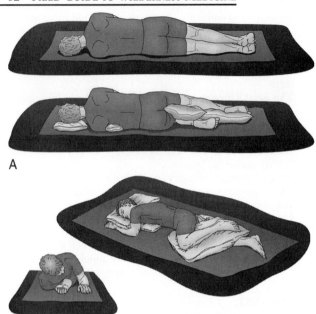

Figure 10-3. A, Patient lying on side with airway/neck in good position and pressure points protected. Flexing the down-side leg stabilizes the torso. The pillow and axillary roll help maintain the spine in good alignment. **B,** Patient positioned semiprone to facilitate gravity drainage of secretions. A pillow under the head keeps the spine in relative alignment. With no pillow under the head, the width of the shoulder inclines the pharynx downward at a steeper angle.

Problems arise if the mouth is closed or soft tissues are folded inward because of the chin lift. In addition, downward pressure on the forehead tends to lift the eyebrows and open the eyelids, so measures may need to be taken to protect the eyes.

2. A second maneuver is the jaw thrust (Fig. 10-4A). Pressure is applied to the angle of the mandible to dislocate it upward while forcefully opening the mouth. This is painful, and the conscious or semiconscious victim will object by clamping down or writhing.

3. A third maneuver is the internal jaw lift (see Fig. 10-4B). The rescuer's thumb is inserted into the victim's mouth under the tongue, and the mandibular mentum (chin) is lifted, thus stretching out the soft tissues and opening the airway. This is the best maneuver for the unconscious victim with a shattered mandible. The internal jaw lift is

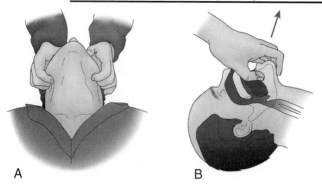

Figure 10-4. A, External jaw thrust. **B,** Internal jaw lift.

dangerous to the rescuer if the victim is semiconscious and can bite.
4. A fourth noninvasive airway maneuver takes some practice but serves several purposes and is the best maneuver if done correctly. In this two-handed triple maneuver, the head is held between two hands to prevent lateral rotation and maintain neck control. The fourth and fifth fingers are hooked behind the angle of the mandible to dislocate the jaw upward, and the thumbs ensure that the mouth is maintained open (see Fig. 10-2). The third finger may be positioned over the facial artery as it comes around the mandible so that the pulse can be monitored at the same time. For greatest stability, the rescuer's elbows should rest on the same surface on which the victim is lying.

Improvised Tongue Traction Technique
If the patient is unconscious, the airway may be opened temporarily by attaching the anterior aspect of the victim's tongue to the lower lip with one or two safety pins (Fig. 10-5). An alternative to piercing the lower lip is to pass a string through the safety pins and exert traction on the tongue by securing the end of the string to the victim's shirt button or jacket zipper (Fig. 10-6).

▶ MECHANICAL AIRWAY ADJUNCTS

The oropharyngeal airway (OPA) is an S-shaped device designed to hold the tongue off the posterior pharyngeal wall (Fig. 10-7). When properly placed, it prevents the tongue from obstructing the glottis. These devices are most effective in unconscious and semiconscious victims who lack a gag reflex

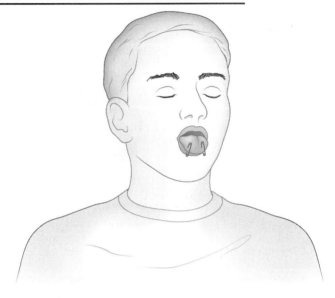

Figure 10-5. Tongue traction. The airway may be opened temporarily by attaching the anterior aspect of the victim's tongue to the lower lip with two safety pins.

or cough. The use of an OPA in a victim with a gag reflex or cough is contraindicated because it may stimulate retching, vomiting, or laryngospasm.

Technique for Insertion of Oropharyngeal Airway

1. Open the mouth and clear the pharynx of any secretions, blood, or vomitus.
2. Insert the OPA upside down or at a 90-degree angle to avoid pushing the tongue posteriorly during insertion. Slide it gently along the roof of the mouth. As the oral airway is inserted past the uvula or crest of the tongue, rotate it so that the tip points down the victim's throat.
3. The flange should rest against the victim's lips, and the distal portions should rest on the posterior pharyngeal wall.

Nasopharyngeal Airway (NPA)

The NPA is an uncuffed trumpet-like tube that provides a conduit for airflow between the nares and pharynx (Fig. 10-8). It is inserted through the nose rather than the mouth. This device is better tolerated than an OPA and is a better choice for wilderness airway management.

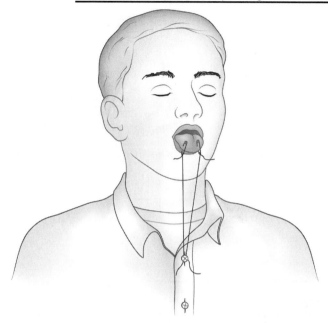

Figure 10-6. Tongue traction. An alternative to piercing the lower lip is to pass a string through the safety pins and exert traction on the tongue by securing the end of the string to the victim's shirt button or jacket zipper.

Technique for Insertion of Nasopharyngeal Airway

1. Lubricate the nasopharyngeal airway with a water-soluble lubricant.
2. Place the NPA in the nostril with the bevel directed toward the nasal septum.
3. Gently push the NPA straight back along the floor of the nasal passage. As the NPA passes through the turbinates, there will be mild resistance, but once the tip has entered the nasopharynx, there will be sensation of a "give."
4. If you meet persistent resistance, rotate the tube slightly, reattempt insertion through the other nostril, or try a smaller-diameter tube. Do not force the tube in.
5. Following insertion, the flange should rest on the victim's nostril and the tube should be visible in the oropharynx as it passes behind the tonsils. The tip should come to rest behind the base of the tongue but above the vocal cords.

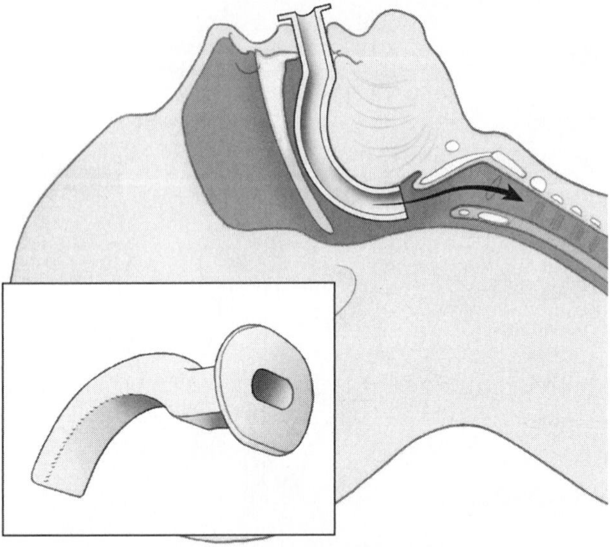

Figure 10-7. Oropharyngeal airway. (Redrawn from Mahadevan SV, Garmel GM [eds]: An Introduction to Clinical Emergency Medicine: Guide for Practitioners in the Emergency Department. Cambridge, UK, Cambridge University Press, 2005. © Chris Gralapp, www.biolumina.com.)

6. Complications of NPAs include failure to pass through the nose (usually resulting from a deviated septum), epistaxis, accidental avulsion of adenoidal tissue, mucosal tears or avulsion of a turbinate, submucosal tunneling (the tube tunnels out of sight behind the posterior pharyngeal wall), and creation of pressure sores.
7. If the NPA or any nasal tube is left in place for more than several days, impedance to normal drainage may predispose the victim to sinusitis or otitis media.

Improvised Mechanical Airways

Any flexible tube of appropriate diameter and length can be used as an improvisational substitute for the NPA. Examples include a Foley catheter, radiator hose, solar shower hose, siphon tubing, or inflation hose from a kayak flotation bag or sport pouch. An endotracheal tube can be shortened and softened in warm water to substitute for a commercial nasal trumpet. The flange can be improvised using a safety pin through the nostril end of the tube (Fig. 10-9).

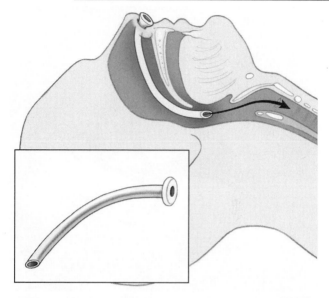

Figure 10-8. Nasopharyngeal airway. (Redrawn from Mahadevan SV, Garmel GM [eds]: An Introduction to Clinical Emergency Medicine: Guide for Practitioners in the Emergency Department. Cambridge, UK, Cambridge University Press, 2005. © Chris Gralapp, www.biolumina.com.)

▶ RESCUE BREATHING AND FOREIGN BODY ASPIRATION

See Chapter 25, Life-Threatening Emergencies.

▶ SUCTIONING

In the wilderness, one must remove secretions without the benefit of electricity, customary suction devices, or aesthetic and sterile protective barriers. A number of innovative products are on the market for the prehospital responder, extended care provider, or potential expedition medic to consider for the expedition first-aid kit (see Chapter 60):

1. Gloves and a face barrier (plastic square with a small one-way valve to place over the victim's face) can be tucked into a 35-mm film container or one of the small pouches marketed specifically for this purpose.
2. A plastic baggie with a slit for the mouth and nostrils can be placed over the victim's face for rescue breathing.
3. Debris can be swept from the mouth with a finger wrapped in a T-shirt or other available cloth.

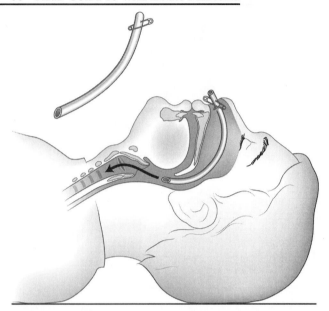

Figure 10-9. Improvised nasal trumpet.

4. The victim can be positioned so that gravity facilitates drainage of blood, vomit, saliva, and mucus. Something absorbent or basin-like can be placed at the side of the mouth to catch drained effluvia.

5. Turkey basters can be included in an expedition first-aid kit for extraction of secretions and for gentle wound irrigation and moisturizing burn dressings or wet compresses. The rubber self-inflating bulbs marketed for infant nasal suctioning can also be used to suction out debris from the mouths and noses of adults.

6. If time permits and the supplies are available, a "mucous trap" suction device can be improvised from a jar with two holes poked in its lid and two tubes or straws duct-taped into the holes. One straw goes to the rescuer, who provides suction, and the other is directed toward whatever has accumulated in the airway. The jar serves to trap the removed secretions so that the rescuer is spared the distasteful experience of suctioning bodily fluids or foreign substances such as mud directly into his or her own mouth.

7. Secretion removal by gravity or suctioning is key to the management of epistaxis and for maintaining the airway of a victim with mandibular fractures (see Chapter 17).

► **AIRWAY EQUIPMENT**

Stethoscope

A stethoscope is a useful addition to the expedition first-aid kit. However, auscultating breath sounds without a stethoscope is easy:

1. Place the ear directly to the chest.
2. Isolate and amplify the breath sounds by listening through a hollow object such as a modified cup, empty water bottle or soda can, or through the cardboard center of a roll of toilet paper.
3. The additional merit of a real stethoscope is that it can be disassembled to harvest compliant tubing that might be used improvisationally to substitute for nasopharyngeal airways, cricothyrotomy tubes or stents, straws for suction devices, chest tubes, restraining tethers, lymphatic constriction bands, or other medical devices.

Masks and One-Way Valves

One-Way Non-Rebreathing Flap-Valve
The purpose of the one-way non-rebreathing flap-valve is to permit air to be pushed into the victim through one aperture while exhaled air and secretions are exhausted through a separate route, thus helping minimize exposure to infectious substances. These one-way valves are small, lightweight, and inexpensive and are easy to tuck into a small container, along with gloves and a face barrier.

Facemasks
Facemasks differ in shape, type of seal, transparency, and materials. For maximum ease of use, a high-volume, low-pressure cushion (the softest, biggest one) should be kept sufficiently inflated so that there is an air-filled buffer yet a smooth contact surface between the cushion and the various contours of the face.

Despite optimal cushion inflation, however, some facial shapes provide special challenges. For example:

1. A seal may be difficult to achieve on the bushy-bearded individual. If the beard cannot be rapidly modified, the rescuer could consider using petroleum jelly, hand lotion, bag balm, or K-Y jelly to try to slick down the beard and seal over areas where air can leak out. This maneuver has the disadvantage of making the rescuer's hands slick and the cushion of the mask slippery, so both of the rescuer's hands will be needed to maintain the mask fit. The rescuer also runs the risk of greasing up everything else

handled during the resuscitation. Alternatively, a large, clear intravenous site dressing (e.g., Tegaderm, 10 to 12 cm, 3M Health Care, St. Paul, MN) can be placed over the mouth and beard. The nostrils are left uncovered, and a slit the width of the mouth permits full mouth opening while sealing over the beard and improving the security of a rescuer's grip.

2. Another challenging facial contour is the prominently chinned, long-faced, and edentulous elder individual. With the facial laxity that comes with age and without bordering teeth, the cheeks tend to cave in. Again, a two-handed mask technique is probably necessary. The thumbs press down on either side of the mask, and the fingers pull up on the jaw and bunch up as much of the cheek tissues as possible. A second pair of hands might be needed to bunch up the tissues around the entire lower perimeter of the mask. The stiffer the cushion, the harder it is to make this seal. Another maneuver to consider in this situation is to roll up two gauze or cloth packs to tuck into the mouth and distend the cheeks. The risks of this maneuver are dislodgment and possible aspiration of the packs and retrograde displacement of the tongue despite a good jaw lift. If there is any choice in the matter, it is almost always easier to mask-ventilate an individual with dentures in place than to ventilate one with dentures removed; thus if intact and secure, dentures should be left in place during field resuscitation.

3. A third challenging facial contour is that of the average infant, any chubby-cheeked, baby-toothed, tonsil-abundant young child, or a moon-faced, short-necked adult. The key to successful mask ventilation in these situations is to keep the victim's mouth open and the soft tissues from folding in on themselves from gravity and extrinsic compression. One approach is to mask-ventilate over a pacifier, oral airway, nasopharyngeal airway, or improvisational hollow object intended to hold the lips apart, mouth open, and tongue pressed down to the floor of the mouth and away from the back of the throat.

To select the most widely adaptable "first-aid kit" mask-and-valve product, look for the following features:

1. Transparent and easily bendable mask body materials that retain little "memory" of residing in their carrying positions and that do not become stiff, brittle, or nondeformable in cold temperatures

2. An inflatable cushion seal that can be adjusted for changes in temperature and altitude

3. A flexible, high-volume, low-pressure cushion seal able to conform to many different face sizes and shapes

4. A mask span that can be used on both small and large victims, tough materials resistant to cracks and punctures, and a compact mask or carrying case that does not take up disproportionate space in the first-aid kit

Other Airway Adjuncts

Other commercial airway adjuncts used in prehospital circumstances include the esophageal-tracheal Combitube, esophageal obturator airway (EOA), esophageal-gastric tube airway (EGA), pharyngotracheal lumen airway (PTLA), and laryngeal mask airway (LMA). Successful insertion of these devices requires formal instruction and practice. Their use in the wilderness setting is appropriately limited to trained and experienced providers.

The LMA is a modified ETT with an inflatable, oval cuff ("laryngeal mask") at its base (Fig. 10-10) that is ideal for

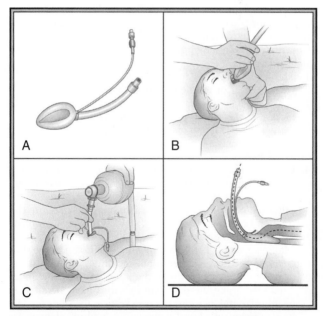

Figure 10-10. Laryngeal mask airway (LMA). **A,** LMA is an adjunctive airway that consists of a tube with a cuffed mask-like projection at the distal end. **B,** LMA is introduced through the mouth into the pharynx. **C,** Once the LMA is in position, a clear, secure airway is present. **D (Anatomic detail),** During insertion, the LMA is advanced until resistance is felt as the distal portion of tube locates in the hypopharynx. The cuff is then inflated. This seals the larynx and leaves the distal opening of the tube just above the glottis, providing a clear, secure airway *(dotted line)*. (Redrawn from Guidelines 2000 for Cardiopulmonary Resuscitation and Emergency Cardiovascular Care. Part 6: Advanced cardiovascular life support. Section 3. Adjuncts for oxygenation, ventilation, and airway control. The American Heart Association in collaboration with the International Liaison Committee on Resuscitation. Circulation 102[8 Suppl]:195-1104, 2000.)

wilderness use. The LMA is inserted blindly into the pharynx and advanced until resistance is felt as the distal portion of the tube locates in the laryngopharynx. Inflation of the collar provides a seal around the laryngeal inlet, facilitating tracheal ventilation. The LMA provides equivalent ventilation to the tracheal tube.

▶ CRICOTHYROTOMY

If the upper airway is completely obstructed and obstruction cannot be relieved or bypassed, the only way to avoid death is to create an air passage directly into the trachea. The most accessible and least complicated access site is through the cricothyroid membrane. Even in experienced hands, the relatively high complication rates (10% to 40%) for emergent cricothyrotomies are still less than those for tracheotomies. Complications include bleeding, puncture of the posterior trachea and esophagus, creation of a false passage, inability to ventilate, aspiration, subcutaneous and mediastinal emphysema, vocal cord injury, and subsequent tracheal stenosis.

1. The cricothyrotomy hole may be made percutaneously with a trocar or needle or surgically with a knife blade.
2. If a syringe containing 1 mL of water or lidocaine is attached to the needle used for puncture, bubbles may be seen as the needle tip enters the trachea.
3. When the trachea is successfully entered, a gush of air will exit, often with a cough.
4. Once the cricothyroid membrane is punctured, it is essential to maintain patency of the tract and identify the hole with a tube, stylet, obturator, tweezers, wire, or another temporary place marker. It is very easy to lose the tract and create a false passage while trying to instrument or cannulate the route.
5. Making a small (1- to 1.5-cm) vertical incision in the skin over the cricothyroid membrane facilitates the ease of the next step: puncture through the lower third of the dime-sized membrane. Vertical skin incisions have advantages over horizontal incisions because vertical incisions tend to be more controlled and better positioned in reference to landmarks.
6. The needle/catheter is advanced in the midline of the neck at a 45-degree angle aiming toward the lower back.
7. Once the needle or introducer aspirates air, the catheter is slid off the stylet and the stylet is withdrawn.
8. Taking care not to kink a flexible catheter at the insertion site, the hub may be secured in place with tape or sutures

or may be attached to a Luer-Lok syringe-adaptor mechanism.

9. With anything other than a commercial cricothyrotomy set or endotracheal tube, provision of positive-pressure ventilation requires creative assembly of an adapter connecting the apparatus in the trachea to the female connector on an Ambu bag. Figure 10-11 shows an example of the step-up series of connections needed for this type of extension.

10. If the catheter in the trachea is to be replaced by a stiffer or bigger cannula, a guidewire is inserted through the catheter several centimeters down the trachea, the catheter is withdrawn with the guidewire remaining, and a dilator is advanced over the guidewire and then withdrawn.

11. Next, the intended cannula is threaded over the guidewire until it is seated with its flanges flush to the skin. The Seldinger technique is the process of identifying a lumen with an introducer, marking the lumen with a guidewire, dilating the entry site, and placing the final apparatus over the guidewire. The procedure of replacing a smaller tube with a larger one is termed a dilational cricothyrotomy.

12. A temporary cricothyrotomy trocar and tube can be fashioned from a tuberculin or 3-mL syringe that has been cut on the diagonal and then forcefully inserted through the cricothyroid membrane (Fig. 10-12). Because the improvised trocar point of the syringe is sharp and irregular, insertion is likely to be traumatic. Care must be taken to not lacerate the posterior tracheal wall or create a tracheoesophageal fistula.

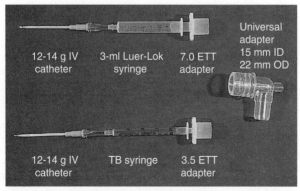

Figure 10-11. Combination of catheter assemblies to allow connection of a needle cricothyrotomy to a 15/22-mm standard adaptor for Ambu ventilation. (Courtesy of Anne E. Dickison, MD.)

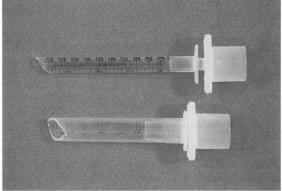

Figure 10-12. A tuberculin or 3-mL syringe can be cut on the diagonal to improvise a combination trocar-cricothyrotomy tube. Caution must be taken with insertion to avoid traumatizing the posterior pharyngeal wall. (Courtesy of Anne E. Dickison, MD.)

13. Even with a universal adapter (15/22-mm) connection, without a jet ventilation device or cricothyrotomy tube of the proper diameter, curvature, and length, it is extremely difficult to positive pressure ventilate a victim through a needle catheter or improvisational substitute. The victim has the best chances at survival if spontaneous respiratory effort can be preserved; it is easier for the victim to draw air in through a critically small opening than it is for a rescuer to generate the pressure needed to force air in through the same aperture. Pressures sufficient to make the chest rise can be generated by a rescuer blowing through the needle catheter, but such efforts rapidly lead to rescuer fatigue.

14. Temporary transtracheal oxygenation and ventilation through a 12- or 14-gauge needle can be provided using a flow rate of 15 L/minute or by jet ventilation (40 psi) at a slow intermittent rate of 6 breaths per minute and an inspiratory-to-expiratory ratio of 1:14. The very long expiratory time is necessary to allow passive expiration through a restrictive channel.

15. Packaged dilator cricothyrotomy sets such as those manufactured by Melker, Arndt, and Corke Cranswick contain a scalpel blade, syringe with an 18-gauge over-the-needle catheter and/or a thin introducer needle, guidewire, appropriately sized dilator, and a polyvinyl airway cannula. The Patil set (Cook Critical Care, Bloomington, IN), the Portex Minitrach II (Concord/Portex, Keene, NH), and

the military version of the Melker set are sold without the guidewire and appeal to prehospital providers unfamiliar with the Seldinger technique. The Pertrach (Pertrach, Inc., Long Beach, CA) is similar in concept except the guidewire and dilator are forged as a single unit so that a finder catheter cannot be used and the introducer must be peeled away. The Nu-Trake device (International Medical Devices, Inc., Northridge, CA) is complicated to use, has a rigid airway that risks trauma to the posterior trachea, and is difficult to secure.

16. In terms of expedition kit portability, three transtracheal puncture emergency airway devices deserve special mention:

   a. Lifestat (New Orleans, LA) manufactures a key-chain emergency airway set that consists of a sharp-pointed metal trocar introducer that fits through a straight metal cannula that screws into a metal extension with a universal 15-mm male adaptor. Lightweight and less than 3 inches long, the three-component apparatus is attached to a separate and detachable key chain (Fig. 10-13).

   b. Cook Critical Care offers a 6-French reinforced-catheter emergency transtracheal airway catheter (order number C-DTJV–6.0–7.5-BTT) with a molded Luer-Lok connection for jet ventilation or added assembly of a 15-mm adaptor for standard modes of positive pressure ventilation.

   c. Cook Critical Care also offers the Wadhwa Emergency Airway Device (order number C-WEAD–100). This

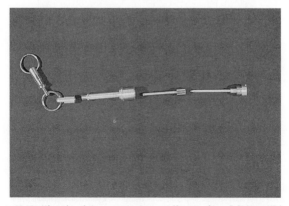

Figure 10-13. Lifestat key-chain emergency airway set. (Courtesy of Anne E. Dickison, MD.)

lightweight, impact-resistant assembly is 7.25 inches long and the diameter of a highlighter pen (Fig. 10-14). It disassembles to yield a 12-French Teflon-coated cricothyrotomy catheter with removable metal stylet (with a molded plastic Luer-Lok connection for oxygen or jet ventilation), plus a flexible nasopharyngeal

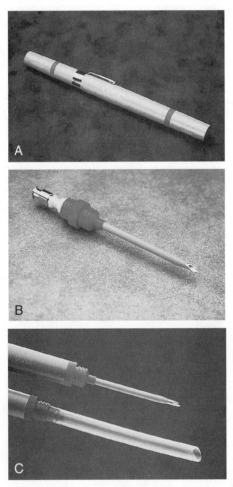

Figure 10-14. A, Wadhwa Emergency Device. **B,** Wadhwa transtracheal catheter with removable stylet and Luer-Lok connection for jet ventilation. **C,** Internal components of the Wadhwa Emergency Airway Device. Both the transtracheal catheter and the nasopharyngeal airway screw into the case for an extension with a 15-mm adaptor. (Courtesy of Cook, Inc.)

airway adhered to a molded plastic flange. Both the cricothyrotomy catheter and the NPA screw into the Wadhwa case to provide a low-resistance extension and a 15-mm (male) connection for standard positive-pressure ventilation equipment.

Emergency Oxygen Administration

11

Emergency medical oxygen (O_2) administration is a critical part of wilderness emergency care. Every provider of wilderness medicine must be familiar with O_2, its therapeutic value, indications, hazards, equipment, and technique of administration.

▶ INDICATIONS

Indications for the use of supplemental O_2 include (but are not limited to) the following:
- Shock
- Hypoxia, hypoxemia
- Trauma
- Medical emergencies (asthma, anaphylaxis, acute myocardial infarction, cerebrovascular accident)
- Decompression illness (DCI) including both decompression sickness (DCS) and arterial gas embolism (AGE)
- Acute mountain sickness (AMS)
- High-altitude pulmonary edema (HAPE)
- High-altitude cerebral edema (HACE)
- Carbon monoxide (CO) poisoning
- Respiratory or cardiopulmonary arrest

▶ CONTRAINDICATIONS

In an acutely hypoxic patient, there is no contraindication to the administration of high concentrations of supplemental O_2 for a limited time. O_2 should not be withheld out of fear of suppressing respiration when hypoxia is suspected. A person with a history of chronic obstructive pulmonary disease (COPD) who is not acutely hypoxic or in need of emergency prehospital care should only be administered his or her prescribed flow rate of supplemental O_2.

Pulmonary Oxygen Toxicity

In situations in which high concentrations of supplemental O_2 administration may be carried out for many hours there exists a concern for possible pulmonary O_2 toxicity. Pulmonary O_2 toxicity only becomes a risk after many (10 to 18) hours and high O_2 concentrations (FIO_2 of 0.5 to 1).

Prolonged exposure to high concentration of O_2 is also associated with the following:
1. Intratracheal and bronchial irritation
2. Substernal or retrosternal burning
3. Chest tightness, cough, and dyspnea

4. Continued prolonged exposure to high O_2 concentrations may result in adult respiratory distress syndrome (ARDS). Early pulmonary changes associated with pulmonary O_2 toxicity are reversible with cessation of O_2 therapy.
5. Avoidance of the onset of symptoms may be accomplished by the use of periodic "air breaks," during which the patient breathes air for 5 to 10 minutes.

Central Nervous System Oxygen Toxicity

Central nervous system (CNS) O_2 toxicity is of concern when a person is exposed to O_2 at ambient pressures greater than 1 atmosphere (sea level) and where FIO_2 exceeds 1, such as while scuba diving or in a hyperbaric O_2 chamber. It is not of concern to persons at normobaric or hypobaric ambient pressure. Signs and symptoms may appear at FIO_2 of greater than 1.6 and include (but are not limited to) the following:
- Sweating
- Bradycardia
- Mood changes
- Visual field constriction
- Twitching
- Syncope
- Seizures

During hyperbaric O_2 therapy, the likelihood of central nervous system O_2 toxicity is reduced by the use of periodic air breaks.

▶ EQUIPMENT

Cylinders

Medical O_2 cylinders or tanks are made of aluminum or steel and come in a variety of sizes (Table 11-1). In the United States, any pressure vessel that is transported on public roads is subject to U.S. Department of Transportation (US DOT) regulations. The US DOT requires that cylinders be visually and hydrostatically tested every 5 years and either be destroyed if they fail or be stamped and labeled appropriately if they pass. Gas suppliers will not fill cylinders that have not been appropriately tested and stamped. The working pressure of steel medical O_2 cylinders is 2015 psi. The working pressure of aluminum O_2 cylinders is either 2015 psi or 2216 psi, depending on the type. High-pressure, lightweight cylinders used for high-altitude climbing are not discussed here. For more information on climbing systems see www.poisk-ltd.ru.

Valves

Valves for medical O_2 cylinders sold in the United States are designed to accept only medical O_2 regulators to avoid the possibility of using a medical O_2 regulator with an incompatible

TABLE 11-1. Common Portable Medical Oxygen Cylinder Specifications

CYLINDER* SIZE	ALLOY	WORKING PRESSURE (LB/SQ INCH OR PSI)	VOLUME (L, CU FT)	LENGTH (IN, CM)	DIAMETER (IN, CM)	WEIGHT (LB, KG)
M9	Aluminum	2015	246.3, 8.7	10.9, 27.7	4.4, 11.1	3.9, 1.8
D	Aluminum	2015	424.71, 15	16.5, 41.9	4.4, 11.1	5.5, 2.5
D	Steel	2015	410.4, 14.5	16.75, 42.5	4.4, 11.1	7.5, 3.4
Jumbo D	Aluminum	2216	648.3, 22.9	17, 43.2	5.3, 13.3	9.0, 4.1
E	Aluminum	2015	679.4, 24	25.6, 65.0	4.4, 11.1	8.0, 3.6
E	Steel	2015	682.0, 24.1	25.75, 65.4	4.4, 11.1	10.5, 4.8

* Aluminum cylinder specifications provided by Luxfer Inc. Steel cylinder specifications provided by Pressed Steel Tank Co.

gas such as acetylene. The two types of valves available in the United States are the CGA-870 and the CGA-540. The CGA-870 is also known as the *pin-index valve* and is used on smaller portable cylinders (e.g., D, E). The CGA-540 is used primarily on larger, nonportable cylinders such as those mounted in ambulances (e.g., H, M).

A number of other valve types are manufactured and used with medical O_2 throughout the world. For example, there are adapters available to make a U.S. pin-index regulator fit on an Australian bull-nose valve, but it must be noted that the use of adapters is discouraged by the U.S. Compressed Gas Association (CGA).

Regulators

The device that mounts directly to the cylinder is the regulator. Its function is to regulate the flow rate of the O_2 by reducing the pressure of the O_2 from either 2015 psi or 2216 psi to a usable flow rate. Regulators are primarily of three types: constant flow only; demand/flow restricted oxygen-powered ventilator (FROPV) only; or multifunction, which has both constant flow and demand/FROPV capability.

The regulator mounts to the cylinder with a matching-type valve. A pressure gauge allows the user to monitor the amount of O_2 in the cylinder.

Devices for Ventilation of Nonbreathing Patients

All of the following devices keep direct patient contact at a minimum to reduce the risk of disease transmission. Other body substance isolation equipment (e.g., gloves, goggles) and practices should be observed as well.

In addition, when used on a nonintubated patient, all of the devices discussed depend on adequate mask seal to be able to deliver adequate ventilations and ensure adequate respiration. The single most common cause of inadequate ventilation and respiration is poor mask seal.

FROPV/Positive Pressure Demand Valve

1. Older style positive pressure demand valves (PPDVs), such as the LSP 063-05 or Elder CPR Demand valve (both manufactured by Life Support Products/Allied Health Care), function both in positive pressure mode (pushing the button to ventilate a nonbreathing patient) and in demand mode.

2. When used in demand mode, the recipient simply holds the mask to his or her face. When he or she inhales, negative pressure in the mask and demand valve opens the valve and gas flows. The flow of gas stops when the person stops

inhaling or exhales, similar to other demand regulators such as scuba and aviation regulators.

3. One misconception is that PPDVs will easily cause pulmonary overpressurization injury, and thus they have fallen out of favor with some health care providers. In fact, in positive pressure mode, all PPDVs manufactured in the United States are required to have an overpressure relief valve that stops the flow of gas at a pressure of 55 to 65 cm H_2O (a little more than half the pressure required to overpressurize a human lung). This is done to avoid pulmonary overpressurization injury. The most recent model, introduced in 1993, the MTV-100 FROPV (LSP/Allied), has two overpressure relief valves, the first set at 60 cm H_2O and the second at 65 to 80 cm H_2O.

4. With respect to the positive pressure mode, earlier PPDVs were originally designed to meet the Emergency Cardiac Care Committee (ECC) cardiopulmonary resuscitation (CPR) guidelines before 1986, which called for "four quick initial breaths and then two quick breaths after every 15 compressions." This faster rate of ventilation was equivalent to 160 L/minute.

5. In 1986, CPR standards were changed to "two slow breaths, each one and one-half seconds in duration." The standard changed again in 1992 to the current one of "two slow, full breaths, with a duration of 1½ to 2 seconds each" (equivalent to 40 L/minute). This was changed to reduce the possibility of gastric insufflation, regurgitation, and aspiration of gastric contents. To meet this guideline of a 1½- to 2-second breath, the manufacturers of PPDVs added a restricting orifice that limited the flow rate to 40 L/minute. Unfortunately, this created increased breathing resistance to the demand feature.

6. In 1993, a new-style PPDV, called the FROPV (MTV-100, manufactured by LSP/Allied), was introduced. Its specifications include a flow rate of 40 L/minute while being used in positive pressure mode and 115 L/minute in demand mode, eliminating the difficulties of the earlier models.

7. The mask adapter is a standard 15-mm fitting that fits a variety of masks and can also be used directly with an endotracheal tube. The disadvantages of the FROPV are that a supply of O_2 is required for its use and that in intubated patients the health care provider will not be able to "feel" decreased lung compliance.

Bag-Valve-Mask

1. The bag-valve-mask (BVM) consists of a mask, bag, and valves that control or direct the flow of air and O_2. Like the FROPV, the mask can be changed to different styles to

accommodate different faces or can be used directly with an endotracheal tube. The volume of the bag is 1000 to 1200 mL, depending on the manufacturer. Some have an outlet and reservoir for use with supplemental O_2.

2. An advantage to the BVM is that although it works best with supplemental O_2, it will function on room air if the O_2 supply is depleted. In addition, in intubated persons, some health care providers are able to "feel" decreased lung compliance.

3. The primary disadvantage is that it requires training and practice to effectively use a BVM, and even with much practice, many find it is difficult to maintain adequate mask seal and ventilate sufficient volumes when only one rescuer is available to use it. Even with proper training, few individuals can maintain adequate mask seal and a patent airway with one hand while squeezing the bag fully to achieve the 800- to 1200-mL standard volume. The US DOT recommends that the BVM be used first with two rescuers (one maintaining mask seal and patency of the airway, the other squeezing the bag). A BVM with one rescuer should be the last choice (after all other devices and techniques) in ventilating a patient. In addition, there is no overpressurization relief valve. This is rarely a concern in nonintubated persons because of the aforementioned difficulties in achieving even minimally acceptable ventilatory volumes, but it is of concern in intubated persons.

Resuscitation Mask

1. The pocket-type resuscitation mask consists of a clear, flexible plastic mask designed to fit over the mouth and nose of the victim while the health care provider ventilates by exhaling through the "chimney." A one-way valve usually directs the rescuer's breath into the victim while at the same time directing the exhaled breath of the victim away from the rescuer. It is a relatively simple device that requires minimal training, is lightweight, and is more likely to be available when equipment is at a minimum. It is available both with and without an outlet for supplemental O_2.

2. The pocket-type mask is most effective when used with supplemental O_2. It will also function on room air and does not have an overpressurization relief valve.

Constant Flow Devices for Adequately Breathing Patients

Non-Rebreather Mask

1. The non-rebreather mask is the first choice when considering constant flow supplemental O_2 in an acute medical

emergency. It consists of a mask, reservoir bag, and two or three one-way valves, one separating the reservoir from the mask and the other one or two on the sides of the mask. Oxygen flows into the reservoir bag so that when the victim inhales, he or she inhales O_2 from the reservoir. The one-way valves on the sides of the mask keep air from coming into the mask and diluting the O_2. When the victim exhales, expired air goes out of the mask through the one or two valves on the face and is prevented from entering the reservoir.

2. The efficiency of this mask depends on the mask fit and seal and proper functioning of the valves. Under ideal conditions this mask (when fitted with all three valves) may deliver an F_{IO_2} of up to 0.95. Field studies show it may deliver an F_{IO_2} as low as 0.60, but it is still the most effective constant flow device available (except for O_2 rebreathers).

3. To use the mask, it is attached to the O_2 supply at a flow rate of 10 to 15 L/minute. The reservoir bag must be inflated or "primed" before placing it on the person. This can be accomplished by placing a thumb or fingers on the valve between the reservoir and mask while the reservoir inflates. Care must be taken to not allow the O_2 supply to be depleted while the mask is on the person. Because of the one-way valves, if there is no O_2 supply, suffocation may result. The mask is available with either two one-way valves on the sides or with only one (labeled as "with safety outlet"). If the mask has only one valve on the side of the mask, it will deliver reduced F_{IO_2}.

4. The advantage of the non-rebreather mask is that it provides the highest F_{IO_2} of the constant flow devices. However, it also wastes O_2 and may not deliver a high F_{IO_2} under less than ideal conditions. Care must be taken to monitor the victim and O_2 supply closely to avoid allowing the tank to empty while the mask is still on the victim's face.

Nasal Cannula

1. The only other recommended constant flow device for prehospital emergency O_2 administration is the nasal cannula. This is recommended when the victim requires lower F_{IO_2} or when the victim will not tolerate any kind of mask such as a person with a long history of COPD. It must be understood that a nasal cannula is capable of only delivering F_{IO_2} of 0.24 to 0.29.

2. Flow rates for a nasal cannula are limited to 1 to 6 L/minute. To use the nasal cannula, place the prongs in the patient's nares and loop the tubing over the top of the ears to hold it in place. Adjust the tightness at the neck to a comfortable

level. Flow rates exceeding 4 L/minute are extremely uncomfortable and may result in drying of the nasal mucosa.

Other constant flow masks such as the partial rebreather mask, simple facemask, and Venturi mask are not recommended for use in prehospital emergency medicine because of low levels of delivered F_{IO_2}.

These masks may be used to deliver supplemental oxygen to climbers on high-altitude expeditions and should not be confused with non-rebreather masks.

Oxygen Rebreathers

1. One of the problems with long transports commonly seen in the case of wilderness or remote emergency medical care is that all of the previously discussed O_2 delivery devices waste O_2 and require multiple portable or large nonportable cylinders if the transport time exceeds 1 hour. Breathing room air, a person inhales 21% O_2 and exhales 16% O_2. If a person inhales (under ideal conditions) 100% O_2, the exhaled gas will contain 95% O_2 and 5% CO_2. The theory of the design of a rebreather is to remove CO_2 from the exhaled gas, supplement for the 5% O_2 that was metabolized, and reuse the exhaled O_2.

2. Several manufacturers produce rebreathers for emergency medical O_2 administration, all of which have the same basic components: a mask; breathing circuit (similar to anesthesia equipment); and canister with an absorbent chemical, usually soda lime or Sodasorb.

3. The soda lime chemically removes CO_2 from the exhaled gas, allowing for the O_2 to be rebreathed. Supplemental O_2 is added at flow rates of less than 2 L/minute to replace the metabolized O_2. Thus a cylinder that can last 45 minutes with a non-rebreather mask or a little more than 1 hour on demand now can last for more than 6 hours, and the victim (with proper technique) will still receive F_{IO_2} of 0.85 to 0.99. In a situation in which equipment is limited because of size and weight, this device may prove invaluable.

4. Different manufacturers recommend beginning the victim on O_2 during assembly or while setting up the unit, then flushing the system of air and applying it to the victim. Others recommend air breaks to minimize the risk of pulmonary oxygen toxicity.

5. Thermal considerations are important because of the chemical reaction that takes place with the soda lime. The reaction produces heat and water, so it provides warmed and humidified O_2. In cold climates this is an advantage, but in hot climates it may be a disadvantage. If one is in a hot climate, it is recommended to pass the breathing circuit

hoses through cold or ice water to cool the gas. Rebreather setups are typically lightweight and allow high FIO_2 (≈ 0.80) at constant flow rates of less than 2 L/minute, thereby extending the life of the cylinder.

6. Disadvantages are the training requirement and that the breathing circuit and absorbent canister containing the soda lime are typically "single-patient use." Like other O_2 delivery devices, the rebreather also depends on an adequate mask seal to function effectively. Poor mask seal results in dilution of inhaled gas with air and lower FIO_2. An increase in breathing resistance may also occur when compared with a constant-flow mask.

7. The most common types of resuscitators available on the market today are the American DAN $REMO_2$ system, two German systems (the Wenoll and the Circulox), and an Australian system (OXI-Saver Resuscitator).

Oxygen Concentrators

An **oxygen concentrator** (also referred to as an *oxygen generator*) is a device that can be used to provide oxygen in a setting where electrical power is available. The power requirement precludes the use of these devices in a true wilderness setting, but practitioners may see these in use on ships, rural communities, or currently by the U.S. military in the conflicts in Iraq and Afghanistan. Oxygen concentrators can be used as an alternative to tanks of compressed oxygen with the caveat that no power equals no oxygen.

Oxygen concentrators vary in their capacity to concentrate oxygen. Most concentrators allow for a continuous supply of oxygen at a flow rate of approximately 3 to 5 L/minute at concentrations from 50% to 95% (FIO_2). They are heavy [about 30 lb (13.61 kg)].

Oxygen-Saving Devices

More than half of the respiratory cycle is spent on expiration, and oxygen that flows during this period is wasted. Devices designed to pulse the delivery during inspiration can save oxygen. Pulse delivery systems monitor micropressure from inspiration efforts, opening an inspiratory valve from the supply. These systems deliver a calibrated pulse of oxygen at the instant negative pressure is detected (and not at any other time). Flow typically continues for up to a second. Pulse delivery can dramatically extend the life of portable cylinders (up to fourfold). Additionally, reservoir systems such as the "moustache"-style nasal canula store oxygen in a chamber (volume ≈ 20 mL). Reservoir systems can reduce oxygen requirements by 50% to 70% at rest. Pulse delivery systems are currently in use by paraglider and glider pilots and gaining popularity among some general aviators. These systems remain a bit too complex for high-altitude mountaineering, where freezing concerns and principles of simplicity prevail.

▶ BREATHING PATIENTS

1. Concerns for ventilating nonbreathing patients include rate (breaths per minute), volume, flow rate or speed, pressure, and oxygenation. The rate of ventilations per minute is 12 breaths per minute for an adult (older than 8 years old) and 20 breaths per minute for children and infants.

2. The recommended volume for ventilations for an adult is 800 to 1200 mL. If a ventilation device or technique does not have an overpressure relief valve and greater volumes are administered, pulmonary barotrauma (pulmonary overpressurization injury) may result. Ventilatory volumes less than 800 mL may not be sufficient to inflate the alveoli, and thus gas exchange will be inadequate. Each ventilation should be at least 1½ to 2 seconds in duration (equivalent to 40 L/minute). Faster ventilation rates or speeds force open the esophagus and then force air into the stomach rather than the lungs. Increased gastric insufflation greatly increases the risk of regurgitation and aspiration of gastric contents.

3. A differential pressure of as little as 90 to 110 cm H_2O is sufficient to rupture alveoli and to allow gas to escape into interstitial spaces. Care must be taken to not exceed these pressures when ventilating a person. Humans can easily generate pressures exceeding 120 cm H_2O by exhaling forcefully, and thus according to ECC CPR guidelines, one should "blow until the chest rises" to accommodate various sizes of individuals. The only device for ventilating adults that has an overpressure relief valve is the PPDV/FROPV.

4. The primary goal of ventilation is oxygenation. With mouth-to-mouth or mouth-to-mask breathing without supplemental O_2, FIO_2 will be the same as exhaled gas, which is 0.16, or 16% O_2. Adding O_2 at a flow rate of 15 L/minute with a pocket mask may increase the FIO_2 to up to 50%. A BVM on room air is 0.21, and with O_2 at 15 L/minute up to 0.9, depending on the equipment and the skill of the ventilator. An FROPV delivers close to 1, or 100% O_2.

5. Both the volume and oxygenation achieved by ventilations depend on the quality of the mask seal and patency of the airway. The single most common cause of inadequate ventilation in a nonintubated person is poor mask seal. Great

care must be taken to ensure that the airway is fully patent and that there is a good mask seal with each ventilation. If the victim is not intubated, an oropharyngeal, nasopharyngeal, or combination airway should be used if available.

6. Because an FROPV delivers the highest F_{IO_2}, is the only device that is limited to 40 L/minute flow rate (1½ to 2 seconds in duration), and has an overpressure relief valve, it may be the best choice for ventilating a person in respiratory arrest, whether or not he is intubated. A BVM unit used by two rescuers (one to maintain the mask seal and the other to squeeze the bag) is the best alternative. This method of ventilation is the first choice for ventilating a person in respiratory arrest, according to the US DOT National Standard Curricula for emergency medical technicians, first responders, and paramedics.

7. According to the previous curricula, the following is the order of preference for ventilating a person in respiratory arrest:
   a. BVM unit with two rescuers and supplemental O_2
   b. Pocket mask with supplemental O_2
   c. FROPV
   d. BVM unit with one rescuer and supplemental O_2
   e. Last choice, and not an option for the professional rescuer, is mouth-to-mouth breathing because of the risk of disease transmission

▶ **HAZARDS**

Oxygen alone or in a vacuum is not flammable. However, in the presence of flammable substances, combustion can be vigorous. It is imperative to use O_2 only in open, well-ventilated areas and not in the presence of burning materials. Care must be taken when handling O_2 equipment to avoid allowing contaminants such as petroleum products to come into contact with the regulator, particularly in or around the orifices on the cylinder or regulator through which O_2 flows. Cylinders should not be exposed to temperatures above 52° C (125° F).

12

Trauma Emergencies: Assessment and Stabilization

▶ DESIGNATE A LEADER

In a group situation, developing a team approach at the site of the accident is vital to the success of the rescue. If there are sufficient people skilled in rescue and medical treatment, begin by designating a leader. This person should direct all first-aid efforts and, when possible, delegate duties rather than perform them. The leader should evaluate the victim's injuries, party size, and terrain and develop a plan for either evacuating the victim or obtaining professional assistance.

▶ PRIMARY SURVEY

Rescuers have nine immediate priorities in managing wilderness trauma, regardless of the injury. The "three ABCs" is a helpful mantra for recalling the nine priorities (Table 12-1).

A1: Assess the Scene
1. Ensure the safety of noninjured members of the party (see Table 12-1).
2. Assess the scene for further hazards such as falling rocks, avalanche, and dangerous animals before rendering first-aid care.
3. Avoid approaching the victim from directly above if falling rock or a snowslide is possible.
4. Do not allow your sense of urgency to transform an accident into a risky and foolish rescue attempt.

A2: Airway
1. If the victim is unresponsive, immediately determine if he or she is breathing.
   a. If the victim's position prevents adequate assessment of the airway, roll the victim onto the back as a single unit, supporting the head and neck (Fig. 12-1).
   b. Place your ear and cheek close to the victim's mouth and nose to detect air movement while looking for movement of the chest and abdomen (Fig. 12-2). In cold weather, look for a vapor cloud and feel for warm air movement.
2. If no movement of air is detected, clean out the mouth with your fingers and use the chin-lift (Fig. 12-3) or jaw-thrust technique to open the airway.
   a. Perform the jaw thrust by kneeling down with your knees on either side of the victim's head, placing your hands on either side of the victim's mandible and pushing the base of the jaw up and forward (Fig. 12-4).

TABLE 12-1. Three ABCs of Emergency First Aid

ABCs	ACTION
A1	Assess the scene
A2	Airway: ensure an open airway
A3	Alert others
B1	Barriers (gloves, mask)
B2	Breathing
B3	Bleeding
C1	CPR and circulation
C2	Cervical spine
C3	Cover and protect victim from environment

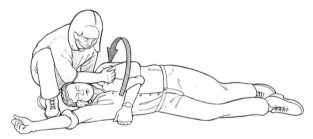

Figure 12-1. One-person roll.

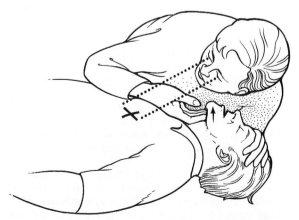

Figure 12-2. Listening for breathing and watching for movement of chest and abdomen.

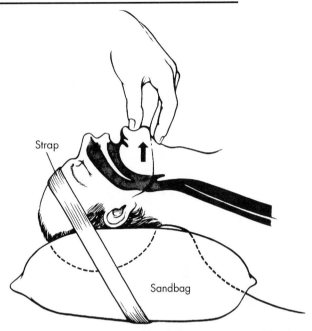

Figure 12-3. Chin lift. This procedure optimally uses two rescuers. One person stabilizes the victim's neck. The other person opens the victim's airway using the thumb to grasp the victim's chin just below the lower lip, while fingers of the same hand are placed underneath the victim's anterior mandible and the chin is gently lifted.

    b. Note that the jaw-thrust and chin-lift techniques are labor intensive and occupy your hands. If you are alone and the situation is critical, you can establish a temporary airway by pinning the anterior aspect of the victim's tongue to the lower lip with a safety pin (Fig. 12-5), noting that this can result in significant bleeding and is perceived by some observers as a maneuver of last resort. An alternative to puncturing the lower lip is to pass a string or shoelace through the safety pin and hold traction on the tongue by securing the other end to the victim's shirt button or jacket zipper.

3. Cricothyroidotomy (cricothyrotomy)—the establishment of an opening in the cricothyroid membrane—is indicated to relieve life-threatening upper airway obstruction when a victim cannot be ventilated effectively through the mouth or nose and endotracheal intubation is not feasible.

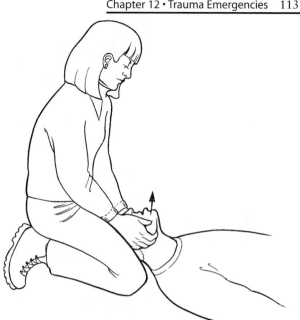

Figure 12-4. Jaw thrust.

a. Locate the cricothyroid membrane by palpating the victim's neck, starting at the top. The first and largest prominence felt will be the thyroid cartilage ("Adam's apple"), whereas the second (below the thyroid cartilage) is the cricoid cartilage. The small space between these two, noted by a small depression, is the cricothyroid membrane (Fig. 12-6A).
b. With the victim lying on his or her back, cleanse the neck around the cricothyroid membrane with an antiseptic.
c. Put on protective gloves. Make a vertical 1-inch incision through the skin with a knife over the membrane (go a little bit above and below the membrane) while using the fingers of your other hand to pry the skin edges apart. Anticipate bleeding from the wound (see Fig. 12-6B and C).
d. After the skin is incised, puncture the membrane by stabbing it with your knife or other pointed object.
e. Stabilize the larynx between the fingers of one hand, and insert an improvised cricothyrotomy tube (Box 12-1) through the membrane with your other hand while aiming

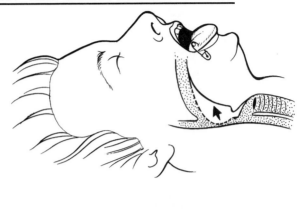

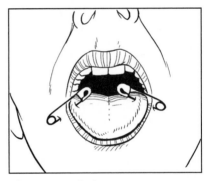

Figure 12-5. Safety-pinning the tongue to open the airway.

caudally (toward the buttocks). Secure the object in place with tape (see Fig. 12-7A and B). You can also insert the improvised tube through the tape before placing it through the cricothyroid membrane.

Complications associated with this procedure include hemorrhage at the insertion site, subcutaneous or mediastinal emphysema caused by faulty placement of the tube into the subcutaneous tissues rather than into the trachea, and perforation through the posterior wall of the trachea with placement of the tube in the esophagus.

A3: Alert Others

Before becoming more involved with the resuscitation, take a moment to alert others about the accident and call or send someone for help.

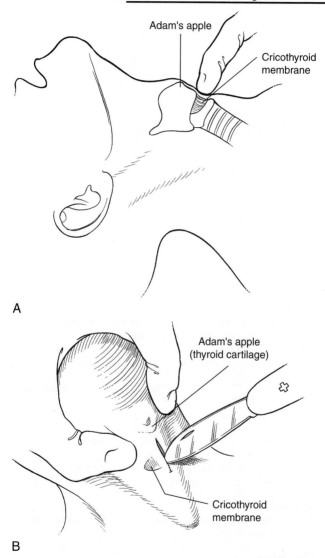

Figure 12-6. Cricothyroidotomy (cricothyrotomy). **A,** Locate the cricothyroid membrane in the depression between the Adam's apple (thyroid cartilage) and the cricoid cartilage. **B,** Make a vertical 1-cm incision through the skin.

Continued

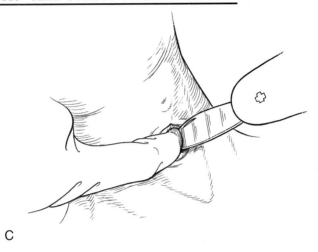

C

Figure 12-6, cont'd. **C,** Locate the cricothyroid membrane with a gloved finger and puncture it with the tip of a knife or other pointed object.

B1: Barriers

1. Protect your hands with surgical gloves. Carry nonlatex gloves to avoid latex allergy in the field.
   a. Surgical gloves can leak, so wash hands or wipe them with an antimicrobial-impregnated towelette after removing the gloves.
   b. Warning: From 5% to 7% of the population and more than 10% of all medical personnel are allergic to latex. Latex allergy can produce rash, severe anaphylactic reaction, or even death. If you suspect that you might have an allergy to latex, use powder-free nonlatex gloves.
2. Use an effective barrier device when performing mouth-to-mouth rescue breathing (see Chapter 25, Fig. 25-1).

B2: Breathing

If the victim is not breathing, initiate ventilation with mouth-to-mouth rescue breathing.

B3: Bleeding

External Bleeding:

1. Carefully check the victim for signs of profuse bleeding. Be sure to feel inside any bulky clothing and check underneath the victim for signs of bleeding.
2. Control bleeding with direct pressure.

Box 12-1. Improvised Cricothyrotomy Tubes

1. Syringe barrel: Cut the barrel of a 1- or 3-mL syringe with the plunger removed at a 45-degree angle at its midpoint. The proximal phalange of the syringe barrel helps secure the device to the neck and prevents it from being aspirated (Fig. 12–7).

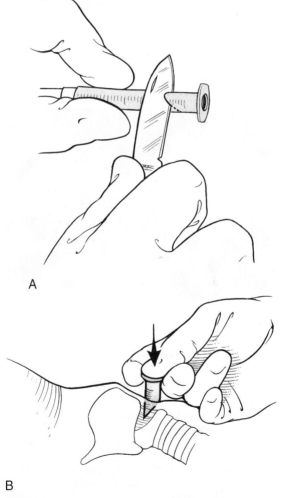

A

B

Figure 12-7. A and **B,** Cut the barrel of a syringe at a 45-degree angle and insert the pointed end through the membrane.

Box continued on following page

Box 12-1. Improvised Cricothyrotomy Tubes—*cont'd*

2. IV Administration Set Drip Chamber: Cut the plastic drip chamber of a macrodrip (15 drops/mL) IV administration set at its halfway point with a knife or scissors. Remove the end protector from the piercing spike and insert the spike into the cricothyroid membrane. The plastic drip chamber is nearly the same size as a 15-mm endotracheal tube adapter and fits snugly in the valve fitting of a bag-valve device (Fig. 12–8).

3. Any small hollow object: Examples include a small flashlight or penlight casing, pen casing, small pill bottle, and large bore needle or IV catheter. Several commercial devices are available that are small and sufficiently lightweight to be included in the first-aid kit.

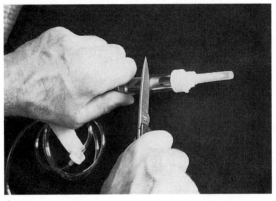

A

Figure 12-8. A, Cut plastic drip chamber at halfway point.

Continued

3. Apply a tourniquet only as a last resort when bleeding cannot be stopped by direct pressure (Box 12-2).

   a. A tourniquet is any band applied around an extremity so tightly that all blood flow distal to the site is stopped.

   b. If the tourniquet is left on for more than 3 hours, tissue distal to the tourniquet may die and the extremity may require amputation.

   c. If you can control the situation, the tourniquet may be loosened every 30 minutes to see if pressure alone will control the bleeding.

Box 12-1. Improvised Cricothyrotomy Tubes—*cont'd*

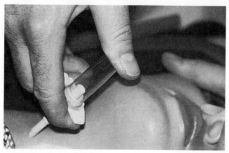

B

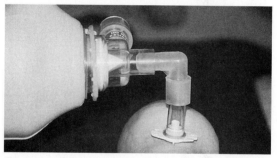

C

Figure 12-8, cont'd. **B,** Insert spike from drip chamber into the cricothyroid membrane. **C,** Bag-valve device will fit over chamber for ventilation.

Internal Bleeding
1. Avoid unnecessary movement of the victim.
2. Splint all fractured extremities.
3. Apply traction to a femur fracture (see Chapter 18).
4. Apply a circumferential compression pelvic sling to a pelvic fracture (Box 12-3).
   a. Unstable pelvic fractures are associated with significant blood loss.
   b. Pelvic reduction and stabilization in the early post-traumatic phase will mitigate venous hemorrhage.
   c. Clothes, sheets, a sleeping bag, pads, air mattress, tent, or tent fly can be used to improvise an effective pelvic sling in the backcountry. The object should be wide enough so that it does not cut into the victim when tightened.

Box 12-2. How to Apply a Tourniquet

1. Tourniquet material should be wide and flat to prevent crushing tissue. Use a firm bandage, belt, or strap 7.5 to 10 cm (3 to 4 inches) wide that will not stretch. Never use wire, rope, or any material that will cut the skin.
2. Wrap the bandage snugly around the extremity several times as close above the wound as possible and tie an overhand knot.
3. Place a stick or similar object on the knot, and tie another overhand knot over the stick (Fig. 12–9A).
4. Twist the stick until the bandage becomes tight enough to stop the bleeding. Tie or tape the stick in place to prevent it from unraveling (see Fig. 12–9B).

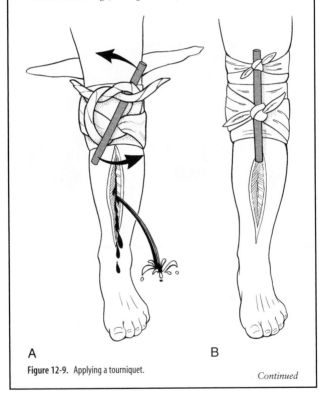

A   B

Figure 12-9. Applying a tourniquet.

Continued

Box 12-2. How to Apply a Tourniquet—*cont'd*

5. Mark the victim with a "TK" where it cannot be missed, and note the time the tourniquet was applied.
6. If you are more than an hour from medical care, loosen the tourniquet very slowly at the end of 45 minutes, while maintaining direct pressure on the wound. If bleeding is again heavy, retighten the tourniquet. If bleeding is now manageable with direct pressure alone, leave the tourniquet in place but do not tighten it again unless severe bleeding starts.

C1: Cardiopulmonary Resuscitation (CPR) and Circulation (see also Chapter 25)

1. If a trauma victim is pulseless and apneic, CPR is not likely to be successful unless the victim has a tension pneumothorax that can be relieved. A short period of CPR (10 to 15 minutes, unless the victim is hypothermic) is recommended.
2. If a pulse is present, vital information can be extrapolated from determining where it can be felt.

Box 12-3. Applying an Improvised Pelvic Sling

1. Ensure that objects have been removed from the patient's pockets and that any belt has been removed so that pressure of the sheet or object doesn't cause discomfort by pressing items against the pelvis.
2. Gently slide the improvised material under the victim's buttocks and center it under the bony prominences of the hips (greater trochanters) (Fig 12-10A).
3. Cross the object over the front of the pelvis and tighten the sling by pulling both ends and securing with a knot, clamp, or duct tape (see Fig 12-10B and C).
4. Another tightening technique is to wrap the sling snugly around the pelvis and tie an overhand knot. Place tent posts, a stick, or similar object on the knot and tie another overhand knot. Twist the poles or stick until the sling becomes tight.
5. If a Therm-a-Rest pad or other inflatable sleeping pad is available, fold it in half so that it approximates the size of the pelvis. Gently slide the pad under the victim's buttocks and center it under the greater trochanters and symphysis pubis. Secure the pad with duct tape, then inflate the pad as you would normally until it produces a snug fit.

Box continued on following page

Box 12-3. Applying an Improvised Pelvic Sling—*cont'd*

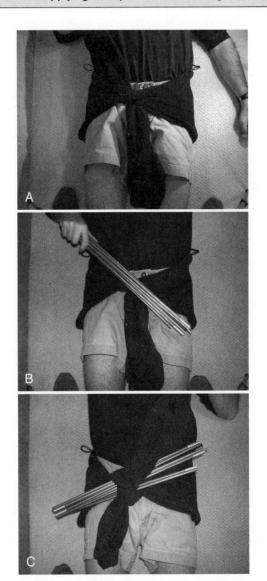

Figure 12-10. Improvised pelvic sling.

a. If a radial artery pulse is palpable, the systolic blood pressure is usually greater than 80 mm Hg.
b. If the femoral artery pulse is palpable, the blood pressure is usually above 70 mm Hg.
c. If the carotid artery pulse is palpable, the blood pressure is usually above 60 mm Hg.

C2: Cervical Spine

1. Initiate and maintain spine immobilization after trauma if some mechanism is responsible for spinal injury and the following:
   - The victim is unconscious.
   - The victim complains of midline neck or back pain.
   - The cervical spine is tender to palpation.
   - Paresthesias or altered sensation exists in the extremities.
   - Paralysis or weakness occurs in an extremity not caused by direct trauma.
   - The victim has an altered level of consciousness or is under the influence of drugs or alcohol.
   - The victim has another painful injury such as a femoral or pelvic fracture, a dislocated shoulder, or broken ribs that may distract the person from appreciating the pain in the spine.
2. If a cervical spine injury is suspected, immobilize the victim's head and neck and prevent any movement of the torso. (See Box 12-4 for immobilization aids.)
3. Avoid moving the victim with a suspected spinal injury if he or she is in a safe location. The victim will need professional evacuation.

C3: Cover and Protect the Victim from the Environment

1. If it is cold, place insulating garments or blankets underneath and on top of the victim. Remove and replace any wet clothing.
2. If it is hot, loosen the victim's clothing and create shade.
3. If the victim is in a dangerous area, move to a safer location while maintaining spine immobilization if indicated.

▶ SECONDARY SURVEY

After the primary survey is complete, perform a comprehensive secondary survey. Begin with a physical examination of the head and move in a systematic fashion through a more detailed physical examination of the face, neck, chest, abdomen, pelvis, extremities, and skin.

Box 12-4. Immobilization Aids

CERVICAL COLLAR

The cervical collar is always viewed as an adjunct to full spinal immobilization and is never used alone.

Properly applied and fitted, the cervical collar is primarily a defense against axial spine loading, particularly in an evacuation that involves tilting the victim's body uphill or downhill.

After the collar is placed around the neck, secure plastic bags, stuffed sacks, socks filled with sand or dirt, or rolled-up towels and clothing on either side of the head and neck to prevent any lateral movement.

SAM SPLINT CERVICAL COLLAR (FIG. 12–11)

Create a bend in the SAM splint approximately 15 cm (6 inches) from the end of the splint. This bend will form the anterior post. Next, create flares for the mandible. Apply the anterior post underneath the chin and bring the remainder of the splint around the neck. Take up circumferential slack by creating lateral posts. Finally, squeeze the back to create a posterior post and secure with tape.

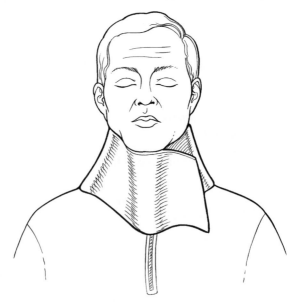

Figure 12-11. SAM splint cervical collar.

Continued

Box 12-4. Immobilization Aids—*cont'd*

CLOSED CELL FOAM SYSTEM

Fold the pad longitudinally into thirds, and center it over the back of the victim's neck. Wrap the pad around the neck and under the chin. If the pad is not long enough, tape or tie on extensions (Fig. 12-12).

Blankets, beach towels, or a rolled plastic tarp can be used in a similar manner. Avoid small, flexible cervical collars that do not optimally extend the chin-to-chest distance.

PADDED HIP BELT

Remove the padded hip belt from a large internal- or external-frame backpack, and modify it to function as a cervical collar. Diminish the width by overlapping the belt and securing the excess material with duct tape.

CLOTHING

Use bulky clothing as a collar.

Prewrap a wide, elastic ("Ace-type") bandage around a jacket to help compress the material and make it more rigid and supportive.

SPINE BOARDS

INTERNAL-FRAME PACK/SNOW SHOVEL SYSTEM

Modify an internal-frame backpack by inserting a snow shovel through the center-line attachment points (the shovel's handgrip may need to be removed first).

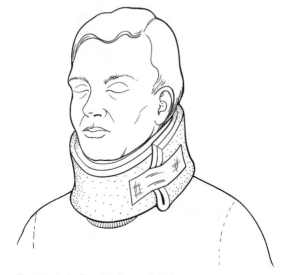

Figure 12-12. Ensolite pad used as a cervical collar.

Box continued on following page

Box 12-4. Immobilization Aids—*cont'd*

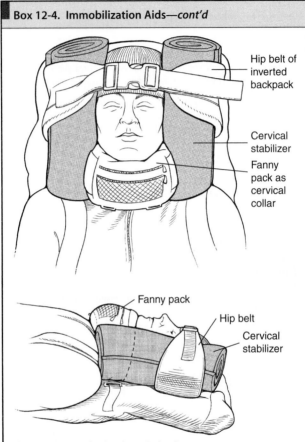

Figure 12-13. Inverted pack used as a spine board.

Tape the victim's head to the lightly padded shovel, which serves as a head bed.

Use the remainder of the pack suspension system to secure the shoulders and torso as if the victim were wearing the pack.

INVERTED PACK SYSTEM
Make an efficient short board using an inverted internal- or external-frame backpack.

Use the padded hip belt as a head bed and the frame as a short board in conjunction with a cervical collar (Fig. 12-13).

SNOWSHOE SYSTEM
Make a snowshoe into a fairly reliable short board.
Be sure to pad the snowshoe first.

Head and Face Evaluation

1. Perform the Glasgow Coma Scale evaluation and repeat as needed (see Appendix B).
2. Perform a more detailed search for focal neurologic signs.
   a. Sensory defects follow the general dermatome patterns shown in Figure 12-14.
   b. Changes in reflexes not accompanied by altered mental status do not mandate evacuation unless the victim also has a spinal cord injury.
3. Palpate the scalp thoroughly, seeking tenderness, depressions, and lacerations.
   a. Immediately evacuate any victim with suspected depressed skull fracture or basilar skull fracture accompanied by penetrating scalp trauma.
   b. Administer a broad-spectrum antibiotic (cefuroxime, adult dose 1.5 g IM).
   c. Do not remove any impaling foreign bodies piercing the head or neck. Pad these to prevent motion.

Evaluation of the Body

1. Undress the victim sufficiently to perform a proper head-to-toe examination. Keep in mind the weather conditions and appropriate concern for the victim's modesty. Check around the victim's neck or wrist for a medical information bracelet or tag and in the victim's wallet or pack for a medical identification card.
2. Remember to ask the victim to move any injured body part before you move it. If the victim resists because of pain or weakness, you should suspect a fracture or spinal cord injury. Never force the victim to move.
3. Examine the victim's skin for sweating, color, and locating injuries such as bruises, rashes, burns, bites, or lacerations. Check inside the victim's lower eyelids for pale color, which can indicate anemia or internal hemorrhage. Note abnormal skin temperature.
4. Examine the chest, watching the victim breathe to see if the chest expands completely and equally on both sides. Examine the chest wall for tenderness and deformities or foreign objects. Auscultate for breath sounds.
5. Gently press all areas of the back and abdomen to find areas of tenderness. Examine the buttocks and genitals.
6. Examine the victim's bony structure. Gently press on the chest, pelvis, arms, and legs to reveal areas of tenderness. Run your fingers down the length of the clavicles and press where they join the sternum. Evaluate the integrity of each rib, and observe for areas of deformation or discoloration.
7. Measure the victim's temperature.
8. Record all findings of your examination.

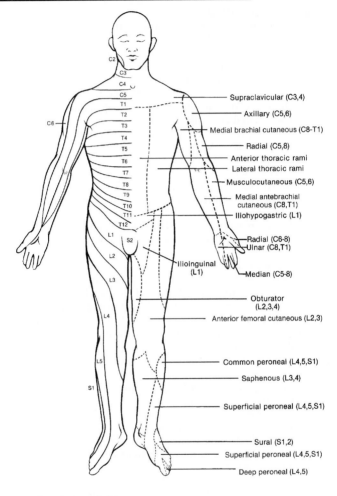

Dermatomes—anterior

Figure 12-14. Dermatome pattern of skin area stimulated by spinal cord elements. Sensory deficits follow general dermatome patterns.

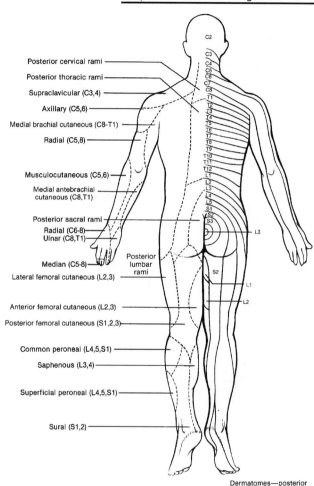

Dermatomes—posterior

Figure 12-14, cont'd.

Shock

13

▶ **DEFINITION**

Shock is a life-threatening condition in which blood flow to body tissues is inadequate and cells are deprived of oxygen. Any serious injury or illness can produce shock. Examples are severe bleeding (either external or internal), femur or pelvis fracture, major burn, dehydration, heart failure from a heart attack, severe allergic reactions, or spinal cord injury with paralysis.

Although shock is often categorized into different types, the signs and symptoms are almost always the same, regardless of the cause. Shock is an emergency that is difficult to treat effectively in the field.

▶ **DISORDERS**

Box 13-1 outlines the types of shock.

Signs and Symptoms
1. Pale, cool, and diaphoretic skin
2. Decreased pulse pressure when blood loss reaches 15% of total blood volume
3. Tachycardia, tachypnea, anxiety, delayed capillary refill, and decreased urine output when blood loss is 15% to 30% of total blood volume (in neurogenic shock, pulse may remain slow)

Hypotension, marked tachycardia, and significant changes in mental status related to blood volume loss greater than 40% of total blood volume; confusion, restlessness, and combativeness possible

Treatment
The rescuer can do little in the field. The important thing is to recognize shock so that transportation to a medical facility is not delayed.
1. Keep the victim lying down on his or her back. If the victim experiences shortness of breath because of heart problems, raise the shoulders or, if tolerated, allow the sitting position.
2. Elevate the legs only if the victim has vasogenic shock or external bleeding that is under control and there is no suspicion of a spinal fracture that might be worsened by leg elevation.
   a. You can elevate the legs by simply allowing the victim to recline with the feet uphill.

Box 13-1. Types of Shock

Hypovolemic Shock
1. External bleeding
2. Internal bleeding
   a. Bleeding from a ruptured or lacerated organ (painful and tender abdomen may be present)
   b. Bleeding from a fractured pelvis or femur
3. Profound dehydration

Cardiogenic Shock
1. Victim may have chest pain or dyspnea
2. Victim may have distended neck veins or swollen ankles

Vasogenic Shock
1. Victim may have bradycardia or "normal" pulse
2. Sometimes called "psychogenic shock"

Neurogenic Shock
1. Caused by a spinal cord injury above the level of the sixth thoracic vertebra (T6)
2. Victim will manifest bradycardia, rather than tachycardia, despite concomitant hypotension
3. Victim is paralyzed
4. Skin may be warm and flushed instead of pale and cool
5. Male victim may have priapism

Septic Shock
1. Fever may be present.
2. The skin may be warm and flushed.
3. Evidence of an infected wound, abdominal pain, pain and frequency of urination, or signs and symptoms of an upper respiratory infection may exist.

Anaphylactic Shock
See Chapter 26.

---

   b. If the victim has internal bleeding, avoid any unnecessary movement.
   c. With cardiogenic shock, the victim may be more comfortable with the head and shoulders raised slightly.
3. Do not elevate the victim's legs if there is a severe head injury, difficulty breathing, a broken leg, neck or back injury, or uncontrolled bleeding, or if doing so causes pain.
4. Keep the victim covered and warm. Particularly try to keep the victim's head, neck, and hands covered. Take the victim out of harsh weather conditions and insulate from

the ground. If you cannot locate sufficient covering for warmth, lie next to the victim and share body heat.

5. Control remediable causes of bleeding.

6. Loosen restrictive clothing.

7. Splint all fractures. If the femur is fractured, apply and maintain traction (see Chapter 18). Apply a pelvic binder for suspected pelvic fractures (see Chapter 12).

8. Administer intravenous (IV) fluid resuscitation.

    a. This is indicated only for a victim with vasogenic shock, one who is dehydrated, or one in whom hypovolemic shock is caused by bleeding from a wound that has been controlled.

    b. Insert an 18-gauge IV line and administer 3000 mL normal saline or lactated Ringer's solution for adults. For children administer 20 mL/kg intravenously initially, over 20 to 30 minutes; amounts approaching 40 to 60 mL/kg IV may be required during the first few hours.

    c. If transport to a medical center will take longer than 6 hours and the victim suffers shock from external bleeding or vasogenic etiology but is alert, oriented, and not vomiting, administer small, frequent sips of fluid. If this causes vomiting, discontinue the attempt at oral rehydration.

9. Do not administer oral fluids to a victim with suspected intraabdominal or thoracic hemorrhage.

10. Administer high-flow oxygen (10 L/minute by facemask) if available.

11. For septic shock, early use of empiric antibiotics that cover the infecting organism is a critical and proven medical treatment. To provide the necessary coverage, start broad-spectrum and/or multiple antibiotics. Combination therapy in adults uses one of the following: a third-generation cephalosporin (ceftriaxone, 1 g intravenously over 3 to 5 minutes) plus anaerobic coverage (clindamycin, 600 to 900 mg intravenously, or metronidazole, 15 mg/kg intravenously over 1 hour) or a fluoroquinolone (ciprofloxacin 400 mg intravenously) plus clindamycin. All initial antibiotics in septic shock should be administered intravenously.

12. For massive soft tissue damage or open fracture, administer a cephalosporin (e.g., cefazolin, 1 g) intravenously over 3 to 5 minutes.

13. In a diabetic person, consider a hypoglycemic reaction (see Chapter 29). If the victim is conscious and can swallow adequately, administer Glutose paste or a sugar-sweetened liquid in small sips. Otherwise, do not give the

victim anything to eat or drink unless he or she is alert and hungry or thirsty.

14. If the victim appears to be suffering from an allergic reaction to a bite or sting (see Chapters 26 and 37), address the cause of that reaction.

15. Because the shock victim cannot be effectively treated in the field, transport him or her to a medical facility as quickly as possible.

Head Injury

14

Head injury assessment begins with the primary survey, in which life-threatening conditions such as airway compromise or severe bleeding are recognized and simultaneous management is begun. For the purposes of wilderness assessment and management, head injuries can be subdivided into three groups: (1) prolonged unconsciousness (more than 5 to 10 minutes), (2) brief loss of consciousness, and (3) no loss of consciousness.

▶ GENERAL TREATMENT

1. Because potential problems include airway compromise from obstruction caused by the tongue, vomit, blood, or broken teeth, make a quick inspection of the victim's mouth as part of the primary survey.
2. Logroll the victim to clear the mouth without jeopardizing the spine (Fig. 14-1). Be aware that the most common associated serious injury is a broken neck or other spinal injury.

▶ DISORDERS

Skull Fracture

Fracture of the skull is not in itself life threatening, unless associated with underlying brain injury or severe bleeding.

Signs and Symptoms
1. Severe headache
2. Deformity, step-off, or crepitus on palpation of the scalp
3. Blood or clear fluid draining from the ears or nose without direct trauma to those areas
4. Ecchymosis around the eyes (raccoon eyes) or behind the ears (Battle's sign)
5. In victim with a skull fracture, possible development of seizures, unequal or nonreactive pupils, weakness, or altered level of consciousness from an underlying brain injury (Box 14-1)

Treatment
1. Evacuate the victim to a medical facility as soon as possible.
2. Keep the victim with the head slightly uphill or elevated to reduce cerebral edema.
3. In any person with a serious head injury, immobilize the cervical spine in anticipation of an injury to this area.

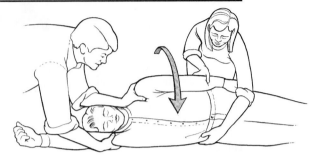

Figure 14-1. Logrolling victim to clear mouth without jeopardizing the spine

Prolonged Unconsciousness

Signs and Symptoms
Loss of consciousness for more than 5 to 10 minutes is a serious warning of significant brain injury.

Treatment
1. Immediate evacuation to a medical center is mandatory.
2. During transport, maintain cervical spine precautions and keep the victim's head uphill on sloping terrain.
3. Be prepared to logroll the victim if the victim vomits.
4. Continually monitor the airway for signs of obstruction and decreasing respiratory rate.
5. Administer high-flow oxygen, if available, at 10 L/minute or by a non-rebreather mask.

Brief Loss of Consciousness

Signs and Symptoms
1. Short-term unconsciousness, in which the victim wakes up after 1 or 2 minutes and gradually regains normal mental status and physical abilities, indicating at least a concussion
2. Confusion or amnesia for the event and repetitive questioning by the victim
3. Headache or nausea

Treatment
1. Be aware that the safest strategy is to evacuate the victim to a medical center for evaluation and observation.
2. Interrupt the victim's normal sleep every 2 to 3 hours briefly to see that the condition has not deteriorated and he or she can be easily aroused.

3. For a victim who is increasingly lethargic, confused, or combative or does not behave normally, immediately evacuate the victim to a medical center.

   a. If the victim develops any signs of brain injury (see Box 14-1), increasing intracranial pressure may have developed. Evacuate the victim immediately.

   b. If the victim has a seizure after a brain injury, even briefly, transport the victim to a medical facility immediately.

No Loss of Consciousness

Signs and Symptoms
Head injury without any loss of consciousness is rarely indicative of a serious injury to the brain.

Treatment
1. Inspect the scalp for evidence of cuts, which generally bleed copiously, and apply pressure as needed.
2. If the victim appears normal (can answer questions appropriately including name, location, and date; walks normally; appears to have coordinated movement; and has normal muscle strength), no immediate evacuation is required.
3. If the victim develops any signs or symptoms of brain injury (see Box 14-1), evacuate the victim immediately.
4. For a child who has had a head injury, then begins to vomit, refuses to eat, becomes drowsy, appears apathetic, or in any other way seems abnormal, evacuate him or her to a medical facility as soon as possible.

▶ GLASGOW COMA SCALE (GCS)

The GCS is the most widely used method of defining a patient's level of consciousness, and it obviates use of ambiguous terminology such as lethargic, stuporous, and obtunded. The

---

Box 14-1. Brain Injury Checklist

- Increasing headache
- Changing level of consciousness
- Persistent or projectile vomiting
- Bleeding from ears or nose (without direct injury to those areas), cerebrospinal fluid rhinorrhea
- Raccoon eyes or Battle's sign
- Seizure

GCS is a neurologic scale that aims to give a reliable, objective way of recording the conscious state of a person, for initial and continuing assessment. A patient is assessed against the criteria of the scale, and the resulting points give the GCS (see below and Appendix B). The patient's best motor, verbal, and eye-opening responses determine the GCS. A patient who is able to follow commands, is fully oriented, and has spontaneous eye opening scores a GCS of 15; a patient with no motor response, eye opening, or verbal response to pain scores a GCS of 3. Patients with a GCS of 8 or less are considered being in "coma." Head injury severity is generally categorized into three levels on the basis of the GCS after initial resuscitation: mild: GCS 13-15, moderate: GCS 9-12, severe: GCS 3-8. Any victim with a GCS score less than 15 who has sustained a head injury should be evacuated as soon as possible. A declining GCS score suggests increasing intracranial pressure.

Elements of the Glasgow Coma Scale

Best eye response (E)
    Four grades exist:
4—Eye(s) opening spontaneously
3—Eye opening to speech (not to be confused with awaking of a sleeping person; such patients receive a score of 4, not 3)
2—Eye opening in response to pain (patient responds to pressure on the patient's fingernail bed; if this does not elicit a response, supraorbital and sternal pressure or rub may be used)
1—No eye opening
Best verbal response (V)
    Five grades exist:
5—Oriented (patient responds coherently and appropriately to questions such as the patient's name and age, where he or she is and why, the year, month, etc.)
4—Confused (patient responds to questions coherently but there is some disorientation and confusion)
3—Inappropriate words (random or exclamatory articulated speech, but no conversational exchange)
2—Incomprehensible sounds (moaning but no words)
1—None
Best motor response (M)
    Six grades exist:
6—Obeys commands (patient does simple things as asked)
5—Localizes to pain (purposeful movements toward changing painful stimuli; e.g., hand crosses midline and gets above clavicle when supraorbital pressure applied)
4—Withdraws from pain (pulls part of body away when pinched; normal flexion)

3—Flexion in response to pain (decorticate response)

2—Extension to pain (decerebrate response: adduction, internal rotation of shoulder, pronation of forearm)

1—No motor response

The GCS has limited applicability to children, especially younger than the age of 36 months (because the verbal performance of even a healthy child would be expected to be poor).

Epidural Hematoma

Signs and Symptoms

1. Victim who wakes up and appears completely normal, then becomes drowsy or disoriented or lapses back into unconsciousness (usually within 30 to 60 minutes)

2. Unconscious victim with one pupil significantly larger than the other

Treatment

Because these are indications of bleeding from an artery inside the skull, causing an expanding blood clot (epidural hematoma) that is compressing the brain, evacuate the victim immediately and rush to a medical facility.

Scalp Wounds

Scalp lacerations are common after head injuries and tend to bleed vigorously because of their rich blood supply.

Treatment

1. Apply direct pressure to the wound with your gloved hand. It might be necessary to hold pressure for up to 30 minutes.

2. If you are faced with a bleeding scalp laceration and the victim has a healthy head of hair, tie the wound closed using the victim's own hair (see Chapter 20). This should not be expected to control the bleeding but will approximate the edges of the wound.

Scalp Bandaging

Wounds to the scalp often require a dressing placed over hair, making adhesion very difficult. The dressing can be secured with a triangular bandage in a method that allows for considerable tension should pressure be necessary to stop bleeding (see Fig. 20-6).

Head Injury and Scuba Diving

Any significant head injury that increases the risk of late seizures is a contraindication for scuba (self-contained underwater breathing apparatus) diving. Such injuries include a significant brain contusion, subdural hematoma, skull fracture, or loss of consciousness or amnesia for greater than 24 hours. In case of minor head injury that does not have any associated symptoms and that does not require anticonvulsant medication, scuba diving can be considered after 6 weeks.

Chest Trauma

15

In the wilderness environment, blunt thoracic injuries usually result from falls or direct blows to the chest. Penetrating injuries result from gun, knife, or arrow wounds; impalement after a fall; or a rib fracture. Immediate, life-threatening thoracic injuries include flail chest, pneumothorax/hemothorax, tension pneumothorax, open ("sucking") chest wound, and pericardial tamponade.

▶ DISORDERS

Rib Fracture

Signs and Symptoms
1. Pain in the chest after blunt chest trauma
2. Pain that worsens with inspiration
3. Point tenderness over the fractured rib(s)
4. Crepitus and displacement, occasionally detected on palpation
5. Fractured ribs usually occur along the side of the chest. Pushing on the sternum while the victim lies supine will produce pain at the fracture site, instead of where you are pushing.

Treatment
1. Care for any open chest wounds.
   a. Cover the wound quickly, especially if there is air bubbling, to avoid "sucking" chest wound (see "Open ['Sucking'] Chest Wound" later).
   b. Use a petrolatum-impregnated gauze, heavy cloth, or adhesive tape for the dressing.
2. Treat an isolated rib fracture.
   a. Administer an oral analgesic, and instruct the victim to rest.
   b. Note that thoracic taping and splinting are not necessary or helpful.
   c. Encourage the victim to cough or deep-breathe at least once per hour.
3. Treat multiple rib fractures.
   a. Be aware that these are significant because of the potential for serious underlying injuries.
   b. Cushion the victim in a position of comfort and frequently reevaluate the victim's ability to breathe.
   c. Do not tape or tightly wrap the ribs because this might prevent complete reexpansion of the lung with inspiration,

leading the victim to take only shallow, inadequate breaths and possibly leading to pneumonia. Encourage the victim to take at least one deep breath or give one good cough every hour.

d. Evacuate the victim as soon as possible. If the chest injury is on one side, transport the victim with the injured side down to facilitate lung expansion and oxygenation of the blood within the uninjured side.

Flail Chest

Signs and Symptoms
1. A portion of the chest wall that is mechanically unstable, indicating that a series of three or more ribs is fractured in both the anterior and posterior planes
2. Unstable segment that paradoxically moves inward during inspiration, thereby inhibiting ventilation

Treatment
1. Immediately evacuate the victim. A small or moderate flail segment can be tolerated for 24 to 48 hours, after which it may need to be managed with mechanical ventilation.
2. Administer an intercostal nerve block to assist in short-term management of pain and pulmonary toilet.
3. Place a bulky pad of dressings, rolled-up extra clothing, or a small pillow gently over the site, or have the victim splint the arm against the injury to stabilize the flail segment and relieve some of the pain.
    a. Use soft and lightweight materials.
    b. Use large strips of tape to hold the pad in place.
    c. Do not tape entirely around the chest because this will restrict breathing efforts.
    d. Do not allow the object to restrict breathing in any manner.
4. If the victim is unable to walk, transport him or her lying on the back or injured side.
5. If the victim is severely short of breath, assist with mouth-to-mouth rescue breathing. Time your breaths with those of the victim, and breathe gently to provide added air during the victim's inspirations.

Pneumothorax/Hemothorax

Signs and Symptoms
1. Pain that may be worse with inspiration
2. Tachypnea
3. Unilateral decreased or absent breath sounds

4. Resonance on percussion with a pneumothorax; flat or dull on percussion with a hemothorax
5. Tactile fremitus

Treatment
1. Evacuate the victim immediately.
2. Monitor closely for the development of a tension pneumothorax.

Tension Pneumothorax

Signs and Symptoms
1. Distended neck veins (may not be present if victim is hypovolemic)
2. Tracheal deviation away from the side of the pneumothorax
3. Unilateral, absent or grossly diminished breath sounds
4. Hyperresonant hemithorax to percussion
5. Subcutaneous emphysema
6. Respiratory distress, cyanosis, cardiovascular collapse

Treatment
Use rapid pleural decompression if the victim appears to be decompensating (Box 15-1; Fig. 15-1). Possible complications include infection and profound bleeding from puncture of the heart, lung, major blood vessel, liver, or spleen.

Open ("Sucking") Chest Wound

Signs and Symptoms
A chest wound in which air is sucked into the pleura on inspiration is usually caused by penetrating injury.

Treatment
1. Place a petrolatum-impregnated gauze pad on top of the wound, cover it with a 4- × 4-inch gauze pad, and tape it on three sides (Fig. 15-2).
2. Allow the untaped fourth side to serve as a relief valve to prevent formation of a tension pneumothorax.
3. If a penetrating object remains impaled in the chest, do not remove it. Place a petrolatum gauze dressing next to the skin around the object, and stabilize it with layers of bulky dressings or pads.
4. A victim with an open chest wound below the nipple line may also have an injury to an intraabdominal organ (see Chapter 16).

Pericardial Tamponade

Blunt or penetrating cardiac injury leading to pericardial tamponade is uncommon but life threatening. A small amount of intrapericardial blood can severely restrict diastolic function.

Box 15-1. How to Perform Pleural Decompression

1. Swab the entire chest with povidone-iodine or other anti-septic.
2. If sterile surgical gloves are available, put them on after washing hands.
3. If local anesthesia is available, infiltrate the puncture site down to the rib and over its upper border.
4. Insert a large-bore (14-gauge) intravenous catheter, needle, or any available pointed, sharp object into the chest just above the third rib in the midclavicular line (midway between the top of the shoulder and the nipple in a line with the nipple approximates this location) (Fig. 15-1A). If you hit the rib, move the needle or knife upward slightly until it passes over the top of the rib, thus avoiding the intercostal blood vessels that course along the lower edge of every rib (see Fig. 15-1B). The chest wall is 3.75 to 6.25 cm

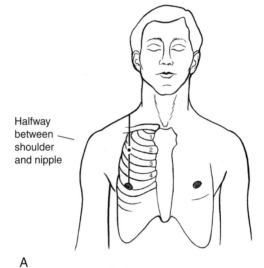

Halfway between shoulder and nipple

A

Figure 15-1. Pleural decompression. **A,** Insertion point for pleural decompression.

Box 15-1. How to Perform Pleural Decompression—*cont'd*

(1½ to 2½ inches) thick, depending on the individual's muscularity and the amount of fat present. A gush of air signals that you have entered the pleural space; do not push the

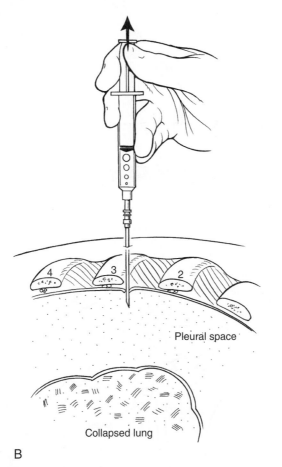

Pleural space

Collapsed lung

B

Figure 15-1. *Continued* **B,** "Walk" needle over top of rib to avoid intercostal vessels.

Box continued on following page

Box 15-1. How to Perform Pleural Decompression—*cont'd*

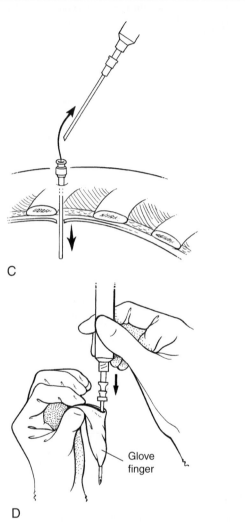

C

D

Glove
finger

Figure 15-1. *Continued* **C,** Catheter in place. **D,** Finger of glove is attached to needle or catheter to create flutter valve.

Box 15-1. How to Perform Pleural Decompression—*cont'd*

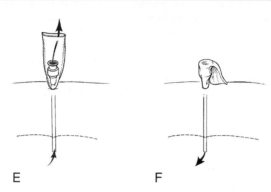

E   **F**

Figure 15-1. *Continued* **E,** Flutter valve allows air to escape. **F,** Flutter valve collapses to prevent air entry.

penetrating object in any further. Releasing the tension converts the tension pneumothorax into an open pneumothorax.
5. Leave the needle or catheter in place (see Fig. 15-1C) and place the cut-out finger portion of a surgical glove with a slit cut into the end over the external opening to create a unidirectional flutter valve that allows continuous egress of air from the pleural space (see Fig. 15-1D to F).

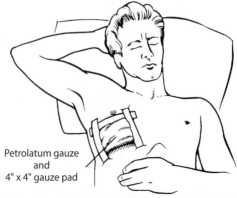

Petrolatum gauze
and
4" x 4" gauze pad

Figure 15-2. Treatment of sucking chest wound. Sealing wound with gel defibrillator pad works best because this pad adheres to wet or dry skin. Petrolatum gauze or plastic wrap also works well.

Signs and Symptoms
1. The triad of distended neck veins, hypotension, and muffled heart sounds are present in only one third of victims.
2. Pulsus paradoxus, an increase in the normal physiologic decrease in blood pressure with inspiration, may be present.

Treatment
1. The only temporizing measure pending evacuation is pericardiocentesis. This procedure should be done in the wilderness only if there is a high index of suspicion, coupled with shock and impending death unresponsive to other resuscitative efforts.
2. Advance a long ($\approx$15 cm [6 inches]), 16- to 18-gauge needle with an overlying catheter through the skin 1 to 2 cm (0.5 to 0.75 inches) below and to the left of the xiphoid. The needle is advanced at a 45-degree angle with the tip directed at the tip of the left scapula.
3. After the pericardial sac is entered, aspirate blood with a syringe until the victim's condition improves. Repeat aspiration as the victim's condition warrants.
4. Immediately evacuate the victim.

Intraabdominal Injury

16

Intraabdominal injury may be penetrating or blunt.

▶ PENETRATING INJURY

Gunshot Wound

Signs and Symptoms
1. Low caliber: small entrance and no exit wound
2. High caliber, high velocity: relatively innocuous entrance wound, large disfiguring exit wound, extensive internal injuries

Treatment
1. Immediately evacuate the victim.
2. Anticipate and treat for shock (see Chapter 13).
3. Administer a broad-spectrum antibiotic (e.g., cefoxitin, adult dose: 2 g IM or IV over 3 to 5 minutes).
4. Do not push extruded bowel back into the abdomen. Keep the exteriorized bowel moist and covered at all times (apply sterile wet dressing, and then cover with Saran wrap).
5. Keep victim NPO.

Stab Wound

Signs and Symptoms
Deep wound laceration caused by knife, piton, ski pole, tree limb, or other sharp object

Treatment
1. If the wound extends into subcutaneous tissue, consider immediate evacuation for medical assessment. Determining whether the object penetrated the peritoneum or if there is concomitant internal organ injury is difficult.
2. Control external bleeding.
3. Anticipate and treat for shock (see Chapter 13).
4. Administer a broad-spectrum antibiotic (e.g., cefoxitin, adult dose: 2 g IM or IV over 3 to 5 minutes) if the wound extends into the subcutaneous tissue.
5. Do not push extruded bowel back into the abdomen. Keep the exteriorized bowel moist and covered at all times (apply sterile wet dressing, and then cover with Saran wrap).
6. Keep victim NPO.

Blunt Injury

Signs and Symptoms
1. Signs of shock (tachypnea, tachycardia, delayed capillary refill, weak or thready pulse, cool or clammy skin)
2. Abdominal distention
3. Pain or muscle guarding elicited on palpation
4. Percussion tenderness
5. Pain referred to the left shoulder (ruptured spleen)
6. Gross hematuria
7. Pain in abdomen with movement
8. Fever

Treatment
1. Immediately evacuate the victim.
2. Anticipate and treat for shock (see Chapter 13).
3. Administer a broad-spectrum antibiotic (e.g., cefoxitin, adult dose: 2 g IM or IV over 3 to 5 minutes).
4. Keep victim NPO.

Maxillofacial Trauma

17

Maxillofacial trauma ranges from simple lacerations to massive injuries with extensive bleeding and airway obstruction. In general, the ability to treat these injuries in the wilderness situation is minimal. Among the problems that may be addressed are lacerations, mandibular fracture, midface (Le Fort) fracture, orbital floor fracture, nasal fracture, and epistaxis.

▶ GENERAL TREATMENT

1. Perform a primary survey, paying particular attention to airway compromise from aspiration of blood, avulsed teeth or dental appliance, direct trauma and swelling, or a retrusive tongue secondary to a mobile mandibular fracture (see Chapter 12, Fig. 12-5). The most important part of care for maxillofacial trauma is maintenance of a clear airway. If the airway is threatened by edema or inability of the victim to keep the airway clear, early intubation is recommended. Cricothyrotomy may be necessary (see Chapter 10).

    a. Remove any loose material (teeth, clots, soft tissue, foreign material) from the oropharynx to clear the airway if necessary.

    b. Note any deformity or asymmetry of the facial structures, which may indicate underlying bone fracture.

    c. Enophthalmos may be one sign that an orbital blowout fracture is present.

    d. Look for malocclusion or a step-off in the teeth as an indication of mandibular or maxillary fracture.

    e. Observe the position and integrity of the nasal septum. If the septum is bulging on one side into the nasal cavity, it could indicate a septal hematoma. A septal hematoma can be drained in the field by making a small incision into the septum with a safety pin or point of a knife, allowing the blood to drain out.

    f. Examine soft tissue injuries, looking for foreign bodies.

    g. Test motor and sensory function by checking for sensation on each side of the face and by having the victim wrinkle the forehead, smile, bare the teeth, and close the eyes tightly.

    h. Gently palpate the facial structures, noting areas of tenderness, bony defects, crepitus, and false motion.

    i. Test dental integrity by grasping the front and bottom anterior teeth and checking for motion.

    j. If the victim is unconscious but breathing well and shows no sign of hemorrhaging into the airway, you can use an oropharyngeal or nasopharyngeal airway to ensure airway patency.
2. Anticipate cervical spine trauma and immobilize the spine if indicated. If cervical spine injury is possible and airway protection is required, perform endotracheal intubation or cricothyrotomy while maintaining manual cervical spine immobilization.
3. Control bleeding with direct pressure.
    a. For intraoral bleeding, have the victim bite firmly on a gauze pad.
    b. For bleeding from the nose, squeeze and hold the nostrils together, use nasal packing, or deploy a Foley catheter (see "Nasal Fracture and Epistaxis" later).
4. Treat shock, if present.
5. Recover any completely avulsed tissues or organs, irrigate with normal saline solution, and transport in a soaked gauze sponge. Among the tissues that can be avulsed are teeth, ears, nose, and areas of soft tissue.

▶ DISORDERS

Lacerations
Facial laceration may be complicated by damage to associated structures that requires specialized medical care.

Signs and Symptoms
1. Lacrimal drainage system: injury confirmed if a probe inserted into the punctum at the medial canthus of the eye emerges from the laceration
2. Parotid duct: injury suspected if there is buccal nerve paralysis or leakage from the wound when Stensen's duct is irrigated with saline solution or water
3. Facial nerve: asymmetry when the victim moves the eyebrows, eyelids, and mouth

Treatment
See Chapter 20.

Mandibular Fracture

Signs and Symptoms
1. Inability to occlude the teeth in a normal manner
2. Sublingual hematoma
3. Deformity, crepitus, mandibular mobility
4. Restricted opening or deviation of the jaw when opening
5. Pain elicited by placing one hand over each angle of the jaw and pressing inward

Midface (Le Fort) Fractures

Signs and Symptoms
1. Tenderness, ecchymosis, and swelling over fracture site
2. Le Fort 1 fracture—facial edema and mobility of the hard palate and upper teeth
3. Le Fort II fracture—facial edema, telecanthus, subconjunctival hemorrhage, mobility of the maxilla at the nasofrontal suture, epistaxis, and possible cerebrospinal fluid rhinorrhea
4. Le Fort III fracture—massive edema with facial elongation and flattening. An anterior open bite may be present due to posterior and inferior displacement of the facial skeleton. Movement of the entire upper dental arch or face on grasping the alveolar process and anterior teeth between the thumb and forefinger and rocking gently back and forth, epistaxis, and cerebrospinal fluid rhinorrhea.

Treatment of Mandibular or Midface Fracture
1. Elevate the victim's head to reduce bleeding and swelling.
2. Stabilize the site with bandages.
3. Control epistaxis (see later).
4. Evacuate the victim immediately.
5. Administer antibiotic prophylaxis with phenoxymethyl penicillin (penicillin V, Penapar-VK), 500 mg (clindamycin if penicillin allergic) PO q6h.

Orbital Floor Fracture

Signs and Symptoms
1. Periorbital edema, crepitus, ecchymosis, enophthalmos, and ocular injury can be present
2. Diplopia, worsened with upward gaze
3. Lowering of the globe or decreased upward gaze on the affected side secondary to entrapment of the inferior rectus muscle
4. Decreased facial sensation

Treatment
Evacuate the victim for definitive management.

Nasal Fracture and Epistaxis

Signs and Symptoms
1. Swelling, tenderness, mobility, ecchymosis, or deformity of the nose
2. Evidence of septal hematoma (blue or purplish fluid-filled sac overlying the nasal septum)

Treatment

Treatment of epistaxis depends on whether the source is anterior or posterior.

1. If a septal hematoma is present, make a small incision through the mucosa and perichondrium to allow drainage. Pack the anterior nasal cavity (see later) to prevent reaccumulation of blood.
2. Treat anterior epistaxis.
   a. If bleeding cannot be controlled by firmly pinching the nostrils against the septum for a full 10 minutes, nasal packing may be necessary. Insert a piece of cotton or gauze soaked with a vasoconstricting agent such as oxymetazoline hydrochloride 0.5% (Afrin) or phenylephrine hydrochloride (Neo-Synephrine) into the nose and leave it in place for 5 to 10 minutes. Next, layer-pack petrolatum-impregnated gauze or strips of a nonadherent dressing into the nose so that both ends of the gauze remain outside the nasal cavity to lessen the likelihood that the victim might inadvertently aspirate the packing.
   b. To pack an adult's nasal cavity completely, at least 3 to 4 feet (about 1 m) of ¼-inch material is required to fill the nasal cavity and tamponade the bleeding site. Expandable packing material, such as Weimert Epistaxis packing or the Rhino Rocket, is available commercially. A tampon or balloon tip from a Foley catheter can also be used as improvised packing.
   c. Anterior nasal packing blocks sinus drainage and may predispose the victim to sinusitis. A prophylactic antibiotic (amoxicillin, 500 mg q6h) is recommended until the pack is removed in 48 hours.
3. Treat posterior epistaxis.
   a. Use a No. 14 to 16 French Foley catheter with a 30-mL balloon to tamponade the site. The catheter should be lubricated with either petrolatum or a water-based lubricant. Insert the catheter through the nasal cavity into the posterior pharynx. Next, inflate the balloon with 10 to 15 mL of water and gently draw it back into the posterior nasopharynx until resistance is met. Inflation should be done slowly and should be stopped if painful. Secure the catheter firmly to the victim's forehead with several strips of tape. Finally, pack the anterior nose in front of the catheter balloon with gauze as described earlier.
   b. Administer a prophylactic antibiotic (amoxicillin, 500 mg q6h, or trimethoprim-sulfamethoxazole [Septra DS] bid).
   c. Evacuate the victim.

Foreign Body in Nose

Signs and Symptoms
1. Pain, foul-smelling drainage, sometimes fever
2. Skin extremely sensitive, possibly swollen with accumulation of mucus and blood

Treatment
A foreign body can be difficult to remove because of the sensitivity of the tissues involved. Also, irritation in the nasal area causes swelling that traps the foreign object inside an accumulation of mucus and blood.
1. Attempt to visualize the object and extract it. Do not proceed if you find the object moving deeper into the nostril or the victim is in extreme pain. Leave the object in place and prepare the victim for evacuation.
2. If the victim is a child and develops a fever, administer dicloxacillin, 25 mg/kg/day in equally divided doses qid, or erythromycin, 30 to 50 mg/kg/day q8h in equal divided doses.

Orthopedic Injury, Splints, and Slings

18

FUNCTIONAL CONSIDERATIONS

▶ JOINT FUNCTION

1. Begin palpation of the long bones distally and proceed across all joints.
2. Palpable crepitus at the joint level mandates application of a splint.
3. If the victim is able to cooperate, have him or her move every joint through an active range of motion (ROM). This exercise quickly focuses the examination on the injury's location.
4. When this is not possible, undertake passive ROM of each joint, after palpating the joint for crepitus and swelling.
5. If crepitus, swelling, deformity, or resistance to motion is noted, apply a splint.
6. If a joint is dislocated, promptly reduce it after completing the neurocirculatory examination.
7. Reduction of the joint generally relieves much of the discomfort.
8. After reduction, assess stability of the joint by careful, controlled ROM evaluation.
9. Remember to perform serial neurovascular examinations (i.e., recheck status).
10. A joint with an associated fracture or interposed soft tissue is frequently unstable after reduction. In such circumstances, take great care while applying the splint to prevent recurrent dislocation.
11. Report the details of the reduction maneuver including orientation of the pull, amount of force involved, degree of victim sedation, residual instability of the joint, and prereduction and postreduction neurovascular status to the definitive care physician.

▶ CIRCULATORY FUNCTION

1. Injury to the major vessels supplying a limb can occur with penetrating or blunt trauma.
2. A fracture can produce injury to vessels by direct laceration (rarely) or by stretching, which produces intimal flaps. These flaps can immediately occlude the distal blood flow or lead to delay in occlusion. For this reason, repeated examination of circulatory function is mandatory before and during transport.

3. Assess the color and warmth of the skin of the distal extremity. Distal pallor and asymmetric regional hypothermia may identify a vascular injury.
4. Pulses palpated in the upper extremity include the brachial, radial, and ulnar. If blood loss and hypothermia make pulses difficult to assess, temperature and color of the distal extremity become keys to diagnosis.
5. Any suspected major arterial injury mandates immediate evacuation after splinting.

▶ **NERVE FUNCTION**

1. Nerve function may be impossible to assess in an unconscious or uncooperative victim.
2. Whenever possible, it is important to establish the status of nerve function to the distal extremity after the victim's condition is stabilized.
3. Periodically compare the initial findings with additional examinations during transport of the victim. Deteriorating neurologic findings guide the speed of evacuation and any ameliorating maneuvers. These decisions may greatly affect the final outcome for the victim.
4. Carefully document sensory examination of the peripheral nerves with regard to light touch and pinprick.
5. Assess muscle function by observing active function and grading the strength of each muscle group against resistance.

GENERAL TREATMENT

See Box 18-1.

▶ **EVACUATION DECISIONS**

1. Musculoskeletal injuries that warrant immediate evacuation to a definitive care center include any suspected cervical, thoracic, or lumbar spine injury.

Box 18-1 Indications for Emergent Evacuation

Suspected spine injury
Suspected pelvic injury
Open fracture
Suspected compartment syndrome
Hip or knee dislocation
Vascular compromise to an extremity
Laceration with tendon or nerve injury
Uncertainty of severity of injury

2. A victim who has a suspected pelvic injury with posterior instability, significant suspected blood loss, or injury to the sacral plexus should receive immediate emergency evacuation on a backboard.

3. All open fractures require definitive débridement and care within 18 hours to prevent the development of infection. Emergency evacuation is imperative. If evacuation time exceeds 8 hours, in addition to antibiotic administration and splinting, irrigation and débridement in the field should be attempted. Antibiotic options are listed (Box 18-2).

4. A victim with a suspected compartment syndrome must be evacuated on an emergency basis.

5. A joint dislocation involving the hip or knee warrants immediate evacuation, even if relocated, because of the associated risk of vascular injury or post-traumatic osteonecrosis of the femoral head in the case of the hip.

6. A laceration involving a tendon or nerve warrants urgent evacuation to a center where an experienced surgeon is available.

7. In all but the most remote wilderness expeditions, arrangements should be made to promptly evacuate the victim when treatment or significance of the injury is uncertain.

Box 18-2. Antibiotic Options

INTRAVENOUS
Cefazolin (Ancef) 1 g q8h and gentamicin (5 mg/kg) q24h or piperacillin with tazobactam (Zosyn) 3.375 g q6h

INTRAMUSCULAR
Ceftriaxone (Rocephin) 1 g q24h
Oral ciprofloxacin 750 mg bid and cephalexin (Keflex) 500 mg qid

WATER EXPOSURE
Ciprofloxacin 400 mg IV or 750 mg PO bid or a sulfonamide and trimethoprim combination (Bactrim DS: 800 mg sulfamethoxazole and 160 mg trimethoprim) with either cefazolin (Ancef) 1 g IV q8h or cephalexin (Keflex) 500 mg PO q6h

DIRT OR BARNYARD
Add penicillin 20 million units IV qd or 500 mg PO q6h.

IF PENICILLIN ALLERGY
Use clindamycin 900 mg IV q8h or 450 mg PO q6h in place of penicillins and cephalexin (Keflex).

ALTERNATIVES
Erythromycin 500 mg q6h or amoxicillin 500 mg PO q8h

▶ SPECIAL CONSIDERATIONS WITH OPEN FRACTURE

1. An injury that includes disruption of the skin and a broken bone is an open fracture and is at risk for bacterial contamination. Assume that any deep wound over a known fracture represents an open fracture. If soil or foreign body contamination is severe, the victim is at risk for sepsis.
2. If medical care is realistically less than 8 hours away and the bone (limb) is not severely angulated or malpositioned, treat the injury with a compression dressing, splint, transport, and administer a broad-spectrum antibiotic.
3. If the delay will be more than 8 hours before definitive medical care, irrigation of the open wound is beneficial and may help prevent serious soft tissue and bone infection.
   a. The water used for irrigation does not have to be sterile. Clean tap water, or water disinfected for drinking, can greatly diminish the bacterial count.
   b. Use a syringe from the medical kit as an irrigating tool (see Chapter 20, Fig. 20-1).
   c. Attach an 18-gauge needle (or irrigation tip) to the syringe.
   d. Irrigate the wound copiously with the pressurized stream of water. For a large wound, more than a liter of water may be necessary.
4. Once the wound has been cleaned and irrigated, cover it with a sterile compression dressing.
5. Realign any angulated or malpositioned fractures and apply the required traction. A dilute solution of 10% povidone-iodine solution can be applied as a brief rinse over the visible bone ends. It is less likely that major contamination will occur when the bone fragments slip back into the soft tissue envelope during reduction.
6. Administer a broad-spectrum antibiotic (see Box 18-2) and splint the extremity. If evacuation time exceeds 8 hours, the incidence of osteomyelitis is high.

▶ SPECIAL CONSIDERATIONS WITH AMPUTATION

1. In the wilderness environment, the amputation victim requires immediate evacuation.
2. Control hemorrhage by direct pressure. A tourniquet is usually not indicated. If a tourniquet is applied as a life-saving measure, be prepared to sacrifice the limb. Check at reasonable intervals to see if pressure alone will control bleeding.
3. Without cooling, an amputated part remains potentially viable for only 4 to 6 hours; with cooling, viability may be extended to 18 hours.

4. Cleanse the amputated part with water, wrap it in a moistened sterile gauze or towel, place it in a plastic bag, and transport it on ice or snow, if available. Do not transport it in direct contact with ice or ice water.
5. Make sure the amputated part accompanies the victim throughout the evacuation process.

▶ SPECIAL CONSIDERATIONS WITH COMPARTMENT SYNDROME

A compartment syndrome exists when locally increased tissue pressure compromises circulation and neuromuscular function. In the wilderness setting, this most frequently occurs in association with a fracture or severe contusion. The lower leg and forearm are the most common sites for this syndrome because tight fasciae encase the muscle compartments in these regions and because these areas are frequently involved with fractures or severe contusions. A compartment syndrome can also occur in the thigh, hand, foot, and gluteal regions.

Signs and Symptoms
1. Complaints by the conscious victim of severe pain that seem out of proportion to the injury
2. Extremely tight feel to the muscle compartment, with applied pressure increasing the pain
3. In the cooperative victim, decreased sensation to light touch and pinprick in the areas supplied by the nerve or nerves traversing the compartment, usually noted on the dorsum of the foot in the first web space, caused by pressure affecting the deep peroneal nerve in the anterior compartment of the leg
4. Most reliable signs: pain, tightness to palpation, and pain on passive stretch
5. Never wait for hypoesthesia, absence of a pulse, presence of pallor, or slow capillary refill to make the diagnosis. Even late in the course, there is usually a pulse and normal capillary refill (unless there is an underlying arterial injury).

Treatment
1. Expedite emergency evacuation. The victim must be definitively treated in the first 6 to 8 hours after onset of this condition to optimize return of function to the involved limb. Be sure that there are no tight bandages, dressings, or splints that can exacerbate the condition. Do not elevate the limb; try to keep it at the level of the heart. Elevation reduces mean arterial pressure in the limb, which can reduce blood flow.

2. Perform emergency fasciotomy to relieve the pressure, which, if untreated, can produce nerve and muscle cell death within 12 hours. Limited fasciotomies can be performed in the field by an experienced surgeon if evacuation will take more than 8 hours.

▶ SPECIAL CONSIDERATIONS WITH POTENTIAL BLOOD LOSS FROM FRACTURE

1. Keep in mind the potential volume of blood loss resulting from specific closed fractures:
   - Pelvis: 6 to 10 units
   - Femur: 2 to 4 units
   - Tibia: 1 to 2 units
   - Humerus: 1 to 2 units
2. Be aware that blood loss can be worsened considerably if the skin overlying the fracture is disrupted.

▶ SPLINTING

Improvisation: General Guidelines

1. When working with a complex improvised system, test your creation on an uninjured person (i.e., "work out the bugs") before you use it on the victim.
2. Remember to include improvisation construction materials including a knife, tape, parachute cord or line, safety pins, wire, and plastic cable ties in your survival kit.
3. Maintain a creative approach to obtaining improvisational materials. Much of the victim's gear can be harvested to provide necessary items. (A backpack can often be dismantled to obtain foam pads, straps, etc.)
4. Practice constructing certain items before you must do this in an actual rescue setting.

Extremity Splints

1. Splint the fracture before the victim is moved unless the victim's life is in immediate danger. In general, make sure the splint incorporates the joints above and below the fracture. If possible, fashion the splint on the uninjured extremity and then transfer it to the injured one.
2. Skis and poles or canoe and kayak paddles can be used as improvised splints. Airbags used as flotation for kayaks and canoes can be converted into pneumatic splints for arm and ankle injuries. The Minicell or Ethafoam pillars found in most kayaks can be removed and carved into pieces to provide upper and lower extremity splints. A life jacket can be molded into a cylinder splint for knee immobilization or into a pillow splint for the ankle. The flexible

aluminum stays found in internal-frame backpacks can be molded into an upper extremity splint. Other improvised splinting materials include sticks or tree limbs; rolled-up magazines, books or newspapers; ice axes; tent poles; and dirt-filled garbage bags or fanny packs.

3. Ideally, a splint should immobilize the fractured bone in a functional position. In general, functional position means that the leg should be straight or slightly bent at the knee, the ankle and elbow bent at 90 degrees, the wrist straight, and the fingers flexed in a curve as if one were attempting to hold a can of soda or a baseball. The "soda can" position is appropriate for initial management and transport; however, for long-term splinting, apply a hand splint with the metacarpophalangeal joints flexed at 90 degrees and the interphalangeal joints extended (the "intrinsic positive" position). This position places the collateral ligaments at maximum length and helps prevent joint contracture.

4. Secure the splint in place with strips of clothing, belts, duct tape, pieces of rope or webbing, pack straps, elasticized roller wraps, or gauze bandages.

Ensolite (Closed-Cell Foam) Pads

The era of Therm-a-Rest types of inflatable pads has rendered closed-cell foam pads increasingly scarce; however, closed-cell foam remains the ultimate padding for almost any improvised splint or rescue device. Even die-hard Therm-a-Rest fans should carry a small amount of closed-cell foam, which doubles as a lightweight, comfortable seat cushion. Unlike inflatable pads, Ensolite will not puncture and deflate.

1. A Therm-a-Rest pad can be used as padding for a long-bone splint immobilizer (e.g., an improvised universal knee immobilizer).

2. An inflatable pad can also be used to stabilize a pelvic fracture.
   a. Wrap the deflated pad around the pelvis.
   b. Secure the pad with tape and inflate the pad, thus creating an improvised pelvic sling (see Fig. 18-24).

SAM Splint

Introduced in 1985, the versatile SAM splint (see Chapter 12, Fig. 12-12) has largely filled the niche formerly occupied by military-style ladder splints and wire mesh splints. It is constructed of a thin sheet of malleable aluminum sandwiched between two thin layers of closed-cell foam, weighs approximately 4½ oz, and can be easily rolled into a tight cylinder. Initially the splint has no rigidity, but after structural

U-shaped bends are placed along the axis of the splint, it becomes quite rigid.

1. The SAM splint(s) can be used for splinting virtually any long bone in the body (Fig. 18-1).
2. It can also be used for fabricating an improvised cervical collar (see Chapter 12, Fig. 12-12).

Triangular Bandage

One of the most ubiquitous components of first-aid kits and one of the easiest to replace through improvisation is the triangular bandage.

1. Typically used to construct a sling and swath bandage for shoulder and arm immobilization, a good substitute for this bulky item can be made with two or three safety pins. Pinning the shirtsleeve of the injured arm to the chest portion of the shirt effectively immobilizes the extremity against the body (Fig. 18-2A).
2. If the victim is wearing a short-sleeved shirt, fold the bottom of the shirt up and over the arm to create a pouch. This can be pinned to the sleeve and chest section of the shirt to secure the arm (see Fig. 18-2B).
3. Triangular bandages are also advocated for securing splints and constructing pressure wraps. Common items such as socks, shirts, belts, pack straps, webbing, shoelaces, fanny packs, and underwear can easily be substituted.

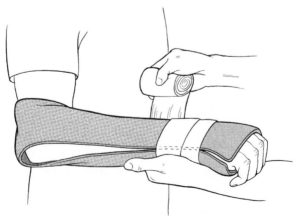

Figure 18-1. SAM sugar tong splint. For a distal radius fracture, the forearm should be placed in a neutral, not pronated, position.

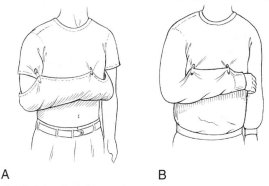

A   B

Figure 18-2. Techniques for pinning arm to shirt as an improvised sling. **A,** With short-sleeved shirt, bottom of shirt is folded up over injured arm and secured to sleeve and upper shirt. **B,** With long-sleeved shirt or jacket, sleeved arm is simply pinned to chest portion of garment.

DISORDERS

▶ UPPER EXTREMITY FRACTURES

Clavicle

A fracture of the clavicle generally occurs in the middle or lateral third of the bone and is typically associated with a direct blow or fall onto the lateral shoulder.

Signs and Symptoms
1. Complaints of shoulder pain, which may be poorly localized and exacerbated by arm or shoulder motion
2. Crepitus at the clavicle confirms the diagnosis
3. Although rare, associated pneumothorax, as the cupola of the lung is punctured
4. Shortness of breath and deep pain on inspiration
5. Associated injury to the brachial plexus, axillary artery, or subclavian vessels

Treatment
1. Localize the pain by gentle palpation to identify the area of maximum tenderness.
2. Auscultate the chest for equal breath sounds if a stethoscope is available.
3. Perform a thorough neurocirculatory examination of the adjacent extremity.
4. Examine the skin carefully for disruption because of the subcutaneous location of the bone.

5. If there is a significant open wound, suspected pneumothorax, or an injury to a nerve or vascular structure, arrange for evacuation.
6. Most clavicle fractures are improved by applying a sling or figure-of-eight type of support, easily improvised with a shirt jacket or cravat. A figure-of-eight support works by pulling the shoulder girdle back, applying longitudinal traction to the clavicle so that the bony fragments are somewhat realigned. Figure-of-eight straps are poorly tolerated by some patients and, if applied too tightly, can cause nerve injury. Usually a simple sling with swath is adequate.
7. Judicious use of ice or snow packs, if available, and analgesics should be used. Elevation may provide added relief during rest. Elevate the victim's upper body and head by 10 to 30 degrees when supine. This is a general rule for any shoulder injury. Supine positioning is generally poorly tolerated by victims after shoulder injury.

Humerus

A fracture of the humeral shaft may be produced by a direct blow or torsional force on the arm. This fracture frequently occurs with a fall, rope accident, or skiing accident.

Signs and Symptoms
1. Fracture of the proximal humerus, often caused by a high-velocity fall onto an abducted, externally rotated arm or a direct blow to the anterior shoulder
   a. Difficult to differentiate from a shoulder dislocation in the acute phase. If there is crepitus or if the upper arm is rotated while palpating the proximal humerus and they do not move as a unit, the humerus is fractured.
   b. Severe pain around the shoulder and with any arm motion
   c. Anterior fullness in the area of the proximal humerus, suggesting associated anterior humeral head dislocation
2. Fracture of the distal humerus
   a. More frequently extraarticular in children and intraarticular in adults, with the child generally sustaining a supracondylar fracture with an extension moment across the elbow in a fall from a height
   b. Peak age of incidence 4 to 8 years, although this can also occur in an adult
   c. Deformity, swelling, pain, and crepitus
3. Radial nerve damage (rare unless the fracture occurs in the mid to distal one third of the humerus)

a. The radial nerve courses around the posterior aspect of the humerus and is occasionally traumatized when the humeral shaft is injured.

b. Numbness over the dorsum of the hand and inability to extend the wrist or fingers

c. Usually caused by contusion or traction injury to the nerve and not to complete disruption

Treatment

1. When a fracture of the humeral shaft is suspected, firmly apply an appropriate splint of fiberglass, wood, or other improvised material with an elastic bandage on the medial and lateral sides of the humerus. Construct the splint so that it reaches proximal to the level of the fracture (Fig. 18-3).

2. Have the victim use a sling for comfort.

a. With suspected proximal humeral injury, use the uninjured side as a reference and palpate the anterior aspect of the injured shoulder firmly while rotating the arm. Palpable crepitus with arm motion confirms the diagnosis. It is unlikely that a combined fracture and dislocation can be reduced in the field. Treat this as a fracture, with splinting of the extremity to the torso with a sling or a sling and swath.

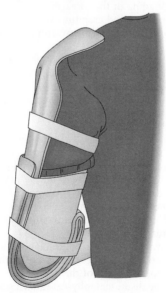

Figure 18-3. Humerus splint. Used in conjunction with a sling and swath, this splint adds extra support and protection for a fractured humerus.

b. Although application of an arm sling is the appropriate field management for a proximal humerus fracture, if associated significant distal nerve or vascular injury exists, arrange for evacuation.

3. For an adult with pain, crepitus, deformity, and swelling after a fall, apply a splint and immobilize the arm to the torso. Be sure to apply the splint with the elbow at 45 to 90 degrees of flexion, depending on the victim's comfort. A splint on the inner and outer surface of the arm that is molded to curve around the elbow provides very satisfactory stabilization. Arrange for prompt evacuation with an open fracture or neurocirculatory deficit.

4. With radial nerve injury, there is a high incidence of spontaneous recovery of function. However, if the victim complains of arm pain associated with deformity and crepitus, carefully check the sensory and motor function of the radial nerve as part of the overall neurocirculatory examination.

Radius

Signs and Symptoms
1. Radial shaft fracture: usually a history of a fall with angular or axial loading of the forearm
   a. Pain, deformity, and crepitus over the radial shaft after a fall or direct blow, with any arm motion exacerbating the pain
   b. Possibly associated with dislocation of the distal radio-ulnar joint (Galeazzi's fracture); tenderness, swelling, and deformity in wrist
   c. If associated with fracture of the ulna, possibly marked forearm instability or tenderness, crepitus, and deformity in the elbow and wrist
2. Radial head fracture: generally occurs in a young to middle-aged adult who falls onto an outstretched hand
   a. Pain around the elbow with loss of full extension
   b. Tenderness at the radial head on the lateral side of the elbow and pain with passive rotation of the forearm
   c. With a more severe, comminuted radial head fracture: pain and crepitus with attempts at motion; ROM severely limited
   d. Frequently, hemarthrosis of the elbow with effusion
   e. Swelling noted as fullness posterior to the radial head and anterior to the tip of the olecranon
3. Fracture of the distal metaphyseal radius: generally associated with a fall onto the outstretched hand from a significant height

a. Obvious pain, deformity ("silver fork deformity"), and crepitus

b. Intra-articular distal radius fracture often associated with fracture of the ulnar styloid

Treatment

1. Carefully examine the wrist and elbow, looking for tenderness, swelling, deformity, and crepitus.

2. Once a shaft fracture of the radius or radius and ulna is identified, splint the wrist, forearm, and elbow in the position of function.

3. For a radial head fracture, move the elbow through gentle ROM and then place it in a posterior splint at 90 degrees of flexion with neutral pronation and supination.

   a. On a prolonged expedition when definitive care cannot be reached, remove the splint at 5 days and perform intermittent active ROM exercises; then reapply the splint for comfort.

   b. With a nondisplaced or minimally displaced radial head fracture, early ROM prevents permanent loss of elbow motion.

   c. If hemarthrosis has occurred and proper equipment is available and you are confident about the diagnosis, aspirate the hemarthrosis and instill 5 mL of lidocaine to facilitate pain relief. This must be done under sterile conditions. This injection should only be attempted in a sterile fashion by persons familiar with shoulder injections.

4. For a distal radius fracture with significant deformity at the wrist, apply longitudinal traction after appropriate sedation (Fig. 18-4). In certain circumstances with a Colles' fracture, simple longitudinal traction will not work

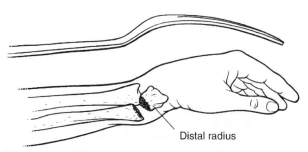

Distal radius

Figure 18-4. Colles' fracture ("dinner fork deformity").

because the fracture is locked dorsally. To effect reduction, reproduce the injury deforming force to unlock the fracture. That is, increase the volar angulation (hyperextend the wrist) at the fracture site, then pull distal traction, reducing the distal fragment volarly with your thumb.

a. Next, apply a splint that immobilizes the wrist and elbow. A U-shaped ("sugar tong") splint, used in conjunction with a sling to limit rotation, is adequate for transport (see Fig. 18-1).

b. With an open fracture, significant neurologic deficits, or abnormal circulatory examination, apply the splints promptly and initiate evacuation. Keep the limb elevated above the heart during transport to minimize swelling.

Ulna

Signs and Symptoms

1. Ulna shaft fracture: when victim attempts to brace a fall with the forearm
   a. Most often associated with fracture of the radial shaft at the same level
   b. When isolated, most often occurs as a result of a direct blow, the so-called nightstick fracture
   c. Can be associated with dislocation of the radial head (Monteggia's fracture), affecting elbow function
   d. Pain, localized swelling, and crepitus
2. Fracture of the proximal ulna (olecranon): result of a fall onto the posterior elbow or from an avulsion after violent asymmetric contraction of the triceps
   a. Inability to extend the elbow actively against gravity if the triceps is dissociated from the forearm with a complete fracture of the olecranon
   b. On initial examination: pain, significant swelling, and ecchymosis; palpable gap in the olecranon, with possible open fracture
   c. With severe trauma, associated with intra-articular fracture of the distal humerus

Treatment

1. For ulna shaft fracture, apply a long-arm splint in the position of function. If the fracture is open, arrange for prompt evacuation.
2. For fracture of the proximal ulna, after the distal neurocirculatory examination and shoulder and wrist assessment, apply a splint in the position of function. A posterior splint at 90 degrees usually works well. If there is an open fracture, absent pulse, severe swelling, or neurologic deficit, arrange for immediate evacuation (Fig. 18-5).

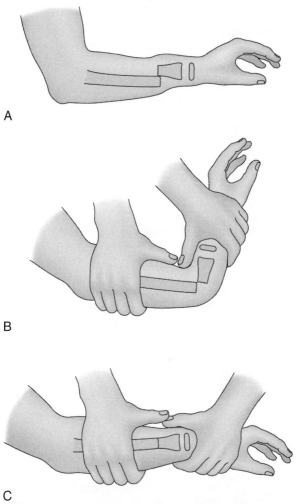

Figure 18-5. Technique for reduction of a complete fracture of the forearm. **A,** Initial fracture position. **B,** Hyperextended fracture to 100 degrees to disengage the fracture ends. **C,** Push with the thumb on the distal fragment to achieve reduction. (**A** to **C** from Green N, Swiontkowski MF: Skeletal Trauma in Children, vol 3, 2nd ed. Philadelphia, WB Saunders, 1998.)

Wrist and Hand

Signs and Symptoms
1. Wrist fracture: history of significant rotational or high axial loading forces such as those occurring with a fall onto the hand
   a. Pain at first, then later swelling of the wrist
   b. Significant pain with any use of the hand or with rotation of the forearm
2. Carpal bone fracture: precise diagnosis impossible without radiographs
   a. Scaphoid most frequently fractured carpal bone
   b. Diagnosis suspected if victim's area of maximum tenderness within the "anatomic snuffbox" (Fig. 18-6)
3. Fracture of the hook of the hamate
   a. Point of maximum tenderness at base of hypothenar eminence
   b. History of using the hand to apply great force to an object with a handle such as an ax or a hammer and meeting great resistance

Treatment
1. Swelling can become severe. Remove all jewelry as soon as possible to prevent constriction as tissue swells.

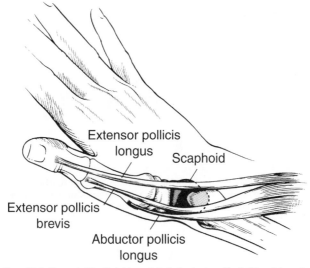

Figure 18-6. The scaphoid (navicular) bone sits in the "anatomic snuffbox" of the radial aspect of the wrist.

2. Make a temporary hand splint with the hand in the position of function, with the wrist straight and the fingers flexed in a curve as if holding a beverage can.

3. Apply a long-term hand splint with the metacarpophalangeal joints flexed 90 degrees and the interphalangeal joints extended, creating the "intrinsic positive position."

4. This position places the collateral ligaments at maximum length and prevents later joint contracture. For an open fracture or one accompanied by median nerve dysfunction, arrange for prompt evacuation.

5. For carpal bone fracture/wrist dislocation, reduce the fracture by grasping the hand in a handshake fashion and pulling with axial traction. Apply a short-arm splint.

6. For suspected scaphoid fracture, if appropriate splinting materials are available, apply a thumb spica splint, immobilizing both the radius and the thumb metacarpal.
   a. Encourage the victim to follow up with an orthopedist as soon as practical.
   b. Lack of appropriate immobilization can result in nonunion and/or avascular necrosis, which can develop into severe osteoarthritis and chronic pain.

7. For fracture of the hook of the hamate bone, use a short-arm splint, which also suffices for other suspected carpal injuries, until definitive treatment can be obtained.

8. Wrist fractures with significant swelling or fractures that have not been anatomically reduced can induce traumatic carpal tunnel syndrome. If there is evidence of median nerve paresthesias, urgent carpal tunnel release may be essential.

Metacarpal

Signs and Symptoms

1. Fracture of the metacarpal base or shaft: result of a crush injury or an axial load when a rock or other immovable object is struck; produces tenderness, crepitus, and deformity

2. Fracture of the metacarpal neck: result of the same mechanism as for the metacarpal base or shaft
   a. Fourth and fifth metacarpals most frequently involved
   b. Occurs at the base of the knuckle and can be associated with significant rotational deformity

3. Fracture of the base of the thumb metacarpal
   a. When an individual falls with an object grasped between the index finger and thumb (a common position with a ski pole)
   b. Difficult to differentiate from an ulnar collateral ligament injury because these injuries often occur simultaneously

Treatment

1. For fracture of the metacarpal base or shaft, apply a short-arm splint (e.g., gutter splint, volar splint, U-splint) extending to the proximal interphalangeal (PIP) joint.
2. For possible fracture of the metacarpal neck, check for rotation of the metacarpal by observing the orientation of the fingernails as the metacarpophalangeal and interphalangeal joints are flexed to 90 degrees.
   a. Make sure that the fingernails are parallel to one another and perpendicular to the orientation of the palm.
   b. Ensure that the terminal portions of each digit point to the scaphoid tubercle.
3. For fracture of the metacarpal neck, if malalignment or significant shortening is noted, attempt rotation and reduction with traction on the involved digit.
   a. For a fractured metacarpal shaft or neck, immobilize by applying an aluminum splint (or stick) to the volar surface and taping the involved digit to the adjacent digit with the metacarpophalangeal joint positioned at 45 to 90 degrees.
   b. If splinting material is available, apply a radial or ulnar gutter splint, with the metacarpophalangeal joint positioned at 45 to 90 degrees. The splint should extend to the end of the fingers.
4. For suspected fracture of the base of the thumb metacarpal, immobilize the thumb and wrist in a thumb spica splint.
5. For open metacarpal fracture, clean the wound, débride as needed, and give presumptive antibiotic therapy for 48 hours or until definitive care can be obtained.

Phalanx

Signs and Symptoms

1. Fracture usually a result of a crush injury or when a digit is caught in a rope
2. Angular rotational deformity and crepitus
3. Without radiography, intra-articular fracture with subluxation or dislocation difficult to differentiate from interphalangeal joint dislocation

Treatment

1. Reduce the fracture by applying traction and correcting the deformity.
2. Immobilize the fracture by taping the injured digit to a volar splint.
3. Cleanse any nail bed fracture or crush site with soap, and then place a sterile dressing and protective volar splint. If

the nail bed is lacerated, suture repair may be necessary to preserve future functional nail growth.

▶ UPPER EXTREMITY DISLOCATIONS

Sternoclavicular Joint

Signs and Symptoms
1. Generally injured by a fall onto an abducted shoulder
    a. Direction of dislocation with the medial head of the clavicle anterior to the manubrium of the sternum
    b. Direct blow to the sternum also possibly causative of this injury, along with rib fracture(s)
2. Pain in the sternum region, frequently accompanied by difficulty taking a deep breath
3. With posterior dislocation, significant pressure placed on the esophagus and superior vena cava
    a. Step-off between the sternum and medial head of the clavicle (compared with the uninjured side)
    b. Difficulty swallowing and engorgement of facial veins, similar to that seen with superior vena cava obstruction syndrome

Treatment
1. Attempt reduction as soon as possible.
    a. Place a large roll of clothing or other firm object between the scapulae, and position the victim on a firm surface.
    b. Apply sharp, firm pressure directed posteriorly to both shoulders.
    c. Repeat this maneuver several times with a larger object placed between the scapulae if reduction attempts are initially unsuccessful.
    d. After reduction, use a sling.
2. With a posterior dislocation, if the victim transcends into extremis, grasp the midshaft clavicle with a towel clip or pliers and forcefully pull it out of the thoracic cavity. Posterior dislocation mandates evacuation (Fig. 18-7).

Acromioclavicular (AC) Joint Separation

Signs and Symptoms
1. Injured by a blow on top of the shoulder
2. First-degree injury (sprain of the AC ligaments): to the capsule between the acromion and the clavicle; no superior migration of the clavicle seen
3. Second-degree injury (complete tear of the AC ligaments and sprain of the coracoclavicular [CC] ligaments): complete capsular disruption, with the CC ligaments remaining

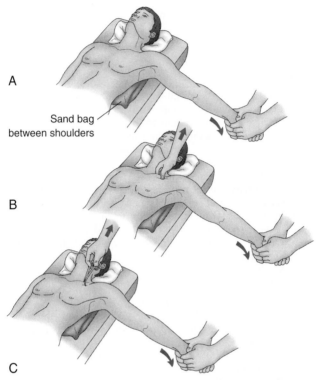

Figure 18-7. Posterior sternoclavicular dislocation. **A,** Place a sand bag between the shoulder blades. **B,** Attempt to pull the clavicle back into position. **C,** If necessary, grasp the clavicle with a towel clip or pliers to accomplish reduction.

intact; superior migration of the clavicle relative to the ac-romion of one half the diameter of the clavicle

4. Third-degree injury (tear of both the AC and CC liga-ments): total disruption of the joint capsule and the CC ligaments, which allows superior migration of the clavicle of up to 2 cm (about 1 inch) (Fig. 18-8). It appears as if the clavicle is superiorly migrated, but actually the scapula (including the glenoid and humeral head) is depressed and the clavicle is in normal position.

5. Type IV is a tear of both the AC and CC ligaments with the distal clavicle displaced posteriorly into the trapezius mus-cle (surgical indication).

6. Type V is a tear of both ligaments with the distal clavicle displaced superiorly into the muscle (surgical indication).

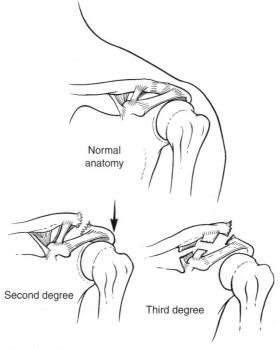

Figure 18-8. Acromioclavicular joint injury.

7. Type VI is a tear of both ligaments with the distal clavicle displaced inferior to the coracoid process (surgical indication and extremely rare).
8. Differentiating between type III and type IV to VI injuries: In a type III the distal clavicle is easily reducible with palpation, but in types IV to VI the clavicle is not reducible.
9. If a separation of type IV or greater is suspected, there is a high incidence of associated injuries (i.e., clavicular fractures, scapular fractures, pneumothorax).

Treatment
1. Because using the arm increases pain, place the arm on the affected side in a sling.
2. As long as the individual can tolerate the discomfort associated with the injury, evacuation is not mandatory. Always rule out more severe associated injuries such as rib fractures and pneumothorax.
3. Apply ice packs and administer appropriate analgesics.
4. Elevate the upper torso to provide additional relief during rest.

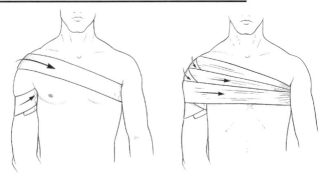

Figure 18-9. Shoulder Spica wrap for support after shoulder dislocation.

Glenohumeral Joint (Shoulder) Dislocation

Signs and Symptoms

1. Generally dislocated anteriorly, or anteriorly and inferiorly; mechanism of injury usually a blow to the arm in the abducted and externally rotated position (e.g., during "high-bracing" in kayaking or other paddle sports, in which extreme abduction and external rotation occur)
2. Recurrent anterior shoulder instability, seen in 30% to 50% of individuals and often easier to reduce than a first-time dislocation
3. Holding the extremity away from the body, unable to bring the arm across the chest
   a. Shoulder that appears square because of anterior, medial, and inferior displacement of the humeral head into a subcoracoid position
   b. No crepitus unless there is an associated fracture
4. With axillary nerve injury, loss of sensation over the mid-deltoid region

Treatment

1. Do a thorough motor, sensory, and circulatory examination of the involved extremity.
2. Carefully assess the axillary and musculocutaneous nerves because they are the nerves most often injured in this dislocation.
3. If within 30 to 60 minutes of definitive medical care, transport the victim with support for the dislocated joint.
4. If skilled individuals are present or if definitive medical care is distant, early reduction of the dislocation can greatly improve the victim's discomfort and enable the victim to function more actively during evacuation (Box 18-3).

Box 18-3. Reduction Techniques

STANDING METHOD
- Have the victim bend forward at the waist while you support the chest with one hand.
- With the other hand, grasp the victim's wrist and apply steady downward traction and external rotation (Fig. 18-10)
- While maintaining traction, slowly flex the victim's shoulder by moving it in a cephalad direction until reduction is obtained.
- If two rescuers are available, one supports the victim at the chest and the other exerts countertraction and flexion at the arm (Fig. 18-11).
- To help with the reduction, apply scapular manipulation by adducting the inferior tip using thumb pressure and stabilizing the superior aspect of the scapula with the cephalad hand.

SITTING METHOD
- Perform the reduction with the victim sitting upright with the elbow on the affected side flexed at a 90-degree angle.
- Form an article of clothing into a 3-foot (90-cm) loop around the proximal forearm.
- Apply downward traction by placing your foot in the loop, freeing your hands to apply gentle rotation (usually slightly external), while maintaining elbow flexion.

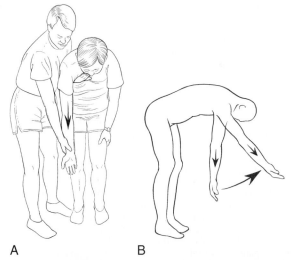

A   B

Figure 18-10. Technique for shoulder relocation with victim standing. **A,** Rescuer supports victim's chest with one hand and pulls down and forward (**B**) with other hand.

Continued

Box 18-3. Reduction Techniques—*cont'd*

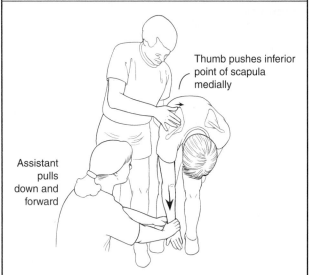

Thumb pushes inferior point of scapula medially

Assistant pulls down and forward

Figure 18-11. If two rescuers are available, scapular rotation to assist shoulder relocation can be performed while second rescuer pulls arm down and forward. Inferior tip of scapula is pushed medially.

- Have an assistant stand on the opposite side of the victim and maintain countertraction by placing his or her arms around the victim's chest, with hands in the axilla.

SUPINE AND PRONE METHODS
- An alternative method is to have the victim lie prone so that the injured arm dangles free.
- A thick pad is placed under the injured shoulder.
- A 10- to 20-lb (4.5- to 9-kg) weight is attached to the wrist or forearm (the victim should not attempt to hold the weight).
- The weight is allowed to exert steady traction on the arm, using gravity to relocate the humeral head.
- The weight can be improvised from a stuff-bag, helmet, or bucket filled with sand (Fig. 18-12).
- Another common method of reduction is linear traction along the axial line of the extremity while stabilizing the torso with a blanket or rope (Fig. 18-13).
- The patient lies supine, on the ground or a makeshift table.
- A sheet or padded belt or strapping can be tied around the caregiver's waist and the victim's bent forearm so that the

Continued

Box 18-3. Reduction Techniques—*cont'd*

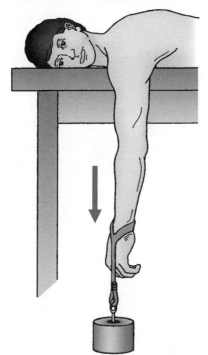

Figure 18-12. Stimson technique. (Redrawn from Rockwood CA, Green CA [eds]: Fractures in Adults, 6th ed, vol 2. Philadelphia, Lippincott Williams & Wilkins, 2001, p 1305.)

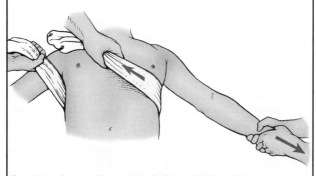

Figure 18-13. Traction and countertraction for dislocated shoulder reduction.

Continued

Box 18-3. Reduction Techniques—*cont'd*

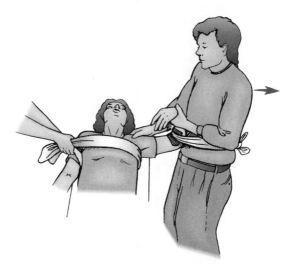

Figure 18-14. Repositioning a dislocated shoulder. Attached to the victim's forearm with a strap, rope, or sheet, the rescuer uses his body weight to apply traction, leaving his hands free to manipulate the victim's arm. A second rescuer applies countertraction, or the victim can be held motionless by fixing the chest sheet to a tree or ground stake. (From Auerbach PS: Medicine for the Outdoors: The Essential Guide to Emergency Medical Procedures and First Aid, 4th ed. Guilford, CT, Lyons Press, 2003.)

caregiver (standing or kneeling) can lean back to apply traction, leaving hands free to guide the head of the humerus back into position (Fig. 18-14).
- Padding is placed in the armpit and bend of the elbow to prevent pressure injury to sensitive nerves beneath the skin.

a. The key element is rapid initiation because the longer a shoulder remains dislocated, the more difficult the eventual reduction.
b. Common to all methods of shoulder reduction are the following: relaxation of muscle spasm, reassurance of the victim, and a method of traction to pass the humeral head over the anterior edge of the glenoid.
c. In some remote settings, it may be easier to apply a method of reduction that can be carried out with the

victim either standing or sitting. This requires access to a flat, comfortable area on which to place the victim in the supine or prone position.

5. After any shoulder reduction, remember to monitor circulation and motor-sensory function to the wrist and hand.
6. Narcotic or benzodiazepine premedication may be helpful if muscle spasm has developed, but avoid these in the multiply-injured victim.
7. If the shoulder cannot be reduced after three vigorous attempts, arrange for evacuation. For a difficult reduction, consider administration of 10 to 15 mL of a local anesthetic into the shoulder joint. This injection should only be attempted in a sterile fashion by someone skilled at shoulder injection.
8. After relocation, to prevent a recurrent dislocation, splint the victim's arm across the chest with a sling or swath or by safety-pinning the sleeve of the arm across the chest. If circumstances require further limited use of the arm (e.g., ski pole use, kayak paddling), partially stabilize the shoulder by wrapping an elastic wrap around the torso and upper arm to limit abduction and external rotation (see Fig. 18-9).
9. Any victim with a first-time dislocation or severe postreduction pain requires evacuation and formal evaluation.

Posterior Shoulder Dislocation

Signs and Symptoms
1. Occurs in less than 5% of shoulder dislocations; caused by a direct blow to the anterior shoulder or may result from marked internal rotation associated with a grand mal seizure.
2. Significant pain and loss of shoulder motion, with external rotation often completely lost; greater range of motion often more possible than with anterior dislocation; diagnosis often missed owing to this motion and the lack of obvious deformity.
3. Using palpation, can usually detect posterior fullness not appreciated on the uninjured (comparison) side.

Treatment
The reduction maneuver, aftercare, and indications for evacuation are similar to those for anterior dislocation.

Shoulder Fracture/Dislocation

Signs and Symptoms
More common with a high-velocity accident (e.g., MVA) or an older victim.
   Crepitus may be noted over fracture site.

Treatment
1. Do not reduce suspected fracture/dislocation in the field.
2. Treat this injury as a fracture, with splinting of the extremity to the torso with a sling or a sling and swath.

Elbow

Signs and Symptoms
1. Occurs with hyperextension or axial loading from a fall onto the outstretched hand; generally posterior and lateral.
2. Signs obvious, with posterior deformity at the elbow and foreshortening of the forearm.

Treatment
1. After careful examination of the distal sensory, motor, and circulatory status, perform reduction.
   a. With countertraction on the upper arm, apply linear traction with the elbow slightly flexed and the forearm in the original degree of pronation or supination (Fig. 18-15).
   b. Premedication with an opiate or benzodiazepine can be extremely helpful.

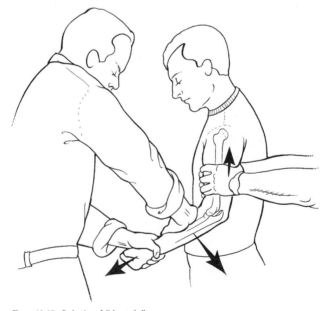

Figure 18-15. Reduction of dislocated elbow.

    c. Reduction (which can be a painful maneuver) leads to nearly complete relief of pain and restoration of normal surface anatomy.
2. After reduction, apply a posterior splint with the elbow in 90 degrees of flexion and the forearm in neutral position (see Fig. 18-3).
    a. Use a sling for comfort.
    b. If reduction is not successful after three vigorous attempts or if a nerve or vascular injury is suspected, apply a splint to the arm in the most comfortable position and initiate evacuation.

Wrist

Signs and Symptoms
1. Frequently associated with carpal fracture(s)
2. Generally produced by a fall onto the outstretched hand
3. Severe pain, swelling, and deformity within the distal wrist
4. Without radiograph, difficult to differentiate from a distal radius fracture

Treatment
1. Carefully assess distal neurocirculatory function, emphasizing median nerve function.
2. For wrist dislocation or fracture, perform a reduction maneuver.
3. Grasp the victim's hand as for a handshake, place countertraction on the upper arm, and apply linear traction. Note that significant force is required, and premedication, if available, may be extremely helpful.
4. If reduction is unsuccessful after three vigorous attempts or if there is median nerve dysfunction, arrange for evacuation.
5. Apply a short-arm (U or volar) splint if reduction is successful (see Fig. 18-1).
6. Elevate the arm as much as possible until the definitive care center can be reached.

Metacarpophalangeal Joint

Dislocation is rare and usually follows a crush injury or occurs when a hand is caught in a rope. The site is usually dorsal, and it may be difficult to reduce in the field.

Signs and Symptoms
1. Finger shortened, deviated to the ulnar side, and positioned in extension
2. Metacarpal head possibly prominent in the palm

3. The thumb metacarpophalangeal joint typically injured
4. Injury to the ulnar collateral ligament of this joint ("skier's thumb") a result of a valgus stress, such as when an individual falls holding an object (e.g., pole) in the first web space

Treatment

Metacarpophalangeal Joint

1. Be aware that dorsal dislocation may be irreducible if the head of the metacarpal becomes trapped between the volar ligaments (Fig. 18-16).
2. Reduction depends on the degree of disruption of supporting structures such as the volar plate and collateral ligaments. Thus this dislocation frequently requires open reduction in an operating room setting.
3. Most dorsal dislocations are easily reduced.
   a. First, the proximal phalanx is hyperextended 90 degrees on the metacarpal.
   b. Then the base of the proximal phalanx is pushed into flexion, maintaining contact at all times with the metacarpal head to prevent entrapment of the volar plate in the joint (see Fig. 18-16).

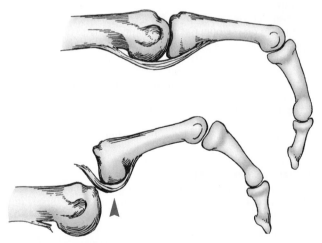

Figure 18-16. The single most important element preventing reduction in a complex metacarpophalangeal (MCP) dislocation is interposition of the volar plate within the joint space. It must be extricated surgically. (From Rockwood CA Jr, Green DP, Bucholz RW [eds]: Rockwood and Green's Fractures in Adults, 3rd ed. Philadelphia, JB Lippincott, 1991.)

   c. Straight longitudinal traction is avoided.

   d. The wrist and IP joints are flexed to relax the flexor tendons.

4. The joint usually reduces easily with a palpable and audible clunk.

5. If reduction of a digital metacarpophalangeal joint dislocation is successful, apply a volar splint with the joint held in 90 degrees of flexion and interphalangeal joints in full extension.

6. If reduction is unsuccessful, splint the joint in the position of comfort and arrange for definitive treatment as soon as possible.

Thumb Metacarpophalangeal Joint

1. The thumb MCP joint is the most commonly injured.

2. Dislocations are reduced as already described.

3. Injury to the ulnar collateral ligament of this joint (skier's or gamekeeper's thumb) results from a valgus stress, as may occur when an individual falls holding an object in the first web space.

4. The patient complains of tenderness over the ulnar aspect of the MCP joint.

5. There may be instability to radial stress with the joint held in 30 degrees of flexion, an indication for surgical repair.

6. Often, the adductor aponeurosis becomes interposed between the ligament and its bony attachment, resulting in a Stener lesion (Fig. 18-17).

7. In the field, a thumb spica splint is applied (Fig. 18-18).

8. If splinting material is not available, the thumb is taped until definitive care can be obtained (Fig. 18-19).

9. When possible, place an ulnar collateral ligament tear in a thumb spica splint (Fig. 18-20). Instability often requires a lateral stress x-ray film for definitive diagnosis and is an indication for surgical repair. Arrange for definitive care within 10 days of the injury.

10. For dorsal dislocation, attempt metacarpophalangeal joint reduction.

   a. Grasp the finger and apply longitudinal traction, moving from metacarpophalangeal joint extension into flexion ("up and over" the metacarpal head).

   b. Splint the thumb in the position of function (see Figs. 18-18 and 18-20).

11. Obtain orthopedic follow-up within 10 days.

Proximal Interphalangeal Joint

PIP joint dislocation is common and occurs with axial loading of a finger.

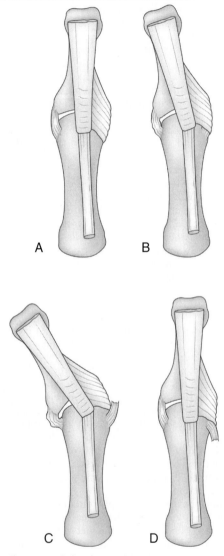

Figure 18-17. *For legend see opposite page.*

Figure 18-17. Diagram of the displacement of the ulnar collateral ligament of the thumb metacarpophalangeal joint. **A,** Normal relationship, with the ulnar ligament covered by the adductor aponeurosis. **B,** With slight radial angulation, the proximal margin of the aponeurosis slides distally and leaves a portion of the ligament uncovered. **C,** With major radical angulation, the ulnar ligament ruptures at its distal insertion. In this degree of angulation, the aponeurosis has displaced distal to the rupture and permitted the ligament to escape from beneath it. **D,** As the joint is realigned, the proximal edge of the adductor aponeurosis sweeps the free end of the ligament proximally and farther away from its insertion. This is the Stener lesion. Unless surgically restored, the ulnar ligament will not heal properly and will be unstable to lateral stress. (Redrawn from Stener B: Skeletal injuries associated with rupture of the ulnar collateral ligament of the metacarpophalangeal joint of the thumb. A clinical and anatomical study. Acta Chir Scand 125: 583-586, 1963.)

Signs and Symptoms
1. Dislocation occurring when an individual attempts to catch an object or a finger becomes entangled in a rope or another piece of equipment
2. Dislocation generally dorsal (middle phalanx in relationship to the proximal)

Treatment
1. Reduction of dorsal PIP dislocations is performed as described for dorsal MCP dislocation (Fig. 18-21).
2. Straight longitudinal traction is avoided to prevent entrapment of the volar plate into the joint.
3. After reduction, do the following:
   a. The finger is taped to an adjacent finger to avoid hyperextension and allow early motion (Fig. 18-22).
   b. Alternatively, apply a volar splint and tape the finger to the splint in slight flexion.
4. Initiate early motion of the joint to regain full extension.
5. Keep the distal interphalangeal (DIP) joint free for active ROM. The active ROM of the DIP encourages the lateral bands to stay dorsal and thus help prevent a boutonniere deformity. Be careful not to hyperextend the PIP, especially with significant swelling, to avoid serious dorsal wound breakdowns.
6. With either volar or distal dislocation, arrange for definitive care as soon as possible.

Distal Interphalangeal Joint
The DIP joint is less frequently injured than the PIP joint.

Signs and Symptoms
1. Volar dislocation or subluxation, resulting in disruption of the terminal extensor mechanism (mallet deformity)

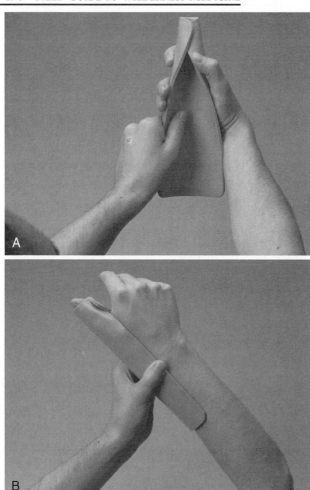

Figure 18-18. Padded aluminum thumb spica.

2. Occasionally, when an object is firmly grasped and then pulled away, rupture of the flexor profundus tendon (jersey finger)
3. Distal interphalangeal joint dislocation: active extension of the distal interphalangeal joint absent
4. Rupture of the flexor profundus tendon: active flexion of the distal interphalangeal joint absent

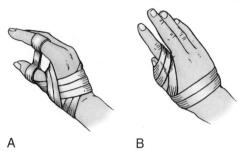

Figure 18-19. Taping the thumb for immobilization. **A,** The buddy-taping method. **B,** A thumb-lock. If possible, padding should be placed between the thumb and forefinger. (From Auerbach PS: Medicine for the Outdoors: The Essential Guide to Emergency Medical Procedures and First Aid, 4th ed. Guilford, CT, Lyons Press, 2003.)

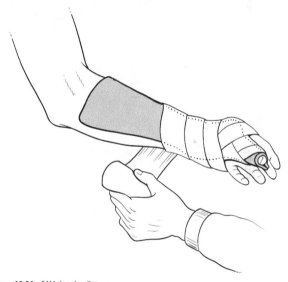

Figure 18-20. SAM thumb splint.

Treatment
1. Reduce a DIP joint dislocation.
   a. Obtain reduction with traction; then examine the joint for full active extension.
   b. Splint the joint in 0 degrees of extension for 3 weeks.
   c. Radiographic examination must be performed to rule out an intra-articular fracture.

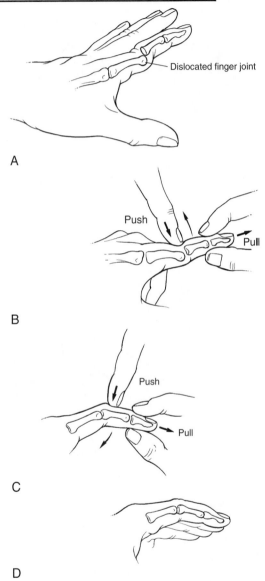

Figure 18-21. Traction method of joint reduction.

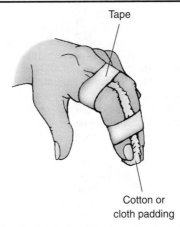

Tape

Cotton or
cloth padding

Figure 18-22. Buddy-taping method to immobilize a finger. (From Auerbach PS: Medicine for the Outdoors: The Essential Guide to Emergency Medical Procedures and First Aid, 4th ed. Guilford, CT, Lyons Press, 2003.)

2. For rupture of the flexor profundus tendon, splint the digit in flexion and instruct the victim to see an upper extremity surgeon within 7 days.

Pelvis Fractures

In the wilderness setting, a pelvis fracture is generally associated with a fall from a significant height or a high-velocity skiing accident.

The key factor in pelvis fracture is identification of posterior injury to the pelvic ring, which is associated with significant hemorrhage, neurologic injury, and mortality.

Bleeding associated with a pelvis injury is from cancellous bone at the fracture sites; retroperitoneal lumbar venous plexus injury; or, rarely, pelvic arterial injuries.

Signs and Symptoms
1. On clinical examination, simple fracture is seen as an area of tenderness not associated with detectable instability.
2. Diagnosis of an unstable pelvis fracture is based on instability of the pelvis associated with posterior pain, swelling, ecchymosis, and motion on examination.
3. To palpate, place hands on each iliac crest. Press outward and then inward to determine whether the pelvis is unstable. An unstable pelvis "gives" with this type of compression or distraction force. This test should only be performed once.

4. Additionally, look for leg-length discrepancy, which can be a sign of a vertically unstable pelvis fracture.
5. Flank, gluteal, perianal, and scrotal swelling with ecchymosis are additional signs of an unstable pelvis fracture.
6. Pelvic hemorrhage may occur rapidly, so identify the injury without delay. Monitor hemodynamic changes.
7. Unstable fractures are associated with a high incidence of significant hemorrhage, neurologic injury, and mortality. Hemorrhage, gastrointestinal, genitourinary, and neurologic injury contribute to mortality rate. An open pelvis fracture has a mortality rate of up to 50%.
8. Anterior-posterior compression injury presents as anterior instability, along with a palpable ramus fracture or gapping of the pubic symphysis ("diastasis").
9. Pelvis fracture may be associated with bladder, prostate, and urethral injury.

Treatment
1. The key factor in initial management of a pelvis fracture is the identification of posterior injury to the pelvic ring. If you find this or any unstable pelvis fracture, arrange for immediate evacuation with the victim on a backboard, taking care to minimize leg and torso motion.
2. Be aware that the victim is usually most comfortable with the hips and knees in slight flexion. Pad the victim generously with blankets or sleeping bags.
3. Attempt to stabilize the pelvis:
   a. Use a SAM sling, or improvise a similar device (Fig. 18-23).
   b. Improvise a MAST garment by wrapping an inflatable mattress around the victim's hips and pelvis, securing it with tape or rolled elastic wrap, and then inflating to a firm, but not rigid, pressure (Fig. 18-24).
   c. If an inflatable mattress or SAM sling is not available, tie a garment securely around the pelvis. A bed sheet or jacket wrapped snugly around the pelvis of an individual with a suspected unstable pelvic fracture may provide stability and accomplish adequate tamponade of bleeding from the fracture.
   d. A standard Sam splint unrolled inside the jacket sling may increase an improvised sling's efficacy.
   e. The applied sling belt or similar contrivance should be left in place until definitive care is available.
4. Be aware that an unstable pelvis fracture can cause significant hemorrhage. If available, arrange for intravenous fluid volume replacement. If possible, start two 16-gauge

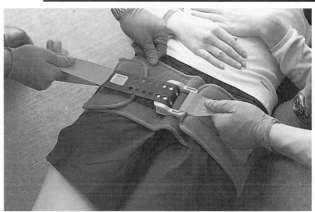

Figure 18-23. SAM sling.

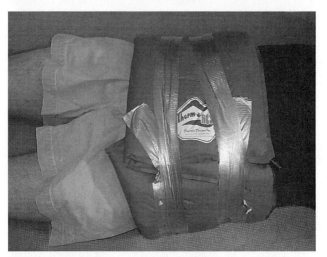

Figure 18-24. Pelvic sling improvised with inflatable sleeping bag and duct tape.

IV catheters in the upper extremities. Do not use the lower extremities because if there is venous disruption in the pelvis, the fluid will extravasate.

▶ LOWER EXTREMITY FRACTURES

Proximal Femur (Hip)
Most hip fractures occur in the femoral neck or intertrochanteric region.

Signs and Symptoms
1. In the absence of head or spinal cord injury, pain around the proximal thigh
2. With some proximal femur fractures, little local reaction in terms of swelling or deformity around the hip region to aid in diagnosis
3. Significant pain from any movement of the affected limb
4. Affected limb often noticeably shortened and externally rotated
5. Victim can rapidly lose 2 units of blood into the proximal thigh

Treatment
1. After doing a careful sensory, motor, and circulatory examination, realign the limb.
2. Light traction with a Kendrick, Thomas, Sager, or improvised splint should be considered for transport.
3. If a traction splint is not available, transport the victim on a backboard, with the limbs strapped together and padding placed between them.
4. Because evidence indicates that emergency treatment of a fracture of the femoral neck decreases the risk of posttraumatic necrosis, arrange for rapid evacuation of any victim in whom this injury is suspected.

Femoral Shaft

Fracture of the femoral shaft follows a fall from a significant height or results from a high-velocity injury.

Signs and Symptoms
1. Crepitus and maximum deformity at midthigh
   a. Severe pain and tenderness
   b. Possible shortening of the injured extremity
2. Often massive swelling

Treatment
1. This may be an open injury; split the victim's clothing open to complete the examination. If you find an open wound, arrange for rapid evacuation.
2. Be aware that there may also be an associated femoral neck fracture.
3. After completing a neurocirculatory examination, place the limb in a commercial or improvised traction device. Box 18-4 lists general principles of traction; Box 18-5 outlines femoral traction systems and discusses the ankle hitch and rigid support; and Box 18-6 lists traction mechanisms, anchors, and method for securing and padding. A number of commercial traction splints are available including the Hare, Klippel, Sager, Thomas, Trac 3,

Box 18-4. General Principles of Traction

WHY USE TRACTION?

In the backcountry environment, traction is essential for two fundamental reasons:

1. A general inability to provide IV volume expansion
2. Prolonged transport time to definitive care. One primary purpose of femoral traction is to limit blood loss into the thigh. For a constant surface area, the volume of a sphere is greater than the volume of a cylinder. Pulling (via traction) the thigh compartment back into its natural cylindrical shape limits blood loss into the soft tissue. Enhanced victim comfort and decreased potential for neurovascular damage are important secondary benefits.

WHAT CRITERIA SHOULD BE USED TO EVALUATE A TRACTION SYSTEM?

Consider five key design principles when evaluating a femoral traction system:

1. Does the splint provide in-line traction, or does it incorrectly pull the victim's leg off to the side or needlessly plantarflex the victim's ankle?
2. Is the splint comfortable? Ask the victim how it feels.
3. Does the splint compromise neurologic or vascular function? Constantly check the victim's distal neurovascular function.
4. Is the splint durable, or will it break when subjected to backcountry stress? Try your traction design on an uninjured victim first.
5. Is the splint cumbersome? Many reasonable splint designs become so bulky and awkward that litter transport, technical rescue, or helicopter evacuation is impossible. For example, a full-length ski splint is not compatible with evacuation in certain small helicopters.

REEL, and Kendrick. The Kendrick traction device is the best suited for wilderness use because of its minimal weight, low volume, and portability.

Distal Femur and Patella

Fracture of the distal end of the femur is frequently intra-articular and occurs with high-velocity loading when the knee is flexed. With axial loading of the femur, the patella becomes the driving wedge and the femoral condyles are impacted.

Signs and Symptoms

1. Crepitus, significant instability (not seen with patellar fracture)
2. Possible patellar fracture or splitting of the distal femoral condyles

Box 18-5. Femoral Traction Systems

Every femoral traction system has six components: ankle hitch, rigid support, traction mechanism, proximal anchor, method for securing, and padding. The ankle hitch and rigid support are outlined next. Box 18-6 lists traction mechanisms, proximal anchoring, method for securing, and padding.

ANKLE HITCH

Various techniques are used to anchor the distal extremity to the splint. Many work well, but some are difficult to recall in an emergency. Choose a technique that is easy to remember, and practice it.

DOUBLE-RUNNER SYSTEM

In this very straightforward technique, lay two short webbing loops ("runners") over and under the ankle (Fig. 18-25A). Pass the long loop sides through the short loop on both sides

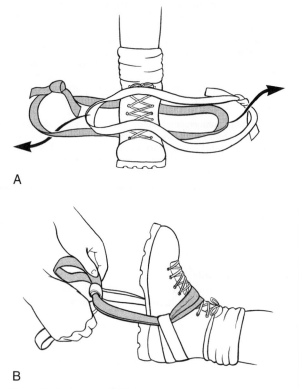

Figure 18-25. Double-runner ankle hitch.

Continued

Box 18-5. Femoral Traction Systems—*cont'd*

and adjust (see Fig. 18-25B). This system is infinitely adjustable, enabling you to center the pull from any direction. Proper padding is essential, especially for a lengthy transport. Use the victim's boot to distribute the pressure over the foot and ankle, although this obscures visualization and palpation of the foot. You can leave the boot in place and cut out the toe section for observation.

VICTIM'S BOOT SYSTEM

Use the victim's own boot as the hitch. Cut two holes into the side walls of the boot just above the midsole, in line with the ankle joint. Thread a piece of nylon webbing or a cravat through to complete the ankle hitch (Fig. 18-26). Because the boot is now

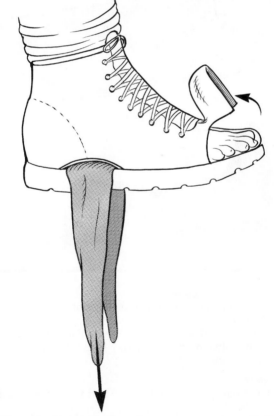

Figure 18-26. Traction using cut boot and cravat.   *Continued*

Box 18-5. Femoral Traction Systems—*cont'd*

functionally ruined, cut away the toe to allow direct neuro-vascular assessment.

Buck's Traction

For extended transport, improvise Buck's traction using a closed-cell foam pad (Fig. 18-27). Duct tape stirrups are added to a small foam pad that is wrapped around the leg. The entire unit is wrapped with an Ace bandage. This system helps distribute the force of the traction over a large surface area.

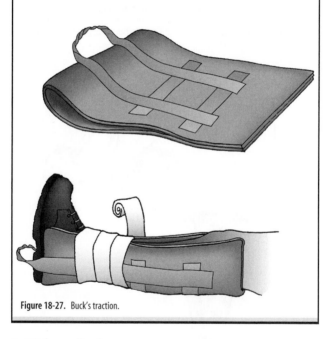

Figure 18-27. Buck's traction.

3. With patellar fracture:
   a. Injury often obvious on deep palpation
   b. If complete fracture of the patella, extensor mechanism will not work and active knee extension will be absent
   c. Injury often open because very little soft tissue overlies this sesamoid bone

Treatment
1. After initial examination of nerve and vessel function, re-align the limb.
2. Apply a posterior splint to the realigned limb for transportation.

3. With an open wound in the region of the fracture or an abnormal nerve or vascular examination, arrange for immediate evacuation.

Rigid Support

This can be fabricated as a unilateral support, similar to the Sager traction splint or Kendrick traction device, or as a bilateral support such as the Thomas half ring or Hare traction splint. Unilateral supports tend to be easier to apply than bilateral support.

Double-Ski Pole System

This is fashioned like a Thomas half ring, with the interlocked pole straps slipped under the proximal thigh to form the ischial support. Some mountain guides carry a prefabricated, drilled ski pole section or aluminum bar that can be used to stabilize the distal end of this system (Fig. 18-28).

Single-Ski Pole System

Use a single ski pole either between the legs, which is ideal for bilateral femoral fractures, or lateral to the injured leg. The ultimate rigid support is an adjustable telescoping ski pole used laterally. You can elongate the pole to the appropriate length for each victim, making the splint very compact for litter work or helicopter evacuation (Fig. 18-29).

Tent Pole System

Fit conventional sectioned tent poles together to create the ideal length for rigid support. Because of their flexibility, make sure the tent poles are well secured to the leg to prevent them from flexing out of position. Place a blanket pin or bent tent stake (Fig. 18-30) in the end of the pole to provide an anchor for the traction system. Alternately, use a Prusik knot to secure the system to the end of the tent pole (Fig. 18-31).

Miscellaneous

You can use any suitable object such as a canoe paddle, two ice axes taped together at the handles, or a straight tree limb to fashion a rigid support. Although skis immediately come to mind as a suitable rigid component, they are often too cumbersome. Because of their length, skis may extend far beyond the victim's feet or require placement into the axilla, which is unnecessary and inhibits the victim's mobility (e.g., sitting up during transport). Premanufactured canvas pockets, available through the National Ski Patrol System, provide a ski tip and tail attachment grommet for use with the ski system.

Tibia and Fibula

Tibial shaft fracture is associated with fibular shaft fracture in 90% of cases. These fractures result from high-impact trauma. The tibial plateau can be fractured with a fall or jump from a height.

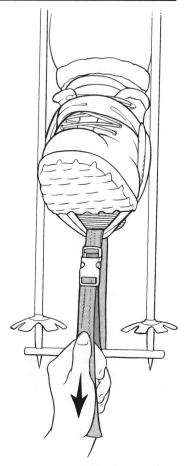

Figure 18-28. Double-ski pole system with prefabricated cross-bar and webbing belt traction. Prefabricated, drilled ski section is used to attach ends of two ski poles. Traction is applied with a webbing belt and sliding buckle.

Signs and Symptoms
1. Pain, swelling, and deformity obvious on initial examination
2. With a tibial plateau fracture, hemarthrosis quickly noted, with significant swelling around the knee
3. Because of anatomic tethering of the popliteal artery by the fascia of the soleus complex, arterial injury possible, especially when associated with a knee dislocation

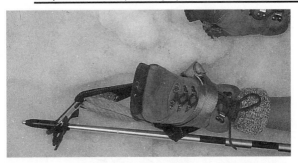

Figure 18-29. Single-ski pole system. An adjustable telescoping ski pole is used as the rigid support. A stirrup is attached to a carabiner placed over the end of the pole. Traction is applied by elongating the ski pole while another rescuer provides manual traction on the victim's leg.

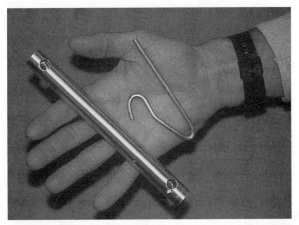

Figure 18-30. Prefabricated, drilled tent pole section, and bent stake, which serves as a distal traction anchor if a tent pole is used as the rigid support.

Treatment
1. When this injury is suspected, the entire limb must be inspected for distal sensory, motor, and circulatory function before realignment. Check distal pulses and capillary refill and for signs of compartment syndrome. Neurovascular checks should be performed every hour.
2. Apply a posterior splint, U splint, or combination, made from fiberglass, plaster, or improvised materials.
3. Use a custom-made or improvised metal splint (e.g., SAM splint) that can be held in place with elastic bandages or

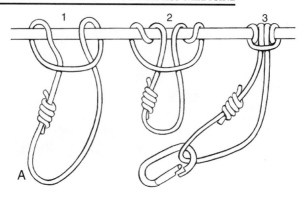

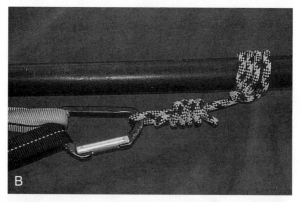

Figure 18-31. **A,** Prusik knot made from a small-diameter cord is used as an adjustable distal traction anchor. **B,** Two Prusik wraps are shown. Three or four wraps provide additional friction and security. If a Prusik knot slips, it can be easily taped in place.

tape. If SAM splints are used, at least two splints are necessary for the medial and lateral component and preferably a third for the posterior section (Fig. 18-32). A foam sleeping pad stabilized with rigid tent poles, ski pole sections, wooden branches, etc. may also be used.

4. Always pad the leg sufficiently before splinting.
5. An air splint also provides adequate immobilization of the tibiofibular fracture.
6. Hold the ankle in neutral position.
7. Strap the injured leg to the noninjured leg to reduce rotational forces during transport.

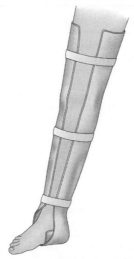

Figure 18-32. Lower leg and/or ankle splint. A sugar-tong splint can be used to immobilize fractures of the tibia, fibula, or ankle.

8. If materials are limited, fashion a crude splint by strapping the injured leg to the noninjured leg with a well-padded tree limb or walking stick placed between them for support.
9. Transport any victim with an unstable lower extremity fracture or dislocation with the limb elevated.

Ankle

The intra-articular distal tibia, medial malleolus, distal fibula, or any combination of these may be involved in an ankle fracture, generally produced by large torsional forces around a fixed foot. With the distal tibia, axial loading from a fall or jump may also be involved.

Signs and Symptoms
1. Significant pain and swelling when the shoe is removed
2. Crepitus and deformity possible

Treatment
1. Palpate along the medial and lateral malleoli to confirm the clinical suspicion.
2. After the shoe is removed to inspect the skin for open wounds, perform a neurocirculatory examination.
3. With rotational deformity in the ankle, realign the ankle with gentle traction before applying a posterior splint with the ankle in neutral position.

Box 18-6. Traction Mechanisms

Historically, the first traction mechanism that comes to mind is the Boy Scout–style "Spanish windlass." A windlass works, but it can be awkward to apply and is often not durable. The windlass can unwind if it is inadvertently jarred and can apply rotational forces to the leg. The amount of traction required is primarily a function of victim comfort. A general rule is to use 10% of body weight or 10 to 15 lb for the average victim. After traction is applied, always recheck distal neurovascular function (circulation, sensation, movement). An improvised traction system invariably relaxes during transport and should be rechecked for proper tension.

CAM LOCK OR FASTEX SLIDER

This is a simple, effective system that uses straps that have Fastex-like sliders and are often used as waist belts or to strap items to packs. Alternatively, use a cam lock with nylon webbing. Attach the belt to the distal portion of the rigid support and then to the ankle hitch. Traction is easily applied by cinching the nylon webbing (Fig. 18-33).

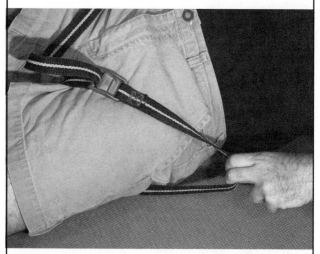

Figure 18-33. Proximal anchor using cam lock belt. The belt is applied as shown. The strap is adjusted loosely to allow the belt to ride up to the point of the hip. If the strap is improperly tightened, it can create pressure over the fracture, and it moves the traction point to a less optimal distal position. Padding is helpful, but not always necessary if the victim is wearing pants and the strap is properly adjusted.

Continued

Box 18-6. Traction Mechanisms—*cont'd*

TRUCKER'S HITCH

Fashion a windlass using small-diameter line (parachute cord) and a standard trucker's hitch for additional mechanical advantage (Fig. 18-34). An adjustable tent pole allows traction to be applied by elongating the pole during manual traction.

PRUSIK KNOT

This is useful with almost any system (see Fig. 18-31A). Prusik knots provide traction from rigid supports with few tie-on points (e.g., a canoe paddle shaft or a tent pole). The Prusik knot can be used to apply the traction (by sliding the knot distally) or simply as an attachment point for one of the traction mechanisms already mentioned.

LITTER TRACTION

If no rigid support is available and a rigid litter (e.g., Stokes) is being used, apply traction from the rigid bar at the foot end of the litter. If this system is used, you must immobilize the victim on the litter with adequate countertraction, such as that using inguinal straps.

PROXIMAL ANCHOR

The simplest proximal anchor uses a single ischial strap, which can be made from a piece of climbing webbing or a prefabricated strap, belt, or cam lock (Fig. 18-35). A cloth cravat can be used in a pinch. On the river a life jacket can be used (Fig. 18-36), and

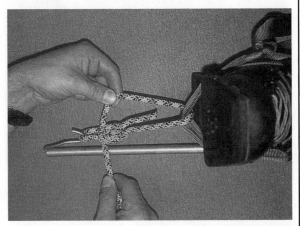

Figure 18-34. Tent pole traction with trucker's hitch. A bent tent stake is placed into the end of the tent pole as the distal traction anchor. A simple trucker's hitch is used to provide traction.

Continued

Box 18-6. Traction Mechanisms—*cont'd*

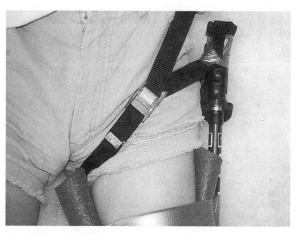

Figure 18-35. Proximal anchor using cam-lock belt. Belt is applied as shown. Ski pole is used laterally as the rigid support. Duct tape is useful for securing components. Padding is helpful but not always necessary if victim is wearing pants.

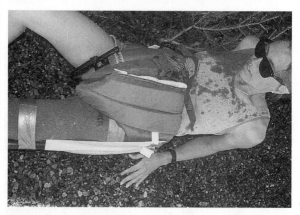

Figure 18-36. Life jacket proximal anchor. An inverted life jacket worn like a diaper forms a well-padded proximal anchor. A kayak paddle is rigged to the life jacket's side adjustment strap.

when climbing, a climbing harness is ideal. The preferred system is a proximal ischial strap, but a padded medial support (analogous to a Sager splint) can also be used. When using a medial traction system (Sager analog), generously pad the inguinal area.

Continued

Box 18-6. Traction Mechanisms—*cont'd*

A folded SAM splint attached to the proximal end of the rigid support works well.

SECURING AND PADDING

All potential pressure points should be checked to ensure that they are adequately padded. An excellent padding system can be made by first covering the upper and lower parts of the leg with a folded length of Ensolite (Fig. 18-37). Folded Ensolite is preferred over the circumferential wrap because the folded system allows for visualization of the extremity if necessary. The victim will be more comfortable if femoral traction is applied with the knee in slight flexion (place padding beneath the knee during transport). The splint must be secured firmly to the leg. Almost any straplike object will work, but a 10- to 15-cm (4- to 6-inch) Ace bandage wrapped circumferentially will provide a comfortable and secure union. Finally, the ankles or feet should be strapped or tied together to give the system additional stability. Tying the ankles together also protects the injured leg from external rotation and jarring during transport.

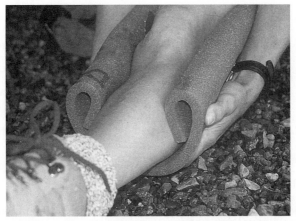

Figure 18-37. Folding Ensolite padding often provides better visualization of extremity than does a circumferential wrap.

4. Apply a U-shaped blanket roll or pillow splint.
5. During transport, elevate the limb above the level of the heart, with the victim supine on a backboard if possible.

Talus and Calcaneus

Signs and Symptoms

1. Fracture of the calcaneus and talus during a fall or jump from a significant height when the victim lands on his or her feet
2. With calcaneus fracture, significant heel pain, deformity, and crepitus immediately evident after the boot is removed
3. Severe swelling within a couple of hours
4. Examine victim for possible lumbar spine fractures
5. With talus fracture, it may be impossible to differentiate clinically from ankle fracture:
   a. Occurs when the foot is forced into maximum dorsiflexion
   b. Tenderness and swelling distal to or at the level of the malleoli
6. With ankle fracture, tenderness and deformity at the level of the malleoli
7. Fractures of other tarsal bones, while exceedingly rare, defined by localizing the tenderness to a specific site

Treatment

1. Apply a short-leg splint with extra padding for all these fractures.
2. Elevate the limb during transportation.
3. If a talus fracture is suspected, expedite evacuation of the victim because posttraumatic necrosis of the talar body is a common complication.

Metatarsal

Fracture at the base of a metatarsal often occurs in combination with a midfoot dislocation. Fractures frequently occur across the entire midfoot joint and are often associated with fractures at the bases of the second and fifth metatarsals. They usually occur with axial loading of the foot while it is in maximum plantarflexion.

Metatarsal shaft fractures occur with crush injuries and with falls or jumps from moderate heights. Midshaft metatarsal fracture also occurs as a stress, or so-called march, fracture. This injury is often the result of prolonged hiking or running.

Signs and Symptoms
1. With metatarsal base fracture
   a. Midfoot pain and swelling
   b. Once the shoe is removed, crepitus and tenderness at the base of the metatarsal
   c. Generally, overall alignment of the foot maintained, but instability is revealed with stressing the midfoot by stabilizing the heel and placing stress across the forefoot in the varus and valgus directions
2. With metatarsal shaft fracture
   a. Dull pain at the midshaft of a metatarsal (often the second or fifth) converted to more severe pain with associated crepitus by a jump from a log or rock
   b. Hallmarks: pain, localized tenderness

Treatment
1. For metatarsal base fracture, place the foot in a well-padded posterior splint and elevate.
2. Do not allow a victim with a suspected midfoot fracture/dislocation to ambulate because swelling will intensify and further injury to the midfoot may result. Beware of compartment syndrome with midfoot or Lisfranc's fracture/dislocation.
3. For metatarsal shaft fracture, manage temporarily by having the victim wear a stiff-soled boot or orthotic insert. If fracture instability or extreme pain is present, apply a short-leg splint and allow no further weight bearing.

Phalanx

The great toe phalanx fracture is a significant problem functionally because of the necessary force placed on the great toe during the toe-off phase of weight bearing. A toe phalanx can be fractured by a crush injury or by having a heavy object drop onto the foot. This injury can be prevented by the use of a hard-toed boot.

Signs and Symptoms
1. Pain
2. Ecchymosis
3. Swelling

Treatment
1. Manage any phalanx fracture by taping the toe to an adjacent uninjured toe with cotton placed in between.
2. Be aware that a stiff-soled boot minimizes the discomfort accompanying weight bearing.

▶ LOWER EXTREMITY DISLOCATIONS

Hip

Posterior hip dislocation is produced by axial loading of the femur with the limb in relative adduction. This injury occurs most commonly with the hip and knee flexed and force applied to the anterior knee or proximal leg. Dislocation may also occur when a large force is applied to the sole of the foot with the knee in extension.

Signs and Symptoms
1. With posterior dislocation, severe pain around the hip
2. Affected limb apparently shortened, adducted, and internally rotated with any hip motion increasing the pain
3. Not clinically possible to determine presence of an associated acetabular fracture
4. With rare case of anterior dislocation, limb abducted and flexed and severely externally rotated. Anterior dislocation is generally produced by wide abduction of the hip from a significant force

Treatment
1. Place the victim in a supine position, and perform a complete survey of all organ systems. Examine the distal limb carefully for associated fracture(s), and perform a careful sensory and motor examination.
2. When the victim is any distance from definitive care, attempt closed reduction.
   a. Place the victim on a flat, hard surface.
   b. Provide analgesia with a narcotic, benzodiazepine, or both if available.
   c. Have an assistant stabilize the pelvis by placing both palms on the anterior iliac crests. Bend the victim's knee, and apply upward linear traction in line with the thigh (with an anterior dislocation) and with the hip flexed 30 degrees (with a posterior dislocation) (Fig. 18-38). If an assistant is available, try pulling a lateral force on the proximal thigh during longitudinal traction.
3. If this maneuver fails to reduce the hip, expedite evacuation because a direct relationship exists between the time to reduction and the incidence of osteonecrosis of the femoral head.

Knee

The tibia may be dislocated in any of four directions relative to the distal femur. The most common direction is anterior (tibia anterior to the femur). This injury represents a true emergency because of the high incidence of associated vascular injury,

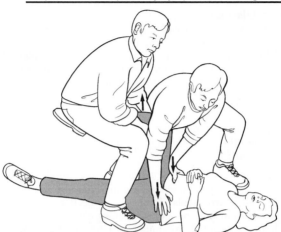

Figure 18-38. Reduction of dislocated hip.

which occurs because of tethering of the popliteal vessels along the posterior border of the tibia by the soleus fascia. Be aware of a spontaneously reduced knee dislocation. If there is a complete rupture of the anterior and posterior cruciate ligaments, assume dislocation with spontaneous reduction until proven otherwise. These injuries may result in intimal tears of the popliteal artery and can lead to loss of a limb.

Signs and Symptoms
1. Knee dislocation obvious because of the amount of deformity involved
2. Intimal flap tears of the popliteal artery, possibly producing delayed arterial thrombosis

Treatment
1. When this injury is suspected, perform a careful neurocirculatory screening examination. Intact distal pulses do not definitively rule out arterial injury.
2. After the initial examination, apply linear traction to the lower limb to reduce the knee. This is generally successful regardless of the direction of dislocation.
3. Immediate evacuation is indicated.
4. Emergency angiography may be indicated.
5. Apply a posterior splint to the limb, and transport the victim on a backboard.
6. Be vigilant for an arterial injury or compartment syndrome. If either is suspected, arrange for emergency evacuation.

Patella Dislocation

Because of the increased femorotibial angle in a female, patella dislocation is much more common in women. Generalized ligamentous laxity may predispose to this problem. Dislocation of the kneecap may result from a twisting injury or asymmetric quadriceps contraction during a fall.

Signs and Symptoms
1. Pain
2. Malposition of patella
3. Large effusion in a spontaneously reduced patella dislocation

Treatment
1. The patella lies lateral to the articular distal femur. Although neurovascular injury rarely occurs in association with this injury, conduct a screening examination.
2. Reduce the patella by simply straightening the knee.
3. If this is not successful, apply gentle pressure to the patella to push it back up onto the distal femoral articular groove.
4. Apply a knee splint with the joint in extension. Encourage the victim to avoid weight bearing, but if this is not possible, be aware that further damage is unlikely.
5. Keep the victim's knee in extension until definitive care can be obtained.
6. Radiography is ultimately required to rule out osteochondral fracture, which is frequently associated with an acute injury.

Ankle

Signs and Symptoms
1. Ankle dislocation is almost always accompanied by fracture(s) of one or both malleoli. This may involve the posterior malleolus from an avulsion fracture of the posterior talofibular ligament ("trimalleolar" fracture/dislocation).
2. Swelling
3. Pain
4. Severe deformity

Treatment
1. Align the ankle joint by grasping the victim's posterior heel, applying traction with the knee bent (to relax the gastrocnemius-soleus complex), and bringing the foot into alignment with the distal tibia.
2. After this maneuver, reexamine the foot, dress any wounds, and apply a posterior splint. Note that a U-shaped blanket roll or pillow splint can also be applied.
3. During transport, keep the limb elevated.

4. Use snow or ice to create cold compresses.
5. This type of inversion injury is infrequently associated with fracture at the insertion of the peroneus brevis tendon. You may identify the presence of this injury with point tenderness at the base of the fifth metatarsal, but a radiograph is required for definitive diagnosis. Early management is the same as for a sprain.

Hindfoot

Signs and Symptoms
Calcaneus dislocated medially or laterally relative to the talus, the latter being slightly more common

Treatment
1. Attempt a reduction if it will be more than 3 hours until the victim can be transported to a definitive care center.
2. If no other injuries are apparent, give the victim a sedative during reduction.
3. Medial dislocation is reduced more easily than lateral dislocation, in which the posterior tibial tendon frequently becomes displaced onto the lateral neck of the talus, blocking the reduction. In either case, the maneuver is the same.
   a. Grasp the heel with the victim's knee flexed (relaxing the gastrocnemius-soleus complex) and apply linear traction to bring the heel over the ankle joint.
   b. Be aware that this maneuver is generally successful for medial dislocation, but lateral dislocation often requires open reduction.
4. After you attempt reduction, apply a posterior splint, U-shaped blanket roll, or pillow splint.
5. Make sure the limb is elevated.
6. Even if the reduction is successful, do not allow the victim to bear weight until definitive care is obtained.

Midfoot

Midfoot (Lisfranc's) dislocation is generally associated with one or more fractures at the base of the metatarsals, usually the second and fifth metatarsals. Midfoot dislocation occurs with axial loading of the foot in maximal plantarflexion.

Signs and Symptoms
1. Forefoot generally displaced laterally relative to the midfoot when the injury is initially unstable; more often the foot is normally aligned.
2. Significant swelling with tenderness at the base of the second and fifth metatarsals

3. Instability and crepitus, with dorsoplantar-oriented force frequent

Treatment
1. After the neurocirculatory examination, stress the forefoot by stabilizing the heel and applying a varus- and valgus-directed force. If the forefoot is unstable and associated with significant swelling, pain, or crepitus, consider a mid-foot dislocation to be present.
2. Apply a short-leg (posterior or U-shaped) splint.
3. Elevate the foot during transport.
4. Do not allow the victim to bear weight.

Metatarsophalangeal and Interphalangeal Joints
Metatarsophalangeal joint dislocation of a toe is relatively uncommon but can occur in the great toe with moderate axial force. An injury of this type at the great toe may be associated with a fracture of the metatarsal or phalanx; the dislocation is generally distal.

The lesser metatarsophalangeal joints are generally dislocated laterally or medially. The most common mechanism for this injury is striking unshod toes on immovable objects.

Signs and Symptoms
1. Open fracture
2. Pain
3. Swelling
4. Ecchymosis

Treatment
1. Because this may be an open fracture, perform a careful inspection of the foot.
2. Relocate the toe by applying linear traction with the victim supine and using the weight of the foot as countertraction.
3. Also, consider reduction of an interphalangeal joint by applying linear traction with gentle manipulation.
4. Once reduced, tape the injured toe to the adjacent toe for 1 to 3 weeks.
5. Have the victim wear a protective boot with a stiff sole and deep toe box.

Firearm and Arrow Injuries/Fishhook Injury

19

▶ FIREARM INJURY

Injuries caused by firearms differ in severity and type according to velocity of the bullet, whether fragmentation occurs, creation of a permanent cavity, presence of powder burns, and type of tissue struck.

General Treatment

1. Follow the basic principles of trauma care and resuscitation including airway, breathing, circulation, control of bleeding, immobilization of the spine and fractured extremities, wound care, and stabilization of the victim for transport (see Chapter 12).
2. Remove the weapon from the vicinity where you are giving medical care. It may be wise to also remove the ammunition and open the firing chamber.
3. Perform endotracheal intubation as soon as possible if the victim has a neck wound and expanding hematoma. If endotracheal intubation is not possible and the airway becomes obstructed, perform a cricothyrotomy.
4. Provide immediate relief of a tension pneumothorax with a needle or tube thoracostomy, or occlusion of a sucking chest wound with petrolatum-impregnated gauze.
5. Control external bleeding by direct pressure and compression wraps.
6. Treat for shock and hypothermia.
7. Do not perform wide débridement of normal-appearing tissue.
8. Monitor the neurovascular status of an extremity wound; keep the extremity elevated to minimize swelling.
9. Remember that the path of the bullet cannot reliably be determined by connecting the entrance and exit wounds.
10. Removal of the bullet or bullet fragments is not necessary unless the bullet is intravascular, intraarticular, or in contact with nervous tissue.
11. Use forceps to remove from the skin any shotgun pellets that have minimal penetration.
12. For powder burns, remove as much of the powder residue as possible with a scrub brush because the powder will tattoo the skin if left in place.

217

▶ ARROW INJURY

Arrowheads used for hunting are designed to inflict injury by lacerating tissue and blood vessels, causing bleeding and shock.

General Treatment

1. Follow the same treatment principles of trauma care and resuscitation as for a firearm injury.
2. Irrigate lacerations inflicted by arrows and remove any foreign material. Close the wound primarily following the guidelines in Chapter 20.
3. Victims pierced by an arrow should be stabilized, and the arrow should be left in place during transport, if possible. Attempts to remove the arrow by pulling it out or pushing it through the wound may cause more injury. Cut the shaft of the arrow and leave about 10 cm (3 or 4 inches) protruding from the wound to make transport easier, if this can be accomplished with a minimum of arrow movement.
4. Fix the portion of the arrow that remains in the wound with a stack of gauze pads or with cloth and tape.
5. Transfer the victim as quickly as possible to a medical care facility for removal of the arrow under controlled conditions.

▶ FISHHOOK INJURY

Fishhooks have a barb or multiple barbs just proximal to the tip that are curved so that the more force that is applied to the hook, the deeper it penetrates. The barb does not allow the hook to be backed out.

General Treatment

1. Clean the skin surrounding the entry point with an antiseptic or with soap and water.
2. Remove the hook using one of the following techniques:
   a. Pass a string or shoelace through and around the bend of the hook; the hook can then be yanked from the skin while the shank of the hook is pressed against the skin surface to disengage the barb (Fig. 19-1). Wear eye protection and be certain that no one is in striking range of a flying hook.
   b. With a steady, firm motion, push the hook through the skin so that the barb completely appears. Cut off the barb or the shaft, and pull the remainder of the hook back out of the skin (Fig. 19-2). When cutting off the barb, take care to wear eye protection and look away at the moment of cutting.

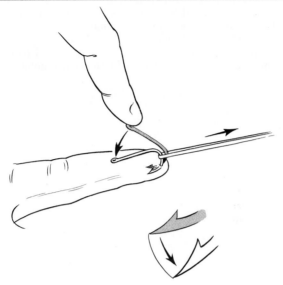

Figure 19-1.   Fishhook removal.

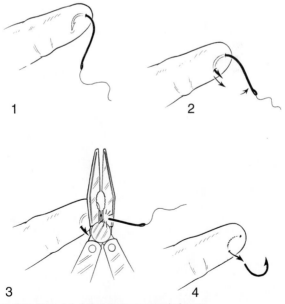

Figure 19-2.   Removal of a fishhook that has penetrated a fingertip.

3. Irrigate the wound with saline solution or water. Inspect the wound daily for signs of infection.
4. For a fishhook embedded in the eye, leave it in place and secure it with tape. Cover the eye with a metal patch or cup, and transport the victim to an ophthalmologist for definitive care.

Wounds (Lacerations and Abrasions) and Dressings

20

▶ **DEFINITIONS**

A laceration, although the most obvious sign of trauma, is rarely life threatening. It represents an injury to the integument and may overlie an occult injury such as a fracture or may extend into the joint space.

General Treatment

The goals of wilderness wound management are to control bleeding, minimize infection, promote healing, and decrease the need for evacuation. Five specific steps should be followed: examination, anesthesia, cleaning and débridement, wound closure or packing, and bandaging (Box 20-1).

Examination

1. For an extremity injury, evaluate distal neurovascular function before administering local anesthesia.
   a. For wrist and hand lacerations, palpate the radial and ulnar pulses.
   b. Compare capillary refill, color, and temperature of each finger to the corresponding finger on the uninjured hand.
   c. Assess sensation of the radial and ulnar aspects of each finger to sharp pain and two-point discrimination.
2. Explore the wound in good light conditions for tendon, muscle, or nerve injury; also look for foreign material. Test the motor function of each joint against resistance by isolating the joint and asking the victim to flex and extend the digit against resistance. A tendon that is 75% lacerated can still have function, but its function may be decreased when it is offered resistance and more painful during movement compared with the uninjured finger on the opposite hand.

▶ **ANESTHESIA**

Topical Anesthesia

1. Mix equal parts of tetracaine 0.5%, adrenaline (epinephrine) 1:2000, and cocaine 11.8% (TAC), and allow the mixture to soak into a 2- × 2-inch sterile gauze pad. Place this directly around and in the wound for 7 to 10 minutes. The maximum dose of the solution is 2 to 5 mL for adults.

Box 20-1. First-Aid Supplies for Wound and Abrasion Care

WOUND MANAGEMENT
10- to 15-mL irrigation syringe with an 18-gauge catheter tip
1 fluid oz povidone-iodine solution USP 10% (Betadine)
Wound closure strips ¼ × 4 inches
Tincture of benzoin
Polysporin, mupirocin, bacitracin, or other antiseptic ointment
Tweezers
Sterile surgical gloves
4- × 4-inch sterile dressings
Nonadherent sterile dressing (Aquaphor, Xeroform, Adaptic, Telfa)
Elastic conforming bandage
Assorted adhesive bandages
Tape
Surgical stapler, suture material, and suturing supplies
Dermabond (2-octyl cyanoacrylate) tissue glue

ABRASION MANAGEMENT
First-aid cleansing pads, 2% to 4% liquid lidocaine, viscous lidocaine jelly
Surgical scrub brush
Spenco 2nd Skin or other nonadherent dressing
Conforming woven bandage or nonwoven adhesive knit bandage
Aloe vera gel
Polysporin, mupirocin, bacitracin, or other antibiotic/antiseptic ointment
Tape

---

2. Do not use TAC on the ear, tip of the nose, or penis, and use it only with caution on highly permeable tissue such as mucous membranes. Eliminating the cocaine, increasing the concentration of tetracaine to 1.87%, and decreasing the concentration of adrenaline to 1:15,000 may achieve an equivalent level of anesthesia.

Local Anesthesia

1. Infiltrate the wound with 1% lidocaine (Xylocaine) without epinephrine or 0.25% bupivacaine (Marcaine) using a 25-gauge needle and syringe.
2. The adult dose of lidocaine should not exceed 300 to 400 mg (30 to 40 mL). The maximum dose for a child is 4 mg/kg or 0.4 mL/kg of a 1% solution.
3. Buffering lidocaine reduces the pain of local anesthetic infiltration. To buffer, add 1 mL of sodium bicarbonate

(1 mEq/mL solution) to 10 mL 1% lidocaine. Once buffered, the shelf life of the product is greatly reduced; discard
the solution after 24 hours.
4. Alternative anesthetic strategies include the following:
   a. Diphenhydramine (Benadryl) has anesthetic properties
      similar to, but less potent than, those of lidocaine. Dilute
      a 50-mg (1-mL) vial in a syringe with 4 mL normal saline
      (NS) solution to produce a 1% solution. Perform local
      infiltration as usual.
   b. Use NS solution alone as the injecting agent. This may
      provide enough anesthesia to suture a small wound.
   c. Place ice directly over the wound to provide a short
      period of decreased pain sensation.

▶ CLEANING AND DÉBRIDEMENT

1. Perform wound cleansing to remove as much bacteria, dirt,
   and damaged tissue as possible. The best method is to use a
   10- to 15-mL syringe with an 18-gauge catheter attached to
   the end as a "squirt gun" to deliver a high-pressure stream.
   If a splash shield is available, use it. Wear eye protection.
2. Make sure the irrigating solution is clean and nontoxic to the
   tissues. Sterile NS solution, disinfected tap water, and 1%
   povidone-iodine solution (not "scrub") are all suitable for
   irrigation.
3. In addition to a vigorous soap and water scrub, use benzalkonium chloride to cleanse wounds inflicted by animals
   suspected of being rabid (see Chapter 41). The quantity of
   irrigation fluid should be at least 400 mL.

▶ IRRIGATION METHOD

1. Draw the irrigation solution into a 10- to 15-ml syringe
   and attach an 18-gauge catheter tip.
2. Hold the syringe so the catheter tip is 2.5 to 5 cm (1 to
   2 inches) above the wound and perpendicular to the skin
   surface. Push down forcefully on the plunger while prying
   open the edges of the wound with your fingers, and squirt the
   solution into the wound (Fig. 20-1A). Be careful to avoid
   being splashed by the irrigant after it hits the skin (put on a
   pair of sunglasses or goggles to protect your eyes from the
   spray or place the catheter through the bottom of an upside
   down plastic or Styrofoam cup, which comprises an improvised splash shield).
3. Repeat this procedure until you have irrigated the wound
   with at least 400 mL of solution.
4. Remove any residual debris or devitalized tissue with
   a tweezers, scissors, knife, or any other sharp object.

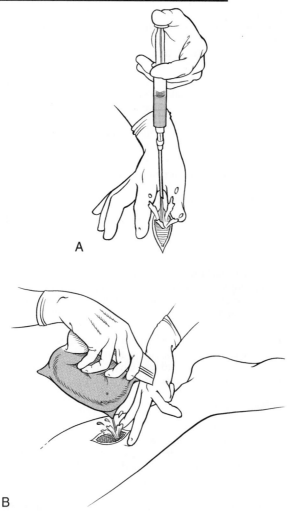

Figure 20-1. Wound irrigation. **A,** Syringe. **B,** Plastic bag.

Any dirt left in a wound increases the likelihood of infection.
5. If the wound edges are macerated, crushed, or necrotic, perform sharp débridement.
6. Improvised wound irrigation can be performed with a puncturable container to hold water such as a sandwich or

garbage bag and a safety pin or 18-gauge needle. Fill the bag with irrigation solution and puncture the bottom of the bag with the safety pin. Enlarge the hole if necessary by puncturing it a second time. Hold the bag just above the wound and squeeze the top firmly to begin irrigating (see Fig. 20-1B). Understand that the pressure generated by this method is far less than that delivered by a syringe and catheter.

▶ DEFINITIVE WOUND CARE

Lacerations that are not at high risk for infection can be safely closed in the backcountry. Time is a critical factor, however, and the longer closure is delayed, the more likely the wound is to become infected after it is closed. The period for safely closing a wound depends on its location. Lacerations on the extremity should be closed within 8 hours of injury. Lacerations on the torso should be closed within 12 hours, whereas wounds on the face and scalp should be closed within 24 hours.

High-Risk Wounds

High-risk wounds that should not be closed in the backcountry include animal or human bites to the hand, wrist, or foot, over a major joint, or through the cheek; any cat bite or scratch wound; deep puncture wounds; deep wounds on the hand or foot; wounds that contain a large amount of crushed or devitalized tissue; and wounds that are older than the periods described earlier.

Treatment
1. Pack the wound open with saline- or water-moistened gauze dressings, after irrigation and débridement.
2. Cover the packed wound with a conforming bandage, and splint the extremity in an elevated position.
3. Start the victim on an immediate course of antibiotic therapy. Options include amoxicillin-clavulanate, 500 mg q6h; cephalexin, 500 mg q6h; or penicillin, 500 mg combined with dicloxacillin, 500 mg q6h.
4. Change the packing at least once a day.
5. Close the wound with sutures, staples, or tape after 4 to 5 days if there is no sign of infection (delayed primary closure).

Low-Risk Wounds

Treatment
Options for closing a wound in the backcountry include taping, suturing, stapling, gluing, and hair-tying.

1. Wound taping: Wound closure tape strips are stronger, longer, stickier, and more porous than are butterfly bandages.
   a. Achieve hemostasis, and dry the wound edges.
   b. Clip off hair near the wound with a scissors so that tape will adhere better. Hair farther from the wound edge can be shaved. Avoid shaving hair directly adjacent to the wound edge because shaving abrades the skin and increases the potential for infection.
   c. Apply a thin layer of tincture of benzoin evenly along both sides of the wound, and allow it to dry (Fig. 20-2A) so that it is tacky, not slippery.
   d. Secure one half of the tape to one side of the wound. Oppose the other wound edge with a finger while using the free end of the tape as a handle to help pull the wound closed (see Fig. 20-2B). Avoid squeezing the wound edges tightly together. They should just touch. Attach the other end of the tape to the skin.
   e. Allow the tape to overlap the wound edge by 2 to 3 cm (¾ to 1¼ inches) on each side, and space the strips 2 to 3 mm apart to allow drainage.
   f. Place cross-stays of tape perpendicular to and over the tape ends to prevent them from peeling off (see Fig. 20-2C).
   g. Note that wound closure strips can be improvised from duct tape or other self-adhering tape. Cut 1-cm (½-inch) strips, and then punch tiny holes along the length of the tape with a safety pin to allow drainage.
2. Improvised wound tape: If no tape is available, glue strips of cloth or nylon from your clothes, pack, or tent to the skin with a "super glue."
   a. Cut 1-cm (½-inch) strips of material, and then punch tiny holes along the length of the material with a safety pin to allow drainage.
   b. Place a drop of glue on the end of material only and hold it on the skin until it dries.
   c. Pull the wound closed, and glue the other end of the material to the skin on the other side of the wound.
   d. Avoid getting any glue into the wound. The glue is generally safe on intact skin but should not be used on the face.
   e. Expect the strips to fall off after about 3 days. The strips can be reapplied with fresh glue.
3. Hair-tying a scalp laceration (assumes the victim has enough hair):
   a. Take a piece of heavy suture material (0-silk works best), dental floss, sewing thread, or thin string and lay it on top of and parallel to the wound (Fig. 20-3A).

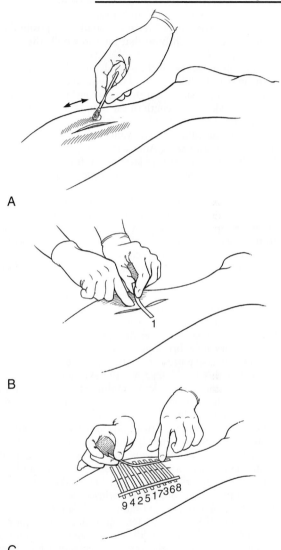

A

B

C

Figure 20-2.   A to C, Wound taping.

   b. Twirl a few strands of hair on each side of the wound, and then cross them over the wound in opposite directions and pull tightly so that the force pulls the wound edges together.
   c. Have an assistant tie the strands of hair together with the material while you hold the wound closed. A square knot works best. Repeat this technique as many times as needed, along the length of the wound, to close the laceration (see Fig. 20-3B).
4. Gluing: Dermabond (2-octyl cyanoacrylate) is approved by the U.S. Food and Drug Administration (FDA) as a topical skin adhesive to repair skin lacerations. It is packaged for a single-use application. Tissue glue is ideal for backcountry use because it precludes the need for topical anesthesia, is easy to use, reduces the risk of needlestick injury, and takes up less room in a backpack than does a conventional suture kit. When applied to the skin surface, tissue glue provides strong tissue support and peels off in 4 to 5 days without leaving evidence of its presence.
   a. Irrigate the wound with copious amounts of disinfected water.
   b. Control any bleeding with direct pressure.
   c. Once hemostasis is obtained, approximate the wound edges using fingers or forceps.
   d. Paint the tissue glue over the apposed wound edges using a very light brushing motion of the applicator tip. Avoid excessive pressure of the applicator on the tissue because this could separate the skin edges and allow glue into the wound. Apply multiple thin layers (at least three), allowing the glue to dry between each application (about 2 minutes).
   e. Glue can be removed from unwanted surfaces with acetone or loosened from skin with petrolatum jelly.
   f. Petroleum-based ointments and salves including antibiotic ointments should not be used on the wound after gluing because these substances can weaken the polymerized film and cause wound dehiscence.
5. Skin staples: Skin staples and sutures are best for large gaping cuts, wounds that are under tension or that cross a joint, or any other wounds that are difficult to keep closed with tape.
   a. Skin stapling is a relatively fast technique for closing wounds and is ideal for use in the wilderness, when evacuation to a medical facility is not readily available.
   b. Staples are as strong as sutures, and, more importantly, they produce less inflammatory response and have less chance of seeding a wound infection.

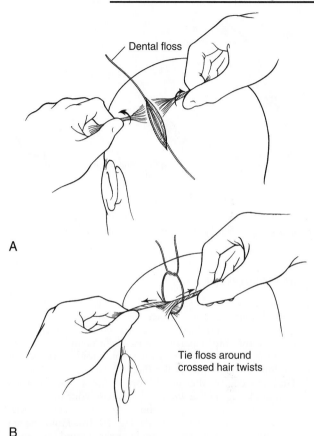

Dental floss

A

Tie floss around
crossed hair twists

B

Figure 20-3. A and B, Scalp laceration closed using dental floss.

c. When used appropriately, staples yield an excellent cosmetic outcome.
d. Staples should not be used on the feet, hands, or face or if the laceration extends into tendons or muscles.
e. Staples are left in place for the same length of time as are sutures in similar anatomic sites.
f. Staple removal requires a special device that is provided by each manufacturer.

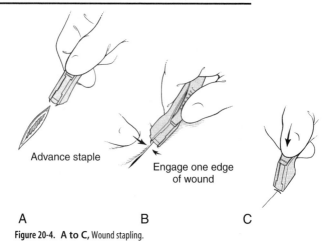

Advance staple

Engage one edge
of wound

A   B   C

Figure 20-4. A to C, Wound stapling.

▶ **STAPLING TECHNIQUE**

1. Stapling devices have evolved significantly in the past several years. A good choice for backcountry use is the 3M Precise Disposable Skin Stapler with 25 staples.
2. Squeeze the stapler partway until it clicks and you feel resistance. The two points of the staple should now be protruding out from the stapler (Fig. 20-4A).
3. Grab one edge of the cut with one of the staples and use it as a hook to pull the wound closed. Use your index finger on the other hand to push the other wound edge in until the wound edges just meet (see Fig. 20-4B). Hold the stapler upright at a 90-degree angle to the wound, and make sure that the stapler is positioned evenly over the cut so that it does not overlap one wound edge more than the other. Gently and evenly squeeze the stapler with your thumb as shown to advance the staple into the tissue (see Fig. 20-4C).
4. Once the staple is seated, relax your thumb pressure fully on the stapler and back out the stapler to disengage it.

▶ **WOUND OINTMENT DRESSING AND BANDAGING**

1. The best dressing is one that does not stick to the wound. Representative dressings are Aquaphor, Xeroform, Adaptic, and Telfa.
2. Apply an antiseptic ointment such as bacitracin or mupirocin to the surface of the wound before bandaging unless the

wound was closed with glue. Honey applied topically on cutaneous wounds has been found to reduce infection and promote wound healing and is a reasonable substitute for a commercial ointment. The antimicrobial properties of honey are attributed to its hypertonicity, low pH, a thermolabile substance called inhibine, and enzymes such as catalase. Inhibines in honey include hydrogen peroxide, flavonoids, and phenolic acids.

3. A bandage is a rolled gauze elastic wrap that secures a dressing in place. A triangular bandage, which is often used to create a sling, can be folded two to three times into a strap, called a cravat (Fig. 20-5). Cravat dressings are useful for applying pressure to a wound that is bleeding in order to promote hemostasis.

   a. Scalp bandaging—wounds to the scalp often require a dressing placed over hair, making adhesion very difficult. The dressing can be secured with a triangular bandage in a method that allows for considerable tension should pressure be necessary to stop bleeding (Fig. 20-6).

   b. Face and ear bandaging—a wound to the face or the pinna of the ear may require a compression dressing. If so,

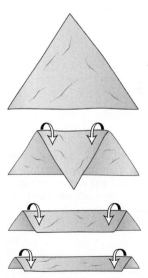

Figure 20-5. Making a cravat from a triangular bandage. (Redrawn from Auerbach PS: Medicine for the Outdoors, 4th ed. Guilford, CT, Lyons Press, 2003, p 262.)

1. Drape a triangular bandage just over the eyes and fold the edge 1 inch under to form a hem. Allow the apex to drop over the back of the neck.

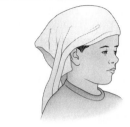

2. Cross the free ends over the back of the head and tie in a half-knot.

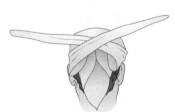

3. Bring the free ends to the front of the head and tie a complete knot. At the posterior aspect of the head, tuck the apex into the half-knot.

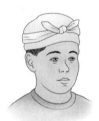

Figure 20-6. Scalp bandaging. (Redrawn from Auerbach PS: Medicine for the Outdoors, 4th ed. Guilford, CT, Lyons Press, 2003, p 265.)

gauze should be placed both anterior and posterior to the ear to allow it to maintain its natural curvature. A cravat is used to secure the dressing (see Fig. 23-9). This method may be used for wounds anywhere along the side of the head or under the chin.

▶ **DEFINITION**

An abrasion is an area of scraped or denuded skin that is often embedded with dirt, gravel, and other debris, which can result in scarring or infection.

General Treatment (see Box 20-1)

1. Apply a topical anesthetic such as 2% to 4% lidocaine or viscous lidocaine jelly over the wound and let it sit for 5 to 10 minutes, or wipe the area with a lidocaine-containing cleansing pad.
2. Vigorously scrub the abrasion with a surgical brush or cleansing pad until all foreign material is removed.
3. Use tweezers to pick out any embedded particles. Irrigate the abrasion with NS solution or water.
4. Apply a thin layer of topical antiseptic ointment, aloe vera gel, or honey to the abrasion.
5. Cover with a nonadherent protective dressing and secure it in place with a bandage. Spenco 2nd Skin works well because it soothes and cools the wound while providing an ideal healing environment. The dressing can also be secured with a woven or nonwoven adhesive knit bandage and left in place for several days, as long as there is no sign of infection.

Sprains and Strains

21

▶ DEFINITIONS

A sprain is the stretching or tearing of ligaments that attach one bone to another. Symptoms include tenderness at the site, swelling, ecchymosis, and pain with movement. Because these symptoms are also present with a fracture, it may be difficult to differentiate between the two.

A strain is an injury to a muscle or its tendon. Strains often result from overexertion or lifting and pulling a heavy object without using good body mechanics. Symptoms are initially the same as for sprains.

▶ GENERAL TREATMENT

1. First-aid treatment for sprain and strain injuries is summarized by the acronym R-I-C-E-S: rest, ice, compression, elevation, and stabilization. Maintain R-I-C-E-S for the first 72 hours after any injury.
   a. Rest. Rest takes the stress off the injured joint and prevents further ligament and tendon damage.
   b. Ice. Ice reduces swelling and eases pain. For ice or cold therapy to be effective, apply ice early and for up to 20 minutes at least three or four times a day, followed by compression bandaging. If a compression wrap is not applied after ice therapy, the joint will swell as soon as the ice is removed.
   c. Compression. A compression wrap prevents swelling and provides some support. Make the wrap by placing some padding (socks, gloves, pieces of Ensolite pad) over the sprained joint and then wrapping it with an elastic bandage. Wrap from distal to proximal. Make sure the wrap is comfortably tight. Monitor the extremity for numbness, tingling, or increased pain, which may indicate that the compression wrap is too tight and should be loosened.
   d. Elevation. Elevate the injured joint above the level of the heart as much as possible to reduce swelling.
   e. Stabilization. Tape or splint the injured part to prevent further injury.
2. Administer an oral nonsteroidal antiinflammatory drug (NSAID) such as ibuprofen, 600 to 800 mg q8h, to reduce pain and inflammation.

235

▶ **DISORDERS**

Ankle Sprain

Signs and Symptoms

1. Ankle sprain: the most commonly injured ligaments are on the lateral aspect of the joint (anterior and posterior talofibular and calcaneofibular ligaments) (Fig. 21-1).

2. A syndesmosis injury, or "high ankle sprain," may also occur. Tenderness occurs over the anterior tibiofibular and deltoid ligaments. A positive squeeze test, in which pain radiates through the interosseous membrane with compression of the tibia against the fibula, exists. The fibula may be fractured. Symptoms of proximal fibular fracture include associated proximal fibular tenderness or crepitus.

3. A midfoot sprain can occur with associated tarsometatarsal fracture (Lisfranc's injury). These injuries present as severe pain and marked swelling along the entire midfoot. This can be a problematic injury associated with compartment syndrome of the foot. Keep the victim non–weight bearing with elevation. Use ice if available. Evacuate the victim for definitive orthopedic reduction.

4. Differentiate ankle sprain from fractures (see also Chapter 18):
   a. Ankle fracture: the victim is unable to bear weight or often has bony tenderness to palpation at the posterior edge or tip of the lateral or medial malleolus.

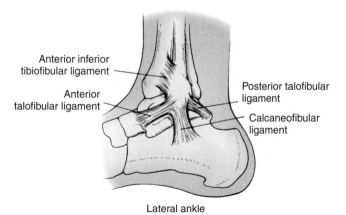

Anterior inferior tibiofibular ligament

Anterior talofibular ligament

Posterior talofibular ligament

Calcaneofibular ligament

Lateral ankle

Figure 21-1. Ligament complexes of the ankle.

b. Foot fracture: the victim is unable to bear weight and often has point tenderness to palpation at the base of the fifth metatarsal or navicular bone. Other metatarsal and phalanx fractures can also occur with associated tenderness.

Treatment
1. Use R-I-C-E-S therapy.
2. If the victim can walk, tape the ankle for support with an "open basket cross-weave stirrup pattern" to prevent further injury (Fig. 21-2). A SAM splint can also be wrapped around the foot and ankle with the shoe in place and secured with tape (Fig. 21-3).
3. To more securely tape an ankle:
   a. Apply an adhesive tape anchor strip halfway around the lower leg about 15 cm (6 inches) above the malleoli.

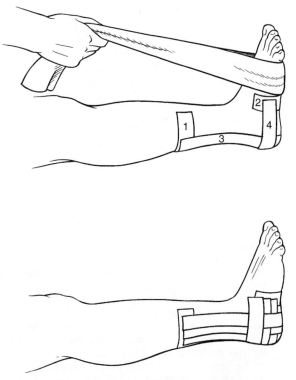

Figure 21-2. Sprained ankle taped using an "open basket cross-weave stirrup pattern."

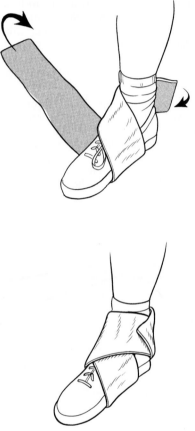

Figure 21-3. SAM splint on ankle.

Leave a 2.5- to 5-cm (1- to 2-inch) gap in front to allow for swelling.
b. Apply an additional anchor strip at the instep of the foot. Leave a 1- to 2-inch gap on the top of the foot.
c. Apply the first of five stirrup strips. Begin on the inside of the upper anchor, and wrap a piece of tape down the inside of the leg, over the inside medial malleolus, across the bottom of the foot, and up the outside part of the leg over the lateral malleolus, ending at the outer aspect of the upper anchor. Apply proper tension to prevent the ankle from inverting.

d. Apply the first of six to eight interconnecting horseshoe strips. Begin at the anchor on the inside of the foot, and wrap below the medial malleolus around the heel, below the lateral malleolus, and ending at the anchor on the outer part of the foot.

e. Repeat steps c and d. Remember to overlap the tape one-half its width. These interlocking strips should provide excellent support for a walking person. At the end of these vertical and horizontal strips, a 1- to 2-inch gap on the top of the foot and ankle will allow for swelling.

f. On both sides, secure the tape ends with two vertical strips of tape running from the foot anchor to the calf anchor.

g. Beginning at the toes, wrap an elastic rolled bandage around the foot and ankle.

Acute Rupture of the Peroneal Retinaculum

Signs and Symptoms
1. Swelling posterior to the lateral malleolus extending proximally over the peroneal tendon
2. Audible and tactile "click" or "snap" over the lateral malleolus with walking
3. Focal tenderness along the posterior edge of the lateral malleolus

Treatment
1. Immobilization (see earlier discussion on ankle sprain)
2. Partial weight bearing with improvised crutch or ski pole assist
3. Orthopedic follow-up
4. Often requires surgical repair if immobilization is ineffective

Ruptured Achilles Tendon

This injury is generally caused by an eccentric stress such as suddenly running hard from a standing position or trying to jump over an obstacle.

Signs and Symptoms
1. An audible "pop," with a sensation similar to being kicked in the calf
2. Difficulty plantarflexing the foot, although the plantaris muscle can plantarflex the foot as well. The only reliable sign is Thompson's test.
3. Thompson's test: The victim is placed in a prone position with the foot hanging free. If there is no plantarflexion of the foot as the calf is squeezed, Thompson's test is positive.

4. Swelling of the distal calf
5. Sometimes, a palpable defect in the tendon 2 to 6 cm (1 to 2½ inches) proximal to its insertion can be appreciated within the first hour. After that, if there is significant bleeding, the defect can be more difficult to detect.

Treatment
1. If the tendon is strained and not completely torn or ruptured, follow R-I-C-E-S.
2. Have the victim gently stretch the tendon to keep it flexible, then gradually put weight on the foot, with walking as pain allows.
3. In-shoe, firm heel lifts should be used in both shoes. The goal of using a heel lift is to reduce the strain on the Achilles tendon while allowing one to remain mobile; to permit the tendon to be less stretched and relaxed while healing slowly occurs. Because tendons have no blood supply, this healing typically requires weeks or months, and the tendon can easily be re-injured if it is stressed during this time.
4. If the Achilles tendon is ruptured, walking will be difficult. Splint the ankle in slight plantarflexion and evacuate the victim. Surgery is generally necessary to repair the torn tendon.
5. Use improvised crutches.

Patellofemoral Syndrome

Patellofemoral syndrome encompasses many diagnoses also known as "anterior knee pain." These can include anterior fat pad syndrome, plica syndrome, patellofemoral maltracking, patellar instability, and chondromalacia patellae.

Signs and Symptoms
1. A dull, aching pain under the patella or in the center of the knee that is aggravated by climbing or descending a hill or by sitting for a long period with the knee bent (the "theater sign").
2. Swollen knee
3. Crepitus, often heard when knee is flexed and extended

Treatment
1. Apply ice, and allow the victim to rest.
2. Administer an NSAID, such as ibuprofen, 600 to 800 mg q8h.
3. Place a wide-supporting elastic band around the leg below the patella to help prevent pain during walking. This should not be overly tight.
4. Use two trekking or ski poles while hiking to help absorb impact and reduce pain.

5. Prevention is important to prevent future recurrences. The best prevention is aggressive lower extremity balancing (hamstring flexibility, hip abductor strengthening, and orthotics if pronated feet are present).

Iliotibial Band Syndrome
This is irritation of the connective tissue along the outside of the thigh.

Signs and Symptoms
1. Stinging pain along the outside of the knee aggravated by running downhill or jumping
2. Pain reproduced by pressing on the outside of the upper knee

Treatment
1. Apply ice and allow the victim to rest.
2. Administer an oral NSAID such as ibuprofen, 600 to 800 mg q8h.
3. Aggressive stretching.

Ligament Sprain
Twisting, rotating, hyperextending, or falling in an awkward position is more likely to produce a sprain injury to one of the major ligaments that support the knee than to create a fracture.

Terminology
ACL: anterior cruciate ligament
MCL: medial cruciate ligament
PCL: posterior cruciate ligament

Signs and Symptoms
1. An audible "pop" at the time of the injury is common with ACL injuries and less common with MCL and lateral collateral ligament (LCL) injuries.
2. Immediate pain that soon becomes a dull ache
3. Often marked swelling with joint effusion
4. For a severe sprain, instability of the knee while walking or turning
5. Severity based on percentage of ligament injured
   a. First-degree sprain: pain but no instability when the knee is stressed
   b. Second-degree sprain: pain and slight instability when the knee is stressed
   c. Third-degree sprain: significant instability, often less pain when the knee is stressed than with lower-grade sprains. A third-degree sprain is a completely torn ligament.

Treatment
1. For first-degree sprain, use R-I-C-E-S. Walking can usually be resumed with little or no additional support.
2. For second-degree sprain, use R-I-C-E-S. Ensure that the victim wears a knee immobilizer while walking. This device should be cylindrical and extend from midthigh to midcalf. Improvised materials that can be used include an Ensolite or Therm-a-Rest pad, life jacket, or internal-frame pack stays held in place with tape or bandannas (Fig. 21-4).
3. For third-degree sprain, use R-I-C-E-S. Do not allow the victim to walk without a knee immobilizer. Use improvised crutches or ski poles for additional support. If, after applying a knee immobilizer, the victim's knee still feels unstable and is prone to buckling with weight, evacuate the victim without allowing walking.

Knee Taping
For first- or second-degree sprains, the knee can be taped for added support while ambulating. Underwrap should not be used because adequate traction to support the joint can only be achieved by taping directly to the skin. Three-inch elastic tape is recommended (Fig. 21-5).

Torn Meniscus (Cartilage)
Menisci are crescent-shaped pieces of cartilage situated between the femur and tibia that act as shock absorbers for the knee. Partial or total tears of the meniscus often occur at the same time that ligaments are torn. They can also occur as an isolated injury with the following:
1. Significant axial compression (big ski jump landing flat on skis)
2. Squatting injuries (lifting up a heavy object from a squatting position or rotating/twisting while in the squatted position, especially in someone who may have an underlying knee ligament deficiency (i.e., old ACL injury).

Signs and Symptoms
1. Pain localized along the joint line after injury. Tenderness is usually medial, lateral, or posterior
2. Catching, clicking, or locking of the knee
3. Occasionally, joint painfully locked in a partially flexed position
4. Pain with squatting
5. Mild swelling

Treatment
1. Apply ice and allow the victim to rest.
2. Administer an oral NSAID such as ibuprofen, 600 to 800 mg q8h.

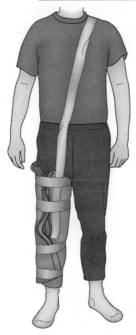

Figure 21-4. Functional knee and lower leg immobilizer. Wrap a sleeping pad around the lower leg from the midthigh to the foot. Fold the pad so that the top of the leg is not included in the splint. This provides better visualization of the extremity and leaves room for swelling. A full-length pad forms a very bulky splint and may need to be trimmed before rolling. Because of the conical shape of the lower extremity and the effects of gravity, foam pad lower extremity splints tend to work their way inferiorly when the victim ambulates. A simple solution is to use "duct tape suspenders" to keep the splint from migrating downward.

3. If the knee feels unstable, apply a complete immobilizer.
4. If the victim has a locked knee, attempt to unlock it by positioning the victim with the leg hanging over the edge of a table or flat surface with the knee in approximately 90 degrees of flexion. After a period of relaxation, apply gentle longitudinal traction to the knee with internal and external rotation. Parenteral or oral pain medication and a muscle relaxant may facilitate the reduction. If the injury does not reduce easily, immobilize the victim and transport.

Finger Sprain
Finger sprains are caused by violent overstretching and tearing of one or more ligaments involving the finger joints.

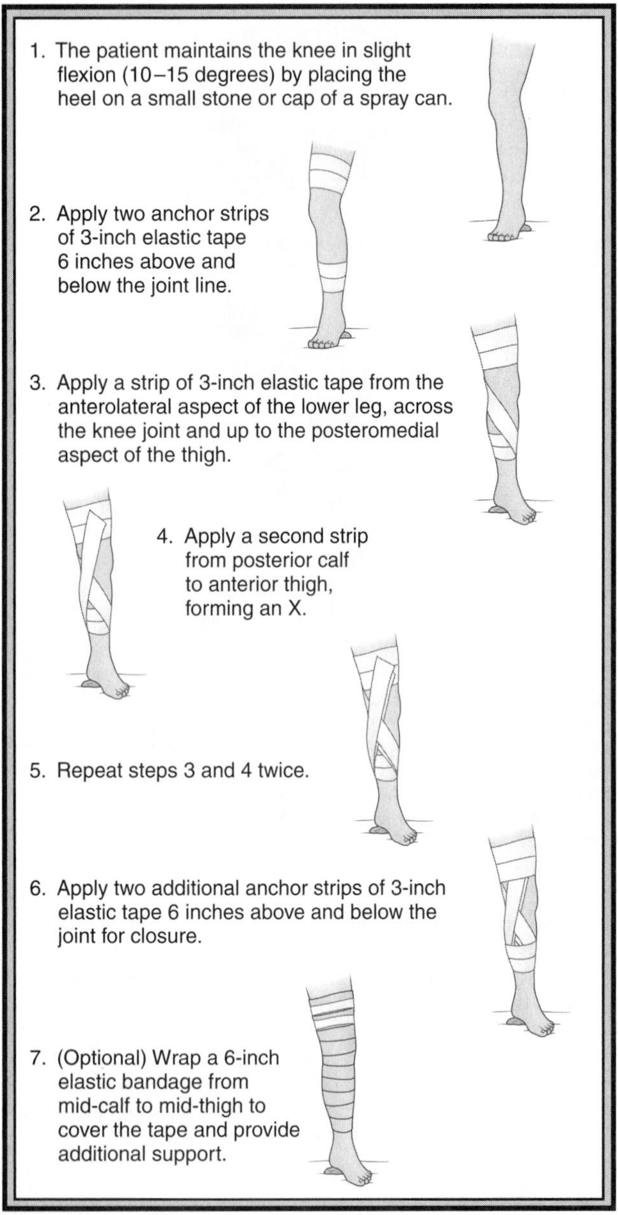

1. The patient maintains the knee in slight flexion (10–15 degrees) by placing the heel on a small stone or cap of a spray can.

2. Apply two anchor strips of 3-inch elastic tape 6 inches above and below the joint line.

3. Apply a strip of 3-inch elastic tape from the anterolateral aspect of the lower leg, across the knee joint and up to the posteromedial aspect of the thigh.

4. Apply a second strip from posterior calf to anterior thigh, forming an X.

5. Repeat steps 3 and 4 twice.

6. Apply two additional anchor strips of 3-inch elastic tape 6 inches above and below the joint for closure.

7. (Optional) Wrap a 6-inch elastic bandage from mid-calf to mid-thigh to cover the tape and provide additional support.

Figure 21-5. Knee taping.

Signs and Symptoms
1. Severe pain at the time of injury
2. Often, a feeling of popping or tearing inside one or more fingers
3. Tenderness, swelling, and later bruising of the finger
4. Impaired use of the injured finger

Treatment
1. Initially, ice, rest, and compressive bandage to reduce swelling and discomfort.
2. Buddy tape the injured finger to the adjacent finger as a natural splint. The second and third fingers and fourth and fifth fingers are always paired. A small piece of gauze, cotton, or cloth should be placed between the fingers to avoid blistering or pressure on a tender joint. Strips of tape should be applied around fingers, but not over the joints (Fig. 21-6).
3. Administer an NSAID such as ibuprofen 600 to 800 mg q8h.

Thumb Sprain

The thumb (ulnar collateral ligament) is frequently injured when placed in extreme extension or abduction, such as occurs when it is caught in the strap of a ski pole when falling. Taping can prevent reproducing the mechanism of injury, particularly when grasping an object (Fig. 21-7).

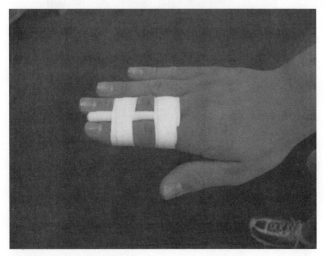

Figure 21-6. Buddy-taping of fingers.

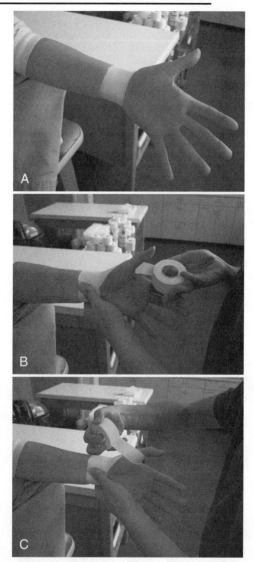

Figure 21-7.   Thumb taping. **A,** Using 1.5-inch athletic tape, wrap an anchor strip around the wrist. **B,** Using 0.75-inch tape, start at the volar aspect and continue along the dorsal aspect of the thumb toward the first web space. **C,** Allow the patient to crimp the tape as it comes across the web space and continues around the base of the thumb.

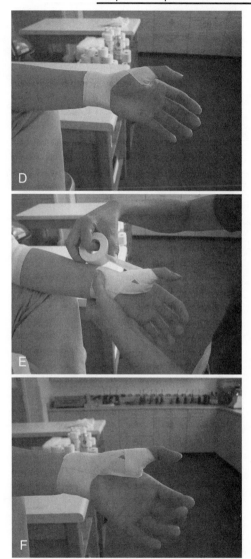

Figure 21-7. *Continued* **D,** Bring the tape around to the volar aspect of the wrist and tape at that point. To complete a thumb spica, apply several more strips in succession. To reinforce, rather than repeating a series of strips, continue as follows. **E,** Apply an anchor strip from volar to dorsal aspects of the wrist through the first web space (note crimping). **F,** Apply strip from the dorsal to volar aspect of the anchor strip.

Continued

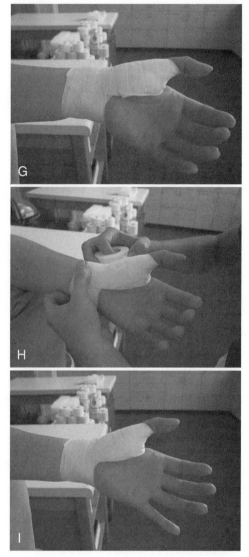

Figure 21-7. *Continued* **G,** Apply successive strip until at wrist. **H,** Add a finishing anchor strip though first web space. **I,** Complete with anchor strip.

Wrist Sprain

Wrist sprains generally occur during falls and initially can be difficult to distinguish from fractures.

Signs and Symptoms
1. Pain and swelling at the wrist
2. Increase in pain with flexion or extension of the wrist

Treatment
1. Initially, ice, rest, and compressive bandage to reduce swelling and discomfort.
2. Administer an NSAID, such as ibuprofen 600 to 800 mg q8h.
3. Although splinting is initially the most desirable treatment, there are two basic taping approaches that can be used, depending on the nature of the injury. Anchors are placed around the palm and distal wrist, while support strips to prevent undesirable movements are placed on the palmar aspect for hyperextension injuries or dorsal aspect for hyperflexion injuries (Fig. 21-8).

Plantar Fasciitis

Plantar fasciitis is inflammation of the fascia on the sole of the foot.

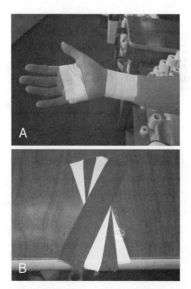

Figure 21-8. Wrist taping. **A,** With the hand wide open, apply one anchor across the palm of the hand and two to three anchors across the distal forearm. **B,** Measure out the distance between the two anchors and construct a fan of three strips of varying angles on a smooth surface.

Continued

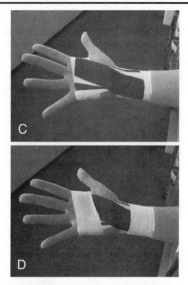

Figure 21-8, *Continued* **C,** For hyperextension injuries, apply these support strips to the palmar aspect. For hyperflexion injuries, apply them to the dorsal aspect. **D,** Apply another set of anchors over the support strips.

Signs and Symptoms
1. Pain at the origin of the plantar fascia, which is located at the most anterior aspect of the heel pad
2. Activities that stretch the plantar fascia elicit pain
3. Pain is worst when first getting up in the morning or after resting

Treatment
1. Heel cord stretching 20 minutes twice a day
2. NSAIDs such as ibuprofen 600 to 800 mg q8h
3. Wearing an orthotic that cups the heel, has a soft spot under the tender area, and supports the arch
4. Wearing an ankle-foot splint at night while sleeping

Blisters and Hot Spots

22

▶ **DEFINITIONS**

Hot spots are produced by friction. If the rubbing continues unabated, a blister forms, characterized as a raised, fluid-filled bubble of skin.

▶ **DISORDERS**

Hot Spots

Signs and Symptoms
Painful area of erythema

Treatment
1. Take a rectangular piece of moleskin or molefoam and cut an oval hole in the middle the size of the hot spot.
2. Center this over the affected area and secure it in place, making sure that the sticky surface is not on irritated skin (Fig. 22-1).
3. Reinforce the moleskin or molefoam with tape or a piece of nonwoven adhesive knit dressing.
4. If moleskin or molefoam is not available, place a piece of tape over the hot spot. You can also improvise moleskin from the cuff of a sweatshirt or flannel shirt and molefoam from a piece of padding from a backpack shoulder strap or hip belt. The improvised moleskin can be secured in place with a "super glue" or Dermabond.
5. If available, apply a Blist-O-Ban bandage to the hot spot.

Blisters

Signs and Symptoms
1. A bubble or pocket of fluid develops over the irritated area. The bubble can be small or quite large and will eventually break and release the fluid.
2. Pain and erythema occur at the site.

Treatment
1. If the blister is small and still intact, do not puncture or drain it.
2. Place a piece of moleskin or molefoam, with a hole cut out slightly larger than the blister, over the site. Make sure it is thick enough to keep the shoe from rubbing against the blister. This may require several layers. Secure this with tape.

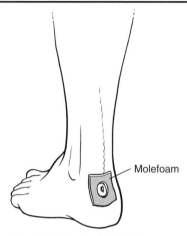

Figure 22-1. Hot spot treated with molefoam.

3. If the blister is large but still intact, puncture it with a clean needle or safety pin at its base and massage out the fluid.
4. Débride any necrotic skin with scissors.
5. Clean the area with an antiseptic towelette or with soap and water.
6. Apply antiseptic ointment or aloe vera gel, and cover with a nonadherent dressing.
   a. An excellent dressing for a blister is Spenco 2nd Skin. Made from an inert, breathable gel of 4% polyethylene oxide and 96% water, it absorbs anything oozing from the wound, helps prevent infection, relieves pain, and reduces further friction. It comes packaged between two sheets of cellophane.
   b. First, remove the cellophane from one side and apply the gooey side against the blister.
   c. Once it is adherent to the skin surface, remove the cellophane from the outside surface.
   d. Secure it in place with the adhesive knit bandage that comes with the product.
   e. Replace the entire dressing daily.
   f. Other excellent dressings for a blister are PolyMedica's Spyroflex, Compeed's Hydrocolloid Dressing, and Southwest Technologies' Elasto-Gel.

7. Place a piece of molefoam, with a hole cut out slightly larger than the blister, around the site. Secure this with tape or a piece of nonwoven adhesive knit dressing. Benzoin applied to the skin around the blister site will help hold the molefoam in place.

8. When supplies are limited, improvise by draining the fluid from the blister with a pin or knife and injecting a small amount of a "super glue" or benzoin into the evacuated space.

   a. Press the loose skin overlying the blister back in place, and cover the site with tape or a suitable dressing.

   b. This can initially be quite painful, but it should allow the victim to continue hiking out of the wilderness.

Improvised Blister Management

1. To dress a blister without moleskin, molefoam, or other commercial blister dressing, you can improvise with a piece of duct tape. Duct tape's smooth outer surface provides protection from friction, while its adhesive side adheres strongly to skin.

2. A sandwich bag can be used to improvise another type of blister dressing. It simulates the Blist-O-Ban, which was developed by SAM Medical Products as an innovative technique (Bursa Tek technology) to prevent blisters. The smooth, gliding surface of the bag helps to stop friction and reduce development of hot spots and blisters. Cut the corner of the sandwich bag, and apply a lubricant between the two surfaces. Secure the piece of bag to the blister site with tape or glue (Fig. 22-2).

3. You can improvise a blister dressing from a piece of gauze, antibacterial ointment, and water.

   a. Moisten the gauze with water.

   b. Squeeze out any excess water, then smear the ointment onto both sides of the gauze. Apply this to the blister.

4. A small square of silk can be glued to the heel or other pressure point.

5. Methyl acrylate–based glue can be used to repair skin fissures.

Prevention

1. Make sure that shoes fit properly. A shoe that is too tight causes pressure sores; one that is too loose leads to friction blisters.

2. Wear a thin liner sock under a heavier one. Friction will then occur between the socks instead of between the boot or shoe and foot.

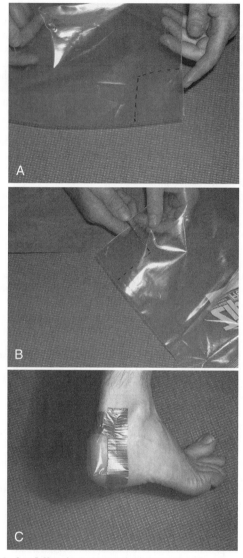

Figure 22-2. A to **C,** Blister dressing improvised with plastic sandwich bag.

3. Dry feet regularly, and use foot powder.
4. Apply moleskin to sensitive areas where blisters typically occur before hot spots develop.
5. Petroleum jelly or a gauze pad, covered by duct tape, is a reliable method of preventing blisters.
6. Duct tape placed on the inner lining of shoes decreases friction between the sock and shoe.

Bandaging and Taping Techniques

23

▶ TAPING

1. In general, taping requires practice, but some simple techniques can be easily mastered.
2. It is most often used in mild to moderate sprains and strains, where some functional capacity such as weight bearing and lifting are maintained.
3. Although taping offers dynamic support, it is in no way comparable with splinting, which can immobilize an extremity.
4. The most common tape applied is white athletic (or adhesive) tape, often used by trainers in organized sports.
5. Athletic tape may be applied to skin, although it may lose adhesion if the body part is not shaved and tape adhesive not applied.
6. Circumferential wrapping techniques should be used with considerable caution with acute injuries. Marked swelling may cause severe constriction when tape encircles the extremity. Always monitor distal neurovascular status.

Some keys to successful taping include the following:
1. Avoid leaving any gaps in the tape because these will lead to blisters.
2. Avoid excessive tension on tape strips that serve to fill these gaps.
3. Apply tape in a manner that follows the skin contour to avoid wrinkles.
4. Try to overlap a half-width on successive strips.

▶ TYPES OF TAPE

1. Athletic tape
   a. Although the major advantage of athletic tape is versatility, its major disadvantage is the tendency of zinc oxide to lose adhesive properties with heat and moisture, thus resulting in loss of support when the patient sweats.
   b. A variety of techniques are used to increase the durability of athletic tape under these conditions, described later in this section.
2. Elastic tape
   a. Elastic tape (e.g., Elastikon by Johnson & Johnson) is cotton elastic cloth tape with a rubber-based adhesive.
   b. The elasticity of the tape allows for greater flexibility and is particularly useful for large joints such as the knees or shoulders.

▶ SKIN PREPARATION

1. Skin preparation involves measures meant to increase longevity of tape adhesion and patient comfort.
2. If tape is to be applied directly to the skin, the area is usually shaved to remove hair that may interfere with direct contact.
3. Care must be taken to avoid small abrasions in the skin when shaving because these can serve as sites of infection.
4. Any obvious abrasion should be covered with a thin layer of gauze or small adhesive strip before taping.
5. A variety of commercially available skin adhesives are available in aerosolized form.
   a. These preparations use benzoin as the adhesive. One example is Cramer's Tuf-Skin.
   b. Skin adhesives are applied after the skin has been shaved and abrasions dressed.
   c. In the wilderness environment, a small plastic bottle of tincture of benzoin is more practical. It can be applied with a sterile applicator or gauze pad.
6. If the area is not shaved, a foam underwrap or prewrap is used to protect body hair. Prewrap is generally supplied in 3-inch rolls in a variety of colors.
7. After applying a topical skin adherent such as Tuf-Skin, prewrap is applied over the part to be taped in a simple, continuous circular wrap.
8. The prewrap is sufficiently self-adherent that it does not need to be taped down.
9. Heel-and-lace pads and foam pads are used to provide greater comfort by relieving potential pressure points.
10. When tape is applied over bony prominences, it can create tension on the skin surface that leads to blistering.
11. Heel-and-lace pads are prefabricated pieces of white foam that are stuck together with petroleum jelly and then applied to the anterior and posterior aspects of the talus when the ankle is taped.
12. Pads of foam can be cut to size to fit over painful areas that need to be taped, as in medial tibial stress syndrome, or they can be used for support in special cases such as taping for patellar subluxation.

▶ ANKLE TAPING

1. The most common injury to the lower extremity while hiking is a sprained ankle.
2. It is usually the result of inverting the ankle on an unstable surface.
3. Pain and swelling linger for several days, and taping can help offer support if the patient is able to bear weight.

4. Because most injuries occur to the lateral ligaments, taping supports the lateral surface by restricting inversion.

5. In general, taping of the ankle consists of anchor strips on the lower leg and foot, stirrups that run in a medial to lateral direction underneath the calcaneus, and support from either a figure-eight or heel-lock technique (Fig. 23-1).

6. The heel lock requires some expertise to perform, so most operators are more comfortable with the figure eight initially.

7. Caution with swelling.

▶ TOE TAPING

1. Taping toes that are sprained or fractured is simple and effective.

2. This treatment involves "buddy-taping" to the adjacent toe with one or two pieces of tape to provide support.

3. A piece of gauze, cotton, or cloth can be placed between the toes to avoid skin breakdown.

4. A sprain of the first metatarsophalangeal joint, also known as *turf toe*, can be a chronic and painful condition.

▶ LOWER LEG TAPING

1. Medial tibial stress syndrome, commonly referred to as "shin splints," can be taped for support and comfort.

2. Tape is brought from a lateral to medial direction, and a small foam pad can be cut to cover the area of tenderness.

3. Underwrap should be used over a foam pad to secure it in place (Fig. 23-2).

▶ KNEE TAPING

1. Because it is a large joint, taping the knee requires expertise and special consideration. Underwrap should not be used because adequate traction to support the joint can only be achieved by taping directly to the skin.

2. The patient's knee should be shaved 6 inches above and below the joint line.

3. In addition, standard athletic tape should not be used because it cannot provide enough support.

4. Three-inch elastic tape provides the foundation.

5. Taping for injuries to the medial aspect of the knee is described in Figure 21-5, Chapter 21.

▶ PATELLA TAPING

1. Subluxation of the patella is exacerbated by the stress of walking long distances across uneven terrain.

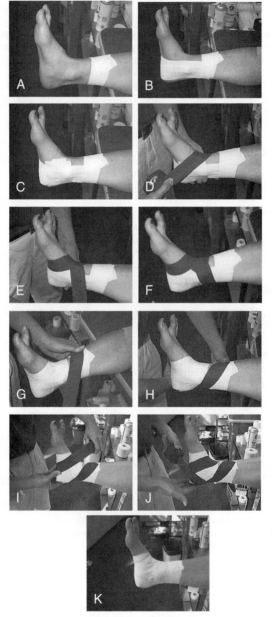

Figure 23-1. For legend see opposite page.

Figure 23-1. Ankle taping. **A,** (1) Ankle at 90 degrees; (2) apply anchors of 1.5-inch tape at the lower leg and distal foot. **B,** (3) Apply three stirrups from medial to lateral in a slight fan-like projection. **C,** (4) Fill in gaps with horizontal strips. **D,** (5) Begin figure eight. Apply tape across front of ankle in left-to-right direction. **E,** (6) Continue under the foot to the opposite side and cross back over the top of the foot. **F,** (7) Complete by wrapping around the leg and end at the anterior aspect of the ankle. **G,** (8) Apply heel locks for both feet (omit if not familiar with this technique). Start in left-to-right direction and apply tape across front of joint. **H,** (9) Wrap around the heel (bottom margin of tape should be above the superior edge of the calcaneus) to form the first heel lock. **I,** (10) Continue under the foot to the opposite side and cross back over the top of the foot. **J,** (11) The tape is then brought back around the superior margin of the calcaneus and down and around the heel. **K,** (12) Finish by wrapping around the ankle. Repeat figure eight or heel lock as desired.

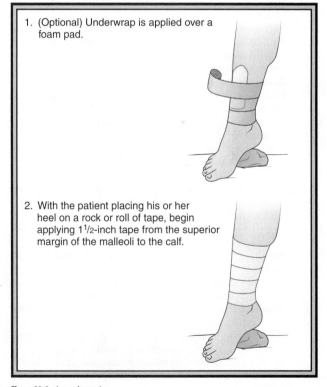

1. (Optional) Underwrap is applied over a foam pad.

2. With the patient placing his or her heel on a rock or roll of tape, begin applying 1 1/2-inch tape from the superior margin of the malleoli to the calf.

Figure 23-2. Lower leg taping.

2. Incorporating a piece of foam into taping the knee can help relieve symptoms.
3. As with all taping around the knee, underwrap should not be used (Fig. 23-3).

▶ FINGER TAPING

Injuries to the fingers are common in a variety of outdoor settings. Both simple fractures and sprains can be initially treated by taping.

1. The most common scenarios involve fingers that are hyper-extended or "jammed."
   a. Injuries in this scenario are often to the palmar ligaments and tendons.
   b. Patients may find it difficult to flex the finger against the resistance of an examiner's finger or may demonstrate tenderness over the palmar aspect of the finger.
   c. Swelling is almost always present and may be difficult to localize.
   d. This presentation is also seen after reduction of a dorsal dislocation of the proximal interphalangeal joint.
   e. In all these cases, it is always best to splint or tape the finger in slight flexion to avoid further injury to the flexor apparatus.
   f. Fingers are buddy-taped to the adjacent finger as a natural splint (see Fig. 21-6, Chapter 21).
   g. The second and third fingers and fourth and fifth fingers are always paired.
   h. If the third and fourth fingers are paired, this makes injury to the second and fifth fingers more likely with subsequent activity.
   i. A small piece of gauze, cotton, or cloth should be placed between the fingers to avoid blistering or pressure on a tender joint.
   j. Strips of tape should be applied around fingers but not over the joints.
2. Although not as common, injuries to the extensor tendons can occur.
   a. Typically these occur with hyperflexion, but they can also occur with hyperextension and axial loading.
   b. A mallet finger results from fracture of the base of the distal phalange, the site of attachment for the extensor tendon.
   c. The resulting inability of the distal phalange to extend fully results in a partially flexed "mallet" finger.
   d. Injuries in which the extensor mechanism is clearly disrupted should be treated with the finger taped in full extension.

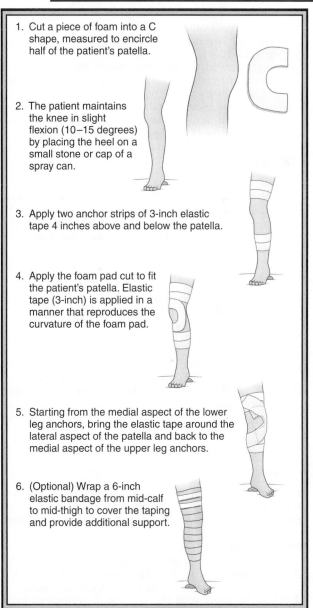

1. Cut a piece of foam into a C shape, measured to encircle half of the patient's patella.

2. The patient maintains the knee in slight flexion (10–15 degrees) by placing the heel on a small stone or cap of a spray can.

3. Apply two anchor strips of 3-inch elastic tape 4 inches above and below the patella.

4. Apply the foam pad cut to fit the patient's patella. Elastic tape (3-inch) is applied in a manner that reproduces the curvature of the foam pad.

5. Starting from the medial aspect of the lower leg anchors, bring the elastic tape around the lateral aspect of the patella and back to the medial aspect of the upper leg anchors.

6. (Optional) Wrap a 6-inch elastic bandage from mid-calf to mid-thigh to cover the taping and provide additional support.

Figure 23-3. Patella taping.

e. Often a straight splint such as a tongue blade or smooth stick can be placed on the dorsal surface and the finger taped to it for additional extensor support (Fig. 23-4).

f. Any injury to the fingers or hands should always be evaluated by a physician, who can determine whether radiographs are necessary.

g. Given the importance of maintaining optimal function of the hands for one's personal and professional activities, this point cannot be overemphasized.

▶ THUMB TAPING

1. The thumb is frequently injured when placed in extreme extension or abduction, such as occurs when it is caught in the strap of a ski pole when falling.

2. Taping can prevent reproducing the mechanism of injury, particularly when grasping an object (see Fig. 21-7, Chapter 21).

▶ WRIST TAPING

1. Wrist sprains generally occur during falls and initially can be difficult to distinguish from fractures.

2. Although splinting is initially the most desirable treatment, there are two basic taping approaches that can be used, depending on the nature of the injury.

3. As with the finger, the most important factor is whether the injury occurred in hyperextension or hyperflexion.

4. Anchors are placed around the palm and distal wrist, whereas support strips to prevent undesirable movements are placed on the palmar aspect for hyperextension injuries or the dorsal aspect for hyperflexion injuries (see Fig. 21-8 in Chapter 21).

▶ BANDAGING

Bandaging may be used to wrap and support an injury or help dress a wound. Many of the techniques described in the section on taping, such as figure-eight patterns, are used in bandaging.

Types of Bandages

1. The type of bandage used depends on its purpose.

2. Elastic bandages (e.g., Ace wrap) come in a variety of widths and are used to wrap injuries such as sprains and strains.

3. These bandages generally come with separate clips or clips built into the bandage to secure it.

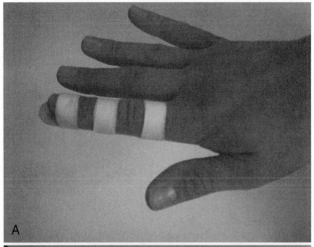

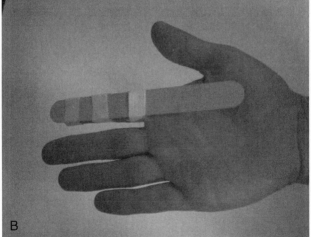

Figure 23-4. A and **B,** Extension taping of finger with small splint. Primarily used for extensor injuries.

4. Of note is the double-length 6-inch elastic bandage that is useful for wrapping large joints such as the knee and shoulder.
5. Bandaging wounds generally involves rolled gauze or cotton-based wraps that secure a dressing in place.

6. These wraps are more desirable than elastic bandages in wound care because they do not place as much tension on the wound dressing.
7. A triangular bandage, which is often used to create a sling, can be folded two to three times into a strap, called a *cravat.*
8. Cravat dressings are useful for applying pressure to a wound that is bleeding to promote hemostasis.
9. In the discussion of bandaging different parts of the body later in this chapter, the method for using an elastic bandage is described.
10. When securing a wound dressing, the same methods may be used, except that rolled gauze or cotton bandages should be substituted.
11. If there is a special technique for wound care, it will be described separately.

Securing Bandages

Because bandages are not adhesive, they must be secured with tape or clips or by tying them to the body. Two techniques for tying off a bandage are as follows:
1. As you finish wrapping with a bandage, bend the free end backward over your fingers, creating a loop. Now double back around the body part and tie the remaining free end to the loop to secure the bandage.
2. As you finish wrapping, tear or cut the remaining portion of bandage lengthwise down the middle. Double back with one of the resulting strips and tie off.

Ankle and Foot Bandaging

1. Ankle bandaging with a 2- to 3-inch elastic wrap can be used to support a sprain. The bandage can be applied over a sock or directly to the skin.
2. It is usually simplest to use a series of figure-eight wraps or, if preferable, a series of heel locks as described in the section on ankle taping.
3. Anchors and stirrups are not used.
4. When bandaging the foot, the same technique should be carried out to the metatarsophalangeal (MTP) joint.
5. Circumferentially bandaging the foot by itself will result in the bandage slipping, as opposed to bandaging the ankle as well.

Knee Bandaging

1. A double-length, 6-inch elastic bandage can provide support to the knee. Ask the patient to hold the knee in slight flexion by placing his heel on a small stone or piece of wood (see Fig. 21-5 in Chapter 21).

2. The elastic wrap is then applied circumferentially from midquadriceps to midcalf (see Fig. 21-5, Chapter 21).
3. If using gauze to secure a dressing or a smaller elastic wrap, then a series of figure-eight wraps can be applied, leaving the patella exposed.

Thigh and Groin Bandaging

1. Quadriceps, hamstring, and hip adductor ("groin") strains can all be treated with an elastic bandage in a hip spica.
2. The bandage is modified slightly for the groin strain (Fig. 23-5).
3. Although the quadriceps and hamstring can be supported by wrapping only the leg with a 6-inch elastic bandage, the hip spica helps prevent slipping and provides additional support.

Wrist and Hand Bandaging

1. Support to the wrist can be supplied by a 2- to 3-inch elastic wrap using a continuous technique (Fig. 23-6).
2. This same technique can be used with gauze to secure a dressing to a wound that can occur when falling on an outstretched hand.
3. A hand cravat bandage can be used for wounds that continue to bleed despite manual pressure.

Finger Bandaging

1. Finger wounds are generally easily treated with adhesive bandages.
2. However, if size or degree of bleeding necessitates a larger dressing, then the following method may be used:
   a. Fold a 1-inch rolled gauze back and forth over the tip of the finger to cover and cushion the wound (Fig. 23-7).
   b. Then wrap the gauze around the finger until the gauze is snug.
   c. On the last turn around the finger, pull the gauze over the top of the hand so that it extends beyond the wrist.
   d. Split this lengthwise; tie the ends around the wrist to secure the bandage.

Thumb Bandaging

1. Application of a bandage or dressing to the thumb usually involves a thumb spica, as described in the taping section. Rather than apply individual strips, the gauze or elastic bandage is looped continuously.

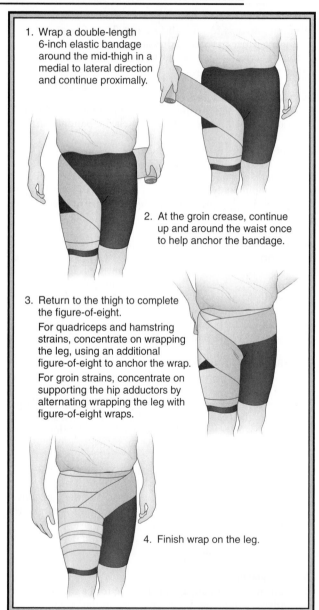

1. Wrap a double-length 6-inch elastic bandage around the mid-thigh in a medial to lateral direction and continue proximally.

2. At the groin crease, continue up and around the waist once to help anchor the bandage.

3. Return to the thigh to complete the figure-of-eight.

   For quadriceps and hamstring strains, concentrate on wrapping the leg, using an additional figure-of-eight to anchor the wrap.

   For groin strains, concentrate on supporting the hip adductors by alternating wrapping the leg with figure-of-eight wraps.

4. Finish wrap on the leg.

Figure 23-5. Thigh and groin bandaging.

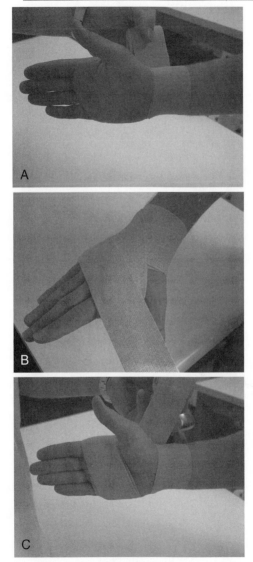

Figure 23-6. Wrist bandaging. **A,** (1) Begin by encircling the wrist two to three times. **B,** (2) Continue across the dorsum of the hand, through the first web space and around the base of the proximal phalanges. **C,** (3) Continue down and across the dorsum of the hand.

Continued

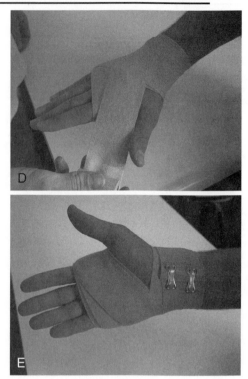

Figure 23-6, cont'd. **D,** (4) Circle the wrist and bring across the dorsum of the hand to form a figure eight. **E,** (5) Repeat, alternating figure-eight patterns on the dorsum of the hand and secure at the wrist.

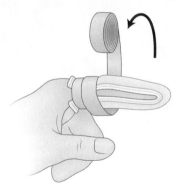

Figure 23-7. To begin a finger bandage, place layers of gauze over the fingertip. (Redrawn from Auerbach PS: Medicine for the Outdoors, 4th ed. Guilford, CT: Lyons Press, 2003, p 263.)

Shoulder Bandaging

1. A shoulder spica is used to support shoulder sprains, strains, and subluxations (Fig. 23-8).

1. Begin by encircling the mid-humerus with a double-length 6-inch elastic bandage and continue proximally while wrapping. Once near the axilla, wrap over the acromio-clavicular joint and around the posterior thorax.

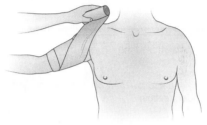

2. Continue under the opposite axilla, across the chest and bring down over the acromioclavicular joint and onto the upper arm.

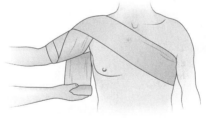

3. Repeat the figure-of-eight pattern as the length of the bandage allows and finish on the upper arm.

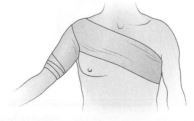

Figure 23-8. Shoulder bandaging.

2. A triangular bandage can be used to dress a shoulder wound.

Scalp Bandaging

1. Wounds to the scalp often require a dressing placed over hair, making adhesion difficult.
2. The dressing can be secured with a triangular bandage in a method that allows for considerable tension should

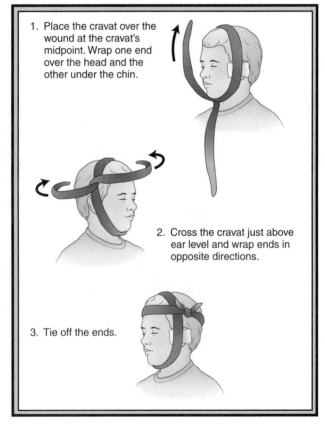

1. Place the cravat over the wound at the cravat's midpoint. Wrap one end over the head and the other under the chin.

2. Cross the cravat just above ear level and wrap ends in opposite directions.

3. Tie off the ends.

Figure 23-9. Ear bandaging. (Redrawn from Auerbach PS: Medicine for the Outdoors, 4th ed. Guilford, CT, Lyons Press, 2003, p 266.)

pressure be necessary to stop bleeding (see Fig. 20-6, Chapter 20).

Ear Bandaging

1. A wound to the pinna may require a compression dressing.
2. If so, gauze should be placed both anterior and posterior to the ear to allow it to maintain its natural curvature.
3. A cravat is used to secure the dressing (Fig. 23-9).
4. This method may be used for wounds anywhere along the side of the head or under the chin.

Eye Bandaging

1. When bandaging an eye, a shield is placed over the eye socket to protect the globe, followed by application of a bandage over the shield.
2. The shield may be commercially available sterile pads, cut foam or felt, stacked gauze, or a shirt or cravat fashioned into a doughnut shape (Fig. 23-10).
3. The bandage is fashioned from a cravat and a spare piece of 15-inch cloth or shirt.
4. The spare cloth is placed over the top of the head from posterior to anterior such that the anterior portion lies over the unaffected eye.
5. A cravat is then applied horizontally to hold the shield over the injured eye.
6. To expose the uninjured eye, pull up both ends of the spare cloth and tie at the top of the head (Fig. 23-11).

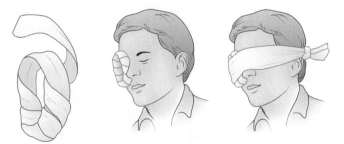

Figure 23-10. Bandage for the injured eye. A cravat or cloth is rolled and wrapped to make a doughnut-shaped shield, which is fixed in place over the eye. (Redrawn from Auerbach PS: Medicine for the Outdoors, 4th ed. Guilford, CT, Lyons Press, 2003, p 175.)

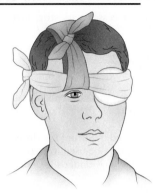

Figure 23-11. Holding an eye patch in place with a cravat. Hang a cloth strip over the uninjured eye. Hold the patch in place with the cravat. Tie the cloth strip to lift the cravat off the uninjured eye. (Redrawn from Auerbach PS: Medicine for the Outdoors, 4th ed. Guilford, CT, Lyons Press, 2003, p 262.)

Pain Management

24

Effective pain management can dramatically enhance a rescue effort and minimize morbidity and mortality. Any health care worker providing medical support to a backcountry trip or expedition should be adequately prepared to provide pain relief. This may be the only therapeutic modality available for the victim.

▶ EVALUATION OF PAIN

The basis of the wilderness pain evaluation should include the following:
1. Location of the pain
2. Time of onset
3. Precipitating or aggravating factors
4. Frequency and duration
5. Character
6. Severity
   a. Historically, visual analog pain scales have been used in an attempt to quantify the intensity of pain.
   b. Many scales exist, but all generally place the pain on a scale from 1 to 10. One represents mild pain, which can easily be ignored. Ten represents the worst pain imaginable, such that bed rest is required and the victim is completely incapacitated.
7. Previous treatment (i.e., prior response to pain medications)

Also determine the following:
1. Past medical and surgical history (including history of substance abuse and/or dependence)
2. Environmental exposures
3. Diet and medications
4. Associated symptoms (e.g., nausea, vomiting, fever, vertigo, dyspnea)

▶ PHYSICAL METHODS FOR TREATMENT OF PAIN

Compression Analgesia
Although compression is taught more as a method for establishing hemostasis than for pain management, compression can reduce pain.
1. An injured extremity is wrapped distal to proximal, with a cloth wrap, rubber Esmarch bandage, or an elasticized ("Ace") wrap.
2. Resultant mild anesthesia may occur because of compression of peripheral nerves.

3. If pain increases, discontinue this method.
4. Compression anesthesia may be safe and appropriate in a wilderness setting if other methods or pharmacologic agents are unavailable or contraindicated.

Cryoanalgesia

1. Wilderness cryoanalgesia may be applied with ice, snow, or frigid water.
2. Cryoanalgesia requires a 20- to 30-minute minimum duration for adequate therapeutic effect.
3. Prevention of iatrogenous frostbite and generalized hypothermia while using cold therapy is critical. How long a tissue will tolerate a cold compress before experiencing cellular damage depends on preexistent tissue hypothermia, peripheral versus central nature of the tissue, and temperature and pressure of the cold compress.
4. Cold water immersion may exacerbate injury in persons with snakebite because of venom-compromised tissues.
5. Cold packs may be beneficial for certain marine coelenterate (e.g., jellyfish) envenomations, which may benefit equally from application of heat (see Chapter 52).
6. Commercial cold packs typically contain a gel of water and propylene glycol, or other similar antifreeze and heat exchange substances, which may be cooled in cold water or snow to prolong their effectiveness.
7. A reasonable practice is to place a dry, thin cotton cloth or piece of foam between the skin and cold metal cylinders, ice, snow, or cold packs. Remove cold therapy every 15 minutes to assess tissue status.

Heat Therapy

1. Heat application is not usually recommended for initial (up to 48 hours after the injury) pain management of acute trauma because it may lead to increased edema and bleeding.
2. Heat can be used for pain management in the wilderness, especially for patients with chronic pain conditions.
3. Heat applied to the skin of the abdomen may markedly reduce gastrointestinal peristalsis and uterine contractions and thus decrease pain associated with these organs.
4. Application of heat need not be extreme. Temperatures of 37.8° C to 40° C (100° F to 104° F) for 10 to 20 minutes generally provide comfort without thermal injury.
5. Heat therapy should be avoided in cognitively impaired persons and for tissue that is anesthetic or ischemic, to prevent further unintended tissue injury.

6. Heat therapy may improve or worsen certain marine envenomations. It is generally helpful for spine (e.g., sea urchin, starfish, scorpionfish, stingray) punctures and perhaps helpful for jellyfish stings. See Chapter 52.
7. Liniments and balms are not true heat transfer agents but consist of multiple botanical or chemical substances that make the tissue feel warm through counterirritant effects and subsequent vasodilation. These substances may help abate a traveler's soreness and stiffness. Common ingredients include menthol, camphor, mustard oil, eucalyptus oil, methyl nicotinate, methyl salicylate, and wormwood oil. These products are generally only recommended on intact skin with a light cloth or plastic covering and should not be placed on mucous membranes. They should not be used with tight compresses or external heat sources. Topical capsaicin in low concentration is used to relieve pain from arthritis, but its application may cause a marked sensation of skin burning.

Splinting
Splinting allows positioning and immobilization of injured body parts and prevents further damage to soft tissues, blood vessels, nerves, and bones. Preventing bony fragments from damaging surrounding tissue diminishes pain and often facilitates mobilization and extrication of a victim.
1. Splints (see Chapter 18) should be well padded to prevent further surface trauma.
2. Splints may be accompanied by pressure dressings or cold compresses for additional pain management.
3. Regular reevaluation of tissue circulatory status is critical to prevent damage from swelling, frostbite, or ischemia in immobile, splinted limbs.

Transcutaneous Electrical Nerve Stimulation
TENS units are so commonly used that wilderness physicians will probably encounter persons using these devices.
1. Wilderness physicians familiar with TENS units may find them useful to treat acute traumatic pain, but, more likely, a traveler will have a TENS unit.
2. Most persons have developed personal preferences for TENS unit settings and skin electrode placement.
3. Rigorous physical activity may cause difficulty maintaining electrode placement. Application to clean, dry skin is important. Preparing the skin with topical benzoin may significantly increase the duration of adhesiveness. Because benzoin is an iodine-based topical solution, avoid it in persons with sensitivity or allergy to iodine.

Topical Anesthetics

1. A local anesthetic may provide relief in a topical application before more invasive cleansing and débridement.
2. The local anesthetic EMLA is a mixture of 5% lidocaine and prilocaine. After this cream is applied to intact skin under a nonabsorbent dressing for at least 45 minutes, an invasive procedure such as intravenous (IV) needle insertion may be more easily tolerated.
3. Lidocaine gel can also be used for this purpose (Table 24-1).

▶ LOCAL ANESTHETIC PHARMACOLOGY

Anesthetic Toxicity

1. Infiltration into a highly vascular site such as around an intercostal nerve leads to more rapid escalation of blood level than does injection into less vascular subcutaneous tissues. Use of an anesthetic/epinephrine mixture leads to slower absorption but must be avoided when injecting distal extremities and digits, where epinephrine-induced vasoconstriction may lead to acute ischemic injury. Because of the possibility of unintentional direct intravascular injection, all local and regional anesthetic infiltrations should be made after negative aspiration for blood and in small aliquots between aspiration attempts.
2. As anesthetic toxicity levels are approached, common early symptoms include circumoral numbness, tinnitus, and cephalgia. Central nervous system (CNS) toxicity in the form of seizures occurs at lower anesthetic blood levels than does

TABLE 24-1. Comparable Anesthetic Dosages* for Peripheral Blocks and Local Infiltration

	DOSAGE (mg/kg)
Amide Anesthetics	
Lidocaine	5
Prilocaine	5
Etidocaine	4
Mepivicaine	5
Bupivacaine	2
Ester Anesthetics	
Procaine	5
Tetracaine	1-2
2-Chloroprocaine	5

*No epinephrine included.

cardiotoxicity, seen as ventricular arrhythmias and cardio-vascular collapse. Generally, cardiotoxicity is achieved at approximately 150% of the blood level concentrations required for anesthetic CNS toxicity. Bupivacaine has demonstrated increased cardiotoxicity relative to lidocaine.

3. Anesthetic allergy per se is uncommon, with perhaps 99% of all adverse anesthetic reactions actually related to pharmacologic toxicity of the anesthetic or to epinephrine mixed with the agent.

Anesthetic Infiltration Techniques and Nerve Blocks

1. Soft tissue analgesia is accomplished with local injection of 1% lidocaine. Generally, the maximum injectable dose for lidocaine is 4 mg/kg. In larger wounds, injections proceed from an area previously anesthetized to lessen discomfort from subsequent injections.

2. Local anesthetic injection typically causes temporary pain resulting from the solution's pH. Buffered solutions are available or may be created by adding sodium bicarbonate (1 mEq/mL) to lidocaine or other anesthetic in a 1:10 ratio, bicarbonate to anesthetic. Tolerance to the injection is improved by gentle and slow injection, allowing prudence with the total dose of anesthetic.

3. Epinephrine may provide useful hemostasis, especially in head and scalp lacerations. Avoid using epinephrine on nose tips, ear lobes, distal extremities, and digits to avoid ischemic injury or even subsequent necrosis.

4. Many central and regional nerve blocks require special training including a thorough knowledge of anatomy and management of potential complications, but several blocks can be appropriate in a wilderness setting if the physician is cautious and limits the amount of anesthetic injected. Make all infiltrations after aseptic preparation of the skin, whenever possible.

Digital Nerve Blocks (Fig. 24-1)

Anesthesia to the digits is easily accomplished with a low-volume field block to the medial and lateral aspects of the digit at the base of the respective phalanx.

1. Approach the digital nerves from the dorsum of the hand or foot rather than from the palm or sole.

2. The dorsal digital nerves and proper digital nerves course along the medial and lateral aspects of the digits roughly at the 10 and 2 o'clock and 4 and 8 o'clock positions, respectively.

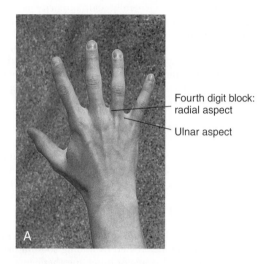

Fourth digit block:
radial aspect

Ulnar aspect

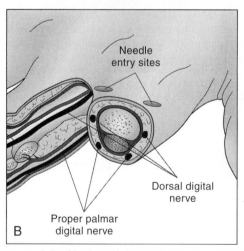

Figure 24-1. **A,** Site of digital nerve block. **B,** Digital nerve anatomy. (**A,** Courtesy of Bryan L. Frank, MD.)

3. From 3 to 5 mL of lidocaine 0.5% to 1.0% injected as a field block with a 25-gauge (or 27-gauge) needle to the medial and lateral aspects of the proximal digit provides a satisfactory digital block.
4. Do not use an epinephrine-containing anesthetic because this could lead to circulatory compromise and possible necrosis of the digit.

Wrist Blocks (Fig. 24-2)

The entire hand may be anesthetized by blocking the nerves at the wrist. The radial nerve supplies the cutaneous branches of the dorsum of the hand and thumb and distally to the distal interphalangeal joints of the index, long, and radial aspect of the ring fingers. Median nerve sensory distribution includes the palmar surface of the hand, ulnar aspect of the thumb, palmar aspect of the index finger, and long and radial portions of the ring finger. The median nerve innervation extends dorsally over the index, long, and ring fingers to the distal interphalangeal joint. The ulnar nerve gives sensation to the palmar and dorsal surfaces of the lateral hand, the fifth finger, and the ulnar half of the ring finger.

1. Using a 25- or 27-gauge needle, inject 2 to 4 mL of lidocaine 1% in the subcutaneous tissue overlying the radial artery. A superficial subcutaneous injection from this point

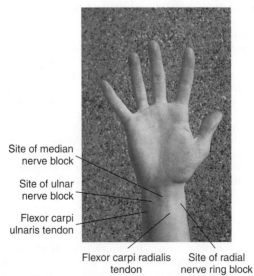

Site of median nerve block

Site of ulnar nerve block

Flexor carpi ulnaris tendon

Flexor carpi radialis tendon

Site of radial nerve ring block

Figure 24-2. Landmarks for wrist block. (Courtesy of Bryan L. Frank, MD.)

and over the radial styloid anesthetizes cutaneous branches from the proximal forearm and extending into the hand.

2. Block the median nerve with 2 to 4 mL of lidocaine 1% just proximal to the palmar wrist crease between the tendons of the palmaris longus and the flexor carpi radialis muscles. Make the injection deep to the volar fascia.

3. If a paresthesia is elicited (resulting from contact with the nerve), withdraw the needle slightly before injection.

4. Block the ulnar nerve with 2 to 4 mL of lidocaine 1% injected just lateral to the ulnar artery, which is radial to the flexor carpi ulnaris tendon at the level of the ulnar styloid.

Ankle Blocks (Fig. 24-3)

Anesthesia of the foot is easily accomplished with blocks of the sensory nerves at the ankle.

1. Using a 25-gauge needle, block the deep peroneal nerve, which provides sensation between the great and second toes, with 5 mL of lidocaine 1% between the tendons of the tibialis anterior and the extensor hallucis longus at the level of the medial and lateral malleoli. The needle may be passed to the bone just lateral to the dorsalis pedis artery. Inject the superficial peroneal nerve with 5 mL of lidocaine 1% with a superficial ring block between the injection of the deep peroneal nerve and the medial malleolus. This blocks sensation to the medial and dorsal aspects of the foot.

2. Inject the posterior tibial nerve with 5 mL of lidocaine 1% just posterior to the medial malleolus, adjacent to the posterior tibial artery.

3. Block the sural nerve, which provides sensation to the posterolateral foot, with a similar volume of lidocaine 1% between the lateral malleolus and Achilles tendon, followed by a subcutaneous infiltration from this site and over the lateral malleolus.

4. Paresthesias are sought in these blocks and will increase the likelihood of success. Posterior tibial nerve distribution includes the heel and plantar foot surface. Follow paresthesias by a slight withdrawal of the needle before injection.

Trigger Point Injections

Persons who suffer from neck and shoulder or lower back strain may benefit greatly from deactivation of myofascial trigger zones. The pain relief may be profound and enable an adventure to continue without disruption. Successful deactivation of trigger zones may be accomplished with either dry needling (acupuncture) or injection of lidocaine 1%. In the

Site for sural   Site for superficial
nerve block   peroneal nerve block

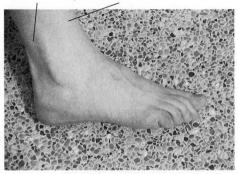

Site for superficial
peroneal nerve block

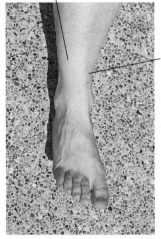

Site for saphenous
nerve block

Figure 24-3. Landmarks for ankle block. (Courtesy of Bryan L. Frank, MD.)

absence of anesthetic or acupuncture needles, trigger point deactivation may be accomplished with a 27-gauge needle.

1. Injection of a trigger zone is typically performed directly into the painful myofascial point and in a four-quadrant zone from the center of the trigger point, advancing 1 to 2 cm into the adjacent tissue at a 45- to 60-degree angle from the skin surface.
2. Muscle twitches or fasciculations may accompany the injections.

3. A volume of 1 to 2 mL of lidocaine 1% is usually ample for each trigger zone.
4. There is no benefit to adding corticosteroids to the anesthetic.
5. Using an acupuncture needle (or a 27- or 30-gauge needle) may deactivate the trigger zones nicely using a similar four-quadrant pecking of the myofascial zone, without injection of anesthetic. A 1- to 1½-inch needle may be used to peck briskly several times in each direction, also at a 45- to 60-degree angle from the center of the trigger zone.
6. Depth of insertion is typically 1 to 2 cm.
7. Soiled skin should be prepared similarly to how it is for an intramuscular injection.

▶ COMPLEMENTARY AND ALTERNATIVE MEDICINE THERAPIES

"Complementary and alternative" denote therapies and modalities that may not be supported by Western-designed prospective, randomized studies; that are not commonly taught in U.S. medical colleges; or that are not generally covered by traditional health insurance plans. Some may contribute significantly to wilderness pain management.

Acupuncture

Properly administered acupuncture should have a very low risk of morbidity and may be extremely effective in alleviating pain and even restoring function to an injured wilderness traveler.

1. Sterile acupuncture needles are compact, lightweight, and easy to include in a day pack or first-aid kit. Integration of acupuncture into the biomedical care of wilderness trauma, pain, and illness may dramatically enhance patient comfort and facilitate extrication from a remote setting.
2. Most acupuncture treatment requires substantial training to be responsibly integrated with conventional Western therapies. National and international standards of training have been established for Western-trained physicians who desire to incorporate acupuncture into their traditional medical practices.
3. The American Academy of Medical Acupuncture (AAMA) represents physician acupuncturists whose training meets or exceeds standards established by the World Health Organization.
4. Physicians interested in learning acupuncture may contact the AAMA for information on training programs designed specifically for physicians.

Herbal/Botanical Remedies

The term *herb* is broadly defined as a nonwoody plant that dies down to the ground after flowering. Combinations of several herbs are often more effective than a single herb, and common formulas have been recorded worldwide for centuries. Appropriate application or prescription of botanical products rarely leads to toxicity or adverse reactions, although such are possible if botanicals are used excessively or carelessly.

Certain botanical products used for pain include the following:

1. Morphine, isolated from the opium poppy.
2. Cocaine, from coca leaves *(Erythroxylon coca)*.
3. Often used as a seasoning or food, oregano *(Origanum vulgare)* has been beneficial for rheumatic pain.
4. Sunflower *(Helianthus annuus)* is a source of phenylalanine, useful for general pain.
5. Turmeric *(Curcuma longa)* contains curcumin, an antiinflammatory substance beneficial for rheumatoid arthritis.
6. Ginger *(Zingiber officinale)* is beneficial for rheumatoid arthritis, osteoarthritis, and fibromyalgia.
7. Clove *(Syzygium aromaticum)* is endorsed by the German botanical resource, Commission E, topically for dental pain.
8. Red peppers (*Capsicum* species) contain substance P–depleting capsaicin and also salicylates.
9. Often taken as an infusion or decoction, kava kava *(Piper methysticum)* contains both dihydrokavain and dihydromethysticin, which have analgesic effectiveness similar to that of aspirin.
10. Evening primrose *(Oenothera biennis)* is a source of tryptophan, which has been recommended to relieve pain associated with diabetic neuropathy.
11. Lavender (*Lavandula* species) contains linalool and linalyl aldehyde, which appear to be useful for pain of burns and other injuries in topical and aromatherapy form.
12. Willow (*Salix* species), used to treat pain since 500 BC, contains salicin and other salicylate compounds. The German Commission E has recognized willow as an effective pain reliever for headaches, arthritis, and many other pains. Salicylate-containing plants include red peppers, wintergreen, and birch bark. Avoid all botanicals containing salicylates in persons who are sensitive or allergic to aspirin products. Furthermore, children who have viral infections such as a cold or influenza should avoid these products because salicylates have been implicated in the development of Reye's syndrome.

13. Chamomile *(Matricaria chamomilla)* contains chamazulene, which is reportedly beneficial for abdominal pain related to gastrointestinal spasm or colic; as an antihistaminic, it has mild calming or sedative properties. It is used in Europe to treat leg ulcers and may be beneficial for painful, irritated bites and stings.

14. Plantain major *(Plantago major)* is also commonly used for bites and stings, poison ivy discomfort, and toothache and has been used traditionally by Native Americans as a wound dressing.

15. Aloe gel *(Aloe vera)* has been used since ancient times to treat burns and sunburn and to promote wound healing.

16. Especially useful for sprains and strains is the mountain daisy or arnica *(Arnica montana),* which is also endorsed by Commission E. Arnica was in the U.S. Pharmacopoeia in the early 1800s to 1960s and has long been used by Native Americans and others for relieving back pain and other myofascial pains and bruising. It is used topically or internally, often in homeopathic form.

17. Comfrey *(Symphytum officinale)* has been used since ancient Grecian times for skin problems. It contains aloin, which is antiinflammatory, and is endorsed by Commission E to topically treat bruises, dislocations, and sprains. Comfrey has experienced a controversial safety record because oral ingestion of its pyrrolizidine alkaloids has been associated with hepatotoxicity and/or carcinogenicity. For this reason, only topical use of comfrey is recommended.

▶ PHARMACOLOGIC TREATMENT OF PAIN

Non-narcotic Analgesics

Non-narcotic analgesics provide mild to moderate pain relief and are generally safer than narcotics.

1. Acetylsalicylic acid (aspirin)
   a. In addition to analgesia, aspirin reduces fever, inhibits platelet function, and diminishes inflammation.
   b. It is generally quite safe but can produce gastrointestinal side effects including gastric irritability, mucosal erosion, and bleeding ulcers.
   c. It is often better tolerated in an enteric-coated formulation. Persons with a history of gastrointestinal ulcers or severe indigestion should avoid aspirin. Dosage should not exceed 650 mg orally every 4 hours.
   d. Other salicylate analgesics include diflunisal, choline magnesium trisalicylate, and salsalate. The latter two

have minimal gastrointestinal toxicity and antiplatelet effects.

e. Salicylates are contraindicated in persons with known allergy to the class of drugs and in children younger than age 15 years with viral respiratory illnesses because their use has been linked to Reye's syndrome.

2. Acetaminophen

a. Acetaminophen is a mild analgesic and antipyretic.

b. Contrary to popular belief, as an analgesic, it has equal efficacy to ibuprofen.

c. It has no antiplatelet, antiinflammatory, or antiprostaglandin effect and is less likely to cause serious gastric irritation.

d. The typical dose is 500 mg PO q4–6h.

e. The dose should not exceed 650 mg every 4 hours.

f. Ingestion of more than 10 g over 24 hours may lead to severe hepatic damage; the drug should be used with extreme caution in anyone with preexisting liver disease.

g. Many over-the-counter medications contain acetaminophen, so these should not be used in combination with pure acetaminophen or in persons with liver disease.

3. Nonsteroidal antiinflammatory drugs (NSAIDs)

a. The first-line NSAID for safety, efficacy, and cost is ibuprofen in doses of 400 to 800 mg PO q6h.

b. Its analgesic and antipyretic properties are similar to those of aspirin and acetaminophen.

c. Its antiinflammatory properties are especially useful for prostaglandin-mediated diseases such as renal colic, biliary colic, dysmenorrhea, and gout.

d. It shows advantages for women with dysmenorrhea because the antiprostaglandin effects somewhat relax the uterus.

e. Increased doses of NSAIDs further inhibit prostaglandin synthesis and increase the antiinflammatory effect; however, used for analgesia, NSAIDs have a ceiling effect (i.e., little additional analgesic effect will occur with increasing dose).

f. Like aspirin, ibuprofen can be a gastric irritant and should be avoided in persons with a history of gastrointestinal ulcer, indigestion, or hiatal hernia.

g. Oral or rectal administration leads to rapid absorption.

h. Ibuprofen has been reported to cause nonspecific fluid retention.

i. Other propionic acid derivatives include naproxen, fenoprofen, oxaprozin, ketoprofen, and flurbiprofen.

5. Cyclooxygenase-2 (COX-2) inhibitors
   a. The newest class of nonsteroidal antiinflammatory drugs (NSAIDs) currently available in the United States is the cyclooxygenase-2 (COX-2) inhibitor.
   b. COX-2 inhibitors directly target cyclooxygenase-2, an enzyme responsible for inflammation and pain. Selectivity for COX-2 reduces the risk of peptic ulceration and bleeding.
   c. These medications inhibit inflammation and also demonstrate analgesic and antipyretic properties.
   d. COX-2 inhibitor medications may be taken orally once a day and are not yet cleared for persons younger than age 18 years or with advanced renal disease. Side effects primarily include gastrointestinal distress, hypertension, rashes, and peripheral edema.
   e. Celecoxib (Celebrex) may be given either 100 mg twice daily or 200 mg daily, with no clinical advantage seen with either method of administration.
   f. Another COX-2 inhibitor is Etoricoxib (Arcoxia).
   g. Comparative trials have confirmed that COX-2 inhibitors are no more or less effective than NSAIDs.
   h. COX-2 inhibitors generally should be reserved for patients who have a history of gastrointestinal bleeding and have failed treatment with acetaminophen.
   i. The debate about the propensity for COX-2 inhibitors to increase the likelihood of adverse cardiac events is ongoing. If there is any concern regarding this possibility, these agents should not be used.

▶ **NARCOTIC ANALGESICS**

Injectables

Opiates are potent and appropriate analgesics for moderate to severe pain in the wilderness. They can easily be combined with NSAIDs and other adjuvants as needed.

1. Despite the plethora of alternative drugs available, none offers superior safety or efficacy to morphine.
   a. Morphine is a potent analgesic with sedative and euphoric effects.
   b. Morphine will also depresses the CNS and respiratory drive.
   c. Although morphine is typically given intravenously, oral forms exist.
   d. Injectable morphine is preferred because of its rapid onset and the ability to titrate response.
   e. The standard dose is 10 to 20 mg IM or 2.5 mg IV q3.5h.

   f. Experienced practitioners often give higher doses, titrating carefully to effect.

   g. For example: Loading dose of 1 to 2 mg q 10 min up to 0.2 mg/kg IV. Maintain analgesia with 2 to 10 mg IV q½–6h.

   h. Morphine and other analgesics are often underdosed. A reasonable approach is to titrate administration to response, being vigilant for side effects and adverse physiologic response such as respiratory depression or hypotension. One should observe subjective pain score and objective physiologic manifestations including degree of sedation, mental status, heart rate, and respiratory rate.

2. Meperidine (Demerol) has a relatively short clinical half-life; however, the inactive metabolite, normeperidine, has a long half-life. If normeperidine accumulates, it can produce CNS excitation, tachycardia, and a decreased seizure threshold. Meperidine also inhibits shivering. Better choices exist (e.g., morphine).

3. Fentanyl is an excellent alternative to morphine, especially in hemodynamically unstable patients or those with an exaggerated histamine response to morphine.

   a. The onset is very rapid.

   b. The loading dose is 1 to 2 μg per kg body weight q5–10 min titrated to effect. The standard dose for a 70-kg person is 50 to 100 μg IV q30-60 min.

   c. Smaller doses can be used initially and titrated to effect.

   d. Fentanyl (Fentanyl Oralet) or "lollipops" are a reasonable choice but require a long time to administer (i.e., lick) and often cause nausea.

   e. A promising recent development is Fentora (fentanyl buccal tablet) intended for buccal mucosal administration. Fentora is designed to be placed and retained within the buccal cavity for a period sufficient to allow disintegration of the tablet and absorption of fentanyl across the oral mucosa. This may become a popular wilderness potent analgesic.

   f. Some rescue teams are administering standard IV formulations of fentanyl administered via nasal "acorn" style nebulizers, Manufacturers are now developing dedicated delivery systems for this use (e.g., "Go Medical" nasal PCA device [www.gomedical.com.au], "MAD" Nasal Drug Delivery Device [http://www. wolfetory.com/nasal.html]).

   g. Fentanyl transdermal system (Duragesic) patches have limited utility for wilderness pain control. Patches have slow onset and may be ineffective in vasoconstricted and/or hypovolemic patients with reduced cutaneous circulation. They are also difficult to titrate.

Side Effects and Overdosage

1. Critical patient assessment is required when using narcotic analgesics to detect respiratory depression, hypotension, and other potential side effects.
2. Potential adverse side effects for all narcotics may include anaphylaxis, nausea, vomiting, rash, respiratory depression, urinary retention, and hypotension. To prevent or treat nausea, consider administering an antiemetic such as ondansetron prior to narcotic administration.
3. Narcotic antagonists such as naloxone and other emergency resuscitative medications should be available when using narcotics in the wilderness.
   a. Naloxone (Narcan) is a narcotic antagonist that may reverse narcotic effects. Doses of 0.2 mg IV or 0.4 mg IV, IM, or SC may be given and repeated every 2 to 5 minutes until CNS, respiratory, or hypotensive narcotic symptoms are reversed, to a maximum dose of 10 mg.
   b. Do not give potent narcotic analgesics to victims with suspected head injury or neurologic illness.
   c. The primary treatment of a relative overdose of narcotics is airway support and stimulation. In the acute pain environment, simply performing a jaw thrust along with verbal stimulation will typically arouse the patient sufficiently to avoid narcotic antagonist administration.
   d. Naloxone should be given only after the victim's airway is secured so that, in the event of vomiting, the risk of aspiration is minimized.
   e. Initially, give enough naloxone to reverse respiratory depression, not enough to reverse analgesia. In an acute pain setting, 0.2 mg is appropriate.
   f. Continuous monitoring of blood pressure, mental status, and respiratory status is critical, with possible repeat doses necessary in 1 to 2 hours. Pain may return with aggressive narcotic reversal, and a balance between pain alleviation and physiologic stability is desired. Additionally, narcotic antagonists may lead to acute narcotic withdrawal symptoms in persons with a tolerance to and dependence on narcotics.

Oral Agents

1. Hydrocodone is generally considered the most potent oral narcotic analgesic that does not require specialized prescribing documentation. This makes hydrocodone an

appropriate choice in the wilderness environment for moderate pain.
2. The typical formulation of hydrocodone is combined with acetaminophen (e.g., Vicodin).
3. The standard dose is 5 to 10 mg hydrocodone PO q4–6h.
4. Oxycodone (Roxicodone) is another good choice but is tightly controlled and requires specialized prescribing documentation.
5. Tramadol, propoxyphene, and codeine provide inferior analgesia to other recommended agents and should not be first choices for wilderness pain control.

▶ ADDITIONAL AGENTS

Narcotic Agonist-Antagonist Combinations
1. Drugs in this class include buprenorphine, butorphanol, and nalbuphine.
2. In the wilderness setting a drug worth noting is transnasal butorphanol (Stadol NS).
   a. The usual recommended dose for initial nasal administration is 1 mg (1 spray in *one* nostril).
   b. Adherence to this dose reduces the incidence of drowsiness and dizziness. If adequate pain relief is not achieved within 60 to 90 minutes, an additional 1 mg dose may be given.
   c. Stadol offers good analgesia, with a low respiratory depression ceiling, but can cause significant sedation and often considerable dysphoria.
   d. It is fast acting and can be given without IV access.

Ketorolac (Toradol)
1. Many clinicians administer ketorolac because it is nonsedating. Ironically, by the time one is giving IV analgesia in the wilderness, some degree of sedation is a usually a welcome side effect.
2. Ketorolac inhibits prostaglandin synthesis and can disrupt the stomach's mucosal barrier. Even though the drug is not taken orally, gastrointestinal toxicity is still possible.
3. It can be useful in the care of patients with acutely painful conditions that involve a prostaglandin-mediated process. Examples of such conditions include renal colic, biliary colic, dysmenorrhea, and gout.
4. It may be used in conjunction with narcotics.
5. Ketorolac is contraindicated in patients with renal impairment or severe volume depletion.

6. Recommended dosage is 60 mg IM or 30 mg IV q4-6h. Use half this dose if the patient is older than 65 years or weighs less than 50 kg. Oral dose is 10 mg.

Ketamine

1. Ketamine should only be used by personnel familiar with airway management and procedures.
2. Ketamine is a dissociative anesthetic agent that also provides significant analgesia.
3. Ketamine possesses sympathomimetic activity that may prove useful in injured persons with depressed cardiac function or shock and may also provide bronchodilation for victims with reactive airway disease.
4. It is contraindicated with head injury because it increases intracranial pressure. Intracranial pressure increase results from augmented cerebral blood flow and direct cerebral vasodilatation. Cerebral metabolic oxygen requirements increase as well.
5. An IV dose of 0.2 to 0.4 mg/kg ketamine provides analgesia, and 1 to 2 mg/kg IV or 2 to 4 mg/kg IM leads to profound analgesia and a dissociative state.
6. A quiet and calm setting diminishes unpleasant dissociative experiences for the recipient.

Muscle Relaxants

1. The term *muscle relaxants* refers to a diverse group of drugs with similar clinical effects but different pharmacologic properties. They are not true skeletal muscle relaxants in the sense of blocking neuromuscular transmission but act by depressing reflexes, generally in the CNS. They are indicated for the relief of muscle spasm related to acute, painful musculoskeletal injuries.
2. Side effects include decreased alertness, motor coordination, and physical dexterity.
3. The specific mechanism of action is unknown but appears to be related to centrally acting sedation. See Table 24-2 for a list of common centrally acting muscle relaxants.

TABLE 24-2. Skeletal Muscle Relaxants

DRUG	DOSAGE (mg)	INTERVAL (hr)	RISKS, PRECAUTIONS
Baclofen	3-5 start, increase 5 mg every 3 days	8	Dizziness, ataxia, confusion, severe abrupt withdrawal

TABLE 24-2. Skeletal Muscle Relaxants—cont'd

DRUG	DOSAGE (mg)	INTERVAL (hr)	RISKS, PRECAUTIONS
Carisoprodol	350	4-6	Dizziness, ataxia, headache, tremor, syncope, severe abrupt withdrawal, contraindicated with acute intermittent porphyria
Chlorphenesin	400	6-8	Confusion, headache, dizziness (8 weeks or less); avoid in patients with hepatic disease
Chlorzoxazone	250-750	4-6	Dizziness, paradoxical stimulation, rare severe hepatotoxicity
Cyclobenzaprine	10	12-24	Anticholinergic; may cause hypotension, arrhythmias; avoid with MAOI use and in patients with hypertension, CHF, arrhythmia, glaucoma, urinary retention, severe depression, or suicide attempts
Diazepam	2-10	6-8, variable	Dizziness, paradoxical stimulation, cardiopulmonary depression; use only in patients with severe anxiety
Metaxalone	800	6-8	Hepatic impairment, rash, dizziness, headache; avoid with drug-induced anemia
Methocarbamol	1000-1500	4-6	Dizziness, headache, rash
Orphenadrine	100	8-12	Anticholinergic; headache, dizziness

CHF, congestive heart failure; MAOI, monoamine oxidase inhibitor.

Life-Threatening Emergencies (Rescue Breathing/CPR/Choking)

25

▶ **RESCUE BREATHING**

Adult

1. Check for breathing (see Chapter 12, Fig. 12-2). If the victim is not lying on his or her back, gently roll him or her over, moving the entire body as a unit while maintaining spine precautions (see Chapter 12, Fig. 12-1).
2. If no breathing is detected, open the airway with the head-tilt maneuver.
   a. Place the palm of one hand on the victim's forehead and tilt the head back while the fingers of the other hand grasp and lift the chin.
   b. If a cervical spine injury is suspected, use the chin-lift or jaw-thrust technique to open the airway (see Chapter 12, Figs. 12-3 and 12-4). Sweep two fingers through the victim's mouth to remove any foreign material or broken teeth.
3. If spontaneous breathing does not resume, pinch the victim's nostrils closed and place your mouth over the victim's mouth. Use a CPR Microshield or improvised barrier during mouth-to-mouth breathing to prevent physical contact with the victim's mouth. A glove can be modified and used as a barrier shield for performing rescue breathing. Cut a slit into the distal part of the middle finger of the glove and insert it into the victim's mouth. Stretch the glove across the victim's mouth and nose and blow into the glove as you would to inflate a balloon. After each breath, remove the part of the glove covering the nose to allow the victim to exhale. The slit creates a one-way valve, preventing backflow of the victim's saliva (Fig. 25-1).
4. Blow air into the victim until you see the chest rise. Remove your mouth to allow the victim to exhale. Give two initial breaths.
5. Repeat this procedure, giving a vigorous breath every 5 seconds until the victim begins to breathe spontaneously, help arrives, or you are too exhausted to continue.
6. If air does not move in and out of the victim's mouth easily or chest movement is not detected, first try tilting the head farther back or, if a cervical spine injury is suspected, repeat the jaw-thrust technique, pushing the victim's jaw farther out. If breathing still does not occur, the airway may be obstructed by a foreign body.

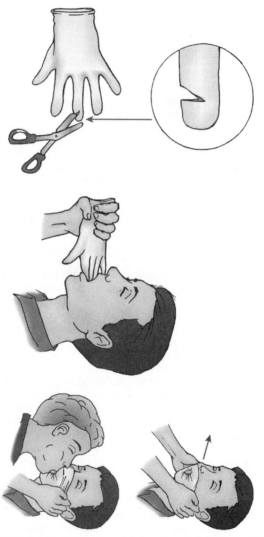

Figure 25-1. An improvised CPR barrier is created using a latex or nitrile glove. Make a slit in the middle finger of the glove.

7. During mouth-to-mouth breathing, the victim's stomach will often fill with air, eventually resulting in vomiting. If vomiting occurs, log-roll the victim in a manner that maintains cervical spine alignment (see Chapter 14, Fig. 14-1) and clear the airway.
8. Check for a pulse by palpating the carotid artery in the victim's neck.
   a. If the victim is hypothermic, spend 1 full minute trying to detect a carotid pulse before assuming the person has no effective cardiac activity.
   b. If a pulse is present, continue rescue breathing.
   c. If no pulse is present, start chest compressions.

Child (Older Than 1 Year)
1. Cover the child's mouth with your mouth.
2. Pinch the child's nose closed with the thumb and forefinger of the same hand that is placed on the forehead for the head tilt. Use your other hand to lift the chin.
3. Breathe two slow (lasting 1½ seconds) breaths into the child's mouth, with a 2-second pause between breaths. You should breathe in enough air to allow the child's chest to rise.
4. If the child does not start to breathe on his or her own, check for a pulse.
   a. If a pulse is present, continue rescue breathing with 20 breaths per minute.
   b. If no pulse is present, start chest compressions.

Infant (Younger Than 1 Year)
1. Do not pinch the nose closed, but cover the infant's nose and mouth with your mouth. Apply the head-tilt maneuver, or use the jaw thrust if you suspect a cervical spine injury (Fig. 25-2).
2. Breathe two slow (lasting 1½ seconds) breaths (use only light puffs of air) into the infant's mouth, with a pause between breaths. You should breathe in enough air to allow the infant's chest to rise.
3. If the infant does not start to breathe on his own, check for a pulse.
   a. If a pulse is present, continue rescue breathing with 20 breaths per minute.
   b. If no pulse is present, start chest compressions.

▶ CARDIOPULMONARY RESUSCITATION

Definition
CPR is the combination of rescue (mouth-to-mouth) breathing and chest compressions in a nonbreathing victim who has no pulse.

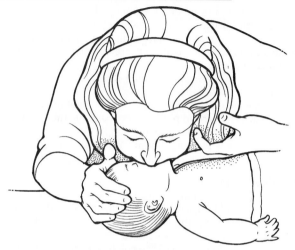

Figure 25-2. Rescue breathing: infant.

When to Start CPR

1. Do not be afraid to initiate CPR, thinking you might be criticized for not continuing it indefinitely. People may blame themselves and each other for not doing extraordinary and heroic resuscitative measures. It is reasonable to give a victim the benefit of the doubt and start CPR, even if he or she has been without a heartbeat or breath for a prolonged time. It is difficult to know exactly how long a person found unconscious has actually been in cardiac arrest.
2. After assessing and initially managing the airway, take 10 seconds (60 seconds if the victim is hypothermic) to feel for a carotid pulse to determine if the heart is beating. If there is no pulse, begin chest compressions along with mouth-to-mouth breathing.

▶ CHEST COMPRESSIONS

Adults

1. Place the victim on his or her back on a firm surface. Position the heel of one hand over the center of the victim's breastbone and the heel of your other hand over the bottom hand, interlocking the fingers (Fig. 25-3).
2. Be certain your shoulders line up directly over the victim's breastbone with elbows held straight.

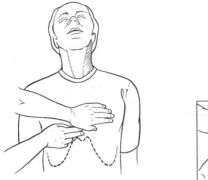
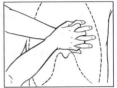

Figure 25-3. Hand position for chest compressions in CPR.

3. Using a stiff-arm technique, compress the breastbone 4 to 5 cm (1½ to 2 inches) and then release. Push hard and push fast—give two compressions per second, or about 100 compressions per minute. Do not remove your hands from the victim's chest between compressions (Fig. 25-4).
4. After 30 compressions, tilt the head back and lift the chin up to open the airway. Prepare to give two rescue breaths. Pinch the nose shut and breathe into the mouth for 1 second. If the chest rises, give a second rescue breath. If the chest does not

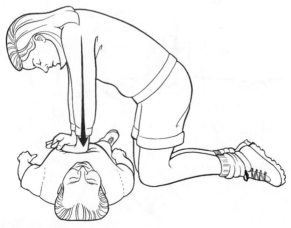

Figure 25-4. Chest compressions: adult.

rise, repeat the head tilt-chin lift and then give the second rescue breath. That is one cycle. If someone else is available, ask that person to give two breaths after you do 30 compressions.

5. During CPR, check every few minutes for the return of a carotid pulse or spontaneous breathing.

6. If the person has not begun moving after five cycles (about 2 minutes) and an automated external defibrillator (AED) is available, open the kit and follow the prompts.

Child (Older Than 1 Year)

The procedure for giving CPR to a child age 1 through 8 is essentially the same as that for an adult. The differences are as follows:

1. Perform five cycles of compressions and breaths on the child—this should take about 2 minutes.

2. Use only one hand to perform heart compressions.

3. Breathe more gently.

4. Use the same compression/breath rate as is used for adults: 30 compressions followed by two breaths. This is one cycle. Following the two breaths, immediately begin the next cycle of compressions and breaths (Fig. 25-5).

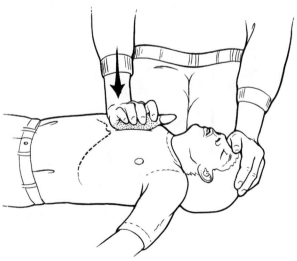

Figure 25-5. Chest compressions: child.

Infant (Younger Than 1 Year)

Most cardiac arrests in infants occur from lack of oxygen such as from drowning or choking. If you know the infant has an airway obstruction, perform first aid for choking. If you do not know why the infant is not breathing, perform CPR.

1. Place your middle and ring fingers on the lower part of the breastbone (Fig. 25-6).
2. Compress the breastbone about one third to one half the thickness of the chest (1.25 to 2.5 cm [½ to 1 inch]).
3. Compress the chest at a rate of approximately 100 per minute.
4. Give 2 breaths after every 30 chest compressions. Use this same ratio whether one or two persons are doing the resuscitation. Stop to check for spontaneous breathing and a pulse after 1 minute, and then after every few minutes.

When to Stop CPR

1. It has often been stated that, "Once started, CPR should never be terminated in the field." To adhere to this dictum is not only impractical—it is potentially hazardous to rescuers.
2. It is well established that after 10 to 15 minutes of CPR, if a victim does not respond, he or she probably never will. The rare exceptions have been victims who were profoundly hypothermic.
3. If CPR is not successful in resuscitating a victim after 15 to 30 minutes, and the victim is not profoundly hypothermic, then it is usually reasonable to discontinue CPR.

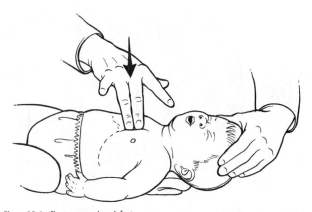

Figure 25-6. Chest compressions: infant.

▶ **CHOKING/OBSTRUCTED AIRWAY**

Choking is a life-threatening emergency that occurs when something obstructs the victim's airway so that he or she cannot breathe.

Signs and Symptoms
1. Suddenly agitated, clutching the throat, especially while eating
2. Inability to speak
3. Cyanosis

Treatment
1. For a choking adult or child, perform the Heimlich maneuver, as follows:
   a. Stand behind the victim and wrap your arms around the victim's waist.
   b. Make a fist with one of your hands and place it just above the victim's navel and below the rib cage, with the thumb side against the abdomen.
   c. Grasp your fist with the other hand and pull your hands forcefully toward you, into the victim's abdomen and slightly upward with a quick thrust.
   d. If unsuccessful, repeat the procedure to achieve a total of four or five thrusts (Fig. 25-7).

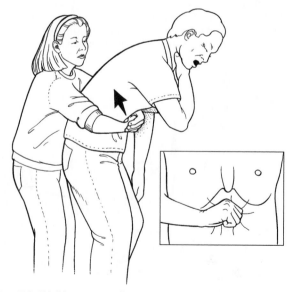

Figure 25-7. Heimlich maneuver: standing.

2. If the adult or child becomes unconscious, do the following:
   a. Lay the victim on his or her back and attempt rescue breathing.
   b. If rescue breathing is unsuccessful because of an airway obstruction, perform the Heimlich maneuver while kneeling down and straddling the victim's thighs. Use the heel of the hand instead of a fist (Fig. 25-8).
   c. If still unsuccessful, sweep the mouth with one or two fingers to try to remove any foreign material.
   d. Continue to perform the Heimlich maneuver, and periodically attempt rescue breathing (Fig. 25-9).
   e. If multiple attempts at clearing the airway and ventilating the victim are unsuccessful, perform a cricothyrotomy (see Chapter 12, Fig. 12-6).
3. For a choking infant (younger than 1 year), do the following:
   a. If the infant is coughing and appears to be getting sufficient air, do not interfere with his or her attempts to cough the obstruction out of the airway.
   b. If the infant cannot cough, cry, or get sufficient air, lay him or her face down, supported by and straddling your forearm, while resting your forearm on your thigh. Support the infant's head by grasping under the chin and holding onto the jaw. Make sure the infant's head is lower than the rest of the body.
   c. Using the heel of your free hand, give up to five firm back blows between the infant's shoulder blades.
   d. If the obstruction is not cleared, place your free hand on the infant's back, holding the back and head so that they are sandwiched between both of your arms.

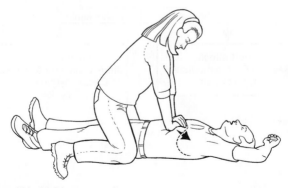

Figure 25-8. Heimlich maneuver: supine.

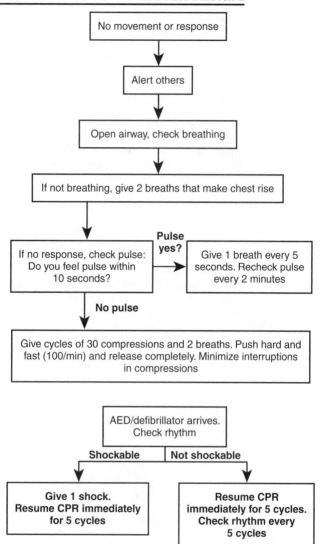

Figure 25-9. Flow chart depicting next stages after unsuccessful Heimlich maneuver is performed.

e. Carefully support the trunk and head while flipping the infant over to a supine position. Support the infant on your thigh, keeping the infant's head lower than the rest of the body. Give five quick, downward chest thrusts with two fingertips positioned over the infant's lower breastbone 1.3 cm (½ inch) below the nipples.

f. Look into the infant's mouth for a foreign object, and try to remove it.

g. If the infant becomes unconscious, try mouth-to-mouth rescue breathing. If you are unsuccessful at getting air into the infant's lungs, repeat steps a through e until you have removed the object or the child has started to breathe on his or her own.

Allergic Reaction

26

▶ **ANAPHYLAXIS**

Signs and Symptoms
1. Urticaria (hives), diffuse epidermal erythema, soft tissue edema
2. Wheezing, stridor, cough, chest tightness, hoarseness, dyspnea
3. Dysphagia, nausea and vomiting, diarrhea, abdominal pain
4. Hypotension and tachycardia (shock), seizures
5. Edema involving the face, lips, tongue, pharynx, and larynx, producing an obstructed airway and respiratory arrest
6. Cardiovascular collapse with shock can occur rapidly, without any other antecedent symptoms. The more immediate the reaction, the more severe the degree of anaphylaxis.
7. Most anaphylactic reactions occur within 5 minutes to 2 hours after exposure to an inciting agent.

Treatment
In the event of anaphylactic shock, there is no time to get the victim to medical facilities from the wilderness. The definitive treatment is epinephrine.
1. Place the individual in the Trendelenburg position.
2. Obtain and maintain the airway, administering oxygen as needed.
3. Place a venous tourniquet above the reaction site (e.g., insect sting) to decrease systemic absorption of the antigen.
4. Administer epinephrine.
   a. Begin with aqueous epinephrine 1:1000 IM in the deltoid region.
   b. The dose for an adult is 0.3 to 0.5 mL (0.3 to 0.5 mg), and for a child it is 0.01 mL/kg, not to exceed a total dose of 0.3 mL. Repeat in 10 to 15 minutes in adults and in 20 minutes in a child if relief is partial.
   c. Epinephrine is available in a spring-loaded injectable cartridge called the EpiPen (Meridian Medical Technologies). This allows for self-administration of the medicine without dealing with a needle and syringe. The device contains 2 mL of epinephrine in a disposable push-button, spring-activated cartridge with a concealed needle. It delivers a single dose of 0.3 mg of epinephrine injection, USP 1:1000 (0.3 mL) in a sterile solution intramuscularly. A child who weighs less than 30 kg (66 lb) should be injected with an EpiPen Jr., which

delivers 0.15 mg epinephrine, USP 1:1000 (0.15 mL) in a sterile solution. Another autoinjector is the Twinject (Verus Pharmaceuticals), which can deliver two doses, either 0.3 mg or 0.15 mg depending on the injector, per device.

d. If the reaction is life threatening and if the patient does not respond to intramuscular epinephrine, administer epinephrine intravenously. Mix 0.1 mL (0.1 mg) of 1:1,000 aqueous epinephrine in 10 mL of normal saline (final dilution, 1:100,000) and infuse over 10 minutes. In an infant or child, the starting dose is 0.1 μg/kg/minute up to a maximum of 1.5 μg/kg/minute. This solution can also be injected under the tongue if an intravenous line cannot be established.

e. Use epinephrine with caution in a person older than age 40 because it can produce cardiac ischemia and arrhythmias.

f. In a refractory case in which the individual is not responsive to epinephrine (e.g., an individual on a beta-blocker medication), administer glucagon at a dose of 1 to 5 mg intravenously over 2 minutes, or intramuscularly.

5. If the reaction is limited to pruritus and urticaria with no wheezing or facial swelling, administer an antihistamine such as diphenhydramine (Benadryl), 50 mg q4–6h for an adult; for children, give 1 mg/kg. Reserve epinephrine for a worsened condition.

6. Additionally, consider adding a histamine-2 blocker such as cimetidine, 400 to 800 mg PO.

7. Victims may use aerosolized epinephrine via a metered-dose inhaler (Primatene Mist, Medihaler-Epi) to counteract the effects of bronchoconstriction and laryngeal edema.

8. Treat bronchospasm and wheezing with albuterol, via a handheld, metered-dose inhaler with a spacer (adult dose: 200 to 400 μg [2 to 8 full inhalations, depending on the preparation] q15 to 20 min prn).

9. Administer a corticosteroid. If IV access is available, administer 125 mg methylprednisolone (Solu-Medrol) or 15 mg dexamethasone. If therapy is initiated orally, administer prednisone, 60 to 100 mg for adults and 2 mg/kg for children.

10. If a stinger remains after an insect sting, remove it by the most rapid means possible.

11. Note that in severe cases, endotracheal intubation may be necessary. Be sure to visualize the vocal cords with a rigid laryngoscope because of the distortion caused by laryngeal

edema. If an airway cannot be obtained immediately, perform a needle cricothyrotomy; for a child, perform a tracheostomy if oral intubation is not successful.

12. After treatment, be prepared to transport the victim immediately for medical evaluation because an anaphylactic reaction can recur as the effects of the epinephrine diminish.

▶ **ALLERGIC RHINITIS**

Signs and Symptoms
1. Sneezing, nasal congestion, rhinorrhea
2. Pruritus of the nose and eyes
3. Coughing, wheezing
4. Urticaria (hives)

Treatment
1. Administer an antihistamine such as cetirizine (Zyrtec) 10 mg qd. The dose for children younger than 12 years of age is 2.5 to 10 mg qd.
2. In some individuals, addition of a decongestant such as pseudoephedrine (Sudafed) 60 mg PO q4–6h to the antihistamine may be helpful.
3. Leukotriene-receptor antagonists (LTRAs) are now approved for use in allergic rhinitis. Montelukast and zafirlukast are two currently available oral LTRAs. The dose of montelukast for adults and adolescents 15 years of age and older is 10 mg at bedtime. Pediatric dose is 5 mg and 4 mg at bedtime for ages 6 to 14 years and 6 months to 5 years, respectively.
4. Nasal corticosteroids are the gold standard of treatment for allergic rhinitis. Several preparations are available; all are equally effective. An example is fluticasone (Flonase) 1 to 2 sprays in each nostril qd. Because of their relatively slow onset of action, the maximal benefit of nasal corticosteroids may not be realized until 1 to 3 weeks after the initiation of therapy.

Cardiopulmonary Emergencies

27

▶ **CARDIAC EMERGENCIES**

Acute Coronary Syndromes (Unstable Angina and Acute Myocardial Infarction)

Signs and Symptoms
1. Chest pain that is often described as a pressure, heaviness, tightness, or crushing or squeezing sensation and located in the center of the chest. The pain may be poorly localized or of a sharp, stabbing nature. It may radiate into the neck, jaw, or shoulders or down the inner aspect of the arms (left more frequent than right). Sometimes there is only mild chest pain, a burning sensation in the lower chest or upper abdomen, or a feeling of indigestion.
2. Diaphoresis, eructation, nausea, vomiting, anxiety, or dyspnea may be present.
3. Pain is often preceded or exacerbated by physical exertion.

Treatment
1. The victim should discontinue all exertion.
2. Administer oxygen if available.
3. Administer aspirin, 325 mg, if the victim is not allergic to it and has no history of significant bleeding.
4. Consider giving nitroglycerin sublingually at a dose of 0.4 mg every 5 minutes for three doses. Nitrates should be withheld if the victim is suspected of being hypotensive (systolic blood pressure lower than 100 mm Hg). In the absence of a blood pressure cuff, hypotension can be recognized by the inability to palpate a strong radial pulse in the wrist or dorsalis pedis pulse in the foot.
5. Consider giving a beta-blocker such as metoprolol, 5 mg, every 5 minutes IV over 1 to 2 minutes for three doses unless systolic pressure is below 100 or the heart rate is less than 60. Other contraindications include a history of heart block, asthma, chronic obstructive pulmonary disease, or congestive heart failure.
6. Keep the victim in a comfortable position.
7. Evacuate the victim immediately to the closest medical facility with the victim exerting as little as possible.
8. Notify the emergency department regarding your estimated time of arrival as soon as possible to facilitate their readiness.

Heart Failure

Many of the signs and symptoms of congestive heart failure are similar to those of high-altitude pulmonary edema (HAPE). Victims of HAPE, however, do not commonly have jugular venous distention and orthopnea.

Signs and Symptoms
1. Dyspnea, which is often worsened by exertion or lying flat (orthopnea)
2. Tachycardia, tachypnea
3. Fatigue
4. Paroxysmal nocturnal dyspnea
5. Peripheral edema
6. Jugular venous distention
7. Pulmonary rales and wheezes
8. Cyanosis and diaphoresis

Treatment
1. Keep the victim sitting up, unless he or she is more comfortable lying on his or her back.
2. Administer 100% oxygen.
3. Administer nitroglycerin sublingually at a dose of 0.4 mg every 5 minutes for three doses. Nitrates should be withheld if the victim is suspected of being hypotensive (systolic blood pressure lower than 100 mm Hg). In the absence of a blood pressure cuff, hypotension can be recognized by the inability to palpate a strong radial pulse in the wrist or dorsalis pedis pulse in the foot.
4. Consider administering furosemide, 20 to 40 mg IV, IM, or PO.
5. Treat wheezing with albuterol, via a handheld, metered-dose inhaler with a spacer (adult dose: 200 to 400 µg [2 to 8 inhalations, depending on the preparation] q15 to 20 min prn).
6. Evacuate the victim immediately to the closest medical facility with the victim exerting as little as possible.

▶ PULMONARY EMERGENCIES

Pulmonary Embolism

A pulmonary embolus is a blood clot that has traveled from a vein somewhere in the body to lodge in the circulation of the lungs. The most common sources of the original blood clot are the veins of the pelvis or legs. Predisposing factors to pulmonary embolism include dehydration, periods of prolonged rest in a single position (sitting in a plane or in a car), recent surgery, pregnancy, cancer, cigarette smoking, and medications (e.g., birth control pills).

Signs and Symptoms
1. Sudden, sharp chest pain that is often pleuritic (worse with deep breathing)
2. Dyspnea
3. Cough (occasionally with hemoptysis)
4. Tachypnea and tachycardia
5. If the clot is large, the victim may become hypotensive and cyanotic and expire rapidly.

Treatment
1. Administer 100% oxygen.
2. Consider administering enoxaparin (Lovenox) 1 mg/kg SC q12h or 1.5 mg/kg SC qd.
3. Immediately evacuate patient to the closest medical facility.

Asthma

Generally, most people know that they are prone to asthma attacks; however, first-time episodes may occur in persons exposed to cold, emotional stress, or exertion or during an allergic reaction.

Signs and Symptoms
1. Dyspnea
2. Wheezing
3. Cough
4. Prolongation of the expiratory phase of breathing
5. Use of accessory muscles of inspiration (neck muscles are most prominent)
6. In severe cases, wheezing may diminish because the lungs become so "tight" that there is not enough air movement to create the abnormal sounds and the victim will appear cyanotic.

Treatment
1. Administer 100% oxygen.
2. Administer an inhalable bronchodilator such as albuterol, via a handheld, metered-dose inhaler with a spacer (adult dose: 200 to 400 µg q2 to 6h prn).
3. Administer diphenhydramine, 50 mg IV, IM, or PO, if the attack is associated with an acute allergic reaction.
4. Administer a corticosteroid (prednisone, 60 to 100 mg for adults and 2 mg/kg for children).
5. In severe cases, intubation and assisted ventilation may be necessary.
6. A person with asthma who is in severe distress or who does not have rapid and marked improvement with medication should be transported rapidly to the nearest medical facility.

Pneumonia

Signs and Symptoms
1. Cough that may be productive of green or yellowish sputum
2. Fever and shaking chills
3. Chest pain that may be pleuritic (worse with breathing)
4. Dyspnea, tachypnea, and tachycardia may be present

Treatment
1. Administer oxygen to maintain SaO_2 greater than 90%.
2. Administer a broad-spectrum antibiotic. Excellent choices include the following:
   a. Azithromycin (Zithromax) (adult dose): 500 mg day one, then 250 mg/day for 4 additional days.
   b. Levofloxacin (Levaquin) (adult dose): 500 mg/day.
   c. Amoxicillin/clavulanate (Augmentin) (adult dose): 500 to 875 mg bid.
   d. Erythromycin (adult dose): 250 to 500 mg q6h.

Neurologic Emergencies

28

▶ STROKE

Stroke is the third leading cause of death and the leading cause of disability in the United States. It is a disease process that disrupts vascular blood flow to a distinct region of the brain. Although the etiology of strokes is diverse, ranging from cardiac emboli to rupture of a congenital aneurysm, there are two major mechanisms of brain injury: (1) ischemia due to vessel occlusion and (2) hemorrhage due to vessel rupture. From 80% to 85% of all strokes are ischemic. Effective treatment for one stroke type may be disastrous when applied to the other type. A victim in the backcountry suspected of having a stroke should be transported immediately to the nearest medical facility because the anatomic location of the lesion and the mechanism of the stroke must be known before effective treatment can be given. Ischemic (thrombotic) strokes can be effectively treated in many cases with intravenous (IV) tissue plasminogen activator (t-PA) if symptoms have been present for less than 3 hours. Mechanical clot removal (e.g., Merci retrieval device) and intra-arterial t-PA may be effective in reversing stroke manifestations up to 8 hours after symptom onset.

A review of the victim's demographics and past medical history may suggest the etiology of the stroke. A 40-year-old, otherwise healthy victim with a stroke-like syndrome is more likely to have a hemorrhagic stroke. A 65-year-old victim with a history of hypertension, coronary artery disease, and diabetes is more likely to have a thrombotic stroke. Stroke in a victim with underlying atrial fibrillation suggests a cardioembolic source. Stroke in an individual with previous transient ischemic attack (TIA)-like symptoms suggests a thrombotic etiology.

Signs and Symptoms
Any or all of the following signs and symptoms may be present:
1. Victim may be alert, drowsy, lethargic, obtunded, or comatose
2. Visual field deficit or gaze preference
3. Sudden onset of unilateral weakness and numbness
4. Unilateral facial motor weakness (facial droop)
5. Dysarthria and/or aphasia
6. Sudden onset of dizziness, vertigo, diplopia, and ataxia
7. Sudden onset of severe headache ("the worst headache of my life")

Treatment
1. Maintain an adequate airway and administer oxygen.
2. Dehydration should be corrected with IV normal saline.
3. Assess the victim for hypoglycemia and give dextrose if indicated (see later). Otherwise, dextrose-containing solutions should be avoided.
4. Keep the victim's head and torso slightly elevated (at least 30 degrees).
5. Transport the victim immediately to the closest medical facility. Continuously assess the victim's airway and level of consciousness because the condition can worsen dramatically during transport.
6. If the victim's primary symptom is dizziness or vertigo, consider giving an antihistamine (diphenhydramine, 50 mg PO q6h, or meclizine, 25 mg PO q6h), anticholinergic (scopolamine, 0.5 mg patch behind ear), or sedative (diazepam, 2 to 10 mg PO q6–8h) medication.

▶ TRANSIENT ISCHEMIC ATTACK

A TIA is a neurologic deficit that resolves within 24 hours (although most resolve within 30 minutes) and is most commonly associated with thrombotic stroke. Signs, symptoms, and treatment are the same as for stroke.

▶ SEIZURE

Seizure can result from head injury, heat illness, infection, hyponatremia, hypoglycemia, stroke, epilepsy, drugs, and other causes.

Signs and Symptoms
1. A generalized (grand mal) seizure begins abruptly with loss of consciousness as the victim suddenly becomes rigid, with trunk and extremities extended, and falls to the ground. As the rigid (tonic) phase of the seizure subsides, there is increasing coarse trembling that evolves into rhythmic (clonic) jerking of the trunk and extremities. The eyes may deviate to one side, there is difficulty breathing, and occasionally there is loss of bladder and/or bowel control and tongue biting.
2. Most seizures last only 1 or 2 minutes.
3. After most seizures, the victim will be confused or combative (postictal) for a period of time (10 to 30 minutes) and then slowly return to normal.

Treatment
1. Protect the victim from injury during the seizure. This may be done with cushions, with a sleeping bag, or by moving hard objects away from the victim.

2. If possible, the victim should be turned to one side to reduce the risk of aspiration should vomiting occur.

3. Do not attempt to place a bite block or any object between the teeth or into the mouth.

4. Keep the victim NPO until he is awake and lucid.

5. If the victim is suffering from hypoglycemia, administer sugar as soon as possible.

   a. If the victim is conscious and able to swallow, give him or her something containing sugar to drink or eat. This could be fruit juice, a banana, candy, or a nondiet soft drink. As soon as the victim feels better, have him or her eat a meal to avoid a recurrence.

   b. If the victim is unconscious, place tiny amounts of sugar granules, cake icing, or Glutose paste (one tube contains 25 g glucose) under the victim's tongue, where it will be passively swallowed and absorbed.

   c. If available, administer 1 to 3 ampules of IV 50% dextrose in water while completing the ABCs (airway, breathing, circulation) of resuscitation. In a child younger than 8 years of age, give 25% dextrose in water in a dose of 2 to 4 mL/kg or even 10% dextrose in water in a dose of 0.5 to 1 g/kg. As an alternative in a victim for whom you cannot quickly obtain IV access, give 1 to 2 mg of glucagon intramuscularly or subcutaneously. This dose may be repeated as needed.

6. If the victim has continuous seizure activity for 10 minutes or more, or two or more seizures that occur without full recovery of consciousness between the attacks (status epilepticus), administer the following:

   a. 100% oxygen

   b. Dextrose, 25 to 50 g IV

   c. Diazepam (adult dose): 5 mg IV/IM or 10 mg PR (repeat as needed q 5 min to total of 20 mg) or lorazepam up to 0.1 mg/kg

▶ **HEADACHE**

Headaches stem from innumerable causes including tension and stress, migraine, dehydration, altitude illness, alcohol hangover, carbon monoxide poisoning, brain tumor, stroke, aneurysm, intracranial hemorrhage, fever, flu, meningitis and other infectious diseases, high blood pressure, sinus infection, and dental problems. Suddenly going "cold turkey" without caffeine during a backpacking trip, especially if you regularly drink more than three cups of coffee a day, can also precipitate a headache (Box 28-1).

> ## Box 28-1. Headaches—"When to Worry"
>
> Some headaches may signal a life-threatening illness. Someone with any of the following symptoms should seek medical attention as soon as possible:
> 1. The headache is the worst of one's life and came on suddenly and severely (aneurysm or intracranial bleeding).
> 2. The headache is associated with extremity numbness or weakness, or there is unilateral facial paralysis (facial droop) (stroke).
> 3. The headache is associated with an altered level of consciousness, aphasia, dysarthria, or ataxia.
> 4. There is fever, stiff neck, or any rash (meningitis).
> 5. The headache grows steadily worse over time.
> 6. There is repetitive or projectile vomiting.

Tension Headache (Stress or Muscle Contraction Headache)

This is the most common type of headache and affects people of all ages. The pain is related to continuous contractions of the muscles of the head and neck. Tension headaches have gradual onset and worsen as the day progresses.

Signs and Symptoms
1. The headache is typically bilateral and often described as tight or vise-like, especially in the back of the head and neck.
2. The pain is not made worse by walking, climbing, or performing physical activity.
3. Sensitivity to light may occur, but nausea and vomiting are not usually present.
4. Pain can last from 30 minutes to 7 days.

Treatment
1. Loosen any tight-fitting pack straps or hat, and adjust your pack so that it rides comfortably.
2. Administer a nonsteroidal antiinflammatory drug (NSAID) such as ibuprofen (Motrin), 800 mg PO q8h, or acetaminophen (Tylenol), 1 g PO q6h prn.
3. For severe pain, administer hydrocodone, 5 mg, and acetaminophen, 500 mg (Vicodin), 1 to 2 tablets PO q4–6h prn.

Migraine Headache

Signs and Symptoms
1. Recurrent headaches that involve usually (but not always) one side of the head
2. Nausea and vomiting common

3. Photosensitivity
4. Walking or physical exertion makes the pain worse.
5. About 15% of individuals with migraine headaches experience an aura (flashing lights, distorted shapes and colors, blurred vision or other visual apparitions) before the onset of the headache.

Treatment
1. Administer an NSAID such as ibuprofen (Motrin), 800 mg PO q8h, or acetaminophen (Tylenol), 1 g PO q6h prn.
2. Caffeine-containing beverages such as coffee may help relieve symptoms, especially if taken early.
3. Consider administering sumatriptan succinate (Imitrex), 6 mg SQ by autoinjector or 25 mg PO, or as a 5- or 20-mg nasal spray. Doses may be repeated in 1 hour if not effective to a total of 12 mg SC, 200 mg PO, or 50 mg nasally in 1 day.
4. Consider administering a stronger pain medication such as hydrocodone, 5 mg, and acetaminophen, 500 mg (Vicodin), 1 to 2 tablets PO q4–6h prn.
5. Administer an antiemetic. Examples include: prochlorperazine (Compazine 5 to 10 mg PO/IM/IV every 6 hours or as a 25 mg rectal suppository; promethazine (Phenergan) 12.5 to 25 mg PO/IV/IM/rectally every 6 hours. Ondansetron (Zofran) 4 mg may be given PO or IV every 8 hours and is very effective with fewer side effects. It is also available in a wafer form that easily dissolves when placed on a person's tongue.

Cluster Headache

Signs and Symptoms
1. Headache is unilateral, severe, and short, lasting 30 to 90 minutes.
2. Eye redness and tearing, nasal congestion, rhinorrhea, and eyelid edema are often present.
3. Attacks may occur multiple times daily and are not usually associated with nausea or vomiting.

Treatment
1. Oxygen by face mask at 8 to 10 L/minute is helpful.
2. Administer an NSAID such as ibuprofen (Motrin), 800 mg PO q8h, or acetaminophen (Tylenol), 1 g PO q6h prn.
3. Migraine treatments (see earlier) have been shown to help some patients.

Meningitis
An infection in the CSF surrounding the brain that often occurs after colonization of the nasopharyngeal tissues by the infecting organism.

Signs and Symptoms
1. Severe headache and photophobia
2. Fever
3. Neck stiffness
4. Nausea and vomiting
5. Mental status changes or focal neurologic signs may occur. Confusion may be the sole presenting complaint, especially in the elderly.
6. A rash with petechiae and purpura may occur.

Treatment
1. Evacuate the victim immediately to the nearest medical center.
2. Administer antibiotics. A third-generation cephalosporin such as ceftriaxone (1 g IV every 8 hours adult dose and 50 mg/kg pediatric dose) with the addition of ampicillin (2 g IV every 4 hours adult dose and 50 mg/kg pediatric dose) is an adequate choice to use during transport to definitive medical care. In addition, acyclovir 10 mg/kg IV should be given every 8 hours for empirical treatment of herpes simplex virus meningitis or encephalitis.
3. Administer dexamethasone (0.4 mg/kg IV) 15 to 20 minutes before first dose of antibiotics.

Dehydration Headache
Headache can be a symptom of dehydration.

Signs and Symptoms
1. The pain is felt on both sides of the head.
2. The pain is usually made worse when the victim stands from a lying position.

Treatment
1. Administer at least 1 to 2 quarts of water or oral rehydration solution.
2. Administer an NSAID such as ibuprofen (Motrin), 800 mg PO q8h, or acetaminophen (Tylenol), 1 g PO q6h prn.

Bell's Palsy
Bell's palsy is the most common form of facial paralysis, involving paralysis of the facial muscles innervated by the seventh (facial) nerve. Bell's palsy is rapidly progressive, with maximum weakness present within 24 to 48 hours.

Signs and Symptoms
1. Almost 50% of patients experience pain in the mastoid region behind the ear when symptoms are first noted.
2. Weakness and/or paralysis of the muscles (upper and lower) of one side of the face. It is important to differentiate

Bell's palsy from a stroke. Bell's palsy should cause weakness on one side of the face including the forehead. A stroke will not produce weakness of the forehead (the victim will still be able to wrinkle his or her forehead when looking upward).
3. Taste may be reduced or lost on the anterior two thirds of the tongue on the same side as the facial weakness.

Treatment
1. Administer acyclovir (800 mg PO five times daily for 7 days).
2. Administer prednisone 40 to 60 mg/day PO for 5 to 10 days.
3. The victim should wear an eye patch to protect the eye.
4. Lacri-Lube or other eye lubricant should be applied every 3 to 4 hours to provide moisture when the eye is not patched.

Diabetic Emergencies

29

▶ **DEFINITIONS AND CHARACTERISTICS**

Insulin is a hormone that allows the body to use and store sugar. In diabetes, either the pancreas is unable to produce enough insulin to be physiologically useful (type I, insulin-dependent diabetes) or the insulin produced is ineffective (type II, non–insulin-dependent diabetes). Some diabetic patients need to take insulin injections to control their disease; others can control their blood sugar levels by diet and oral hypoglycemic medications. Anyone with diabetes should wear appropriate identification in case assistance is necessary. Physiologic derangements seen with diabetes include high blood sugar levels, kidney failure, skin ulcers, bleeding into the vitreous of the eye, and other disorders associated with deterioration of the small blood vessels. If a diabetic person becomes confused, weak, or unconscious, he or she may be suffering from insulin-induced hypoglycemia or lapsing into a diabetic coma.

▶ **DISORDERS**

Insulin-Induced Hypoglycemia

If a diabetic person takes too much insulin or, while taking an appropriate dose of insulin or a glucose-lowering agent, either fails to eat sufficient carbohydrate to match the insulin level or exercises at a greatly increased rate, a rapid drop in blood sugar level can occur.

Signs and Symptoms
1. Altered level of consciousness, possibly confusion, nervousness, belligerence, fainting, seizures, unconsciousness, or coma
2. Weakness, tremor, sweating, hunger, abdominal pain, ataxia, slurred speech, tachycardia
3. Minimal to absent prodrome so that the victim becomes unarousable without warning

Treatment
1. If possible, obtain a blood glucose reading before beginning therapy. Dipstick readings are helpful in permitting rapid, reasonably accurate blood glucose estimates. Check with the victim or others to see if glucagon has already been given because it will alter the blood glucose reading.
2. If the victim is still conscious and able to swallow, give him or her something containing sugar to drink or eat as soon as possible. This could be fruit juice, a banana, candy, or a

nondiet soft drink. As soon as the victim feels better, have him or her eat a meal to avoid a recurrence.

3. If the victim is unconscious:
   a. Place tiny amounts of sugar granules, cake icing, or Glutose paste (one tube contains 25 g glucose) under the victim's tongue, where it will be passively swallowed and absorbed.
   b. If available, administer 1 to 3 ampules of IV 50% dextrose in water while completing the ABCs (airway, breathing, circulation) of resuscitation. In a child younger than 8 years of age, give 25% dextrose in water in a dose of 2 to 4 mL/kg or even 10% dextrose in water in a dose of 0.5 to 1 g/kg.
   c. As an alternative in a victim for whom you cannot quickly obtain IV access, give 1 to 2 mg of glucagon intramuscularly or subcutaneously. This dose may be repeated as needed.
   d. Be aware that families of insulin-dependent diabetic persons are often taught how to administer intramuscular glucagon at home. In addition, an intranasal form is available. Check with the victim or others to see if glucagon has already been given because it has a slightly delayed (up to minutes) onset of action. It is virtually impossible to overdose on glucagon, so if an additional injection is given, there is no need to worry.
4. Provide supportive care including airway management, aspiration and seizure precautions, administration of oxygen, and treatment of shock.

Diabetic Ketoacidosis

In diabetic ketoacidosis (DKA), blood sugar levels become dangerously high. The blood becomes acidotic as the byproducts of metabolism (ketones) accumulate, dehydration occurs, and body chemistry falls out of balance.

Signs and Symptoms
1. History of recent polydipsia, polyuria, polyphagia, visual blurring, weakness, weight loss, nausea, vomiting, and abdominal pain
2. Early symptoms: polyuria, polydipsia, nausea and vomiting
3. Later symptoms: tachycardia, tachypnea with Kussmaul's breathing, hyperventilation, and possibly fruity odor of ketones on the breath
4. Abdominal pain, especially in children
5. Skin dry with little sweating, hypotension, or orthostatic blood pressure changes

6. Eventually, confusion, combativeness, or coma with signs of profound dehydration
7. Possibly an elevated temperature, resulting from sepsis

Treatment
1. If unsure whether the victim has hyperglycemia or hypoglycemia, assume it is hypoglycemia and administer sugar.
2. If the victim can drink, encourage him or her to consume large quantities of unsweetened fluids. Otherwise, administer IV NS solution (2 L over 2 hours). Fluid resuscitation alone may help considerably in lowering hyperglycemia.
3. Provide supportive care including airway management, administration of oxygen, and treatment of shock while transporting the victim to a medical center.
4. If insulin is available, administer it as an IV infusion at a rate of 0.1 unit/kg/hr or as appropriate for the measured blood sugar level.

Hyperglycemic Hyperosmolar Nonketotic Coma

Hyperglycemic hyperosmolar nonketotic coma (HHNC) represents a form of acute diabetes-related decompensation.

Signs and Symptoms
1. Prodrome significantly longer than that for diabetic ketoacidosis
2. Extreme dehydration, hyperosmolarity, volume depletion, altered level of consciousness
3. Fever, thirst, polyuria, oliguria
4. Orthostatic hypotension or frank hypotension, tachycardia, depressed sensorium, seizures, other changes in neurologic function

Treatment
1. Administer fluids rapidly. Give 2 to 3 L of NS solution over the first several hours.
2. Supplement the insulin levels using regular insulin, 0.1 unit/kg/hr IV. Careful monitoring is required.
3. Correct electrolyte abnormalities including sodium, potassium, phosphorus, and magnesium.
4. Correct acidosis cautiously.
5. Transport to a medical facility.

Insulin Allergy

Signs and Symptoms
1. Local itching or pain
2. Delayed edema, urticaria, or anaphylaxis
3. Systemic reactions when the victim has discontinued insulin and then resumed therapy

Treatment
1. For mild reaction, administer diphenhydramine, 50 mg q6h for adults and 1 mg/kg for children.
2. For anaphylactic reaction, administer epinephrine (see Chapter 26).
3. Evacuate the victim immediately to a medical facility.

Genitourinary Tract Disorders

30

In the wilderness, genitourinary tract disorders are common and urinary tract infections (UTIs) usually comprise the majority of complaints. Also included in this chapter are pyelonephritis, urethritis, cervicitis, epididymitis, prostatitis, testicular torsion, and urinary tract obstruction.

▶ URINARY TRACT INFECTION

1. UTIs are more common in women.
2. The incidence increases in postmenopausal women and women with histories of recent frequent sexual intercourse.
3. In women the primary cause of UTI is invasion of the urinary tract by bacteria that have ascended the urethra from the introitus.
4. Most of these infections are caused by gram-negative aerobic bacteria, most often *Escherichia coli*.
5. UTIs are rare entities in men younger than 50 years of age.
6. Despite the difference in prevalence, symptoms in men and women are similar.
7. Infection of the urinary tract in a male is often associated with prostatic enlargement or infection.

Lower UTI (Uncomplicated UTI)

Signs and Symptoms
1. Bladder irritation (dysuria, frequency, urgency)
2. May lead to hematuria
   Confirmation of the diagnosis by examination of urine is typically impossible in the wilderness. Other genitourinary processes that may mimic UTI include the following:
1. Chills and fever, suggestive of upper UTI (pyelonephritis)
2. Presence of risk factors in sexual history suggestive of chlamydial urethritis; more probable in sexually active women with multiple partners; chlamydial or gonococcal cervicitis is often associated with cervical discharge
3. Vaginal discharge, external irritation, or pain with intercourse suggests a vaginal etiology, specifically vaginal infection
4. Dysuria with flank pain, restlessness, and costovertebral angle (CVA) tenderness suggests urinary tract stone(s)
5. In a male with dysuria, urethritis or prostatitis is possible

Treatment
1. Perform a physical examination including determination of temperature, abdominal examination, and assessment for CVA tenderness.
2. Perform a pelvic (bimanual) examination in a woman whose symptoms are associated with pelvic pain or vaginal bleeding. Although a formal pelvic examination using a speculum with the individual in a lithotomy position is virtually impossible in the wilderness, a simple bimanual examination can easily be performed to help identify an adnexal or uterine process (e.g., ectopic pregnancy, pelvic inflammatory disease [PID]).
3. Give oral antibiotic therapy (standard 3-day treatment) using one of the following:
   a. Trimethoprim/sulfamethoxazole (Co-trimoxazole, Bactrim, Septra), one double-strength tablet bid for 3 days
   b. Ciprofloxacin (Cipro), 500 mg bid for 3 days
   c. Cephalexin (Keflex) 250 to 500 mg for 7 to 10 days recommended for pregnant women
4. If symptoms persist after standard therapy:
   a. Consider a resistant organism.
   b. In a male, consider a relapse caused by prostatitis. Extend treatment for 10 to 14 days or change to an extended-spectrum antibiotic (e.g., change from trimethoprim/sulfamethoxazole to ciprofloxacin).
5. In addition to the antibiotic therapy, provide for pain relief.
   a. When dysuria is a major component, give phenazopyridine (Pyridium) as a urinary anesthetic (200 mg PO tid for a maximum of 2 days). Warn the victim that the urine will turn orange.

Upper UTI (Pyelonephritis)
Pyelonephritis is an infection of the upper urinary tract (kidney) most often caused by ascending infection from the lower urinary tract.

Signs and Symptoms
1. Fever greater than 102° F (38.9° C), chills, CVA tenderness
2. Urinary frequency and dysuria
3. Malaise, abdominal pain

Treatment
1. Administer an oral antibiotic if the victim is immunocompetent, without evidence of toxicity (fever, chills, or malaise), and can tolerate oral medication.
   a. Reasonable antibiotic choices include the same medications recommended for lower tract infection (see earlier) but require a full 10- to 14-day course.

2. For a toxic victim, initiate therapy with a parenteral anti-biotic such as a third-generation cephalosporin (ceftriax-one [Rocephin], 1 g IM or IV q12h).
3. Treat nontoxic victims with a single parenteral dose, followed by 10 to 14 days of oral therapy.
4. When a high fever is present:
    a. Routinely administer acetaminophen or aspirin to make the victim more comfortable.
    b. If the fever persists, consider the possibility of a resistant organism, UTI, or an abscess.
5. Arrange for evacuation when protracted vomiting makes oral therapy impossible or when generalized toxicity (volume depletion, fever greater than 102° F [38.9° C] or marked CVA tenderness) is present. Additional risk factors include immunocompromise and extremes of age.
6. Instruct all victims to seek medical follow-up on return, even if symptoms resolve fully.

Urinary Stones

Signs and Symptoms
1. Pain, with location depending on stone's location, but typically felt in flank
    a. May radiate to groin as stone migrates distally
    b. Other causes for pain considered at this point: acute aortic dissection, back strain, herniated lumbar disk
2. Nausea and vomiting
3. Restlessness and inability to lie still
4. CVA tenderness
5. Absence of peritoneal signs; if these develop, they indicate a possible intraperitoneal process (e.g., appendicitis)
6. Absence of fever unless an associated UTI is present (which may develop in an obstructed ureter)
7. Gross hematuria possible, but microscopic hematuria more likely (urine dipstick test required for detection)

Treatment
1. Consider evacuation for severe nausea and vomiting (inadequate oral intake), fever (suggestive of an infection proximal to the obstruction), or the presence of an intraperitoneal process.
2. Arrange for adequate hydration to help move the stone.
3. Although not usually practical in the wilderness, filtering the urine for stones is helpful for diagnosis.
4. Administer an antiinflammatory medication such as ketorolac (Toradol), 60 mg IM or 30 mg IV q6-8h, or an oral non-steroidal antiinflammatory drug (NSAID) such as ibuprofen,

600 to 800 mg q6-8h, to reduce the pain of renal colic. You may also use these in addition to narcotic analgesia.

5. Administer a narcotic analgesic if needed.
   a. Use an oral narcotic combination drug such as hydrocodone bitartrate, 5 mg, with acetaminophen, 500 mg (Vicodin), 1 or 2 tablets q4-6h.
   b. For more severe pain, administer a parenteral narcotic such as morphine sulfate, 2 to 5 mg IV q 5 min, titrated for pain relief. Make sure that naloxone (Narcan) is available.

6. For additional narcotic analgesics see Chapter 24.

7. Administer an antiemetic drug if nausea and vomiting are factors.

8. Encourage the victim to seek medical follow-up even if symptoms resolve fully.

Acute Scrotal Pain

When palpation of the scrotum including the testes, epididymis, and cord structures reveals no abnormality or tenderness, consider referred pain as a possible consequence of renal, ureteral, or prostate disease.

Epididymitis

Epididymitis is abrupt inflammation of the epididymis that spreads rapidly and can appear as generalized inflammation of the entire hemiscrotum (Fig. 30-1). The differential diagnosis includes torsion of the testis, acute orchitis, or tumor of the testis with hemorrhage or hydrocele. Most cases of

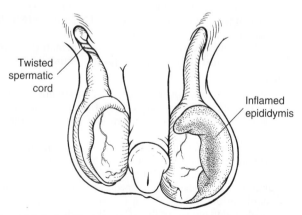

Twisted spermatic cord

Inflamed epididymis

Figure 30-1. Testicular disorders: twisted (torsed) spermatic cord and inflamed epididymis.

epididymitis in young men are caused by *Chlamydia trachomatis*. At any age, UTI caused by gram-negative rods can spread to the epididymis.

Signs and Symptoms
1. Acute scrotal pain in men older than age 20 years (infectious epididymitis)
2. Testicular torsion in men younger than age 30 years (usually)
3. Gradual (over days) onset of pain
4. Dysuria or urethral discharge
5. Normal urinalysis in torsion, but pyuria in epididymitis (if urinalysis can be done, i.e., access to a urine dipstick)
6. Fever possible
7. Recent history of a UTI
8. Tenderness and swelling localized to one epididymis (usually at the superior pole of the testis)
9. Prehn's sign: relief of pain when elevating the testis (suggestive of epididymitis rather than torsion)

Treatment
1. Administer an antibiotic that covers *Neisseria gonorrhoeae* and *C. trachomatis.*
   Ceftriaxone (Rocephin) 125 mg IM in a single dose and the following:
   a. Azithromycin 1 g in a single dose or
   b. Doxycycline, 100 mg PO bid for 10 days
   Alternatively (if lacking ceftriaxone), consider ciprofloxacin (Cipro), 500 mg PO × 14 days, or ofloxacin (Floxin), 300 mg bid for 14 days in combination with a or b mentioned earlier, but these quinolones have inconsistent activity against *N. gonorrhoeae.*
2. Allow the victim to rest supine with the scrotum elevated.
3. Administer analgesic medication.
4. Arrange for the victim to wear men's supportive briefs or an athletic supporter to offer pain relief if the victim is expected to ambulate.
5. Be aware that relief after therapy usually occurs within 24 hours.
6. Inform the victim that induration and edema in the region of the epididymis may persist for 6 to 8 weeks.

Testicular Torsion

Signs and Symptoms
1. Rare in males older than 30 years of age
2. May or may not occur during physical exertion
3. Nausea and vomiting

4. No preceding urethral discharge or fever
5. Testis that rides high in the upper part of the scrotum
6. Relief of pain when the affected testis is elevated (Prehn's sign) is suggestive of epididymitis rather than torsion, but this is not absolute (see Fig. 30-1)

Treatment
1. Be aware that testicular torsion of the spermatic cord requires surgical intervention. Therefore consider immediate evacuation if this diagnosis is suspected.
2. Attempt manual correction.
   a. Torsion most often occurs with the anterior portion of the testis rotating from its lateral aspect to its medial aspect.
   b. To correct the torsion manually, attempt to turn the right testis clockwise and the left testis counterclockwise, when viewed from above.
   c. Be aware that extreme tenderness may make manual correction difficult.
   d. Relief of pain suggests that torsion has been corrected.
3. Advise the victim that evaluation by a urologist is indicated after successful detorsion.
4. Be aware that if the torsion is not corrected, loss of the affected testis is likely.

Acute Bacterial Prostatitis

Signs and Symptoms
1. Abrupt onset, associated with systemic signs of infection
2. Fever, chills, perineal pain, low back pain, dysuria, frequency, and urgency
3. Hematuria possible
4. Tender, swollen ("boggy") prostate on palpation during rectal examination
5. Resultant acute urinary retention

Treatment
1. Initiate oral antibiotic treatment with a fluoroquinolone such as ciprofloxacin, 750 mg bid.
2. Alternatively, administer ampicillin (500 mg PO qid).
3. Alternatively, administer trimethoprim/sulfamethoxazole, one DS tablet PO bid.
4. Continue therapy for at least 14 days.
5. If urinary retention is present, catheterization or suprapubic aspiration may be necessary.
6. Arrange for "bed rest" if conditions permit.

Male Urethritis

Male urethritis is typically sexually transmitted. It may be caused by *N. gonorrhoeae* (gonococcal urethritis) but more often is caused by *C. trachomatis* (the major cause of nongonococcal urethritis). *Ureaplasma urealyticum* and *Mycoplasma hominis* are thought to be responsible for most other cases.

Signs and Symptoms
1. Urethral discharge (mucopurulent with chlamydial and frankly purulent with gonococcal urethritis), dysuria, meatal pruritus
2. Flank or abdominal pain, fever, or hematuria is not usually found; if present, another etiology is suggested
3. Difficult to differentiate from a UTI in the field

Treatment
1. Administer an antibiotic that covers *N. gonorrhoeae* and *C. trachomatis*:
   a. Ceftriaxone (Rocephin) 125 mg IM in a single dose and
   b. Azithromycin 1 g in a single dose or
   c. Doxycycline, 100 mg, PO bid for 10 days
2. Alternatively (if lacking ceftriaxone), give azithromycin (Zithromax) 2 g in a single dose (covers *N. gonorrhoeae* and *C. trachomatis*).
3. Consider ciprofloxacin (Cipro) 500 mg PO × 14 days, or ofloxacin (Floxin), 300 mg PO bid for 14 days, in combination with b or c mentioned earlier. These quinolones have shown inconsistent activity against *N. gonorrhoeae* and should only be used in the absence of other antibiotics (above).
4. Treat suspected nongonococcal urethritis with doxycycline, 100 mg bid for 7 to 14 days. Alternatively, administer azithromycin 1 g as a single dose.·
5. In the absence of azithromycin or doxycycline, substitute tetracycline, 500 mg, or erythromycin, 500 mg qid for 7 days.
6. Notify any current sexual partners of the victim, and treat them with an appropriate regimen.

Urinary Retention

Signs and Symptoms
1. Principle symptoms are bladder distention and pain that may mimic an acute abdomen
2. Overflow incontinence

3. Dribbling and hesitancy
4. On examination:
   a. Prostatic enlargement in men
   b. Lower midline abdominal tenderness and distention

Treatment

1. Bladder decompression should be initially attempted with a standard Foley catheter.
2. In men with prostatic hypertrophy, passage of the catheter may be challenging, and a large catheter or coudé catheter should be used if a standard Foley catheter cannot be passed.
3. Instrumentation of the urethra with hemostats or dilators is dangerous and should not be attempted in the field.
4. Recently introduced are the OPTION-*vf* (Fig. 30-2A) and OPTION-*vm* (See Fig. 30-2B) (Option Medical, Dublin, OH) catheters, which are valved urinary catheters that eliminate the need for urine drainage bags and connecting tubes normally required with Foley catheters. These catheters

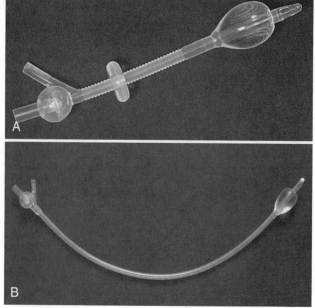

Figure 30-2. A, OPTION-*vf* (female) catheter. **B,** OPTION-*vm* (male) catheter. (Courtesy Option Medical, Dublin, OH.)

incorporate a manually activated valve at the end of the catheter that allows the patient to store urine in the bladder and
to mimic normal voiding behavior. The catheters may be
used with a continuous drainage adapter when appropriate
so that a bag may be placed and urination rate and volume
assessed.

Gynecologic and Obstetric Emergencies

31

▶ **PATTERNS OF MENSTRUAL BLEEDING**

1. Normal cycle: every 28 days ± 5 days with a duration of 3 to 6 days
2. Normal menstrual flow: 80 mL or 3 to 5 pads or tampons per day with a duration of 3 to 5 days
3. Menorrhagia: extended duration
4. Metrorrhagia: continuous duration or with no identifiable pattern
5. Menometrorrhagia: increased quantity and duration
6. Hypermenorrhea: increased quantity
7. Intermenstrual spotting: small amounts of vaginal bleeding that may occur before or after menstruation or midcycle

▶ **VAGINAL BLEEDING ASSOCIATED WITH PREGNANCY**

Ectopic Pregnancy
Ectopic pregnancy is a medical emergency that requires prompt evacuation of the victim to a surgical facility.

History
1. Any history of prior ectopic pregnancy, salpingitis, pelvic inflammatory disease, tubal surgery, or use of fertility agents or intrauterine device (IUD) should increase clinical suspicion.
2. Prior bilateral tubal ligation does not exclude the diagnosis.
3. History is usually suggestive of early pregnancy and includes nausea, amenorrhea, and breast tenderness.
4. A prior seemingly normal or abnormal menstrual period is also possible.

Signs and Symptoms
1. An ectopic pregnancy may rupture as early as 5 weeks' gestation but most commonly ruptures after 7 weeks' gestation.
2. Ectopic rupture is generally preceded by abnormal vaginal bleeding and unilateral lower abdominal pain.
3. A triad exists of vaginal bleeding, adnexal mass, and lower abdominal pain that is usually unilateral and may radiate to the shoulder.
4. Cervical motion tenderness may be present on pelvic examination.
5. Dizziness, syncope, and unstable vital signs may be present if blood loss is substantial.
6. Rebound tenderness and rigidity are signs of rupture.

7. Any patient with a positive pregnancy test and lower abdominal pain, usually unilateral, should be assumed to have an ectopic pregnancy until proven otherwise.
8. Urine pregnancy test
   a. This test is currently sensitive enough to detect levels of urinary beta-human chorionic gonadotropin (beta-hCG) as low as 20 mU/mL from the third to fourth week after the first day of the last menstrual period.
   b. This test should be included in remote expedition medical supplies. To ensure adequate performance of the test, use a test with an internal reference.

Treatment
1. Immediate evacuation
2. Treat for shock (see Chapter 13)

Spontaneous Abortion
Early pregnancy loss before 20 weeks' gestation

Types
Threatened
1. Closed internal cervical os on pelvic examination
2. Progressive bleeding and cramping
3. Occurs in 25% of normal pregnancies
4. 50% progress to termination, regardless of management
Inevitable
1. Cervix dilated on pelvic examination
2. Products of conception (POC) not yet passed, despite vaginal bleeding
Incomplete
1. Dilated cervical os with partial passage of POC
2. Accompanied by increased bleeding and persistent pain
Complete
1. Diagnosis based on pathologic examination of all POC and cannot be made in the wilderness.
2. A presumed complete abortion is handled as an incomplete abortion.
Missed
1. Closed internal os despite retained POC
2. May lead to subsequent infection and hemorrhage if uterine contents not evacuated
Septic
1. Associated with lower abdominal pain, tenderness, and fever
2. Endometritis or parametritis after a spontaneous or therapeutic abortion
3. Can lead to septic shock

Signs and Symptoms
1. History suggestive of early pregnancy including late or missed period and breast tenderness
2. Positive urine pregnancy test with above signs and symptoms
3. Spontaneous abortion presents as abnormal vaginal bleeding, followed by uterine cramping.
4. Bleeding can vary from dark red spotting to bright red clots.
5. Consistency may be gritty, with passage of products of conception.
6. Cervix may be dilated or closed.

Treatment
1. Unless a pretrip ultrasound has verified an intrauterine pregnancy, immediately evacuate the victim to rule out ectopic pregnancy.
2. Keep the victim at "bed rest."
3. Direct all field treatment to volume replacement.
4. Evacuation of uterus to prevent further hemorrhage or infection will be necessary once transported to medical facility.
5. Treatment of septic abortion will involve broad-spectrum intravenous antibiotics.
6. Treatment of shock until evacuated.
7. Under wilderness conditions, control of significant maternal hemorrhage accompanying miscarriage may be difficult. Once the uterus is empty, uterine involution, spontaneous or aided by uterine massage, is usually sufficient to impede bleeding from the implantation site. In the absence of the ability to perform curettage, treatment with methylergonovine, 0.2 mg PO or IM, can enhance uterine contractions, accelerate expulsion of products of conception, and promote uterine involution to maintain hemostasis while plans are being made for evacuation of the victim. Methylergonovine should not be used in persons with hypertensive disorders or vascular disease unless the benefits outweigh the risks of generalized vasoconstriction. As an alternative, carboprost tromethamine 250 micrograms IM, or misoprostol 100 micrograms PO or vaginally, can be administered to stop uterine bleeding with less risk for cardiovascular compromise.

Placenta Previa
Painless vaginal bleeding secondary to improper placental implantation at the lower uterine segment. Placental implantation may completely obscure the cervical os or just rim the edge of the internal os.

History
1. Suggestive of pregnancy (see earlier)
2. History of painless bleeding
3. Endometrial trauma or uterine surgery a risk factor

Signs and Symptoms
1. Definitive diagnosis impossible in the field
2. Positive urine pregnancy test
3. Painless vaginal bleeding (spotting to bright red blood with clots)
4. May lead to uterine contractions
5. Can occur as early as 20 weeks' gestation

Treatment
1. "Bed rest"
2. Volume replacement if indicated
2. Immediate evacuation
3. Vaginal/pelvic or rectal examination contraindicated

Placental Abruption
1. Rupture of the placenta from the wall of the uterus
2. Separation partial to complete
3. History of painful bleeding in late pregnancy or after trauma

History
1. A history suggestive of pregnancy (see earlier)
2. Most common in the third trimester of pregnancy
3. Vaginal bleeding usually accompanied by pain
4. Any history of trauma, maternal hypertension, cocaine abuse, or advanced maternal age should warrant suspicion.

Signs and Symptoms
1. Definitive diagnosis impossible in the field
2. Positive pregnancy test
3. Vaginal bleeding. In some cases the hemorrhage is concealed internally and vaginal bleeding is minimal.
4. Lower abdominal pain
5. Uterine tenderness
6. Uterine contractions

Treatment
Same as for placenta previa

Bleeding Not Associated with Pregnancy
Abnormal Uterine Bleeding in a
Nonpregnant Woman
Abnormal bleeding that occurs in a nonpregnant woman is referred to as dysfunctional uterine bleeding (DUB).

1. Includes bleeding between normal menstrual cycles, change in normal pattern of menstrual cycle, increased or decreased amount of menstrual bleeding
2. Consider other systemic or structural processes:
   a. Complications of pregnancy: threatened, incomplete, or spontaneous abortion; ectopic or molar pregnancy
   b. Infectious: vaginitis, cervicitis, pelvic inflammatory disease (PID)
   c. Coagulopathy
   d. Medications: aspirin, warfarin, oral contraceptives, tricyclic antidepressants, major tranquilizers
   e. Systemic illness: hepatic, thyroid, and adrenal dysfunction
   f. Polycystic ovarian syndrome and other endocrinopathies
   g. Anatomic lesions: fibroids, polyps, ovarian cysts, endometriosis, endometrial hyperplasia, neoplasm
   h. Intrauterine device
   i. Vaginal or pelvic trauma
   j. Often associated with:
      • Intense exercise
      • Low-calorie diet
      • Rapid weight change
      • Increased psychologic stress
   k. Common in perimenopausal women
   l. Common in adolescence secondary to immaturity of the hypothalamic-pituitary-ovarian axis

Treatment
1. Perform a urine pregnancy test to reach the diagnosis, ruling out the possibility of a complication of pregnancy.
2. In the wilderness, modern, low-dose oral contraceptive pills can be safely used whether the bleeding is caused by estrogen or progestin deficiency or excess.
3. High doses of oral contraceptive pills of the combination monophasic type, such as Lo/Ovral (norgestrel, 0.3 mg, and ethinyl estradiol, 30 μg), are usually effective.
4. The usual dose for this purpose is three pills/day for 7 days (i.e., one complete pack over a single-week course).
5. Bleeding is typically controlled within 12 to 36 hours.
6. Side effects such as nausea, headache, fluid retention, and depression sometimes occur.
7. After completion of the oral contraceptive pills (i.e., after 7 days), expect significant withdrawal bleeding.
8. A nonsteroidal antiinflammatory agent may be started for pain management.

9. If abdominal or pelvic pain develops or if heavy bleeding persists, arrange for immediate evacuation of the victim. It is highly unusual for the bleeding to progress to massive hemorrhage.
10. Note that any victim with DUB in the field should seek definitive follow-up as soon as is practical.

▶ **VAGINAL DISCHARGE**

Normal vaginal discharge is usually odorless, nonirritating, and white to transparent.

Bacterial Vaginosis

This is a non–sexually transmitted disease, usually with a polymicrobial cause. Pathogens include *Gardnerella vaginalis, Bacteroides non-fragilis, Mobiluncus, Peptococcus,* and *Mycoplasma hominis.*

Signs and Symptoms
1. Copious amounts of thin gray or yellow discharge
2. Malodorous fishy odor secondary to the release of amines
3. Minimal to no vulvar irritation

Treatment
1. Metronidazole (Flagyl), 2 g; single-dose oral treatment is practical in the wilderness setting.
2. Metronidazole, 500 mg, orally bid or tid for 5 to 7 days is more effective.
3. Metronidazole, 250 mg, orally tid for 7 days in second and third trimester of pregnancy. Avoid in the first trimester of pregnancy.
4. Consider clindamycin, 300 to 600 mg, bid for 7 days as an alternative. Clindamycin may also be administered as 2% vaginal gel once daily for 7 days.

Candida Vulvovaginitis

Candida albicans is the most common pathogen, responsible for 80% to 90% cases.

Signs and Symptoms
1. Increased thick, white vaginal discharge
2. Odorless
3. Vulvar itching or burning
4. Dysuria and dyspareunia

Treatment
1. Fluconazole (Diflucan), 150 mg single oral dose
2. Alternatives: azole derivatives (clotrimazole, miconazole, butoconazole, tioconazole, or terconazole) available as

intravaginal creams, tablets, and suppositories; treatment of at least 3 days found to have lower immediate recurrence rates (e.g., clotrimazole, 200 mg intravaginally for 3 days or 100 mg for 7 days)
3. Prophylactic suppressive therapy with clotrimazole, 500 mg vaginal tablet weekly, or fluconazole, 100 mg oral tablet weekly

Trichomonas Vaginitis

This is a sexually transmitted disease caused by *Trichomonas vaginalis*.

Signs and Symptoms
1. Copious and adherent, frothy discharge that is yellowish gray or green
2. Malodorous if mixed with bacterial vaginosis
3. Severe pruritus
4. Intense vulvovaginal erythema
5. Strawberry cervix: petechial lesions of the cervix
6. Dysuria and dyspareunia

Treatment
1. Metronidazole, 2 g single oral dose or 500 mg bid for 7 days. Tinidazole, 2 g single oral dose may also be used. Avoid in first trimester. Metronidazole 0.75% vaginal gel is not appropriate for treatment.
2. Take with plenty of water and avoid alcohol to minimize gastrointestinal side effects.
3. Treat partner simultaneously.

▶ GONORRHEA/CHLAMYDIA

This sexually transmitted disease causes a concomitant infection that warrants treatment of both *Chlamydia trachomatis* and *Neisseria gonorrhoeae* simultaneously.

Signs and Symptoms
1. Gonorrhea is usually accompanied by urinary frequency, dysuria, and vaginal discharge.
2. *Chlamydia* infection is often asymptomatic.
3. Definitive diagnosis requires special cultures not available in the wilderness.

Treatment
1. Ceftriaxone, 125 mg IM single dose, with azithromycin, 1 g single oral dose.
2. Alternatively, administer ceftriaxone, 125 mg IM single dose, with doxycycline, 100 mg PO bid for 7 days.

▶ PAIN: VULVAR/VAGINAL

Vulvovaginal Abscess and Cellulitis/Bartholin's Abscess

This usually results from polymicrobial infection and duct obstruction of Bartholin's gland. The causative organisms include *Neisseria gonorrhoeae* and *Chlamydia trachomatis*.

Signs and Symptoms
1. Severe localized vulvar pain and tenderness just lateral to the posterior vaginal introitus
2. Unilateral vulvar erythema and edema
3. Tender, fluctuant palpable mass lateral to the posterior introitus

Treatment
1. Incision and drainage if adequate equipment is available
2. Make the incision over the medial aspect of the mucosa, at the point of maximal fluctuance
3. Insert a hemostat through the mucosal incision and spread the tips into the deeper tissue. Ensure there is entrance into a true cavity.
4. Irrigate with a syringe and catheter technique.
5. Apply gauze packing to maintain drainage for 24 to 48 hours.
6. With evidence of cellulitis, administer cephalexin, 500 mg orally bid to tid until resolved.
7. If the availability of water and conditions permit, arrange for a sitz bath daily.
8. Change the dressing once to twice daily until the wound is well healed without drainage.
9. Recurrence is common after simple incision and drainage, warranting follow-up treatment on return.

▶ HERPES SIMPLEX VIRUSES (HSV-1 AND HSV-2)

Signs and Symptoms
1. Prodrome of hypesthesia and localized pain preceding eruption of multiple vesicles
2. Vesicles coalesce into ulcerations
3. Initial outbreak may be accompanied with fever and malaise

Treatment
1. Acyclovir, 200 mg, orally 5 times daily for 7 to 10 days in victims with an initial outbreak
2. Acyclovir shortens the ulcerative phase.

▶ PAIN: PELVIC/LOWER ABDOMINAL

Pelvic Inflammatory Disease

PID is a syndrome caused by pathogens ascending from the lower genital tract to the fallopian tubes and adjacent structures.

Risk Factors
1. Other sexually transmitted diseases
2. Previous episode of PID
3. Multiple sexual partners
4. IUD placement

Signs and Symptoms
1. Fever, vaginal discharge, unilateral or bilateral lower abdominal pain
2. Yellowish endocervical discharge on pelvic examination accompanied by cervical motion tenderness

Treatment
1. Differential diagnosis includes appendicitis, septic abortion, pyelonephritis, as well as other entities in this category
2. Pregnancy test to rule out ectopic pregnancy
3. If available, test for gonorrhea and chlamydia.
4. For severe symptoms, treat with ceftriaxone, 250 mg IM single dose, followed by doxycycline, 100 mg PO bid for 10 to 14 days.
5. Alternative treatment: ofloxacin, 400 mg PO bid, with metronidazole, 500 mg bid for 14 days
6. Evacuate immediately if there is a positive pregnancy test, adnexal mass, peritoneal signs, toxic appearance, presence of an IUD, or fever greater than 102.2° F (39° C).

Ectopic

See "Ectopic Pregnancy," earlier.

Mittelschmerz

Pain associated with ovulation

Signs and Symptoms
1. Sudden onset of right lower quadrant (RLQ) or left lower quadrant (LLQ) abdominal pain occurring midcycle (between days 12 and 16) in a reproductive woman at the time of ovulation
2. The presentation is not associated with marked gastrointestinal, genitourinary, or systemic symptoms.
3. Symptoms usually last less than 8 hours.
4. Not associated with vaginal bleeding or spotting
5. Associated with mild referred pain and rebound tenderness

6. Pelvic examination to rule out PID (often less adnexal tenderness than with PID)
7. Negative urine pregnancy test and urinalysis
8. Rule out appendicitis if pain is right sided.

Treatment
1. Bed rest for 12 to 24 hours
2. Administer a mild non-narcotic analgesic for pain relief

Ovarian Torsion
This may be complete or incomplete. It may occur during pregnancy involving the corpus luteum and result in adnexal torsion.

Signs and Symptoms
1. RLQ or LLQ pain that is sharp, localized, and sudden in onset
2. Pain is usually intermittent and may be accompanied by low-grade fever, nausea, and vomiting.
3. Unilateral adnexal tenderness, which may or may not be accompanied by a palpable mass
4. Rule out appendicitis if pain is right sided.
5. Negative or positive pregnancy test results, depending on the cause of the torsion.

Treatment
1. Immediate evacuation
2. Laparotomy once transported to a medical facility

Ovarian Cyst
1. Rupture usually occurs after ovarian torsion or trauma
2. May involve hemorrhage

History
Onset of symptoms may occur shortly after intercourse or exercise.

Signs and Symptoms
1. Sudden onset, unilateral sharp pain
2. May or may not be accompanied by rebound tenderness
3. Enlarging adnexal mass is ominous for hemorrhage
4. May spontaneously resolve
5. Rule out appendicitis if pain is right sided
6. Negative or positive pregnancy test, depending on type of ovarian cyst

Treatment
1. Immediate evacuation to surgical facility if symptoms persist

2. If hemorrhage is suspected, direct all field treatment to volume replacement.
3. Treat for shock, if indicated.

▶ EMERGENCY WILDERNESS CHILDBIRTH

To the extent possible, a clean, comfortable, and quiet site is prepared for the delivery. If clean and sterile supplies and medications are available, these should be brought to this location and inventoried. Otherwise, clean towels, clothing, bedding, soap, and water should be made readily accessible.

Vertex Delivery (Fig. 31-1)
1. When the perineum begins to distend, instruct the woman to bear down with each contraction.
2. Support the perineum between the rectum and introitus, using your index finger and thumb.
3. Control the delivery of the head, keeping it in flexion until it clears the symphysis pubis.
4. Once the head is cleared, ask the woman to stop pushing.
5. Exert steady inward and upward pressure at the perineum, against the chin with countertraction on the occiput. Allow for controlled extension of the head.
6. Once delivered, the head will automatically rotate laterally to align itself with the shoulders.
7. Suction the nose and mouth, using gauze or a cloth if a suction bulb is not available.
8. Palpate the fetal neck for a nuchal cord. If present, undo the nuchal cord by slipping it over the fetal head. The cord may also be clamped twice and cut.
9. Instruct the woman to resume bearing down steadily and cup both sides of the fetal head.
10. Apply gentle downward pressure on the head, until the anterior shoulder is visible.
11. Apply upward traction, until the posterior shoulder is delivered. The rest of the body will quickly follow.
12. Hold the baby below the perineum. Towel dry and suction the oropharynx.
13. Clamp or tie the umbilical cord twice and sever between the clamps or ties.
14. After a wilderness delivery, administer a broad-spectrum antibiotic to the mother for 24 to 48 hours.
15. If the mother is Rh negative and the baby's blood type is Rh positive or unknown, administer Rh immune globulin, 300 μg IM, to the mother.

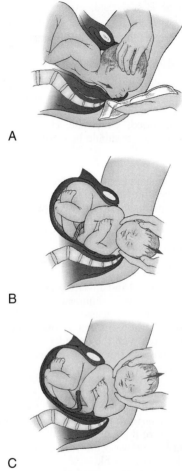

A

B

C

Figure 31-1. Management of vaginal vertex delivery. **A,** Control delivery of fetal head by upward pressure on chin with countertraction on occiput until symphysis is cleared. **B,** Delivery of anterior shoulder by downward traction on fetal head. **C,** Delivery of posterior shoulder by upward traction on fetal head. (Modified from Pritchard JA, MacDonald PC: Williams Obstetrics, 16th ed. New York, Appleton-Century-Crofts, 1980. Courtesy McGraw-Hill, New York.)

Breech Delivery (Fig. 31-2)

Because most wilderness deliveries will be "unexpected" and more likely to be premature, the baby also will more likely be in a breech lie. Under the best of circumstances, delivery of a breech carries a threefold to fourfold greater risk than a vertex presentation for morbidity resulting

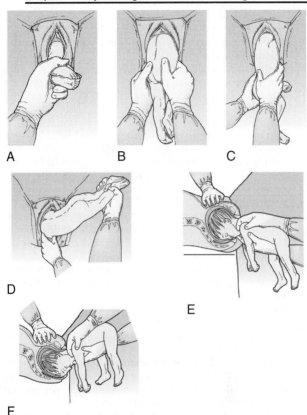

Figure 31-2. Management of vaginal breech delivery. **A,** Downward traction at ankles until buttocks clear the introitus. **B,** Traction on pelvic girdle until an axilla becomes visible. **C,** Delivery of posterior shoulder and arm. **D,** Delivery of anterior shoulder and arm with downward traction. **E,** Cradling the baby on forearm, finger is inserted into mouth or against chin. **F,** Delivery completed by outward traction while maintaining fetal head in flexed position. (Modified from Pritchard JA, MacDonald PC: Williams Obstetrics, 16th ed. New York, Appleton-Century-Crofts, 1980. Courtesy McGraw-Hill, New York.)

from prematurity, congenital abnormalities, and trauma at delivery.

1. Breech babies come in many forms: frank breech (hips flexed, knees extended, buttocks presenting); complete breech (both hips and both knees flexed, buttocks and feet presenting); incomplete breech (one hip flexed, one hip partially extended, both knees flexed, buttocks and feet presenting); and footling breech (hips and knees extended, feet presenting).

2. The approach in a wilderness setting demands patience. No effort should be made to deliver a breech baby until the presenting part is visible at the introitus and the cervix is completely dilated.

3. Membranes should not be artificially ruptured in breech presentations.

4. When the cervix is completely dilated, the woman is instructed to push.

5. Regardless of the type of breech presentation, the safest course is to allow the body to be extruded to at least the level of the umbilicus by maternal efforts alone.

6. A baby in a frank or complete breech lie should have the posterior leg delivered by gently grasping the thigh and flexing the leg at the knee as it is rotated medially and toward the introitus.

7. The baby should then be rotated to the sacrum anterior position, then another 45 degrees in the same direction to facilitate delivery of the other leg using the technique described for the first.

8. The legs and buttocks can be wrapped in a clean towel to provide a firmer grip and decrease trauma to the baby.

9. The delivery from this point is the same as for footling breech presentations. The upper legs should be grasped on each side with the index fingers crossing the infant's pelvic girdle and both thumbs positioned just above the crease of the buttocks.

10. Using gentle side-to-side rotational motion over an arc of 90 degrees outward and downward, traction should be applied while the mother pushes, until the upper portion of a scapula is visible at the introitus.

11. With the baby's body rotated 45 degrees toward the opposite side, the arm is delivered by flexion and medial rotation across the chest.

12. The baby is rotated to the opposite side in the same position, and the other arm is then delivered.

13. If assistants are present, the woman should be helped into the McRobert's position, with hyperflexion at the hips to maximize the space between the symphysis and the sacrum.

14. Maintaining the baby in the same plane as the vagina, the birth attendant reaches palm up between the baby's legs and into the vagina, supporting the baby's entire body on the forearm while placing the second and fourth fingers over the infant's maxillae and placing the middle finger into the mouth or on the chin.

15. The other hand is positioned over the infant's upper back so that the fingers are overlying each shoulder.

16. If there is sufficient room, the middle fingers can be applied to the fetal occiput. Then with the woman pushing, the baby's head is flexed downward, completing the delivery.
17. Firm suprapubic pressure can help to maintain the head in flexion. During this final stage the baby's body should not be elevated more than 45 degrees above the plane of the vagina to avoid hyperextension of the head.
18. If the fetal head cannot be delivered because the cervix is incompletely dilated, the cervix can be cut at the 2 and 10 o'clock positions (Dührssen incisions) to provide sufficient room to complete the delivery.
19. Once delivered, if the baby breathes and cries spontaneously or with minimal stimulation, cutting the umbilical cord can be delayed while the baby is dried. This allows some of the blood retained in the placenta from umbilical vein compression (common with breech deliveries) to return to the baby.
20. On the contrary, if the baby is clearly depressed, the umbilical cord should be immediately clamped and cut and neonatal resuscitation begun.

Delivery of the Placenta
1. Place the heel of your hand just above the symphysis to hold the uterus in place.
2. Apply fundal pressure with the tips of the same hand.
3. Simultaneously, apply steady downward traction of the umbilical cord with the other hand. Do not use excessive traction.
4. A gush of blood and lengthening of the cord signify separation.
5. Once separated, rotate the placenta several times as it passes through the introitus.
6. Massage the uterus to promote contraction.
7. Assess for lacerations to the perineum and repair accordingly.
8. Apply pressure to control small amounts of bleeding.
9. Place ice packs to the perineum for the first 12 to 24 hours if available.

Breastfeeding
1. During the first 24 hours after delivery, feed every 2 to 3 hours; 5 minutes on each breast, alternating first breast.
2. As milk production is established over the next 2 to 3 days, advance the feeding schedule to 10- to 15-minute periods on each breast 8 to 12 times per day.
3. Have the mother drink at least 2 L of fluids each day; increase caloric intake and consume foods rich in calcium.

4. For engorgement, apply cool compresses after nursing, wear a nursing bra, and use acetaminophen for pain.
5. For mastitis, administer a course of antibiotics (e.g., dicloxacillin or cephalexin) for 10 to 14 days. In an appropriate circumstance, suspect methicillin-resistant *Staphylococcus aureus*.

Preeclampsia

The diagnosis is based in the field on the basis of hypertension (140 mm Hg systolic or 90 mm Hg diastolic measured on two separate occasions 6 or more hours apart; severe preeclampsia is defined by the values of 160 mm Hg systolic or 110 mm Hg diastolic), decreased urine output, persistent epigastric pain, shortness of breath, and seizures (eclampsia). With any sign or suggestion of preeclampsia including peripheral edema, visual disturbances, severe headache, irritability, epigastric or right upper quadrant pain, or persistent nausea and vomiting, it is best to seek prompt evacuation.

▶ EMERGENCY CONTRACEPTION

Emergency contraception is defined as a method of contraception that women can use after unprotected intercourse or contraceptive failure to prevent pregnancy.

1. Two doses of levonorgestrel pills (Plan B) taken 12 hours apart within 72 hours of unprotected intercourse
2. Two doses of estrogen-progestin combination oral contraceptive pills (for this purpose, each dose: Ovrette 20 tablets; Ovral 2 white tablets; Lo-Ovral 4 white tablets; Nordette 4 orange tablets; Levelen 4 orange tablets; Levora 4 white tablets; TriLevelen 4 yellow tablets; Triphasil 4 yellow tablets; Trivora 4 pink tablets; Alesse 5 pink tablets) taken 12 hours apart within 72 hours of unprotected intercourse

▶ IMMUNIZATIONS DURING PREGNANCY (Table 31-1)

Medication Use In Pregnancy

The Food and Drug Administration (FDA) has developed a set of guidelines to categorize drugs with regard to developmental toxicity and adverse fetal outcome (Box 31-1). Medication use during pregnancy and lactation is guided by these recommendations (Table 31-2).

TABLE 31-1. Immunizations during Pregnancy

VACCINE/ IMMUNOBIOLOGIC AGENT	TYPE OF VACCINE	ISSUES IN PREGNANCY
Measles-mumps-rubella (MMR) Live attenuated	Contraindicated; delay pregnancy for 1 mo after MMR is given; if exposed, check titer if immunity unknown; may give immune globulin for exposure	
Polio	Inactivated virus	Use if indicated
Varicella	Live attenuated	Contraindicated in pregnancy; check titer if exposed to varicella during pregnancy; give varicella zoster immune globulin if not immune by history or titer
Tetanus-diphtheria	Combined toxoid	Safe in pregnancy
Influenza	Inactivated vaccine	Recommended for all pregnant women in second and third trimester; indicated for pregnant women in any trimester if history of high-risk medical condition
Pneumococcal	Polysaccharide	Vaccine used only in high-risk pregnancies; after splenectomy
Meningococcal	Polysaccharide	Administer for high-risk exposure
Typhoid (Ty21a)	Live attenuated bacterial, oral	No data in pregnancy; avoid in pregnancy on theoretical grounds (live vaccine)

Continued

TABLE 31-1. Immunizations during Pregnancy—cont'd

VACCINE/ IMMUNOBIOLOGIC AGENT	TYPE OF VACCINE	ISSUES IN PREGNANCY
Typhoid Vi	Vi capsular polysaccharide, parental	No data in pregnancy; use only if clearly indicated
Hepatitis A	Formalin-inactivated vaccine	Use if clearly indicated; risk for complications of hepatitis A increased in pregnancy; consider checking titer if prior exposure
Hepatitis B	Recombinant or plasma derived	Pre-exposure and postexposure prophylaxis indicated in pregnant women at risk for infection
Yellow fever	Live attenuated	Indicated if exposure unavoidable; give letter of waiver for travel to low-risk area
Japanese encephalitis (JE)	Inactivated virus	Data on safety in pregnancy not available. Theoretical risk of vaccination should be weighed against risk for disease. JE virus infection acquired during first or second trimester of pregnancy may result in uterine infection and fetal mortality.
Tick-borne encephalitis	Inactivated	Not recommended in pregnancy; practice strict tick bite precautions
Rabies	Killed virus	Postexposure prophylaxis is indicated during pregnancy

TABLE 31-1. Immunizations during Pregnancy—cont'd

VACCINE/ IMMUNOBIOLOGIC AGENT	TYPE OF VACCINE	ISSUES IN PREGNANCY
	Human diploid cell rabies	Pre-exposure prophylaxis only when substantial risk for exposure exists; HDCRV or rabies vaccine adsorbed (RVA)
Immune globulins (IGs) Pooled or hyperimmune	IGs or specific antitoxic serum including antivenom for snakebite, spider bite, diphtheria antitoxin, hepatitis B IG, rabies IG, tetanus IG, varicella zoster IG	Give appropriate IG or antitoxin as indicated for exposure
Cholera	Killed oral cholera toxin B	No live organisms. May be efficacious in high-risk situations but not recommended during pregnancy at this time. Not available in subunit whole cell (BS-WC) in United States
	Live attenuated oral cholera vaccine	Not recommended in pregnancy; not available in United States
	(CVD 103 HgR strain)	Available in Canada and Europe

Modified from Centers for Disease Control and Prevention: Health Information for International Travel 2005-2006. Atlanta, U.S. Department of Health and Human Services, Public Health Service, 2005, pp. 494-495.

Box 31-1. U.S. Food and Drug Administration Use-in-Pregnancy Classifications

Category A: Adequate and well-controlled studies in women show no risk to the fetus.

Category B: No evidence of risk in humans. Either studies in animals show risk, but human findings do not, or, in the absence of human studies, animal findings are negative.

Category C: Risk cannot be ruled out. No adequate and well-controlled studies in humans, or animal studies are either positive for fetal risk or lacking as well. Drugs should be given only if the potential benefit justifies the potential risk to the fetus.

Category D: There is positive evidence of human fetal risk. Nevertheless, potential benefits may outweigh the potential risks.

Category X: Contraindicated in pregnancy. Studies in animals or humans or investigations or postmarketing reports have shown fetal risk that far outweighs any potential benefit to the patient.

TABLE 31-2. Medication Use during Pregnancy and Lactation

MEDICATION	CATEGORY	ISSUES DURING PREGNANCY	ISSUES DURING LACTATION
Analgesics/ Antipyretics		Try nonpharmaceutic methods such as rest, heat, and massage first to treat pain	
Acetaminophen	B	Safe in low doses short term	Compatible
Aspirin	C/D	Avoid first and last trimester. Has been associated with premature closure of ductus and excessive bleeding. Low-dose aspirin (60-80 mg) may be used for pre-eclampsia	Use caution

TABLE 31-2. Medication Use during Pregnancy and Lactation—cont'd

MEDICATION	CATEGORY	ISSUES DURING PREGNANCY	ISSUES DURING LACTATION
Nonsteroidal antiinflammatory (ibuprofen, naproxen)	B/D	Should not be used in first and last trimester owing to effects on premature closure of ductus and effects on clotting. Not teratogenic	Safe
Codeine	C/D	Use cautiously. May cause respiratory depression and withdrawal symptoms in fetus if used near term	Compatible
Hydrocodone	C	Use cautiously. May cause respiratory depression in infant if used near term	Use caution. Probably compatible
Antibiotics for URI, UTI, GI, Skin, Other		Use antibiotics only if strong evidence of bacterial infection	
Amoxicillin, amoxicillin + clavulanic acid (Augmentin) Amoxicillin + sulbactam (Unasyn)	B	Safe. Use for treatment of otitis media, sinusitis, and strep throat	Safe

TABLE 31-2. Medication Use during Pregnancy and Lactation—cont'd

MEDICATION	CATEGORY	ISSUES DURING PREGNANCY	ISSUES DURING LACTATION
Azithromycin	B	Safe. Use for bronchitis, pneumonia, *Campylobacter, Shigella, Salmonella, Escherichia coli*	Safe
Cephalosporins	B	Safe. Use for otitis, streptococcal infections, sinusitis, pharyngitis	Safe. Can be used to treat mastitis
Clindamycin PO or clindamycin vaginal cream	B	Safe. Treat bacterial vaginosis (BV) orally or locally in second or third trimester. Avoid first trimester	Safe
Ciprofloxacin, other quinolones	C	Controversial. Sometimes used short term in severe infections and/or long term in life-threatening infections (e.g., anthrax). May be used if potential benefit justifies risk to fetus	Safe
Dicloxacillin	B	Safe. Used for skin infections	Safe. Used to treat mastitis

TABLE 31-2. Medication Use during Pregnancy and Lactation—cont'd

MEDICATION	CATEGORY	ISSUES DURING PREGNANCY	ISSUES DURING LACTATION
Doxycycline, tetracycline	D	May cause permanent discoloration of the teeth during tooth development including the last half of pregnancy, infancy, and childhood to the age of 8 yr	Avoid
Erythromycin (base or stearate)	B	Safe. Treatment of bacterial causes of URI	Safe
Nitrofurantoin	B	Drug of choice for UTI in pregnancy	Safe
Penicillin	B	Safe	Safe
Sulfonamides	C/D	Safe. Not recommended in third trimester owing to risk for hyperbilirubinemia	Avoid owing to risk for kernicterus
Trimethoprim	C	Safe	Safe
Gastrointestinal			
Antidiarrheal		Replace fluids	
Atropine sulfate and diphenoxylate hydrochloride (Lomotil)	C	Avoid during pregnancy	Avoid
Loperamide (Imodium)	B	Use if severe symptoms	Compatible

Continued

TABLE 31-2. Medication Use during Pregnancy and Lactation—cont'd

MEDICATION	CATEGORY	ISSUES DURING PREGNANCY	ISSUES DURING LACTATION
Antiemetics for nausea, heart-burn, esopha-geal reflux		Encourage supportive measures first rather than medications: crackers upon arising, frequent small meals, protein meal at bedtime	
Antacids	B	May use sparingly for symptoms as needed	Safe
Bismuth sub-salicylate (Pepto-Bismol)	D	Avoid. Contains salicylate	Avoid
Cimetidine, ranitidine, omeprazole	B	Safe. Study during the first trimester found not associated with an increase in congenital malformations	Safe
Metoclo-pramide (Reglan)	B	Safe in small doses	Safe
Dimenhydri-nate (Dramamine)	B	Safe for severe nausea	Safe
Phenothiazines (Compazine)	C	Rare cases of congenital malformations have occurred after use dur-ing pregnancy.	Avoid
Promethazine (Phenergan)	C	Used for nausea	Probably compatible
Acupressure (Sea Bands)		Safe	Safe
Emetrol (fluid replacement)	B	Safe. Oral solution	Safe

TABLE 31-2. Medication Use during Pregnancy and Lactation—cont'd

MEDICATION	CATEGORY	ISSUES DURING PREGNANCY	ISSUES DURING LACTATION
Ginger	B	Safe	Safe
Meclizine	B	Safe for treatment of severe nausea and vomiting	Safe
Pyridoxine (B6)	A	Safe. Used for nausea	Safe
Constipation		Increase fiber + fluid in diet first	
Bisacodyl	B	Safe to use occasionally	Safe
Milk of magnesia	B	Safe in small amounts	Safe
Psyllium hydrophilic mucilloid	B	Safe	Safe
Hemorrhoids		Increase fiber + fluid in diet	
Anusol HC suppositories	B	Safe	Safe
URI, Congestion, Cough		Symptomatic Rx: steam, rest, fluids	
Antihistamines			
Chlorpheniramine	B	Use cautiously for severe symptoms	Unknown
Cetirizine (Zyrtec)	B	Safe. Nonsedating. Use cautiously	Unknown
Diphenhydramine (Benadryl)	B	Safe. Use cautiously	Avoid
Loratadine (Claritin)	B	Safe. Nonsedating. Use cautiously	Unknown
Dextromethorphan	C	Probably safe. Use in small amounts	Unknown
Guaifenesin	C	Probably safe. Use only if needed	Unknown

Continued

TABLE 31-2. Medication Use during Pregnancy and Lactation—cont'd

MEDICATION	CATEGORY	ISSUES DURING PREGNANCY	ISSUES DURING LACTATION
Pseudoephedrine (Sudafed)	C	Avoid first trimester. Use cautiously	Unknown
Saline nasal spray	A	Safe	Safe
Topical nasal deconges- tants Oxymetazoline (Afrin)	C	Safe. Do not use for more than 3 days	Safe
Asthma, Allergy			
Inhaled bron- chodilators	C	Safe for use of wheezing dur- ing pregnancy	Unknown
Inhaled steroids	C	Use if indi- cated	Safe
Nasal steroids	C	Use if indi- cated	Safe
Antimalarials			
Mefloquine (Larium)	C	Avoid during first trimester unless un- avoidable travel to high- risk area. Safe in second and third trimester for high-risk travel	Excreted in breast milk. Infant still needs own chemopro- phylaxis
Chloroquine	C	Avoid in first trimester unless travel to high- risk area	Safe. Ex- creted in milk in small amounts. Infant still needs chemopro- phylaxis

TABLE 31-2. Medication Use during Pregnancy and Lactation—cont'd

MEDICATION	CATEGORY	ISSUES DURING PREGNANCY	ISSUES DURING LACTATION
Atovaquone, proguanil	C	Avoid in first trimester. Not recommended for prophylaxis at this time due to insufficient data. Used for treatment of malaria	Safe if infant is > 11 kg (24 lb) or if benefit for mother outweighs possible risk
Doxycycline	D	Contraindicated for malaria prophylaxis. May be considered for treatment of severe infections	Avoid
Primaquine	C	Do not administer during pregnancy because of the possibility the fetus may be G6PD deficient. If a cure with primaquine is indicated, continue to suppress with chloroquine (or other chemoprophylaxis) until delivery	Avoid
Proguanil	C	Not associated with teratogenicity. Not effective as single agent	Probably compatible

Continued

TABLE 31-2. Medication Use during Pregnancy and Lactation—cont'd

MEDICATION	CATEGORY	ISSUES DURING PREGNANCY	ISSUES DURING LACTATION
Insect Repellent			
DEET		Safe. Use sparingly as directed	Compatible
Antiparasitics			
Albendazole	C	Teratogenic in animal studies. Avoid during first trimester. Treat after delivery if possible. May be indicated for serious infections	Probably compatible
Metronidazole	B	Contraindicated during first trimester. Use in second and third trimesters only if clearly indicated	Single dose: hold breastfeeding 12-24 h. Use caution
Antivirals			
Acyclovir	B	Use when indicated	Compatible
Altitude Sickness			
Acetazolamide (Diamox)	C	Do not use during first trimester Use only if benefit outweighs risk	Compatible
Dexamethasone (Decadron)	C	May use if needed for treatment for altitude illness	Avoid breastfeeding during use

TABLE 31-2. Medication Use during Pregnancy and Lactation—cont'd

MEDICATION	CATEGORY	ISSUES DURING PREGNANCY	ISSUES DURING LACTATION
Calcium channel blockers (Nifedipine)	C	Use only to treat severe symptoms of pulmonary edema	Probably compatible
Water Disinfection		Boil water, use filters	
Iodine	D	Avoid. May lead to goiter and fetal hypothyroidism	Avoid

GI, gastrointestinal; URI, upper respiratory infection; UTI, urinary tract infection.

Data from Briggs G, Freeman R, Yaffe S: Drugs in Pregnancy and Lactation. Baltimore, Lippincott Williams & Wilkins, 2005; Micromedex Online; American Academy of Pediatrics, 2005; and Lexi-Comp Online UptoDate.

Wilderness Eye Emergencies

32

▶ **WILDERNESS EYE KIT**

See Box 32-1 and Appendix G.

▶ **OCULAR PROCEDURES**

Examination of Vision

Any victim with ocular complaints should have his or her vision evaluated in each eye separately.

1. Have the victim cover one eye and read any fine print available (persons older than age 40 may require reading glasses).
2. If the victim is unable to read print, try to determine the level of visual acuity (count fingers, hand motion, light perception, no light perception).

Examination of Pupils

Examine the pupils for size, equality, shape, and reaction to light.

1. Approximately 10% of the population has pupils of unequal size (anisocoria).
2. If light is shined in either eye, both pupils should constrict equally (consensual response). If one pupil is seen to be dilated when a penlight is rapidly alternated from one eye to the other, this may indicate retinal or optic nerve dysfunction.
3. An irregularly shaped, tapered "teardrop pupil" suggests ocular penetration.
4. When evaluating a red or painful eye, a significant difference in size between pupils may provide a clue to diagnose iritis (constricted) or glaucoma (dilated).
5. Although somewhat rare, mid-dilation is noted in angle-closure glaucoma.
6. A widely dilated, nonreactive pupil is suggestive of contact with medicine (e.g., scopolamine patch) or a cerebral aneurysm.

Estimation of Anterior Chamber Depth (i.e., rule out narrow angle, a contributing factor to glaucoma)

Shine a small flashlight obliquely from the temporal side of the eye (Fig. 32-1A).

1. If the nasal iris is well illuminated, it suggests a normal anterior chamber.

> ### Box 32-1. Wilderness Eye Emergency Kit
>
> **MEDICATIONS**
> Moxifloxacin 0.5% drops
> Tetracaine 0.5% drops
> Prednisolone 1% drops
> Moxifloxacin 400-mg tabs
> Levofloxacin 500-mg tabs
> Bacitracin ointment
> Prednisone 20-mg tabs
> Artificial tears
> Scopolamine 0.25% drops
> Diclofenac 0.1% drops
> Pilocarpine 2% drops
>
> **MISCELLANEOUS**
> Penlight with blue filter
> Fluorescein strips
> Cotton-tipped applicators
> Metal eye shield
> Eye patches (gauze)
> Tape (1 inch, plastic or nylon)
> Near vision card
> Wound closure strips (¼ inch)
> Magnifying glass

2. If the nasal iris lies in shadow, it suggests a shallow anterior chamber (narrow angle) (See Fig. 32-1B).
3. This may be a difficult test to interpret. It is helpful to compare one eye with the other or the victim's eye with that of another person.
4. A history of being farsighted should raise suspicion; narrow angles accompany hyperopia and small anterior chambers (usually these individuals wear thick glasses that magnify their eyes on direct inspection).

Extraocular Muscle Testing

Have the victim follow a flashlight or finger through the extremes of gaze in six directions. Ask if one image or two are seen.

1. Double vision in any field of gaze may represent extraocular muscle palsy.
2. Grossly limited extraocular motion with bulging of the eye from the orbit suggests acute orbital inflammation or retrobulbar hemorrhage.
3. If the eye appears sunken within the orbit and the victim exhibits limited upward gaze, suspect a blowout fracture of the orbital floor.

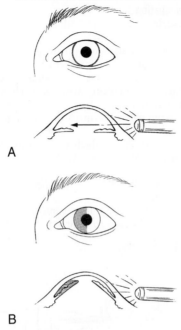

Figure 32-1. Estimating depth of anterior chamber.

Visual Field Testing

1. Ask the victim to cover one eye completely and look directly at your opposing eye from a distance of about 1 m (3 ft).
2. Place your fingers outside the victim's field of peripheral vision and slowly move them centrally.
3. Ask the victim to inform you when he or she can see your fingers. The victim's fields are generally normal when they correspond with those of the examiner.

Upper Eyelid Eversion

1. Place the end of a cotton-tipped applicator horizontally above the tarsal plate while you pull the eyelashes and the lid margin down and out (Fig. 32-2A).
2. Flip the lid up to evert it. Hold the everted lid in position by pressing the lashes against the superior orbital rim (see Fig. 32-2B).

Fluorescein Examination

1. Use fluorescein staining to evaluate any red or painful eye.
2. Wet the fluorescein strip with a drop of saline (artificial tears) or a drop of topical anesthetic.
3. When examining an eye with a possible infection, always use a separate fluorescein strip for each eye to avoid cross-contamination.
4. Next, apply the wetted strip to the inside of the victim's lower lid.
5. Ask the victim to blink, which will spread the fluorescein over the surface of the eye. Areas of corneal disruption stain brilliant green.
6. Use a small, blue filter placed over a penlight, which works well in the dark.
7. Outside during the day, simple sunlight often causes any significant corneal lesion to fluoresce.

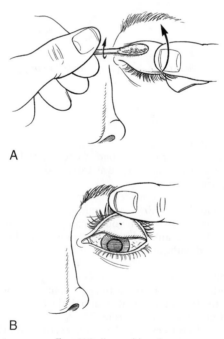

A

B

Figure 32-2. Upper eyelid eversion.

8. Fluorescein permanently stains soft contact lenses, so instruct victims to remove these lenses before the fluorescein examination and leave them out for several hours after the examination.

9. If there is concern regarding a penetrating injury, fluorescein can be used to paint the area of concern. Observe if fluorescein dilutes by pinpoint leak of aqueous fluid (a positive Seidel test indicates an open globe).

Eye Patching

1. Use a pressure patch to hold the eyelid closed and thereby facilitate healing of a corneal defect. Protect the injured eye from bright light.

2. A (light) pressure patch is indicated in many common eye emergencies and whenever the surface of the cornea has been injured, especially with a large corneal defect. The patient will be more comfortable; however, pressure patching probably does not speed up corneal healing.

3. Small corneal defects may heal rapidly without patching.

4. After patching, the victim often experiences less pain and tearing.

5. Do not use patching when the corneal epithelial defect is secondary to an infection (e.g., conjunctivitis, corneal ulcer) or if injury was caused by or contaminated with organic matter.

6. Use caution if the victim is a contact lens wearer, especially extended-wear lenses, which contribute to an increased risk of infection.

7. Never apply a pressure patch to an eye after a penetrating injury. After eye penetration or trauma, tape a protective cup (e.g., padded drinking cup) over the eye or fashion a cloth "donut" from a cravat or other cloth to avoid placing pressure on the eye or inflicting any further trauma during evacuation (see Fig. 23-10).

8. "Plano" (non-corrective) soft contact lenses are often used by ophthalmologists for patching corneal lesions. These might be considered if available.

Equipment
Two gauze eye patches (gauze 2- × 2-inch or commercial patches)
1-inch (2.5-cm) tape
Antibiotic ointment
Mydriatic-cycloplegic eye drops

Procedure
1. Before patching a corneal abrasion, apply both a drop or two of a mydriatic-cycloplegic solution and a thin ribbon of antibiotic-antiseptic ointment.
   a. The cycloplegic relaxes ciliary muscle spasm that accompanies corneal abrasion.
   b. Check the victim for a narrow anterior chamber before instilling the drops (see Estimation of Anterior Chamber Depth), although this is usually not realistic in the field.
2. Use antibiotic ointment for prophylaxis, although corneal abrasions rarely become infected.
3. For the patch to be effective, you must put it on just tightly enough to keep the eyelid shut, but do not put undue pressure on the eye.
4. Use two patches.
   a. Double the first patch by folding vertically, and place it over the closed lid. If a second patch is not available, this patch can be held in place with a single piece of tape.
   b. Put the unfolded second patch over the first folded patch.
5. Prepare the skin near the eye with tincture of benzoin (if available) to help the tape adhere. Be careful to keep benzoin out of the eye.
6. Place the tape diagonally from the center of the forehead to the cheekbone. Make sure the tape completely covers the patch to minimize slippage but does not extend onto the angle of the mandible.
7. Remove the patch every 24 hours so that the eye can be reexamined and the patch changed. Using a clean patch every 24 hours helps to prevent infection.
8. Instruct the victim with an eye patch to rest the uninjured eye. Discourage reading because rapid involuntary movement of the patched eye occurs.

Locating a Displaced Contact Lens
Soft contact lens wearers may occasionally have one of their lenses become displaced, causing blurred vision and a foreign body sensation. Once the lens is displaced, it may be difficult to locate.
1. The conjunctival fornix of the lower lid is easily examined by distracting the lens from the globe with gentle downward finger pressure applied to the lower lid.
2. If the contact lens has been displaced into the superior conjunctival fornix (usually the case), it may be more difficult to locate.
3. If visual inspection with a penlight and a handheld magnifying lens is not successful in finding the lens, gentle digital

massage over the closed upper lid directed toward the medial canthus often results in the contact lens emerging at that location. Several minutes of massage may be required. A few drops of artificial tears often facilitate the process.

4. If this maneuver is unproductive, the eye may be anesthetized with a drop of topical anesthetic, the upper lid distracted from the globe with upward finger pressure, and the fornix swept with a moistened cotton-tipped applicator.

5. Alternatively, using a paper clip opened to a right angle to create a simple retractor, evert the eyelid after proparacaine (or other topical anesthetic) instillation, and then lift the edge of the tarsus with the rounded edge of the paper clip.

6. If the lens is not the last and can be discarded, it can often be easily localized with fluorescein (Fig. 32-3).

DISORDERS

▶ SUDDEN LOSS OF VISION IN WHITE, "QUIET" EYE
(Box 32-2)

Acute and significant visual loss is an emergency. The common causes of acute visual loss include the following:

1. Retinal detachment
2. Central retinal artery occlusion
3. Arteritic ischemic optic neuropathy (giant cell/temporal arteritis)
4. Nonarteritic ischemic optic neuropathy
5. Optic neuritis
6. Central retinal vein occlusion
7. Vitreous hemorrhage
8. High-altitude retinal hemorrhage

Each of these conditions requires immediate evacuation and definitive follow-up. However, giant cell or temporal arteritis (a type of arteritic anterior ischemic optic neuropathy) requires immediate field treatment to avoid bilateral loss of vision.

Giant Cell (Temporal) Arteritis
Signs and Symptoms
1. Rapid, painless vision loss
2. Rare in persons younger than age 50
3. Associated with temporal headache
4. Jaw claudication
5. Low-grade fever
6. History of associated weight loss

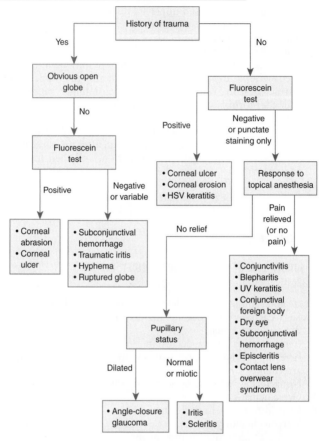

Figure 32-3. Algorithm showing wilderness diagnostic procedure for the acute red eye.

Box 32-2. Differential Diagnosis of Acute Loss of Vision in White, "Quiet" Eye

Retinal detachment
Central retinal artery occlusion
Anterior ischemic optic neuropathy
Optic neuritis
Central retinal vein occlusion
Arteritic anterior ischemic optic neuropathy
Vitreous hemorrhage
High-altitude retinal hemorrhage

7. History of polymyalgia rheumatica
8. Transient visual obscurations
9. Usually affects one eye first, then the second eye within hours to days

Treatment
1. Because this disease can cause significant visual loss in the absence of effective treatment, initiate care immediately with a high-dose corticosteroid (e.g., prednisone, 80 to 100 mg/day PO).
2. Evacuate the victim so that a high-dose steroid can be administered intravenously.
3. When treated, symptoms often improve within 1 to 3 days. However, steroids are typically continued for many weeks.

▶ RED EYE (Box 32-3)

Acute Angle-Closure Glaucoma
Acute angle-closure glaucoma results from a sudden rise in intraocular pressure (IOP). Patients at risk include elders and far-sighted individuals.

Box 32-3. Differential Diagnosis of the Acute Red Eye

Obvious open globe
Corneal abrasion
Corneal ulcer
Subconjunctival hemorrhage
Traumatic iritis
Hyphema
Occult open globe
Herpes simplex virus keratitis
Corneal erosion
Acute angle-closure glaucoma
Iritis
Scleritis
Conjunctivitis
Blepharitis
Ultraviolet keratitis
Episcleritis
Conjunctival foreign body
Dry eye
Contact lens overwear syndrome

Signs and Symptoms
1. Acute onset of severe pain and blurred vision
2. A red eye, often with the pupil slightly dilated and a "steamy" (edematous) cornea
3. The affected eye often feels appreciably harder than the unaffected eye (palpate through the lid gently and with extreme caution)
4. Symptoms beginning in low light
5. Possible nausea, vomiting, and generalized head pain
6. Person may complain of colored halos around lights
7. May be intermittent

Treatment
1. Instill timolol 0.5% (Timoptic), 1 drop bid (caution if patient has asthma, chronic obstructive pulmonary disease, or history of heart block).
2. Instill pilocarpine 2% (Pilocar), 1 drop q 15 min × 4, then qid.
3. Administer acetazolamide (Diamox), 250 mg PO qid. This is key because when intraocular pressure rises dramatically, topical drops do not penetrate and become ineffective.
4. Arrange for immediate evacuation for emergency ocular surgery (laser iridotomy).
5. The other eye is also at risk; it is prudent to treat this eye with pilocarpine bid, prophylactically.

Corneal Abrasion

Signs and Symptoms
1. Intense pain localized to the cornea after an injurious event
2. Conjunctival erythema
3. Pain is relieved with a drop of topical anesthetic (topical anesthetic not to be used repeatedly because it increases risk of infection and prolongs wound healing).
   a. Identification of a corneal lesion sometimes made using visible light but often enhanced by fluorescein staining (see Ocular Procedures, earlier)

Treatment
1. Apply a topical antibiotic solution. A solution is preferable to an ointment when the victim is expected to remain active. If the victim is sleeping or if the eye is patched, an ointment has slightly greater effective duration of effect.
2. If the abrasion is extensive (>30% of the corneal surface) or painful, add a mydriatic-cycloplegic agent to the regimen.
3. Instruct the victim to avoid activity requiring frequent active eye movement.
4. Determine whether to patch (see Ocular Procedures, earlier).

5. Be aware that many small (<3 mm) abrasions resolve as quickly with or without corneal (eye) patching.

6. Base the decision to patch the eye on abrasion size and comfort (many victims with severe corneal defects feel more comfortable after patching).

7. NOTE: Do not patch if victim is a contact lens wearer or the corneal epithelial defect was caused by or contaminated with organic matter.

8. If the eye is not patched, apply cool compresses over the eye after the topical antibiotic to soothe the area.

9. Alternatively, a soft contact patch lens (e.g., planar or plus one) instilled with Acular is very comfortable and antibiotic drops can be delivered through the lens.

10. Administer an oral analgesic or antiinflammatory drug to provide symptomatic relief

11. A corneal abrasion typically resolves within 24 to 48 hours, although a large abrasion may take longer. Evacuate promptly any victim with a corneal lesion that does not resolve within 4 days or that is progressing (enlarging or becoming more painful).

Corneal Erosion

This occurs when a small portion of corneal epithelium is torn as the eyelid opens, usually in a person with a prior history of corneal abrasion (can occur months to years after initial injury). The cause of recurrent corneal erosion is failure of complete bonding of the healing corneal epithelium to its basement membrane.

Signs and Symptoms

1. Acute ocular pain, photophobia, and tearing, often occurring at the time of awakening, when the eyes are first opened

2. Typically, bright fluorescein staining of the erosion, but with the erosion sometimes healing before the examination, revealing a normal cornea; erosions often recur

Treatment

1. Apply antibiotic ointment to the eye (above lower eyelid) before patching.

2. Apply the cycloplegic drug one time only.

3. Patch the affected eye for 12 hours, then remove the patch to inspect the eye. If total resolution has not occurred, replace the patch for another 12 hours.

4. If available, use hypertonic ophthalmic saline solution (Muro–128) after the patch is removed, 1 to 2 drops q3–4h.

5. If hypertonic ophthalmic saline solution is not available, instill artificial tears 4 to 8 times per day.

6. If the victim with corneal erosion does not respond to treatment, encourage evacuation.

Contact Lens–Related Corneal Abrasion

A lens-related corneal abrasion is at high risk for transformation into a corneal ulcer.

Signs and Symptoms
Same as for other corneal abrasions

Treatment
1. Discontinue contact lens wear.
2. Do not patch.
3. Apply a fluoroquinolone antibiotic solution (e.g., gatifloxacin (Zymar) ophthalmic solution, 1 to 2 drops q2–4h for 5 to 7 days).

Corneal Ulcer

Ulceration usually occurs after an injury or in a soft contact lens wearer. Soft contact lenses allow pathogens to adhere to the corneal surface, creating deposits of organisms that can invade the stroma. This is especially true if the soft lens is worn continuously.

Signs and Symptoms
1. Red, painful eye
2. A white or gray spot (white cell infiltrate) on the cornea visible without fluorescein
3. Photophobia
4. Decreased visual acuity in the affected eye
5. Discharge may or may not be present

Treatment
1. Instill gatifloxacin ophthalmic solution (Zymar) 1 drop q 15 min for 6 hours, then 1 drop q 30 min, continued during the evacuation. If gatifloxacin or another quinolone is not available, use another ocular antibiotic. These may have reduced efficacy.
2. Apply a cycloplegic agent.
3. Do not patch the eye.
4. Do not wear contact lenses.
5. Administer an analgesic as needed.
6. Be aware that immediate ophthalmologic consultation is required for appropriate cultures and antimicrobial treatment. Do not withhold antibiotics pending evacuation.

Corneal Foreign Body

Signs and Symptoms
1. Pain, irritation, tearing, redness, and a sensation of "something in the eye"

2. Sometimes visualized with the naked eye, often enhanced with fluorescein staining (highlighting any corneal damage)

Treatment
1. A foreign body can often be removed by simple irrigation with a copious amount of the cleanest water available (disinfected drinking water).
2. If simple irrigation is unsuccessful and the foreign body can be visualized, use a moistened cotton swab to gently brush away the foreign body. The corneal epithelium can be easily damaged by forceful or repetitive use of this technique. Do not blindly sweep in hopes of success.
3. After removal of the foreign body, instill topical antibiotic drops. You may apply an eye patch if there is an epithelial defect.
4. Apply a cool compress to ease discomfort.
5. Inform the victim that the foreign body sensation will return after the anesthetic wears off.
6. If the foreign body is metallic, a rust ring may develop. This is not dangerous and can be removed later by an ophthalmologist.
7. If the foreign body cannot be easily removed or if signs and symptoms (pain, irritation, redness) persist for more than a day after removal, initiate evacuation.

▶ CONJUNCTIVITIS

The specific determination of the cause for conjunctivitis can be difficult in the field. Many presentations are viral or allergic. Fortunately, most cases are self-limited or are bacterial and respond to an antibiotic. Visual acuity should always be checked, even though conjunctivitis typically does not cause a change. Any deterioration is cause for concern and potential evacuation.

Acute Bacterial Conjunctivitis (Pink Eye)

Signs and Symptoms
1. Hyperemia of the conjunctiva
2. Irritation and tearing
3. Eyelids that stick together during sleep
4. Purulent discharge

Treatment
1. Apply topical antibiotic solution 1 to 2 drops q2–6h for at least 5 to 7 days.
2. If the infection progresses (increasing symptoms) despite antibiotic therapy, arrange for evacuation.

3. If corneal opacification is noted (e.g., corneal ulcer, more common in a soft contact lens wearer), arrange for evacuation.
4. Do not patch the eye.

Viral Conjunctivitis (Acute Follicular Conjunctivitis)

Signs and Symptoms
1. Redness of the conjunctiva
2. Tearing (with scant or no purulent discharge)
3. Possible history of upper respiratory infection or contact with person with red eye
4. Generally involves one eye, then progresses to other eye several days later
5. Tender preauricular lymph nodes
6. Redness and edema of the eyelids

Treatment
1. Consider instilling a topical antibiotic (because specific diagnosis is difficult in the field), 1 to 2 drops q2–6h for at least 5 to 7 days.
2. Administer artificial tears prn for relief or vasoconstrictive drops qid for 1 to 2 days.
3. Apply cool compresses for symptomatic relief. Be careful not to cross-contaminate the uninvolved eye.
4. Be diligent about hand washing; avoid sharing towels to prevent spread to others.
5. Be aware that viral conjunctivitis may last 2 weeks.
6. Evacuate the victim if the condition is not resolving or if any corneal opacification is noted.
7. Do not patch the eye.

Chemical Conjunctivitis and Chemical Injury to the Cornea

Chemical conjunctivitis may be caused by any irritant (e.g., sunscreen, insect repellent, stove fuel) accidentally introduced into the eye. Caustic substances may cause more serious burns affecting the cornea. Alkali and acid burns are true emergencies.

Signs and Symptoms
1. Immediate pain, tearing, and irritation
2. Redness of the conjunctiva
3. Loss of vascularity (e.g., "whitening") of the conjunctiva is an ominous sign

Treatment
1. Instill a topical anesthetic.
2. Irrigate the eye with a copious amount of the cleanest water available immediately. In most cases, 1 to 2 L of

irrigant is sufficient. However, for an alkali burn, use at least 3 L or 30 minutes of continuous irrigation.
3. If the injury was from an acid or alkali, transport the victim rapidly to definitive care. If possible, continue irrigation during transport.
4. Instill a cycloplegic to reduce ciliary spasm.
5. Instill antibiotic ophthalmic ointment.
6. Cool compresses may provide relief. Be careful not to cross-contaminate the uninvolved eye.
7. Evacuate any victim with a corneal burn associated with corneal opacification or significant defect on fluorescein staining.

Inclusion (Chlamydial) Conjunctivitis

Chlamydial conjunctivitis is usually a sexually transmitted disease (STD), seen most often in young adults. It is a common cause of blindness in the developing world.

Signs and Symptoms
1. Similar to those for acute bacterial conjunctivitis
2. History of urethritis or cervicitis (from an STD)
3. Swollen eyelids
4. Many small follicles (raised pale bumps) in the palpebral conjunctivae (especially of the lower lid)

Treatment
1. Administer doxycycline, 100 mg bid PO for 21 days.
2. Apply cool compresses to provide relief. Be careful not to cross-contaminate the uninvolved eye.
3. Inclusion conjunctivitis may be difficult to differentiate from other, more common forms of bacterial conjunctivitis.

Allergic Conjunctivitis

Signs and Symptoms
1. Itching and tearing (without purulent discharge)
2. At times, swelling and redness of the conjunctivae

Treatment
1. Instill vasoconstrictive drops (e.g., 0.3% pheniramine maleate plus 0.025% naphazoline ophthalmic solution [Naphcon-A]) up to qid for 1 to 2 days.
2. Consider topical ketorolac (Acular) 0.5% ophthalmic solution, 1 drop q6-12h, for 1 to 2 days.
3. Apply cool compresses.
4. Administer an oral antihistamine to relieve itching.

Herpes Simplex Viral Keratitis

Ocular herpes can result from sexually transmitted herpes simplex virus (HSV-2). However, it is usually caused by HSV-1, the virus responsible for cold sores.

Signs and Symptoms
1. Symptoms mimicking those of corneal abrasion
   a. Red eye
   b. Pain, photophobia, tearing, foreign body sensation
   c. Decreased vision
2. History of previous episode
3. In early herpetic infection, only small punctate lesions or a single vesicle of the cornea seen
4. Over time, typical dendritic (branching) pattern of corneal involvement becoming apparent on fluorescein staining
5. Typically unilateral

Treatment
1. If available, instill a topical antiviral agent (trifluridine [Viroptic] 1% ophthalmic solution) q2h while the victim is awake until the corneal epithelium has healed. Instill this agent qid for 1 week.
2. Evacuate the victim.

▶ INFECTION OF THE EYELID

Blepharitis

Signs and Symptoms
1. Itching and burning of the eyelids, often with crusting around the eyes on awakening
2. Red eyelid margins that are crusted and thickened
3. Occasionally, injected conjunctivae

Treatment
1. Gently scrub the eyelid margins with baby shampoo bid using a washcloth or cotton-tipped applicator.
2. Apply warm compresses for 15 to 20 minutes tid to qid.
3. Instill artificial tears for associated mild ocular irritation or dry eyes four to eight times a day.
4. Apply antibiotic ointment qid to the eyelid margin for 1 week, then qhs for 1 more week.

Hordeolum

Hordeolum is a common infection in a gland of the eyelid. A small hordeolum that forms an external pustule and points toward the skin is called a *stye*.

Signs and Symptoms
1. Localized pain, swelling, and redness of the eyelid, often associated with a purulent discharge
2. Infection pointing to either the skin or to the conjunctival side of the lid

Treatment
1. Apply warm compresses for 15 to 20 minutes several times per day.
2. Gently scrub the eyelid with soap and water several times per day.
3. Apply a topical antibiotic such as erythromycin (Ilotycin) ophthalmic solution q4–6h for 7 to 10 days.
4. If cellulitis is present, administer a systemic antibiotic for 7 to 10 days.
5. If the upper and lower lids are involved and there is orbital extension (i.e., extraocular movement limitation), it is an emergency and requires immediate evacuation.
6. Perform incision and drainage only if there is an identifiable pointing lesion and no response to conservative treatment.

Chalazion

Signs and Symptoms
1. Noninflamed, nontender mass in the upper or lower lid
2. May follow a hordeolum
3. Usually points toward the conjunctival side of the lid

Treatment
1. Apply warm compresses.
2. Note that incision and curettage are often necessary if the condition persists (this should only be done by an ophthalmologist).

▶ PERIOCULAR INFLAMMATION (Box 32-4)
Preseptal Cellulitis
Signs and Symptoms
1. Tenderness and redness of the eyelid, often associated with fever
2. Consider using pen to outline the area of erythema for gauging clinical progression

---

Box 32-4. Differential Diagnosis of Acute Periocular Inflammation

Preseptal cellulitis
Orbital cellulitis
Dacryocystitis
Orbital pseudotumor
Insect envenomation

3. Unlike orbital cellulitis, no pain with eye movement or restriction of extraocular movement
4. Inability to open the eye because of marked eyelid edema
5. Appearance resembling and easily confused with an allergic eyelid reaction or insect bite
6. With an allergic or inflammatory process, usually itching without tenderness

Treatment
1. Administer levofloxacin (Levaquin), 500 mg PO bid for 7 to 10 days.
2. Alternatively, administer ciprofloxacin (Cipro), 750 PO bid for 7 to 10 days.
3. Alternatively, administer cephalexin (Keflex), 500 mg PO tid to qid for 7 to 10 days.
4. Apply warm compresses to the inflamed region qid.
5. Re-examine q2h initially.
6. Consider evacuation for any victim with the following conditions:
   a. Toxic appearance
   b. Decreased EOM
   c. Child younger than age 5 years
   d. No improvement or any worsening after 2 to 3 days of oral antibiotics

Orbital Cellulitis

Pathogens that cause orbital cellulitis include *Staphylococcus* and *Streptococcus* species, *Haemophilus influenzae* (common in children), *Bacteroides,* and various gram-negative rods (especially after trauma).

Signs and Symptoms
1. Red eye, blurred vision, diplopia, headache, fever, eyelid edema
2. Erythema, warmth, and tenderness over the affected area
3. Conjunctival chemosis and injection
4. Restricted ocular motility and pain developing on attempted ocular motion
5. Possible coexisting meningitis

Treatment
1. Evacuate the victim immediately.
2. Administer ceftriaxone (Rocephin), 1 to 2 g IV ql2h.
3. Although oral antibiotics are considered suboptimal for this condition, a reasonable regimen initiated during transport might include any of the following:
   a. Levofloxacin (Levaquin), 500 mg bid
   b. Ciprofloxacin (Cipro), 750 mg bid

    c. Absent these drugs, a second- or third-generation oral cephalosporin (e.g., cefpodoxime [Vantin] or amoxicillin with clavulanate [Augmentin]) could be used.

Dacryocystitis (Inflammation of the Lacrimal Sac)

Signs and Symptoms
1. Pain, redness, and swelling over the lacrimal sac (innermost aspect of lower eyelid)
2. Mucoid or purulent discharge expressed from the nasolacrimal punctum when pressure is applied

Treatment
1. Administer ciprofloxacin (Cipro), 750 mg bid for 7 to 10 days.
2. Be aware that topical antibiotics are minimally effective.
3. Apply warm compresses.
4. Administer pain medication as needed.

▶ EPISCLERITIS

Signs and Symptoms
1. Normal vision
2. Localized inflammation and dilation of the episcleral vessels
3. Little discomfort or discharge
4. Often in only one sector of the eye
5. Caused by irritants or is idiopathic
6. Often a history of prior similar episodes

Treatment
1. If irritation exists, use artificial tears or instill 0.3% pheniramine maleate plus 0.025% naphazoline ophthalmic solution (Naphcon-A) up to qid.
2. Consider topical ketorolac (Acular) 0.5% ophthalmic solution, 1 drop q6–12h, or an oral nonsteroidal antiinflammatory drug (NSAID).
3. Systemic ibuprofen may be beneficial, 400 mg PO tid.

▶ IRITIS

Iritis may result from a specific etiology (e.g., infection, trauma, overexposure to ultraviolet [UV] light) or may occur independently.

Signs and Symptoms
1. Moderate to severe pain that does not respond to topical anesthesia
2. Photophobia
3. Blurred vision

4. Pupil of the involved eye constricted and less reactive
5. Redness surrounding the cornea; ciliary vessels running through the sclera beneath the conjunctivae becoming injected, causing a purplish area of injection around the cornea ("ciliary injection")

Treatment
1. Address any specific cause.
2. Instill a mydriatic-cycloplegic agent to reduce pain and ciliary spasm and prevent synechiae.
3. Administer topical prednisolone (Pred-Forte), 1 drop q2–6h for 1 to 3 days.
4. Systemic ibuprofen may be beneficial, 400 mg PO tid.
5. Evacuate the victim if the condition persists or progresses. The iritis associated with UV photokeratitis or corneal abrasion is usually self-limited.

▶ ULTRAVIOLET PHOTOKERATITIS (SNOWBLINDNESS)

UV-induced photokeratitis represents corneal damage. Intense exposure to UV light may cause a corneal burn in 1 hour, although symptoms may not become apparent for 6 to 12 hours.

Signs and Symptoms
1. Pain, although there is typically a 6- to 12-hour symptom-free interval just after exposure
2. Severe gritty sensation in the eyes
3. Photophobia
4. Tearing
5. Marked conjunctival erythema and chemosis
6. Eyelid edema
7. Ciliary injection with iritis
8. Usually bilateral
9. On fluorescein staining, a horizontal band-like uptake that corresponds with the shielding effect of the squinting eyelids

Treatment
1. Spontaneous healing generally occurs in 24 hours. However, take steps to minimize pain and disability.
2. Remove contact lenses.
3. Instill a single dose of a topical anesthetic to help control pain during the examination. Do not use the anesthetic more than once because prolonged use can impair corneal reepithelialization.
4. Consider administering a topical NSAID solution (ketorolac [Acular] 0.5% ophthalmic solution), 1 drop q6–12h.

5. Apply an antibiotic solution. If a pressure patch is used, apply topical antibiotic ointment before patching.
6. Administer an NSAID such as ibuprofen to control symptoms.
7. Administer a systemic narcotic analgesic, if necessary.
8. Apply cold compresses to provide some relief.
9. If needed, instill a mydriatic-cycloplegic agent to reduce pain associated with ciliary spasm.
10. Note that topical steroids are not recommended because of the potential for delayed epithelial healing.
11. Patch the affected eye for 12 hours, and then remove the patch to inspect the eye. If total resolution has not occurred, replace the patch for another 12 hours.

Prevention
1. Wear sunglasses that block more than 99% of UV type B light.
2. Add side shields to sunglasses to prevent reflected UV light from striking the cornea.
3. Always carry spare sunglasses.
4. Create a makeshift shield by cutting narrow horizontal slits in a piece of cardboard, foam padding, or duct tape and securing this over the eyes.

▶ SUBCONJUNCTIVAL HEMORRHAGE

This condition is usually caused by local trauma, coughing, or straining.

Signs and Symptoms
1. Usually asymptomatic
2. Blood seen underneath the conjunctivae, often localized to one sector of the eye
3. After trauma, critical to consider the presence of a conjunctival lesion or a ruptured globe

Treatment
1. In general, no treatment is required.
2. Reassure the victim.
3. Administer artificial teardrops qid to relieve mild ocular irritation.
4. Subconjunctival hemorrhage usually resolves spontaneously in 1 to 2 weeks.
5. If the condition does not resolve or recurs, seek ophthalmologic care.

▶ HYPHEMA

Hyphema usually results from a blunt injury to the eye, resulting in hemorrhage into the anterior chamber.

Signs and Symptoms
1. Meniscus or layering of blood along the lower anterior chamber (in front of the iris) after the victim has been upright for 5 to 10 minutes
2. Decreased vision and eye pain
3. Lethargy and vomiting possible as a result of acutely increased IOP

Treatment
1. Allow the victim to rest in an upright (e.g., sitting) position.
2. Avoid activity.
3. No near work (i.e., avoid the accommodative pupillary response).
4. Place shield over eye; do not patch.
5. Instill an intermediate- to long-acting mydriatic-cycloplegic agent.
6. Do not give aspirin or NSAIDs.
7. If the hyphema is large, arrange for immediate evacuation. A small hyphema may be better treated with rest, avoiding high physical exertion and jostling associated with evacuation.

▶ RUPTURED GLOBE

Signs and Symptoms
1. History of significant trauma or projectile injury
2. Reduced vision, pain (see "Examination of Vision," earlier)
3. Pupil appearing distorted and teardrop shaped, pointing toward the rupture
4. An abnormal anterior chamber (either shallow or deep compared with the contralateral eye)
5. Significant conjunctival hemorrhage or with dark specks of uveal tissue underneath
6. Limited extraocular mobility

Treatment
1. Do not press on the eye.
2. Plan for evacuation.
3. Elevate the victim's head to decrease IOP.
4. Cover the eye with a cup or improvised shield to avoid any pressure on the globe.
5. Avoid any activities (including further ocular examination) that may cause the victim to blink excessively or to strain.
6. Administer a systemic antibiotic such as levofloxacin (Levaquin) 500 mg bid or ciprofloxacin (Cipro) 750 mg PO bid or a third-generation injectable cephalosporin, ceftriaxone (Rocephin) 1 g IV q12h if available.

7. If an extended evacuation is necessary and a small puncture wound can be identified, consider applying a drop or two of superglue to the wound. Although this is a radical maneuver, uninterrupted loss of aqueous or vitreous would otherwise result in permanent blindness.

▶ REFRACTIVE CHANGES AT ALTITUDE AFTER REFRACTIVE SURGERY

1. Acute hyperopic shift has been reported in persons who have had radial keratotomy (RK) and then experienced altitude exposure.
2. The effect of altitude exposure on post-RK eyes is most likely caused by hypoxia rather than by decreased pressure.
3. Breathing a normoxic inspired gas mix does not protect against the development of hypoxic corneal changes.
4. The effect of the post-RK hyperopic shift seen at altitude depends on the postoperative refractive state (undercorrected patients may actually have their vision improve) and the accommodative abilities of the individual.
5. Individuals who have undergone RK and plan to undertake an altitude exposure of 2744 m (9000 ft) or higher while mountaineering should bring multiple eyeglasses with increasing plus lens power.
6. Reports have noted mild myopic shifts at altitude in some individuals after LASIK.

Ear, Nose, and Throat Emergencies

33

▶ EPISTAXIS

1. Epistaxis is a common problem in travelers.
2. Reduced humidity in airplanes, cold climates, and high-altitude environments can produce drying and erosion of the nasal mucosa.
3. Daily applications of a small quantity of petroleum jelly (Vaseline) to the septum can help to keep the nasal mucosa moist.
4. Other etiologic factors include facial trauma, infections, and inflammatory rhinitis.
5. Although most cases of epistaxis are minor, some present life-threatening emergencies (see Chapter 27).
6. Anterior epistaxis from one side of the nasal cavity occurs in more than 90% of cases (i.e., posterior bleeds are rare).

Treatment
1. The existing clot should be completely cleared, "blown out" by the patient.
2. One or two sprays of a topical nasal vasoconstrictor should be inhaled into the affected nostril (e.g., oxymetazoline [Afrin] or phenylephrine [Neo-Synephrine]).
3. The patient should be sitting (i.e., keeping the head elevated and still).
4. The nostrils should be gently compressed for a minimum of 10 minutes.
5. If the measures described earlier do not control the bleeding, nasal packing may be necessary.
   a. Soak a piece of cotton or gauze with a vasoconstrictor such as oxymetazoline (Afrin) nasal spray and insert it into the nose, leaving it in place for 5 to 10 minutes.
   b. Petroleum jelly–impregnated gauze or strips of a nonadherent dressing can then be packed into the nose so that both ends of the gauze remain outside the nasal cavity (Fig. 33-1). This prevents the victim from inadvertently aspirating the nasal packing.
   c. Complete packing of the nasal cavity of an adult victim requires a minimum of 1 m (3 feet) of packing to fill the nasal cavity and tamponade the bleeding site.
   d. Expandable packing material such as Weimert Epistaxis Packing, Rapid Rhino (ArthroCare Corporation, Sunnyvale, CA), or the Rhino Rocket (Shippert Medical Technologies, Centennial, CO) is available commercially. These can be lubricated with K-Y jelly or water before

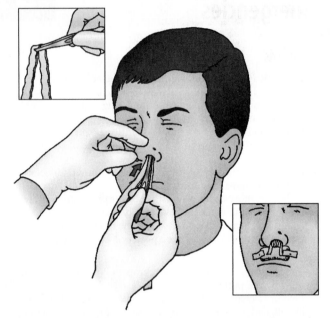

Figure 33-1. Anterior epistaxis from one side of the nasal cavity can be treated using nasal packing soaked in a vasoconstrictor. Petroleum jelly–impregnated gauze or strips of nonadherent dressing can be packed in the nose so that both ends of the gauze remain outside the nasal cavity.

insertion. A tampon or balloon tip from a Foley catheter can also be used as improvised packing.

e. If packing is bulky, consider bilateral packing to reduce asymmetric pressure on the septum.

f. Anterior nasal packing blocks sinus drainage and predisposes to sinusitis. Prophylactic antibiotics are usually recommended until the pack is removed in 48 hours.

7. If the bleeding site is located posteriorly, use a 14- to 16-French Foley catheter with a 30-mL balloon to tamponade the site (Fig. 33-2).

a. Prelubricate the catheter with either petroleum jelly (Vaseline) or a water-based lubricant.

b. Insert it through the nasal cavity into the posterior pharynx. Inflate the balloon with 10 to 15 mL of water, and gently withdraw the catheter back into the posterior nasopharynx until resistance is met.

c. Secure the catheter firmly to the victim's forehead with several strips of tape.

   d. Avoid severe pressure on the nares.

   e. Pack the anterior nose in front of the catheter balloon as described earlier.

▶ ESOPHAGEAL FOREIGN BODIES

1. Esophageal foreign bodies may cause significant morbidity.
2. Respiratory compromise caused by tracheal compression or by aspiration of secretions can occur.
3. Mediastinitis, pleural effusion, pneumothorax, and abscess may be seen with perforations of the esophagus from sharp objects or pressure necrosis caused by large objects.
4. The use of a Foley balloon-tipped catheter can be a safe method for removing blunt esophageal foreign bodies. Success rates of 98% have been cited.
5. Associated complications include laryngospasm, epistaxis, pain, esophageal perforation, and tracheal aspiration of the dislodged foreign body.
6. Sharp, ragged foreign bodies or an uncooperative victim precludes use of this technique.
   a. Lubricate a 12- to 16-French Foley catheter and place it orally into the esophagus while the victim is seated.
   b. After placing the victim in Trendelenburg's position, pass the catheter beyond the foreign body and inflate the balloon with water.
   c. Withdraw the catheter with steady traction until the foreign body can be removed from the hypopharynx or is expelled by coughing.
   d. Take care to avoid lodging the foreign body in the nasopharynx.
   e. Any significant impedance to withdrawal should terminate the attempt.
7. Use of this technique is recommended only in extreme wilderness settings or when endoscopy is not available.

▶ FOREIGN BODIES IN THE EAR

Signs and Symptoms
1. Victims may experience significant discomfort.
2. Nausea or vomiting may occur if a live insect is in the ear canal.
3. Victim may complain of a sense of fullness in the affected ear.
4. Associated hearing loss may occur.
5. Bleeding may occur either from direct trauma or from the victim's attempts to remove the foreign body.
6. Insects can injure the tympanic membrane or external canal.
7. Erythema and swelling of the canal or a foul-smelling discharge may develop over time.

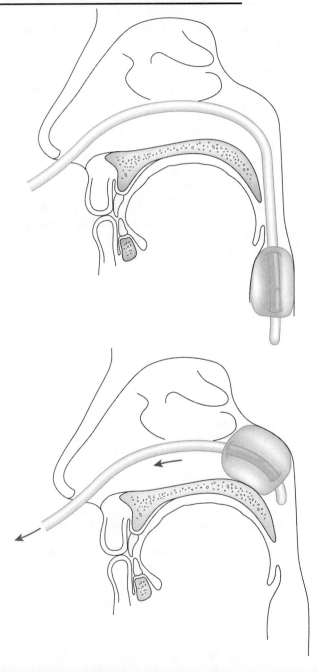

Figure 33-2. Posterior nasal packing using a Foley catheter. Insert a Foley catheter into the nose and gently pass it back until it enters the back of the throat (**A**). After the tip of the catheter is in the victim's throat, carefully inflate the balloon with 10 to 12 mL of air or water from a syringe. Inflation should be done slowly and should be stopped if painful. After the balloon is inflated, gently pull the catheter back out until resistance is met (**B**).

Treatment
1. The insect should be killed before removal. Instill one of the following:
   a. Lidocaine (2%)
   b. Alcohol
   c. Mineral oil
2. Irrigation is the simplest method of foreign body removal.
   a. Do not irrigate if the tympanic membrane is perforated.
   b. An ordinary 20- to 60-cc syringe with an irrigation tip or catheter may be used for irrigation.
   c. Use clean water (i.e., disinfected for drinking).
3. Sometimes the object can be easily extracted with simple forceps.
4. Avoid pushing the object in deeper.
5. Alternatively, form a right-angled hook with a 25-gauge needle. This can be used to get behind and remove a soft foreign body.
6. Mild sedation may be necessary.
7. Analgesics should be given if indicated.
8. Following removal, inspect the external canal.
9. If evidence of infection or abrasion is noted, administer a combination antibiotic and steroid otic suspension (e.g., neomycin and polymixin B and hydrocortisone otic suspension [Cortisporin] or ciprofloxacin with hydrocortisone [Cipro HC]) 4 to 5 times per day for 5 to 7 days.

▶ **OTITIS MEDIA**

Signs and Symptoms
In the wilderness, otoscopic examination is usually not possible. Diagnosis is based on clinical symptoms including one or more of the following.
1. Earache
2. Otorrhea (less common)
3. Fever (not required for the diagnosis)
4. Associated upper respiratory infection
5. Decreased hearing

Treatment

Mild otitis may be managed with a short period of observation without specific treatment. Failure to improve within 48 to 72 hours should prompt initiation of antibiotic therapy.

Treatment is directed toward *Pneumococcus* and *Moraxella*. Less common causes are *Haemophilus influenzae*, *Mycoplasma* species, viruses, and other bacteria. Sterile effusions occur in approximately 20% of cases.

The antibiotic of choice is amoxicillin 250 to 500 mg PO q8h or amoxicillin and clavulanate potassium (Augmentin) 500 to 875 mg PO q12h for 5 to 7 days (in adults). In the wilderness these antibiotics may not be available. An alternative is azithromycin (Zithromax) 500 mg as a single dose on day 1, followed by 250 mg once daily on days 2 through 5. Newer-generation fluoroquinolones (e.g., levofloxacin) may also be used 250 to 500 mg qd for 5 to 7 days.

Perforation of the tympanic membrane may complicate otitis media. Treatment is essentially as described earlier. Appropriate follow-up is indicated following perforation. Perforations generally heal within a few weeks without complications.

▶ OTITIS EXTERNA

See Chapter 54.

▶ SINUSITIS

Signs and Symptoms

Common complaints include the following:

1. Nasal congestion
2. Purulent nasal discharge
3. Facial pain (may be increased by leaning forward or with any head movement)
4. Facial tenderness to palpation
5. Retro-orbital pain (if the ethmoid sinus is involved)
6. Headache
7. Concomitant or preceding upper respiratory infection
8. Dental pain
9. Decreased sense of smell
10. Cough

Fever may be present but is uncommon.

Treatment

Acute sinusitis is usually bacterial in origin.

1. Encourage hydration to promote sinus drainage.
2. Nasal vasoconstrictors (e.g., Afrin) may provide relief during initial management. These should not be used longer than 3 days to avoid rebound phenomenon.

3. Warm facial compresses may provide symptomatic relief.
4. Decongestants and nonsteroidal antiinflammatory drugs (NSAIDs) may be useful in reducing secretions (avoid antihistamines).
5. In severe cases a short course of oral prednisone may be considered.
6. Analgesic medication may be necessary, non-narcotic or narcotic.
7. The organisms most commonly implicated in bacterial sinusitis are *Haemophilus influenzae* and *Streptococcus pneumoniae* (in adults).
8. A higher incidence of anaerobic organisms exists (e.g., *Bacteroides, Peptostreptococcus,* and *Fusobacterium* species are seen in chronic sinusitis).
9. Specific antibiotic treatment involves the following:
   a. Trimethoprim and sulfamethoxazole (Bactrim, Septra) 1 tab (double strength) PO bid for 7 to 14 days.
   b. Amoxicillin and clavulanate (Augmentin) 500 mg PO q12h for 7 to 14 days.
   c. Azithromycin (Zithromax) 500 mg as a single dose on day 1, followed by 250 mg once daily on days 2 through 5.
   d. Levofloxacin (Levaquin) 500 mg PO qd for 7 to 14 days.
   e. NOTE: Longer-duration antibiotic courses are indicated for serious or persistent disease.
10. For worsening or severe toxicity (e.g., lethargy, vomiting, high fever), seek urgent follow-up.

Dental Emergencies

34

The most common dental emergencies result from inflammation, infection, or trauma.

▶ TOOTHACHE (PULPITIS)

The common toothache is caused by inflammation of the dental pulp and is often associated with dental caries.

Signs and Symptoms
1. Pain, which may be severe, intermittent, and difficult to localize. Pain often radiates to the eye or ear region.
2. Pain that is often made worse by hot or cold foods or liquids
3. Carious lesion in the painful tooth; occasionally sensitive to percussion or palpation

Treatment
1. If the offending carious lesion can be localized, first apply a piece of cotton soaked with eugenol (oil of cloves).
2. Place a temporary filling material such as Cavit or zinc oxide-eugenol (ZOE) cement (Intermediate Restorative Material [IRM]) into the lesion to protect the nerve. Softened candle wax can also be used.
3. Administer a nonsteroidal antiinflammatory drug (NSAID) (e.g., ibuprofen, 800 mg PO q6h prn).
4. If the episodes of pain last longer, indicating a moderate pulpitis, fill the lesion as described earlier and give the victim a non-narcotic analgesic.
5. For severe pulpitis, with continuous and severe pain, administer a local anesthetic and then evacuate the victim. You can achieve a nerve block with bupivacaine 2% with 1:200,000 epinephrine (Marcaine) that lasts for about 8 hours and does not produce central nervous system depression. Large doses of narcotics may not provide pain relief and might compromise the victim's ability to participate in evacuation.
6. In extraordinary circumstances, locate the offending tooth, expose the pulp, remove the inflamed tissue with a barbed broach, and cover the lesion with temporary filling material.

▶ PERIAPICAL OSTEITIS

Inflammation of the supporting structures at the root of a tooth

Signs and Symptoms
1. Constant, often throbbing pain
2. Tooth is sensitive to tapping. Area over the apex of the tooth is tender to palpation, but there is no frank swelling.
3. Victim can usually point to the exact source of the pain.

Treatment
1. Administer an NSAID (e.g., ibuprofen, 800 mg PO q6h prn).
2. Place a strip of leather, webbing, or something similar between the teeth on the nonpainful side.
3. Soft diet

▶ CRACKED TOOTH

Signs and Symptoms
1. Sharp pain when chewing certain foods
2. Tooth feels weak or only hurts when the victim bites on something hard

Treatment
1. Avoid chewing on the affected side.
2. See a dentist as soon as possible.

▶ TEMPOROMANDIBULAR DISORDERS

Myofascial Pain and Dysfunction (MPD)
Participants in wilderness activities are exposed to many of the risk factors for MPD (stress-associated grinding of the teeth, increased jaw function from eating jerky and other dried foods).

Signs and Symptoms
1. Pain in the muscles of mastication, which is usually unilateral and increases with chewing
2. Headache or earache
3. Intermittent clicking of the temporomandibular joint (TMJ)
4. Limitation of jaw movement
5. Change in bite
6. Tenderness of the jaw muscles or TMJ to palpation
7. Inability to open the mouth widely or deviation of the chin to one side on opening

Treatment
1. Rest the muscles (soft diet and control of tooth clenching and grinding habits).
2. Apply moist heat.

3. Place a soft material such as a folded piece of gauze between the front teeth to keep the teeth from touching.
4. Administer an analgesic (e.g., ibuprofen, 800 mg PO q6h).

Mandibular Dislocation

Dislocation of the mandible and inability to close the mouth can result from external trauma or sudden wide opening of the mouth, such as occurs with yawning. If there is a history of trauma, a condylar fracture should be suspected.

Signs and Symptoms
1. Inability to completely open or close the mouth
2. Pain at the TMJ

Treatment
1. Place the rescuer's thumbs on the victim's lower molars and move the mandible down, then posteriorly, and then up. The thumbs should be padded to prevent bites as the jaw pops back into its socket.
2. If muscle spasm is severe, sedation might be necessary.
3. After reduction of the mandible, the victim must avoid wide mouth opening.

▶ INFECTIONS

Aphthous Ulcers
Signs and Symptoms
1. Painful, oral mucosa lesions are round, superficial, and have a red halo.
2. The victim usually gives a history of similar ulcerations.
3. The lesions typically last 10 to 14 days.

Treatment
1. Apply a topical steroid (fluocinonide 0.05%) mixed with Orabase over each ulcer six to eight times per day. Do not mix the medications until you are ready to apply them, and do not rub the mixture into the lesions.
2. Other options include premixed preparations such as Kenalog in Orabase.
3. Tincture of benzoin or a topical anesthetic (viscous lidocaine 2%) can be applied to the dried surface of the ulcer before meals and at bedtime.

Viral Infections
Herpes labialis (cold sore, fever blister) is the most common oral viral infection. Use of sun-blocking agents on the lips helps prevent herpes labialis.

Signs and Symptoms
1. Prodrome of tingling or paresthesia in the area
2. Yellow, fluid-filled vesicles that rupture to leave ragged ulcers on the lip, palate, tongue, and buccal mucosa
3. Primary herpetic gingivostomatitis is characterized by a thin zone of red, painful gingiva just next to the teeth. Sore throat, lymphadenopathy, and low-grade fever are also present.

Treatment
1. Administer valacyclovir (Valtrex) 2 g PO twice daily for 1 day, with doses taken about 12 hours apart as soon as the victim becomes aware of a prodromal "tingle" or paresthesia.
2. For herpetic gingivostomatitis, use soothing mouth rinses such as warm saline or a mixture of equal amounts of diphenhydramine (Benadryl) elixir, 12.5 mg/5 mL, kaolin-pectin (Kaopectate) and viscous lidocaine 2% (rinse and expectorate 5 mL q2h).

Apical Abscess and Cellulitis
Signs and Symptoms
1. Dental pain associated with swelling and fluctuance in the gum line at the base of the tooth; swelling much more common on facial side than on lingual side
2. Pain caused by percussion of the offending tooth
3. No sensitivity to hot or cold in the affected tooth

Treatment
1. Incision and drainage is the treatment of choice (Fig. 34-1).
   a. Infiltrate the area with a local anesthetic. Adequate anesthesia may also be obtained by applying cold (ice or snow) to the area to be incised.
   b. Make an incision at the point of maximum fluctuance down to bone in one swift movement.
   c. Spread the incision with a hemostat or knife handle.
   d. Place a T-shaped drain into the wound. Drain material can be improvised from a piece of surgical glove or gauze dressing.
2. Administer warm saline rinses q2h, and an analgesic (ibuprofen 800 mg PO every 6 hours) as needed for pain.
3. If incision and drainage cannot be performed, administer an oral antibiotic (penicillin, 500 mg, or erythromycin, 500 mg, q6h).
4. Make every effort to locate a dentist because this condition can lead to a systemic infection and often requires extraction of the tooth or root canal therapy.

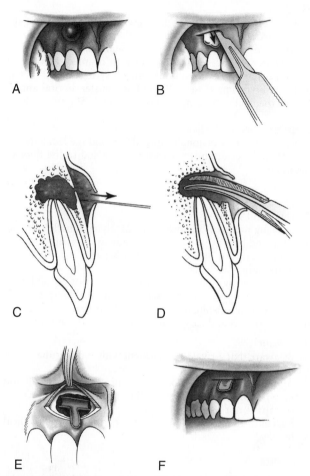

Figure 34-1. Apical dental abscess. **A,** Abscess. **B,** Incision. **C,** Release of pus. **D,** Open cavity. **E,** Drain placement. **F,** Drain in place.

Pericoronitis

Pericoronitis is an infection of the gingival flap around a partially erupted tooth. The most common site is the mandibular third molar.

Signs and Symptoms
1. May mimic streptococcal pharyngitis or tonsillitis
2. Pain at the site of infection
3. Trismus

Treatment
1. Initiate field treatment, which consists of curettage of the area around the tooth and under the flap. In the absence of proper dental instruments, use a small, curved hemostat.
2. Irrigate the space under the flap with disinfected water or sterile normal saline solution using a syringe and catheter.
3. Begin hot saline rinses q2h, and administer an oral antibiotic (penicillin, 500 mg, or erythromycin, 500 mg, q6h).

Deep Fascial Space Infection
Apical infection occasionally spreads beyond the local area to the canine, buccal, and masticator spaces and to the floor of the mouth.

Signs and Symptoms
1. Trismus
2. Fever and sepsis
3. Swelling minimal because of the overlying muscle mass
4. Submandibular space infection (Ludwig's angina) that produces elevation of the tongue and brawny, painful edema of the submandibular area
5. Continued swelling that restricts neck motion and produces dysphonia, odynophagia, and drooling; possible progression to acute airway obstruction and asphyxia
6. Mediastinitis and cavernous sinus venous thrombosis

Treatment
1. Be aware that airway management with early intubation or cricothyroidotomy may be necessary.
2. Administer an intravenous antibiotic (penicillin, 2 million units) or oral antibiotic (penicillin, 1000 mg) if intravenous therapy is not available.
3. Evacuate the victim immediately to the nearest medical facility.

▶ TRAUMA

Uncomplicated Crown Fracture
Signs and Symptoms
1. Fractured tooth, but no pulp tissue visible
2. Possible sensitivity to cold or heat

Treatment
1. Smooth any sharp edges with a fingernail file or cover with wax.
2. If thermal sensitivity is severe, apply ZOE B&T cement (zinc oxide-eugenol with polymer reinforcement), intermediate restorative material (IRM), Cavit, or softened candle wax to the fractured crown.

Uncomplicated Crown-Root Fracture
Signs and Symptoms
Similar to uncomplicated crown fracture, except that the fracture is nearly vertical, leaving a small, chisel-shaped fragment attached only by the palatal gingiva

Treatment
1. Treatment is the same as for an uncomplicated crown fracture.
2. Remove the mobile fragment to make the victim more comfortable.

Complicated Crown Fracture
Signs and Symptoms
1. Tooth fractured
2. Pulp exposed

Treatment
1. Stop the bleeding by placing a moistened tea bag into the socket or next to the bleeding gum.
2. Cap the exposed area with IRM, Cavit, or softened candle wax.

Complicated Crown-Root Fracture
Signs and Symptoms
Obliquely fractured tooth, resulting in pulp exposure and a mobile fragment attached to the palatal gingiva

Treatment
1. Remove the mobile fragment.
2. Cap the exposed area with IRM or Cavit.

Root Fracture
Signs and Symptoms
Slight to severe malposition of the crown

Treatment
1. Reposition the tooth as precisely as possible, and splint the tooth by suturing it to the gum (Fig. 34-2).
2. If the coronal fragment cannot be stabilized and you are days away from a medical facility, remove the mobile fragment. Do not attempt to extract the apical fragment.

Extrusion
Signs and Symptoms
Tooth that is partially displaced from its socket and extremely mobile

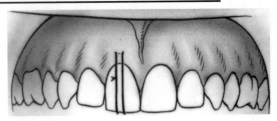

Figure 34-2. Suture used to stabilize a loosened or avulsed tooth.

Treatment
1. Reposition the tooth with gentle, steady pressure, allowing time to displace the blood that has collected into the apical region of the socket.
2. Observe the victim's occlusion as a guide to proper reduction. If the victim bites and contacts only the injured tooth, further positioning is necessary.
3. Splint the tooth for 2 to 3 weeks, if possible.

Lateral Luxation
Signs and Symptoms
1. Tooth displaced but not mobile because the apex is locked into its new position in the alveolar bone
2. High, metallic tone on percussion

Treatment
1. Use one finger to guide the apex gently down and back while another finger repositions the crown (Fig. 34-3). The tooth may snap back into place and be stable or may require splinting.
2. Use a suture to splint the tooth in place (see Fig. 34-2).

Total Avulsion
If a tooth is totally avulsed from the bone, it may be salvageable if replaced within 30 to 60 minutes.

Signs and Symptoms
1. Tooth no longer attached to the bone
2. Bleeding in the socket site

Treatment
1. Clean the debris off the tooth by rinsing gently (do not scrub) with either saline solution or milk. Handle the tooth only by the crown.
2. Remove any clotted blood from the socket with gentle irrigation and suction.

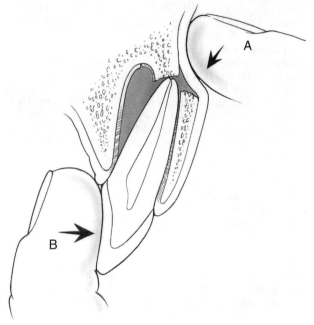

Figure 34-3. Reduction of lateral luxation. Use one finger (**A**) to guide the apex gently down and back while another finger (**B**) repositions the crown. (Modified from Andreasen JO, Andreasen FM: Essentials of Traumatic Injuries to the Teeth. Copenhagen, Munksgaard, 1990.)

3. Gently replace the tooth in the socket with slow, steady pressure.
4. Splint or suture the tooth in place.
5. If the tooth cannot be replaced immediately, store it in balanced Hank's solution, tissue culture medium, physiologic saline solution, white milk, or saliva, in that order of preference.
6. Relieve bleeding by placing a moistened tea bag into the socket that is bleeding.

▶ DENTAL FIRST-AID KIT

Items necessary to manage dental emergencies can be added to a wilderness first-aid kit without a large sacrifice of space or weight.

1. Cavit (Premier, Norristown, PA) is a temporary filling. Squeeze a small amount of the material from the tube and place it in the tooth. Wet a dental packing instrument or cotton-tipped applicator or toothpick to prevent sticking,

and pack the Cavit well. Then remove any excess. Have the victim bite to displace material that would interfere with occlusion. The filling material will set in a few minutes after contact with saliva.

2. Zinc oxide/eugenol cements (Intermediate Restorative Material, L.D. Caulk Company, Milford, DE) consist of a liquid and a powder. Start with two drops of the liquid, and begin mixing in the powder. Keep adding powder to make a dough that is not sticky yet will hold together. Dip the instruments in some powder to keep the mixture from sticking. Insert and shape the filling material as explained earlier.

3. For longer expeditions include the following:
   a. No. 151 universal extraction forceps
   b. Straight elevator
   c. Mouth mirror
   d. Orthodontic wax
   e. Dental floss
   f. Dental syringe
   g. 30-gauge needles
   h. Anesthetic cartridges (4% articaine with 1:100,000 epinephrine or 2% bupivacaine with 1:200,000 epinephrine [Marcaine] for long-term pain relief)

Mental Health

35

▶ **ANXIETY**

Symptoms
1. Excessive worrying out of proportion to the situation, with preoccupying concerns and fears
2. Increased heart rate, blood pressure, and respirations
3. Sweaty palms
4. Nausea and diarrhea
5. Muscular tension
6. Extreme: "fight or flight" with dramatic increase in physical manifestations; altered memory

Treatment
1. Provide ample reassurance.
2. Suggest and support constructive behaviors.
3. Build rapport.
4. Listen uncritically.
5. Administer lorazepam or diazepam.

▶ **PHOBIA (e.g., Fear of Heights or Snakes)**

Treatment
1. Consider alternate routes of travel.
2. Reassure or distract the person.
3. Administer lorazepam or diazepam (use caution if sedation or diminished motor coordination poses a danger to self or others).

▶ **PANIC ATTACK**

Symptoms
1. Typically lasts 10 to 30 minutes
2. With or without obvious cause or trigger
3. Sensation of pounding heart
4. Sweating, trembling, chest pain, nausea, dizziness, numbness, chills, hot flushes, shortness of breath
5. Hyperventilation
6. Desire to flee
7. Fear of dying, having a heart attack, going crazy, or losing control

Treatment
1. Carefully evaluate to identify physical cause.
2. Do not leave victim alone, but do not crowd victim.

3. Administer a benzodiazepine such as alprazolam, lorazepam, or diazepam.
4. Consider the addition of selective serotonin reuptake inhibitor (SSRI) such as fluoxetine or sertraline.

▶ OBSESSIVE-COMPULSIVE DISORDER (e.g., Compulsive Hand Washing)

If this is identified on a wilderness trip, consider tactfully discussing the victim's (odd) behavior with the group in order to allay his or her anxieties and make the afflicted person less likely to be isolated by the group.

▶ DEPRESSION (WITH OR WITHOUT MANIA)

Symptoms
1. Feelings of sadness, uselessness, low self-esteem
2. Failure to believe that the situation will improve
3. Difficulty sleeping
4. Diminished appetite, low energy, failure to concentrate
5. Social withdrawal and lack of enjoyment
6. Diminished sexual drive
7. Crying for no apparent reason; emotional outbursts
8. Psychosis
9. Suicidal ideation

During the early part of the manic phase of bipolar disorder, sometimes known as *hypomania,* the victim may exhibit positive behavior, productivity, hard work, high energy, and expansive thinking. However, as the person becomes manic, he or she may exhibit the following:
1. Rapid, pressured speech that is difficult to interpret
2. Lack of sleep
3. Excessive gregarious behavior
4. Hypersexual behavior
5. Impaired judgment in all matters including risk taking, financial, and social
6. Feeling of superhuman powers
7. Failure to listen to reason

Treatment for Mania
1. Administer lorazepam 4 to 8 mg over the course of 12 hours.
2. Administer risperdal 2 to 6 mg over the course of 12 hours.
3. Avoid confrontation.
4. Protect the victim from hurting himself or others.
5. Remove all weapons from an available situation.
6. Obtain evacuation.

Considerations for the Person Taking Lithium
for Depression
1. Keep the person well hydrated to avoid lithium toxicity.
2. If lithium toxicity (symptoms: tremulousness, seizures) is suspected, stop the medication, enforce hydration, and seek evacuation.

▶ SCHIZOPHRENIA

Symptoms
1. Inability to rationally perceive reality
2. Delusions (false beliefs not based in reality)
3. Hallucinations (sensory perceptions with a sensory stimulus)
4. Awkward behavior and emotional personal distancing
5. Flat affect
6. Jumbled thoughts

Treatment
For florid psychosis:
1. Consider increase in prescribed antipsychotic medications.
2. Consider administration of haloperidol, risperidone 1 to 4 mg PO, or olanzapine 5 mg PO.
3. Consider administration of a benzodiazepine to achieve a calming effect.
4. Keep the victim from hurting himself of others.
5. Achieve evacuation.
6. Consider other causes for the behavior: head injury, illicit drugs, brain tumor, metabolic disturbance, and heat-related illness.

   For acute dystonia (painful involuntary muscle contractions) from antipsychotic medications:
1. Diphenhydramine 25 to 50 mg IM, IV, or PO
2. Diazepam 5 mg IM, IV, or PO

▶ ORGANIC MENTAL DISORDERS

Delirium is a medical emergency and is often associated with fluctuating level of consciousness. Confusion and disorientation are hallmarks; hallucinations may be present. Causes include the following:
1. High-altitude cerebral edema
2. Acute hypoxia
3. Hypoglycemia
4. Dehydration
5. Head injury
6. Heat-related illness
7. Meningitis
8. Encephalitis
9. Metabolic abnormality (e.g., hyponatremia, hypercalcemia)
10. Drug or alcohol intoxication or withdrawal

Snake and Other Reptile Bites

36

▶ **DEFINITIONS AND CHARACTERISTICS**

Two main families of venomous snakes indigenous to the United States are Crotalidae (pit vipers) and Elapidae (coral snakes). Most snake bites are caused by the pit vipers, so called because of a depression, or pit, in the maxillary bone. Rattlesnakes (see Plate 5), the cottonmouth (water moccasin) snake (see Plate 6), and the copperhead snake (see Plate 7) are members of the pit viper family. The major snakes of medical importance outside of North America are the cobras, mambas, kraits, coral snakes, Australian elapids, sea snakes, vipers, rattlesnakes, asps, and colubrids (rear-fanged snakes). The fastest pit viper can crawl at a maximum speed of approximately 3 miles (4.8 km) per hour. The speed of a pit viper's strike has been clocked at 8 feet (2.4 m) per second; the snake can reach distances of approximately one half its body length.

Identifying characteristics of pit vipers include the following (Fig. 36-1):

1. Depression, or pit, in the maxillary bone, located midway between and below the level of the eye and the nostril on each side of the head
2. Vertical elliptical pupils ("cat's eye")
3. Triangular head that is distinct from the remainder of the body
4. Single row of subcaudal scutes, or scales
5. May have rattles on the tails
6. One or two fangs on each side of the head

Two members of the coral snake family, Elapidae, occur in the United States: the western coral snake *(Micruroides euryxanthus)* (see Plate 8), found in Arizona and New Mexico, and the eastern coral snake *(Micrurus fulvius)* (see Plate 9), distributed from coastal North Carolina through the Gulf states to western Texas. The elapids differ from pit vipers in having very short fangs, round pupils, and subcaudal scales in a double row. Because many nonpoisonous mimics occur in coral snake territory, the rule of thumb for identifying a venomous species is that red bands bordered by yellow or white indicate a venomous reptile, whereas red bands bordered by black indicate a nonvenomous reptile. This rule applies to all coral snakes native to the United States but does not apply to species found south of Mexico City and in other non-U.S. countries. A few essentially harmless, rear-fanged colubrid snakes in the United States such as the night snake and lyre snake possess elliptical pupils but lack facial pits.

413

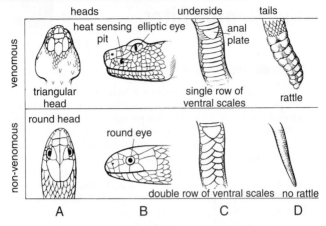

Figure 36-1. Identification of venomous pit vipers. **A,** Triangular head. **B,** Elliptic eye; heat-sensing facial pits on sides of head near nostrils. **C,** Single row of ventral scales leading up to anal plate. **D,** Rattles on tail (baby rattlesnakes have only "buttons" but are still quite venomous).

▶ PIT VIPER ENVENOMATION

Not all bites result in significant, or any, envenomation. Observe the victim closely for signs and symptoms.

Signs and Symptoms
1. Common: local burning pain immediately after the bite, weakness, nausea and vomiting, paresthesias (numbness and tingling of the tongue and mouth or scalp or feet), pain, fang marks, swelling and edema (usually within 5 minutes), faintness, dizziness
2. Less common: ecchymoses, fasciculations, hypotension, bullae, necrosis, thirst, increased salivation, unconsciousness, blurred vision, increased respiratory rate
3. Without treatment
   a. May have rapidly progressing edema that can involve an entire extremity within 1 hour if envenomation is severe (Table 36-1)
   b. Usually spreads more slowly, over 6 to 12 hours
   c. Edema that is soft, pitting, and limited to subcutaneous tissues
4. Hemorrhagic blebs and bullae developing at the site of the bite within 6 to 36 hours; may progress proximally along the involved extremity
5. Paresthesias of the scalp, face, and lips, along with periorbital muscle fasciculations, indicating that a significant envenomation has occurred

TABLE 36-1. Grades of Envenomation

ENVENOMATION	CHARACTERISTICS
None	Fang marks, but no local or systemic reactions
Minimal	Fang marks, local swelling and pain, but no systemic reactions
Moderate	Fang marks and swelling progressing beyond the site of the bite; systemic signs and symptoms such as nausea, vomiting, paresthesias, or hypotension
Severe	Fang marks present with marked swelling of the extremity, subcutaneous ecchymosis, severe symptoms including manifestations of coagulopathy

   a. May be complaints of a rubbery or metallic taste in the mouth
   b. General symptoms: weakness, sweating, nausea, faintness
6. Hemorrhage manifested as skin petechiae, epistaxis, hematemesis, melena, hemoptysis, and blindness; pulmonary edema possible
7. With some Mojave Desert rattlesnakes, bites produce neuromuscular blockade, leading to respiratory paralysis, in the absence of a significant local tissue reaction. Paralysis initially appears as cranial nerve deficits (hoarseness, difficulty swallowing, ptosis) and progresses to involve the diaphragm.

Treatment
1. Direct treatment at reducing venom effects, minimizing tissue damage, and preventing complicated sequelae.
2. Provide prehospital management.
   a. Avoid panic. Instruct the victim to back out of the snake's striking range, which is approximately the length of the snake.
   b. Attempts to secure or kill the snake are not recommended because of the risk of additional bites to the victim or rescuer and because precious time can be lost. Absolute identification of the snake is not necessary for treatment. However, if the snake has been killed and someone decides transport it, do not handle it directly; arrange to transport it in a closed container. Handle the snake using a stick that is longer than the snake. Decapitated head reactions persist for 20 to 60 minutes,

and even the severed head of a snake can envenom a person. If a digital or instant print photograph of a snake can be taken from a safe distance, this can be used for identification.

c. Immobilize the bitten extremity by splinting as if for a fracture. Keep the limb well padded at heart level (neither elevated nor lowered) in a position of function. Measure the bitten limb's circumference at two or more sites every 15 minutes.

d. Obtain medical assistance. Arrange for the victim to be transported to the nearest medical facility, with minimal exertion.

e. Encourage the victim to drink liquids to maintain adequate hydration.

3. The pressure immobilization technique (see later, for coral snake bite treatment) is not routinely recommended. If it is employed, the bandage should not be removed until antivenin is ready to infuse (if asymptomatic) or is infusing (if symptomatic) because of a potential bolus venom release after its removal.

4. The classic recommendation to apply a tourniquet is no longer advised. An arterial-occlusive tourniquet represents a decision to sacrifice a limb to minimize systemic symptoms and save a life, but has not been proven effective, and may be harmful. A lympho-occlusive (a pressure of ≈20 mm Hg) constriction band applied proximal to the bite has been suggested but never proven to be helpful. If this method is chosen, take care to allow arterial inflow to the affected limb.

5. The classic recommendation to incise and suck the wound by mouth is not recommended. Incising the bite site across fang marks is not recommended. With regard to suction, a negative-pressure device called the Extractor (Sawyer Products, Safety Harbor, FL) has been claimed to remove a clinically significant amount of venom if it is applied over the bite site within 3 minutes of the bite and left in place for 30 to 60 minutes. However, it may also promote local necrosis in the pattern of the applied suction; recent studies discourage its use.

6. Electric shock therapy can be dangerous to victims and has no proven value in managing bites by venomous snakes.

7. Immersion cryotherapy is not recommended because freezing or vasoconstricting already compromised tissues may contribute to necrosis. Local application of ice to the bite wound as a first-aid measure has not been proven to be of benefit.

8. Antivenom use in the field can be recommended only when a qualified physician is on the scene and when all equipment (including definitive airway management equipment) and

drugs are available to manage a potential anaphylactic/
anaphylactoid reaction to the serum. Backpacking the extensive equipment and drugs necessary to administer intravenous antivenom is cumbersome, and severe anaphylaxis must
be anticipated. The currently recommended antivenom product, CroFab, poses a lesser risk for severe allergic reaction
and may prove to be safe enough for field use, but it is not
yet recommended for out-of-hospital use.
9. Prophylactic antibiotics are unnecessary in most cases. However, if the delay to definitive care will exceed 5 hours, administer a broad-spectrum antibiotic such as dicloxacillin or
cephalexin, 250 to 500 mg PO qid, for 7 to 10 days.

▶ CORAL SNAKE ENVENOMATION

The coral snake clinical envenomation syndrome is attributed to
the eastern coral snake. The bite of the western coral snake is
generally of lesser severity; no fatal bite has been reported from
this species. The earliest findings may be nausea and vomiting,
followed by headache, abdominal pain, diaphoresis, and pallor.

Signs and Symptoms
1. Little or no pain and no local edema or necrosis; fang
marks may be difficult to see; venom primarily neurotoxic
2. Within 90 minutes of envenomation, weak or numb feeling
in bitten extremity
3. Several hours later, systemic symptoms appear including
tremors, drowsiness or euphoria, and marked salivation;
systemic signs and symptoms may be delayed as long as
13 hours after significant bites and can then progress
rapidly
4. After 5 to 10 hours, slurred speech and diplopia, heralding
the onset of cranial nerve palsies
   a. Bulbar paralysis: manifested as dysphagia and dyspnea
   b. Total flaccid paralysis possible
5. Symptoms possibly delayed as long as 13 hours after the
bite
6. Paresthesias and muscle fasciculations common at the site
of the bite
7. Flaccid paralysis, respiratory failure
8. Nausea and vomiting, weakness, dizziness, difficulty
breathing
9. Less common: local edema, diplopia, dyspnea, diaphoresis,
myalgia, confusion; death extremely rare

Treatment
1. Apply the pressure immobilization technique. This technique (Fig. 36-2) has been used successfully to manage

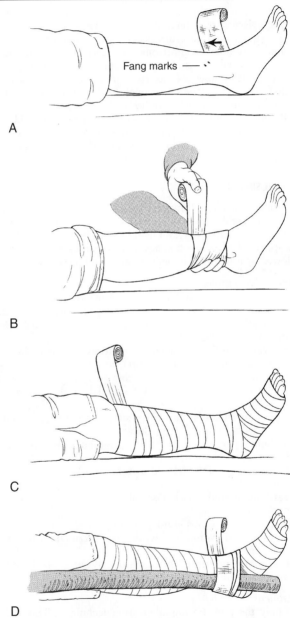

Fang marks

A

B

C

D

Figure 36-2. See legend on opposite page.

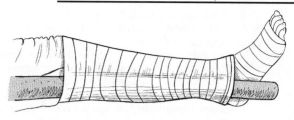

E

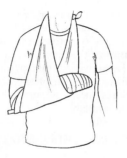

F

Figure 36-2. *Continued* Australian compression and immobilization technique. This technique has proved effective in management of elapid and sea snake envenomations. Its efficacy in viperid (true viper) bites has yet to be evaluated clinically.

certain elapid snakebites and funnel-web spider bites in Australia and marine envenomations. The efficacy of the technique depends on collapsing small, superficial lymphatic and venous vessels to retard venom uptake and distribution. Possible disadvantages include increased local tissue damage in crotalid bites because of the necrotizing effect of the venom if it remains localized to certain sites over time. Therefore it is not recommended for use but might on rare occasion be considered when the deleterious local effects must be balanced against a life-threatening situation that follows the systemic distribution of venom.

a. To apply the pressure immobilization technique for venom sequestration, if the bite location permits, place a cloth or gauze pad ($\approx$6 to 8 cm [2½ to 3 inches] by 6 to 8 cm by 2 cm [1 inch] thick) directly over the area and hold it firmly in place with a circumferential bandage 15 to 18 cm (6 to 8 inches) wide applied at lymphatic-venous occlusive pressure. If the cloth or gauze pad is not available, a rolled bandage may be used alone. Take care not to occlude the arterial circulation, as determined by the detection of arterial pulsations and proper capillary refill.

b. Splint the limb, and do not release the bandage until after the victim has been brought to proper medical attention and you are prepared to provide systemic support, or after 24 hours. Take care to check frequently that swelling beneath the bandage has not compromised the arterial circulation.

2. Note that because it is difficult to ascertain early whether envenomation by a coral snake has occurred, treatment and observation are mandatory. Early treatment with antivenom is advised in any suspected bite with envenomation because signs and symptoms can be delayed in onset. Therefore transport the bitten victim to a medical facility where definitive antivenom therapy can be undertaken.

3. Be aware that management of envenomation by the western coral snake is purely supportive because no antiserum is commercially available.

▶ **ENVENOMATION BY NON–NORTH AMERICAN SNAKES**

Signs and Symptoms

1. For elapids (cobras, mambas, kraits, Australian venomous snakes, coral snakes):
   a. Local: findings absent or minimal; significant pain with some species, regional lymphadenopathy and necrosis with some species, edema with some species
   b. Systemic: neurotoxicity (cranial nerve dysfunction, ptosis, dysphonia, blurred vision, altered mental status, peripheral weakness and paralysis, respiratory failure) with delayed (up to 10 hours) onset possible, hypersalivation, diaphoresis, cardiovascular failure, coagulopathy, myonecrosis, renal failure
   c. Eye exposure to venom from any of the spitting cobras or ringhals: immediate burning pain and tearing, which may lead to corneal ulceration, uveitis, and permanent blindness

2. For sea snakes:
   a. Local: trivial; fang marks difficult to identify
   b. Systemic: neurotoxicity (cranial nerve dysfunction, peripheral weakness and paralysis, respiratory failure); hypersalivation; dysphagia; dysarthria; trismus; muscle spasm; myotoxicity with resulting muscle pain and tenderness; myoglobinemia; myoglobinuria; hyperkalemia

3. For vipers and pit vipers:
   a. Local: pain, soft tissue swelling, regional lymphade-nopathy, ecchymosis, bloody exudate from fang marks, hemorrhagic bullae; early absence of findings does not rule out significant envenomation; local necrosis possi-bly significant
   b. Systemic: essentially any organ system potentially in-volved; cardiovascular toxicity (hypotension, pulmo-nary edema); neurotoxicity (cranial nerve dysfunction, peripheral weakness) with some species; hemorrhagic diathesis; renal failure; altered taste sensation; head-ache; diarrhea; vomiting; fever; abdominal pain; hypo-tension
4. For burrowing asps:
   a. Local: single fang puncture mark common, severe pain, some swelling, lymphadenopathy, occasional local ne-crosis
   b. Systemic: nausea, vomiting, diaphoresis, fever, respira-tory distress, cardiac arrhythmias
5. For colubrids:
   a. Local: mild to moderate local swelling, pain, ecchymo-sis, bloody exudate from fang marks
   b. Systemic: nausea, vomiting, coagulopathy, renal dys-function, headache

Treatment
1. Initiate same field treatment as for North American pit viper envenomation, with the notation to use the pres-sure immobilization technique for bites of elapids, sea snakes, burrowing asps, colubrids, and any unknown snake when the bite does not produce significant local pain.
2. For viper and pit viper bites or when the bite does produce significant local pain, apply a proximal constriction band and local suction. In either case, splint the extremity at heart level.
3. Arrange to transport the victim as quickly as possible to the nearest appropriate medical facility where antivenom therapy can be initiated.

▶ VENOMOUS LIZARD BITES

The Gila monster (see Plate 10) and Mexican beaded lizard (see Plate 11) are found in North America. Both possess venom glands and grooved teeth. Human envenomation most often occurs when the lizard retains its grasp and chews on the victim.

Signs and Symptoms
1. Usually simple puncture wounds, although teeth may break off or be shed during the bite and remain in the wound
2. Pain, often severe and burning, at the wound site within 5 minutes
   a. Pain radiating up the extremity
   b. Intense pain lasting 3 to 5 hours and then subsiding after 8 hours
3. Edema at the wound site, usually within 15 minutes, that progresses slowly in variable degrees up the extremity
4. Cyanosis or blue discoloration around the wound
5. Weakness, fainting, diaphoresis
6. Tenderness at the wound site for 3 to 4 weeks after the bite, but usually little tissue necrosis
7. Hypotension rare; no coagulation defects noted

Treatment
A Gila monster may hang on tenaciously during a bite, and mechanical means may be required to loosen the grip of the jaws.
1. Cleanse the wound thoroughly with a soap and water scrub or with a dilution of povidone-iodine.
2. Infiltrate the puncture wounds with 1% lidocaine using a 25-gauge needle, and then probe the wounds to detect the presence of shed or broken teeth, helping to prevent future infection from a foreign body.
3. Administer an analgesic appropriate for the degree of pain.

Bites and Stings from Arthropods and Mosquitoes

37

The principal disorders involving the bites or stings of arthropods are spider bites; bee, wasp, and ant stings; caterpillar spine irritation; interactions with sucking bugs, beetles, flies and other winged insects, lice, fleas, mites, chiggers, and ticks; and stings from scorpions.

DISORDERS

▶ SPIDER BITES

Spiders use their venom to capture, immobilize, and/or predigest prey. Therefore the bites of many spiders cause local reactions in humans, which may include immediate pain, swelling, erythema, and blisters. The local skin reaction usually lasts from minutes to hours but occasionally may be persistent for days. Unless the venom is from a toxic species, there are few or no systemic symptoms and all treatment is symptomatic or supportive.

Brown ("Fiddle" or "Recluse") Spiders

Necrotic arachnidism, or "loxoscelism," is caused by spiders of the genus *Loxosceles* and other spiders that deposit a venom characterized by its local dermonecrotic activity. The "fiddle-back" spider (see Plate 12) carries the characteristic violin-shaped marking on the dorsum of its cephalothorax. The clinical spectrum of loxoscelism ranges from mild and transient skin irritation to severe local necrosis accompanied by hematologic and renal pathologic conditions.

Signs and Symptoms
1. Most common presentation is an isolated cutaneous lesion
2. Local symptoms beginning the moment of the bite, with a sharp stinging sensation, although some victims report no awareness of having been bitten
3. Stinging subsiding over 6 to 8 hours, then replaced by aching and pruritus
4. Site becoming edematous, with an erythematous halo surrounding an irregularly shaped violaceous center of incipient necrosis; white ring of vasospasm and ischemia may be discernible between the central lesion and the halo
5. Often erythematous margin spreading irregularly, in a gravitationally influenced pattern that leaves the original center near the top of the lesion

6. In more severe cases, serous or hemorrhagic bullae arising at the center within 24 to 72 hours, with an underlying eschar (see Plate 13)
7. Systemic reactions: hemoglobinuria within 24 hours of envenomation; fever, chills, maculopapular rash, weakness, leukocytosis, arthralgias, nausea, and vomiting within 24 hours of the bite

Treatment
1. Apply cold compresses intermittently for the first 4 days after the bite. Do not apply heat.
2. If the wound appears infected, apply a topical antiseptic (mupirocin, bacitracin) under a sterile dressing. Administer an oral antibiotic such as cephalexin, dicloxacillin, or erythromycin.
3. Seek advanced medical care to consider adjunctive measures for the bite wound and to evaluate admission for coagulopathy or renal failure caused by hemolysis and hemoglobinuria.
4. Obtain appropriate tetanus prophylaxis when it becomes available.

Widow Spiders
Female spiders of the genus *Latrodectus* carry the characteristic hourglass marking on the ventral abdomen (see Plate 14).

Signs and Symptoms
1. Initial bite sometimes sharply painful, but often nearly painless, with only a tiny papule or punctum visible; surrounding skin slightly reddened and sometimes indurated; in many cases, no further progression of symptoms occurs
2. Neuromuscular symptoms: can become dramatic within 30 to 60 minutes as involuntary spasm and rigidity affect the large muscle groups of the abdomen, limbs, and lower back; worst pain usually occurs within the first 8 to 12 hours but may remain severe for several days
3. Predominantly abdominal presentation resembling an acute abdomen
4. Priapism, fasciculations, weakness, ptosis, thready pulse, fever, salivation, diaphoresis, vomiting, bronchorrhea, pulmonary edema, rhabdomyolysis, hypertension with or without seizures
5. Characteristic pattern of facial swelling, known as *Latrodectus* facies, possible hours after the bite

Treatment
The natural course of an envenomation is to resolve completely after a few days, although pain may last for a week or more.

1. Cleanse the bite site. Apply a cold pack (ice pack) to the bite site.
2. For muscle spasm, administer diazepam or another benzodiazepine.
3. Administer pain medication.
4. Monitor the victim for hypertension.
   a. Administer a centrally acting or vasodilating antihypertensive if the victim develops urgent hypertension and such a drug is available.
   b. Be alert for a seizure associated with rapid acceleration of hypertension.
5. Antivenom is available in the United States from Merck and Co.; in Australia from Commonwealth Serum Laboratories; and in South Africa from the South African Institute of Medical Research. In general, antivenin is recommended for respiratory arrest, seizures, uncontrolled hypertension, or pregnancy. The usual dose is one to three vials or ampules.

Funnel-Web Spiders

Funnel-web spiders (see Plate 15) are large, aggressive spiders that deliver a potent neurotoxin.

Signs and Symptoms

1. Intense pain at the bite site, with or without a local wheal surrounded by erythema lasting for 30 minutes; localized sweating
2. Phase I
   a. Begins minutes after venom injection, with local piloerection and muscle fasciculation; becomes generalized over the next 10 to 20 minutes
   b. Intense pain at the bite site; perioral tingling, nausea and vomiting, diaphoresis, salivation, lacrimation, diarrhea
   c. Severe hypertension, tachycardia, hyperthermia, and coma developing next
   d. Sporadic apnea and grotesque muscle writhing after the previous symptoms
3. Phase II
   a. Begins 1 to 2 hours after envenomation, as phase I symptoms begin to subside
   b. May be a return of consciousness and the appearance of recovery
   c. In severe cases, gradually worsening hypotension, with periods of apnea and the onset of pulmonary edema

Treatment

1. In the field, apply the pressure immobilization technique for venom sequestration at the bite site (see Chapter 36).

2. Give specific antivenom, which is developed in rabbits and is the mainstay of treatment. Two ampules (100 mg purified IgG per ampule) of antivenom are administered intravenously every 15 minutes until symptoms improve.
3. Be aware that general management, in addition to antivenom administration, is based on symptoms and is supportive.
   a. Give oxygen and intravenous fluid support.
   b. Use atropine, 0.6 to 1 mg IV, to lessen salivation and bronchorrhea.
   c. Administer a beta-adrenergic blocking agent to control severe hypertension and tachycardia.

Banana Spiders

The *Phoneutria* spiders of South America are large nocturnal creatures noted for their aggressive behavior and painful bites.

Signs and Symptoms
1. Severe local pain that radiates up the extremity into the trunk, followed within 10 to 20 minutes by tachycardia, hypertension, hypothermia, profuse diaphoresis, salivation, vertigo, visual disturbances, nausea and vomiting, and priapism
2. If death occurs in 2 to 6 hours, usually a result of respiratory paralysis

Treatment
1. Treat mild envenomation symptomatically by infiltrating the bite site with a local anesthetic.
2. Be aware that narcotics may potentiate the venom's respiratory depressant effect and should not be used.
3. For severe envenomation, administer monovalent antivenom (Belo Horizonte) or polyvalent antivenom (Sero Antiaracidico Polivalente, Instituto Butantan).

Wolf Spiders

Wolf spiders are diurnal predators that are usually a mottled dark gray or brown (Fig. 37-1).

Signs and Symptoms
1. Local pain, swelling, and erythema
2. Rarely, necrosis

Treatment
1. Apply a cold (ice) pack to the bite site.
2. Administer oral pain medication or infiltrate the area with an anesthetic agent.

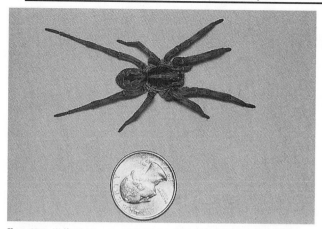

Figure 37-1. Wolf spider (*Lycosa* species). (Courtesy Arizona Poison & Drug Information Center, 1996.)

Tarantulas

Tarantulas are large, slow spiders (Fig. 37-2) capable of inflicting a painful bite when threatened. Several varieties possess urticating hairs, which they flick by the thousands through the air into an attacker's skin and eyes.

Signs and Symptoms
1. Intense inflammation where hairs land, which may remain pruritic for weeks
2. Aching or stinging pain at the bite site
3. Keratoconjunctivitis

Treatment
1. Be aware that therapy is supportive and based on symptoms. To remove urticating hairs, apply and remove sticky tape from the skin in a few repeated applications.
2. Elevate the bitten extremity and immobilize it to reduce pain.
3. Administer pain medication.
4. Note that topical or systemic corticosteroids and oral antihistamines can be used for urticating hair exposure.
5. For eye exposure, irrigate the eyes, and then consider ophthalmic corticosteroid treatment for keratoconjunctivitis.

Hobo Spiders

The bite of the hobo spider, also called the Northwestern brown spider *(Tegenaria agrestis)*, can cause a necrotic reaction similar to that induced by the brown recluse spider.

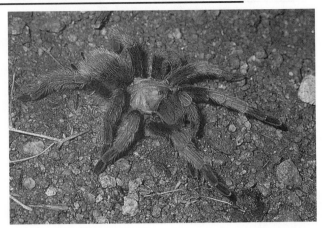

Figure 37-2. Mature female *Aphonopelma iodium*. (Courtesy Michael Cardwell & Associates, 1997.)

Signs and Symptoms
1. Local redness, vesiculation, and necrosis
2. Systemic effects: headache, visual disturbances, hallucinations, weakness, lethargy

Treatment
1. Apply cold compresses intermittently for the first 4 days after the bite. Do not apply heat.
2. If the wound appears infected, apply a topical antiseptic (mupirocin, bacitracin) under a sterile dressing. Administer an oral antibiotic such as cephalexin, dicloxacillin, or erythromycin.

Running Spiders and Sac Spiders
Running and sac spiders are often nondescript spiders with yellow, brown, green, or olive coloration.

Signs and Symptoms
1. Vary with species
2. May include dyspnea, varying degrees of weakness, local redness, pain and edema, headache, fever, nausea, and necrosis

Treatment
1. Be aware that this lesion usually heals without problems provided secondary infection does not develop.
2. Apply cool compresses, elevate the involved area, immobilize the victim, and give analgesics as needed.

▶ BEES, WASPS, AND ANTS

By far the most important venomous insects are members of the order Hymenoptera, including bees, wasps, and ants (Fig. 37-3). The abdomen and thorax are connected by a slender pedicle, which may be quite long in certain wasps and ants.

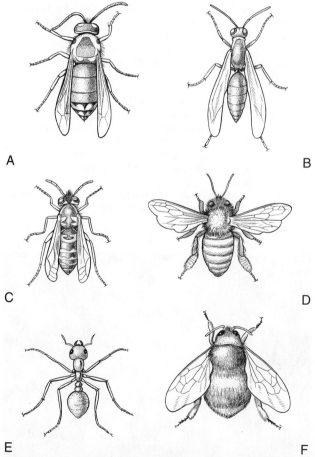

Figure 37-3. Representative venomous Hymenoptera: **A,** Hornet *(Vespula maculata);* **B,** wasp *(Chlorion icheumerea);* **C,** yellowjacket *(Vespula maculiforma);* **D,** honey bee *(Apis mellifera);* **E,** fire ant *(Solenopsis invicta);* **F,** bumblebee *(Bombus species).*

Signs and Symptoms

1. Instantaneous pain, followed by a wheal-and-flare reaction, with variable edema. Most stings are on the head and neck, followed by the foot, leg, hand, and arm. Stings may occur in the mouth, pharynx, or esophagus if the insects are accidentally ingested.

2. With fire ants, vesicles that subsequently become sterile pustules from insects grasping the skin with their mouth parts and inflicting multiple stings (Fig. 37-4)

3. With multiple bee, wasp, yellow jacket, or hornet stings, vomiting, diarrhea, generalized edema, dyspnea, hypotension, and collapse. The lethal dose of honeybee venom has been estimated at 500 to 1500 stings.

4. Large local reactions relatively common, spreading more than 15 cm (6 inches) beyond the sting and persisting longer than 24 hours.

5. Allergic sting reactions
   a. Occur in areas remote from the sting and typically include pruritus, hives, difficulty breathing, nausea, papular urticaria, and angioedema. Other symptoms include abdominal pain and vomiting.
   b. When reaction is life threatening, marked respiratory distress, hypotension, loss of consciousness, and arrhythmias.
   c. Most fatalities occur from anaphylaxis, and most of these occur within 1 hour of the sting.

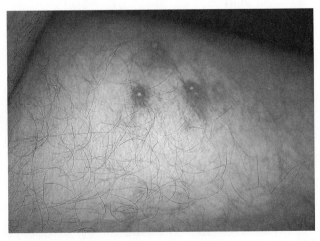

Figure 37-4. Fire ant lesions.

Treatment

1. Be aware that the treatment of anaphylactic reaction follows conventional guidelines, as follows:
   a. Maintain the airway and administer oxygen.
   b. Obtain intravenous access. Administer lactated Ringer's or normal saline (NS) solution to support the blood pressure at a level of 90 mm Hg systolic.
   c. Administer epinephrine. Begin with aqueous epinephrine 1:1000 subcutaneously in the deltoid region. The dose for adults is 0.3 to 0.5 mL, and for children 0.01 mL/kg. An alternative is to inject the contents of an EpiPen or EpiPen Jr intramuscularly into the lateral thigh region. Repeat in 20 minutes if relief is partial. If the reaction is limited to pruritus and urticaria, there is no wheezing or facial swelling, and the victim is older than 45 years, administer an antihistamine and reserve epinephrine for a worsened condition.
   d. If the reaction is life threatening and there is no response to subcutaneous epinephrine, administer epinephrine intravenously. Give an adult a 0.1-mg bolus of 1:1000 aqueous epinephrine (0.1 mL) diluted in 10 mL NS solution (final dilution 1:100,000) infused over 10 minutes. Prepare a mixture for continuous infusion by adding 1 mg 1:1000 aqueous epinephrine (1 mL) to 250 mL NS solution, thus creating a concentration of 4 μg/mL. This infusion should be started at 1 μg/min (15 minidrops/min) and increased to 4 to 5 μg/min if the clinical response is inadequate. In infants and children, the starting dose is 0.1 μg/kg/min up to a maximum of 1.5 μg/kg/min, with the awareness that infusion rates in excess of 0.5 μg/kg/min may be associated with cardiac ischemia and arrhythmias.
   e. Relieve bronchospasm. Administer micronized albuterol or metaproterenol by hand-held metered-dose inhaler.
   f. Administer antihistamines. Manage mild reactions with diphenhydramine, 50 to 75 mg IV, IM, or PO. The dose for children is 1 mg/kg. Nonsedating antihistamines such as fexofenadine, 60 mg, or cimetidine, 300 mg, are adjuncts.
   g. Administer corticosteroids. If the reaction is severe or prolonged or if the victim is regularly medicated with corticosteroids, administer hydrocortisone, 200 mg, methylprednisolone, 50 mg, or dexamethasone, 15 mg, IV with a 10-day oral taper to follow. The parenteral dose of hydrocortisone for children is 2.5 mg/kg. If the therapy is initiated orally, administer prednisone, 60 to 100 mg for adults and 1 mg/kg for children.

2. For mild hymenopteran stings, apply ice packs to provide relief.
3. Be aware that a honeybee or yellow jacket may leave a stinger in the wound. Remove the stinger (and possibly, attached venom sac) as quickly as possible with a sharp edge or forceps. Do not be overly concerned about squeezing the sac—it is more important to remove the stinger and sac as quickly as possible.
4. Note that a home remedy such as a paste of unseasoned meat tenderizer or baking soda is of variable usefulness, although some report the former to be effective. Topical anesthetics in "sting sticks" have limited usefulness.
5. Because infection is common, apply antimicrobial ointment such as mupirocin to cover the wound. Breaking fire ant blisters is not recommended.
6. Be aware that envenomation from multiple hymenopteran stings may require more aggressive therapy including intravenous calcium gluconate (5 to 10 mL of 10% solution) in conjunction with a parenteral antihistamine and corticosteroid to relieve pain, swelling, and nausea and vomiting. A corticosteroid, such as methylprednisolone, 24 mg the first day, then tapered over 5 days, often hastens resolution of a large local reaction to a bee or wasp sting.
7. Manage delayed serum sickness in response to multiple hymenopteran stings with a corticosteroid such as prednisone, 60 to 100 mg for adults and 1 mg/kg for children, tapered over 2 weeks.

▶ CATERPILLARS

Injury usually follows contact with caterpillars and is less frequent with the cocoon or adult stage. The largest outbreaks have been associated with spines detached from live or dead caterpillars and cocoons.

Signs and Symptoms
1. With caterpillars that have hollow spines and venom glands, instant nettling pain, followed by redness and swelling, after direct contact with the live insect
   a. Ordinarily, no systemic manifestations; symptoms subsiding within 24 hours
   b. Possibly intense pain with central radiation, accompanied by nausea and vomiting, headache, fever, and lymphadenopathy
   c. Rarely, coagulopathy
2. With attached or detached spines from certain caterpillars or moths, itching and erythematous, papular, or urticarial rash within a few hours to 2 days after contact

a. Rash persisting for up to 1 week
b. Lesions rarely bullous
c. Conjunctivitis, upper respiratory tract irritation, rare asthma-like symptoms with or without dermatitis

Treatment
1. Apply adhesive tape, a commercial facial peel, or a thin layer of rubber cement to remove spines.
2. Administer an oral antihistamine and/or a nonsteroidal antiinflammatory drug (NSAID). If the dermatitis is severe and persistent, consider administering a corticosteroid such as prednisone, 60 to 100 mg for adults and 1 mg/kg for children, tapered over 10 days. An oral antihistamine such as fexofenadine may be helpful. Pain medication is added as needed to control discomfort.

▶ **SUCKING BUGS**

"Sucking bugs" have sucking mouth parts, generally in the form of a beak. Included are the assassin bugs, kissing bugs, and flying bedbugs. Many of these bugs bite at night on exposed parts of the body. The bites themselves may be painless.

Signs and Symptoms
1. On initial exposure, usually no reaction
2. With repeated bites, reddish itching papules that may persist for up to 1 week; bites often grouped in a cluster or line and may be accompanied by giant urticarial wheals, lymphadenopathy, hemorrhagic bullae, and fever
3. Systemic anaphylaxis possible
4. Possible pain at the sting site
   a. Local swelling that lasts several hours
   b. With bedbugs, usually a pruritic wheal with central hemorrhagic punctum, followed by a reddish papule that persists for days

Treatment
Treatment is supportive and not particularly effective.

▶ **BEETLES**

Several families of beetles such as the blister and rove beetles produce toxic secretions that may be deposited on the skin.

Signs and Symptoms
1. With the blister beetle, contact painless and seldom remembered by the victim; blisters induced by cantharidin toxin appear 2 to 5 hours after contact, generally as single or multiple areas, usually 5 to 50 mm in diameter and thin

walled; unless broken or rubbed, they are not usually painful
2. With the rove beetle, vesicant substance is an alkaloid; if the beetle is crushed or rubbed on the skin, redness occurs after several hours, followed by a crop of small blisters that persist for 2 to 3 days; conjunctivitis occurs if the secretion is rubbed into the eyes

Treatment
1. Treat beetle vesication as a superficial chemical burn.
2. Topical preparations containing corticosteroids and anti-histamines are not particularly effective.

▶ TWO-WINGED FLIES, BITING MIDGES, AND MOSQUITOES (Fig. 37-5)

Signs and Symptoms
1. Immediate pruritic wheals followed after 12 to 24 hours by red, swollen, and itchy lesions; can have blistering or necrosis
2. Rarely, immune response leading to asthma, bullous eruptions, fever, lymphadenopathy, or hepatomegaly

Mosquitoes

Mosquitoes are characterized by scaled wings, long legs, and a slender body. The size of these insects varies, but they rarely exceed 15 mm in length. They can fly at 0.9 to 1.6 miles per hour. Mosquitoes do not sting because there is no stinger; they pierce the skin and suck blood with the mouth parts. They identify victims by scent, as well as by carbon dioxide of exhaled breath and some chemicals found in sweat. The female mosquito requires about 50 seconds to attach and approximately 2 minutes to finish feeding.

Clinical Manifestations of Mosquito Bites
1. Local irritation with soft, pale, pruritic wheal, with itching
2. Papular urticaria, with itching
3. Occasional hive-like skin lesion, with itching
4. Rare blisters, bullae, erythema multiforme, or purpura, with or without itching

Treatment
1. Immediately after the bite, apply a cold (ice) pack.
2. Apply a topical antipruritic lotion or cream.
3. If the reaction is severe or prolonged, consider the administration of a corticosteroid such as prednisone, 60 to 100 mg for adults and 1 mg/kg for children, tapered over 7 to 14 days. A topical corticosteroid cream or ointment may be helpful.

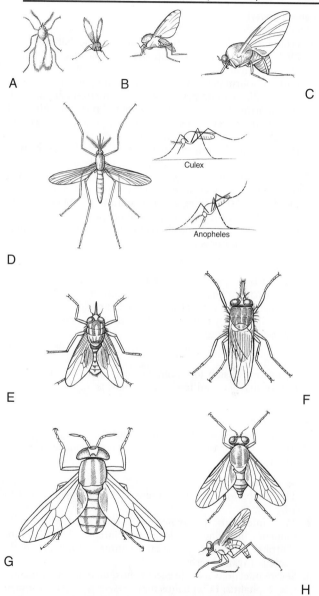

Figure 37-5. Blood-feeding biting flies (not drawn to scale): **A,** Sand fly; **B,** biting midge; **C,** blackfly; **D,** mosquito; **E,** stable fly; **F,** tsetse fly; **G,** tabanid fly; **H,** snipe fly.

Dengue (Fever)

Signs and Symptoms
1. From bite to clinical infection, 4- to 6-day incubation period
2. High fever (>102° F [39° C]), myalgias, headache, arthralgias, and rash
3. Positive tourniquet test for capillary fragility: the appearance of 20 or more petechiae over a square-inch patch on the forearm after deflation of the blood pressure cuff (held for 5 minutes between systolic and diastolic pressures)
4. Irritability, depression, encephalitis, seizures
5. Differentiation between dengue fever and dengue hemorrhagic fever (DHF) is development of plasma leakage in DHF. Following 2 to 7 days of higher fever come bleeding (ranging from petechiae, ecchymoses, epistaxis, and mucosal bleeding to GI bleeding and hematuria), thrombocytopenia (<100,000/mm³), hemoconcentration, and hepatomegaly. Other symptoms include abdominal pain, nausea and vomiting, and restlessness or lethargy.

Treatment
1. Prognosis for patients with dengue fever is generally good, with an acute phase of 1 week and up to 2 weeks of convalescence with general malaise and anorexia. Prognosis is worse if DHF or dengue shock syndrome exists.
2. Resuscitate aggressively with fluid and electrolytes.
3. Use acetaminophen as an antipyretic, and do not use aspirin.
4. Blood transfusion for severe anemia; consider administration of platelets and fresh frozen plasma.

West Nile Virus

West Nile virus is a single-stranded RNA virus. Mosquitoes are the vectors for this virus, and birds are the most common reservoir.

Signs and Symptoms
1. The incubation period from bite to clinical infection is 3 to 14 days.
2. Most infections are asymptomatic or present with a mild influenza-like illness with malaise, fatigue, difficulty concentrating, headache, nausea, vomiting, anorexia, lymphadenopathy, and rash.
3. Severe infections include encephalitis, meningitis, or meningoencephalitis. Encephalitis may present with Parkinsonian features or other movement disorders such as myoclonus or intention tremor or with acute flaccid paralysis or asymmetric weakness.

Treatment

No specific treatment is available. Therapy is symptomatic and supportive.

▶ CUTANEOUS MYIASIS

Parasitism by fly larvae occurs when an insect such as the human botfly deposits an egg on human skin. The egg hatches immediately, and the larva enters the skin through the bite of the carrier or through some other small break in the skin. The larvae grow to 15 to 20 mm under the skin.

Signs and Symptoms

1. As the larva grows under the skin, the initial pruritic papule becomes a furuncle with a characteristic central opening from which serosanguineous fluid exudes (see Plate 16).
2. Pain often accompanies movement of the older larvae, but lesions are not particularly tender to palpation.
3. The tip of the larva may protrude from the central opening, or bubbles produced by its respiration may be seen.
4. Lymphadenopathy, fever, and secondary infection are rare.

Treatment

1. Sometimes, simple pressure will extrude the organism, particularly if it is small.
2. Occlusion of the breathing hole with heavy oil, nail polish, or animal fat (e.g., bacon) may cause the larva to emerge sufficiently for it to be grasped and withdrawn.
3. Alternatively, inject about 2 mL of local anesthetic into the base of the lesion, thus extruding the larva by fluid pressure.
4. If you attempt surgical excision under local anesthesia, take care not to break or rupture the larva because this might result in an inflammatory reaction that leads to infection.

▶ LICE

Lice are very active, but nits (eggs) are easily identified as whitish ovals, about 0.5 mm long, attached firmly to one side of the hair. Machine washing and drying of sheets and clothing at hot settings will kill lice and nits.

Signs and Symptoms

1. Small, red macule in response to secretions released by the louse during biting and feeding
2. Characteristic body louse bite: a central hemorrhagic punctum in many of the macules

3. Excoriations, crusts, eczematization in a parallel pattern from scratching, particularly on the shoulders, trunk, and buttocks (favorite sites for bites)
4. Severe pruritus and inflammation caused by sensitization after repeated exposure to bites; victim possibly infested for weeks before pruritus becomes marked
5. Occipital and posterior cervical adenopathy associated with head lice

Treatment
1. Treat head lice with one application of 1% permethrin cream rinse or 0.5% malathion lotion. Hair should be washed, rinsed, and dried, and the rinse is applied for 10 to 20 minutes before being washed off. A fine-toothed comb may be used to remove nits after rinsing. Combing should be repeated in 1 to 2 days to confirm treatment success. If head lice are resistant, use 0.3% pyrethrins and 3% piperonyl butoxide in combination. Alternatively, use 1% hexachlorocyclohexane (lindane) shampoo, or for someone who is intolerant of permethrin. Note that it is contraindicated in children and should be used only as a last resort for elders. Apply it to the wet hair, lather, and leave it in place for 4 minutes before rinsing. Repeat the treatment 7 to 10 days later as a precaution in case some nits were not killed by the first application.
2. Treat body lice with the same medications, but be aware that parasites and nits are not usually found on the skin. These must be eradicated from the clothing. Take a good bath and launder all clothing.
3. Treat pubic lice with the same medications. One method is to apply permethrin 1% cream rinse for 10 minutes and rinse. Another method is to rub crotamiton lotion into the affected area daily for several weeks to destroy hatching ova and prevent a persistent infection. Manage eyelash infection by careful application of physostigmine ophthalmic ointment, using a cotton-tipped applicator.

▶ **FLEAS** (Fig. 37-6)

Signs and Symptoms
1. Small, central, hemorrhagic punctum surrounded by erythema and urticaria; bullae or even ulceration after bite in highly sensitive individuals
2. Intensely pruritic, with scratching often resulting in crusting and the development of impetigo
3. Tungiasis caused by burrowing flea (jigger, chigo, sand flea), usually on the feet, buttocks, or perineum of a person who wears no shoes or frequently squats

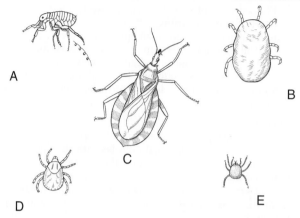

Figure 37-6. Various blood-feeding arthropods (not drawn to scale): **A,** Flea; **B,** kissing bug; **C,** soft tick; **D,** hard tick; **E,** chigger mite.

   a. Firm, itchy nodule with posterior end of the flea visible as a dark plug or spot in the center of the nodule

   b. Numerous papules aggregating into plaques with a honeycomb appearance

   c. Secondary infection around each flea inevitable, resulting in ulceration and suppuration

Treatment

1. Relieve pruritus by applying calamine lotion with phenol.
2. Administer a systemic antihistamine to help control itching.
3. Clean excoriations and apply a topical antiseptic ointment such as mupirocin.
4. With a burrowing flea infestation (tungiasis), remove the burrowing flea or a pustule will rupture, leaving an ulcer.
5. Preparations containing 9.1% imidacloprid eliminate or reduce fleas on dogs when applied to the skin. An oral preparation used for dogs and cats contains lufenuron, an inhibitor of insect development.

▶ MITES

The human scabies mite is *Sarcoptes scabiei* var. *hominis*. The adult female burrows into the epidermis.

Signs and Symptoms

1. Hallmark of scabies: severe nocturnal pruritus
   a. Itching also provoked by any warming of the body

b. Elapsed time of 4 to 6 weeks between infestation and onset of severe pruritus
2. Cutaneous manifestations: an epidermal burrow (a linear or serpentine track, rarely longer than 5 to 10 mm) with a predilection for the interdigital spaces, palms, flexor surfaces of the wrists, elbows, feet and ankles, belt line, anterior axillary folds, lower buttocks, and penis and scrotum

Treatment
1. A single overnight application of 5% permethrin cream is curative. Apply the chemical even beneath the fingernails. Symptoms may persist for more than a month until the mite and mite products are shed with the epidermis. One percent hexachlorocyclohexane (lindane) cream or lotion is curative, although it is contraindicated in infants and pregnant women.
2. Sulfur in petrolatum 5% to 10% or another suitable vehicle applied for 3 consecutive nights is an alternative, as is crotamiton cream 10% or lotion applied for 2 consecutive nights.
3. Treat contacts simultaneously. Clothing and linens should be laundered the morning after treatment to kill mites that may have strayed from the skin.

▶ CHIGGER MITES

In the United States the most important mite species of the family Trombiculidae is *Eutrombicula alfreddugèsi,* known as the red bug, chigger, or harvest mite. Adult mites lay eggs among vegetation, and newly hatched larvae crawl up the vegetation, from which they attach themselves to human skin with hooked mouth parts.

Signs and Symptoms
1. Maddeningly pruritic hemorrhagic punctum that usually becomes surrounded by intense erythema within 24 hours
2. Bites may number in the hundreds and can be associated with an allergic reaction
3. Blisters, purplish discoloration, swelling of feet and ankles, secondary infection in excoriated skin

Treatment
1. Treatment is symptomatic and consists of topical antipruritic agents, corticosteroids, and systemic antihistamines.
2. Consider superpotent topical corticosteroid cream or ointment such as 0.05% clobetasol, applied sparingly several times daily.
3. Phenol 1% in calamine may be effective for itching.

▶ **TICKS** (see Fig. 37-6)

Local Reaction to Tick Bites

Signs and Symptoms
1. Vary from small pruritic nodule to extensive area of ulceration, erythema, and induration
2. Possibly accompanied by fever, chills, and malaise

Treatment
1. If tick mouth parts or the head remain embedded in the wound, remove them surgically using a needle or the sharp tip of a knife or scalpel.
2. Manage wound infection with an antibiotic.

Tick Paralysis

Tick paralysis occurs most frequently during the spring and summer when ticks are feeding. Girls are more often affected than boys because the ticks can hide more easily in girls' longer scalp hair.

Signs and Symptoms
1. From 5 to 6 days after the adult female tick attaches: restlessness, irritability, paresthesias in the hands and feet
2. Over the ensuing 24 to 48 hours: ascending, symmetric, and flaccid paralysis with loss of deep tendon reflexes; weakness usually greater in the lower extremities
3. Within 1 to 2 days: severe generalized weakness possible, accompanied by bulbar and respiratory paralysis
   a. Cerebellar dysfunction with incoordination and ataxia possible
   b. Facial paralysis an isolated finding in persons with ticks embedded behind the ear

Treatment
1. Note that the diagnosis is established when the paralysis resolves after tick removal. In North America, most victims show improvement within hours of tick removal, with a return to normal in several days.
2. Aside from tick removal, treatment is supportive.

Lyme Disease

Lyme disease, caused by *Borrelia burgdorferi*, is transmitted most often by the deer tick *Ixodes scapularis* and the western black-legged tick *Ixodes pacificus*.

Signs and Symptoms
1. Stage I (early localized)
   a. Average 7 to 10 days (range: 3 to 32 days) after inoculation, victim develops an expanding, annular,

and erythematous skin lesion (erythema migrans) (Fig. 37-7; see also Plate 44)

b. Initially, central red macule or papule, but as lesion expands, partial central clearing usually seen while outer borders remain bright red

c. Borders usually flat but may be raised

d. Center of some early lesions intensely red and indurated, vesicular, or necrotic; sometimes area develops multiple red rings within the outside margin, or the central area turns blue before clearing

e. Lesion diameter 15 cm (6 inches) (range: 3 to 68 cm [1 to 27 inches]) and may be anywhere on the body, although most common sites are thigh, groin, and axilla

f. Lesion warm to the touch and usually described as burning, but occasionally as itching or painful

g. Rash fading after an average of 28 days (range: 1 to 14 weeks) without treatment; with antibiotics, lesion resolves after several days

h. Constitutional symptoms accompany erythema migrans, but usually mild and consisting of regional lymphadenopathy, fever, fatigue, neck stiffness, arthralgia, myalgia, and malaise

i. Annular erythematous lesions occur hours after bite, representative of hypersensitivity reaction and not to be confused with erythema migrans

2. Stage II (early disseminated)

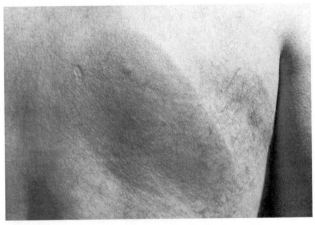

Figure 37-7. Rash of erythema migrans. (Photo courtesy of Paul Auerbach, MD.)

a. During hematogenous spread of microorganisms (a few days to weeks after bite), multiple annular skin lesions in 20% to 50% of victims
   - Generally smaller, migrate less, and lack indurated centers
   - Located anywhere except palms and soles
   - No blistering or mucosal involvement
b. Other skin manifestations: malar rash; rarely, urticaria
c. Most common constitutional symptoms: malaise and fatigue, which may be severe and are usually constant throughout the duration of the illness
d. Fever, typically low grade and intermittent, common
e. Tender regional lymphadenopathy along distribution of erythema migrans or posterior cervical chains
f. Generalized lymphadenopathy and splenomegaly
g. Symptoms of meningeal irritation in some victims including severe intermittent headaches, stiff neck with extreme forward flexion, and lack of Kernig's or Brudzinski's signs
h. Mild encephalopathy with somnolence, insomnia, memory disturbances, emotional lability, dizziness, poor balance, and clumsiness
i. Dysesthesias of the scalp
j. Musculoskeletal complaints including arthralgias; migratory pain in tendons, bursae, and bones; and generalized stiffness or severe cramping pain, particularly in the calves, thighs, and back
k. Symptoms of hepatitis and generalized abdominal pain
l. Conjunctivitis in 10% to 15% of victims
m. Neurologic manifestations an average of 4 weeks after the onset of erythema migrans including meningoencephalitis, with headache as a major symptom; facial nerve palsy (in 11% of Lyme disease patients and 50% of victims with Lyme disease meningitis, but may be an isolated finding); radiculoneuritis (triad of meningitis, cranial neuritis, and radiculoneuritis suggests Lyme disease in the differential diagnosis)
n. Cardiac abnormalities in 4% to 10% of victims including atrioventricular block that can progress to complete heart block
o. Arthritis in about 60% of untreated persons with erythema migrans
   - Develops in a few weeks to 2 years (median 4 weeks) after onset of illness
   - Typical pattern of brief recurrent episodes of asymmetric, oligoarticular swelling and pain in large joints, separated by longer periods of complete remission

3. Knee most frequently involved, followed by the shoulder, elbow, temporomandibular joint, ankle, wrist, hip, and small joints of the hands and feet
4. Stage II (late disease)—begins a year or more after the onset of erythema migrans, although patients may present with stage III disease as the initial manifestation of Lyme disease

Treatment
If the diagnosis of Lyme disease is made by clinical or serologic determination, initiate antibiotic therapy.
1. For stage I disease, give tetracycline (250 mg PO qid), doxycycline (100 mg PO bid), or amoxicillin or cefuroxime (500 mg PO tid) for 14 to 28 days. Another alternative not yet approved by the U.S. Food and Drug Administration is azithromycin, 200 mg PO bid for 3 weeks. Anticipate a Jarisch-Herxheimer reaction within the first 24 hours of therapy.
2. Treat any manifestations of stage II disease with the above agents for 21 to 28 days. Alternatively, administer ceftriaxone, 1 g IV q12h, for 2 to 4 weeks.

Prophylaxis
It is generally believed that a tick must remain attached to a human for 72 hours to effectively transmit the agent of Lyme disease. In the event that prophylaxis is desired, a single dose of doxycycline, 200 mg PO, immediately after the tick is removed has been suggested by one author to be as effective as a 10- to 14-day course of doxycycline.

Relapsing Fever
Relapsing fever is an acute borrelial disease characterized by recurrent paroxysms of fever separated by afebrile periods.

Signs and Symptoms
1. Abrupt onset of fever lasting about 3 days, afebrile period of variable duration (average 6 to 7 days), and relapse with return of fever and other clinical manifestations
   a. Fever usually high, greater than 102.2° F (39° C)
   b. Initial febrile period averaging 3 days but possibly lasting 1 to 17 days
   c. Febrile period terminating with rapid defervescence (the crisis), accompanied by drenching sweats and intense thirst
2. Pruritic eschar at the site of the tick bite possible but usually absent by the onset of clinical symptoms
3. Incubation period of about 7 days, then fever, frequently accompanied by shaking chills, severe headache, myalgias,

arthralgias, muscular weakness, lethargy, upper abdominal pain, nausea, and vomiting

4. Splenomegaly, hepatomegaly, altered sensorium, peripheral neuropathy, pupillary abnormalities, pathologic deep tendon reflexes

5. Rash, ranging from a macular eruption to petechiae and erythema multiforme, developing in about 25% of victims

Treatment
1. Tetracycline and erythromycin are both effective. A 7- to 10-day course (500 mg PO qid) of either drug is recommended.

2. A Jarisch-Herxheimer reaction is common after the first dose of antibiotics. It is often severe and may be fatal.
   a. The reaction begins with a rise in body temperature and exacerbation of existing signs and symptoms. Vasodilation and a fall in blood pressure follow.
   b. Pretreat any victim who will be receiving the initial dose of an antibiotic to treat relapsing fever with an intravenous infusion of isotonic saline solution in anticipation of the Jarisch-Herxheimer reaction.
   c. Note that a lower initial dose of antibiotic may reduce the frequency of this reaction.

Rocky Mountain Spotted Fever

Rocky Mountain spotted fever (RMSF) is caused by *Rickettsia rickettsii*. Most cases in the United States occur between the months of April and September, when the vector ticks are active.

Signs and Symptoms
1. Ranges from mild, subclinical illness to fulminant disease with vascular collapse and death within 3 to 6 days of onset

2. Incubation period 2 to 14 days, with severe disease associated with the shorter incubation period

3. Typically, a sudden onset of fever, chills, headache, and myalgias; fever is usually high, greater than 102.2° F (39° F)

4. Most characteristic feature: rash, which develops 2 to 5 days after the onset of illness
   a. Typically develops first on the wrists, hands, ankles, and feet, spreading rapidly in centripetal fashion to cover most of the body including the palms, soles, and face
   b. Lesions initially pink macules, 2 to 5 mm in diameter, that readily blanch with pressure
   c. After 2 to 3 days: lesions fixed, darker red, papular, and finally petechial

    d. Hemorrhagic lesions coalescing to form large areas of ecchymoses

    e. Unfortunately, rash often absent on initial presentation, making diagnosis more difficult; in 10% to 15% of victims, no rash ever noted ("spotless fever")

5. Other signs and symptoms: abdominal pain, vomiting, diarrhea, confusion, conjunctivitis, peripheral edema
6. Seizures possible during acute phase of illness but rarely persist
7. Lethargy and confusion common, possibly progressing to stupor or coma
8. Cough, chest pain, dyspnea, or coryza also noted

Treatment
1. Initiate antibiotic therapy at the earliest suspicion for RMSF. Unfortunately, the classic triad of rash, fever, and tick bite is rarely present.
2. Give either tetracycline or chloramphenicol, both of which are very effective, although neither drug is rickettsicidal. These antibiotics inhibit the rickettsiae until an adequate immune response by the victim eradicates the infection.
    a. Give tetracycline, 25 to 50 mg/kg/day PO in four divided doses (2 g/day for adults).
    b. Give chloramphenicol, 50 mg/kg/day PO for adults and 75 mg/kg/day for children.
3. Continue treatment until the victim is afebrile for 48 hours, or for a minimum of 5 to 7 days. Be aware that relapses are common but may be treated with the same drug when they occur.

Ehrlichiosis

Ehrlichiae are tick-borne rickettsial organisms that cause disease in humans and animals throughout the world. Human ehrlichiosis has a broad clinical spectrum, ranging from a subclinical infection to a mild viral-like illness to a life-threatening disease.

Signs and Symptoms
1. After an average incubation period of 7 days (range: 1 to 21 days): high fever, headache, chills or rigors, malaise, myalgia, anorexia
2. Rash, which may be maculopapular or petechial, in 20% to 40% of victims about 8 days after onset of illness
3. Severe complications: more likely in older persons and include cough, pneumonitis, dyspnea, respiratory failure, encephalopathy, and renal failure

Treatment
Give tetracycline, 500 mg PO qid, or doxycycline, 200 mg PO bid, for 5 to 10 days.

Colorado Tick Fever

Colorado tick fever is caused by a small ribonucleic acid (RNA) virus that is transmitted by ticks to humans. The incubation period is 3 to 6 days (range: 0 to 14 days).

Signs and Symptoms
1. Usually begins with an abrupt onset of fever
   a. Most characteristic feature of illness (seen in 50% of victims): biphasic, or "saddleback," fever pattern
   b. From 2 to 3 days of fever, followed by 1 or 2 days of remission, then an additional 2 to 3 days of fever
   c. During fever, also have severe headache, myalgias, lethargy
2. Photophobia, ocular pain, anorexia, nausea, vomiting, abdominal pain
3. Macular or maculopapular rash in 5% to 12% of victims
4. Usually mild, but severe complications possible, especially in children younger than age 10 years; include meningoencephalitis or hemorrhagic diathesis
5. Three weeks or longer required for full recovery, with most common persistent symptoms malaise and weakness

Treatment
Treatment is supportive and based on symptoms.

Babesiosis

Babesia organisms are intraerythrocytic protozoan parasites. The vector tick may be the same as that which carries the infectious agent of Lyme disease. The presence of an intact spleen appears to play an important role in resistance to *Babesia* organisms.

Signs and Symptoms
1. Acute babesiosis: gradual onset of malaise, anorexia, and fatigue followed within several days to a week by fever, sweats, and myalgias
2. Less common symptoms: headache, nausea, vomiting, depression, shaking chills, splenomegaly, jaundice, hepatomegaly
3. No rash associated with disease
4. Hemolytic anemia more pronounced in splenectomized victims

Treatment
1. Note that limited or no efficacy has been shown with anti-malarial therapy.
2. Currently, treatment is only recommended for the seriously ill victim or the victim with asplenia, immunosuppression, or elder status. Give a combination of quinine, 650 mg PO, and clindamycin, 600 mg PO q8h. Azithromycin was used as a successful alternative to clindamycin in one treatment failure. Exchange transfusion is sometimes helpful in seriously ill patients with high levels of parasitemia.

Prevention of Tick-Borne Diseases and Tick Removal

Close and regular inspection of all parts of the body should be performed when traveling in tick-infested areas. Protective clothing (long pants cinched at the ankles or tucked into boots and socks) should be worn when in tick-infested areas. Spraying clothes with an insect repellent may provide an additional barrier against ticks (Box 37-1; see also Fig. 38-1). Adult ixodid ticks are generally on the body for 1 to 2 hours before attaching.

Procedure (Fig. 37-8)
1. Grasp the attached tick as close as possible to the skin surface with blunt curved forceps, tweezers, or fingers

---

Box 37-1. Insect Repellents

- Wear proper clothing to prevent the insect from obtaining access to the skin. Light-colored clothing makes it easier to spot ticks and is less attractive to biting flies.
- Use screens over windows, screened enclosures, or bed nets with fine mesh.
- Avoid unnecessary use of lights. Camp in a site that is high, dry, open, and uncluttered.
- Apply a repellent containing N,N-diethyl-3-methylbenzamide, commonly known as DEET (from its former chemical name). Bathing, excessive sweating, wiping, or other abrasive action that depletes the supply of available repellent on skin may justify reapplication. Avoid prolonged use of high concentrations (in excess of 35%) of DEET, particularly with small children.
- Use premethrin-impregnated fabric (see Fig. 38-1). Note that the insecticidal action can noticeably reduce the density of the biting population in the immediate area. After contact, pests drop or fly away from the treated clothing, but they are not necessarily killed.

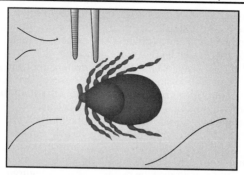

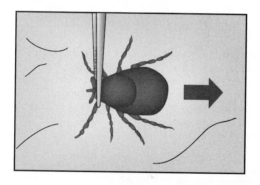

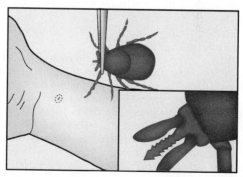

Figure 37-8.   Ideal tick removal method. Grasp the tick near the surface of the skin. Withdraw it from the skin in a steady, constant motion. Do not turn, jerk, or twist. (From Goddard J: Infectious Diseases and Arthropods. Totowa, NJ, Humana Press, 1999, with permission.)

protected with tissue. Note that medium-tipped angled forceps are best because sharp forceps can puncture an engorged tick and straight ones make the angle of approach to grasp the tick more difficult.

2. Pull the tick out counter to the direction that the mouth parts entered the skin; be sure to use steady pressure and take care not to crush or squeeze the tick's body because expressed fluid may contain infective agents.

3. After the tick is removed, disinfect the bite site.

4. Be aware that traditional methods of tick removal such as applying fingernail polish, using isopropyl alcohol, or applying a hot extinguished match do not effect tick detachment and may induce the tick to salivate or regurgitate into the wound.

▶ SCORPIONS

Centruroides exilicauda, the bark scorpion (see Plate 17) of Arizona, is usually less than 5 cm (2 inches) long, yellow to brown, and possibly striped. It carries the identifying subaculear tooth beneath its stinger. Some scorpions fluoresce under a "black light," which can be used to inspect clothing, sleeping bags, etc. Other scorpions worldwide cause similar syndromes.

Signs and Symptoms
1. Begin immediately after envenomation and progress to maximum severity in 5 hours
2. Infants: extreme illness possible 15 to 30 minutes after a sting
3. Improvement without administration of antivenom within 9 to 30 hours
4. Paresthesias and pain persisting for days to 2 weeks
5. Grade I: local pain and paresthesias at the site of envenomation, which can be elicited by tapping on the sting site
6. Grade II: pain and paresthesias remote from the sting bite, along with local findings. The victim may complain of a "thick tongue" and "trouble swallowing." Children and adults frequently rub their nose, eyes, and ears, and infants may show unexplained crying.
7. Grade III: either cranial nerve or somatic skeletal neuromuscular dysfunction
   a. Cranial nerve dysfunction: blurred vision, wandering eye movements (involuntary, conjugate, slow, roving); hypersalivation; difficulty swallowing; tongue fasciculation; upper airway obstruction; slurred speech
   b. Somatic skeletal neuromuscular dysfunction: jerking of the upper extremities, restlessness, arching of the back,

and severe involuntary shaking and jerking that may be mistaken for a seizure (true seizures are caused by other scorpion species)
8. Grade IV: both cranial nerve and somatic skeletal neuro-muscular dysfunction
9. Hypertension, nausea, vomiting, hyperthermia, tachycardia, and respiratory distress also possible

Treatment
1. Control local pain with ice packs, which may be applied for 30 minutes each hour. Give oral analgesics as needed. Infiltration with a local anesthetic or application of a digital or regional nerve block may be used.
2. Observe the victim of a grade I or II envenomation for progression to more severe symptoms.
3. Avoid the use of narcotics, barbiturates, benzodiazepines, or other potent analgesics to control symptoms of agitation or motor hyperactivity unless prepared to definitively manage the airway because these agents may lead to apnea and loss of protective airway reflexes.
4. Manage hyperthermia from uncontrolled muscular activity with administration of acetaminophen or, if extremely severe, physical cooling methods.
5. Atropine may be used for severe bradycardia but should otherwise be avoided because it might exacerbate tachycardia and hypertension.
6. Sublingual (oral) nifedipine (5 to 10 mg by puncturing and swallowing the gelatin capsule) may be used to block excessive adrenergic tone. Another drug that has been used for this purpose is prazosin, a selective alpha-adrenergic blocker.
7. Be aware that antivenom administration worldwide is controversial. Some recommend it for reversal of grade III envenomation with respiratory distress or grade IV envenomation. Administration carries the risk of anaphylaxis. Ideally, it should be administered in a hospital critical care setting. Contraindications include prior administration of antivenom derived from the same species; current beta-adrenergic locker use; history of asthma or atopy; current angiotensin-converting enzyme inhibitor use; history of allergy to the animal species from which the antivenom is derived; allergy to that animal's milk; or prior extensive exposure to the animal, especially its blood. Antivenom against *C. exilicauda* is no longer available in the United States.

Protection from Blood-Feeding Arthropods

38

Of all the hazards, large and small, that may befall the outdoor enthusiast, perhaps the most vexatious comes from the smallest perils—blood-feeding arthropods. Mosquitoes, flies, fleas, mites, midges, chiggers, and ticks all readily bite humans (Box 38-1).

▶ PERSONAL PROTECTION

Personal protection against insect bites can be achieved in three ways:
1. By avoiding infested habitats
2. By using protective clothing and shelters
3. By applying insect repellents

Habitat Avoidance
Avoiding infested habitats reduces the risk of being bitten.
1. Mosquitoes and other nocturnal bloodsuckers are particularly active at dusk, making this a good time to be indoors.
2. To avoid the usual resting places of biting arthropods, campgrounds should be situated in areas that are high, dry, open, and as free from vegetation as possible.
3. Areas with standing or stagnant water should be avoided, as these are ideal breeding grounds for mosquitoes.
4. Attempts should be made to avoid unnecessary use of lights, which attract many insects.

Physical Protection
1. Physical barriers can be extremely effective in preventing insect bites, by blocking arthropods' access to the skin.
2. Long-sleeved shirts, socks, long pants, and a hat will protect all but the face, neck, and hands.
3. Tucking pants into the socks or boots makes it much more difficult for ticks or chigger mites to gain access to the skin.
4. Light-colored clothing is preferable because it makes it easier to spot ticks, and it is less attractive to mosquitoes and biting flies.
5. Ticks will find it more difficult to cling to smooth, tightly woven fabrics (e.g., nylon).
6. Loose-fitting clothing, made out of tightly woven fabric, with a tucked-in T-shirt undergarment is particularly effective at reducing bites on the upper body.

Box 38-1. Mosquito Facts (Family Culicidae)

Mosquitoes are responsible for more arthropod bites than any other blood-sucking organism. They can be found all over the world, except in Antarctica.

1. Mosquitoes rely on visual, thermal, and olfactory stimuli to help them locate a bloodmeal.
2. For mosquitoes that feed during the daytime, host movement and dark-colored clothing may initiate orientation toward an individual.
3. Visual stimuli appear to be important for in-flight orientation, particularly over long ranges.
4. Olfactory stimuli become more important as a mosquito nears its host.
5. Carbon dioxide serves as a long-range attractant, luring mosquitoes at distances of up to 36 m (118 feet).
6. At close range, skin warmth and moisture serve as attractants.
7. Volatile compounds, derived from sebum, eccrine and apocrine sweat, and/or the cutaneous microflora bacterial action on these secretions, may also act as chemoattractants.
8. Floral fragrances found in perfumes, lotions, soaps, and hair-care products can also lure mosquitoes.
9. Alcohol ingestion may increase the likelihood of being bitten by mosquitoes.
10. Significant variability in the attractiveness of different individuals to the same or different species of mosquitoes can exist.
11. Men tend to be bitten more readily than women.
12. Adults are more likely to be bitten than children.
13. Heavyset people are more likely to attract mosquitoes, perhaps because of their greater relative heat or carbon dioxide output.
14. During the day, mosquitoes tend to rest in cool, dark areas such as on dense vegetation or in hollow tree stumps, animal burrows, and caves. To complete their life cycle, mosquitoes also require standing water, which may be found in tree holes, woodland pools, marshes, or puddles. To minimize the chance of being bitten by mosquitoes, campsites should be situated as far away from these sites as possible.

---

7. A light-colored, full-brimmed hat will protect the head and neck.
   a. Deerflies tend to land on the hat instead of the head.
   b. Blackflies and biting midges are less likely to crawl to the shaded skin beneath the brim.
8. Mesh garments or garments made of tightly woven material are available to protect against insect bites.

a. Head nets, hooded jackets, pants, and mittens are available from a number of manufacturers in a wide range of sizes and styles (Box 38-2).

b. With a mesh size of less than 0.3 mm, many of these garments are woven tightly enough to exclude even biting midges and ticks.

c. As with any clothing, bending or crouching may still pull the garments close enough to the skin surface to enable insects to bite through.

d. One manufacturer (Shannon Outdoors, Louisville, GA) addresses this potential problem with a double-layered mesh that reportedly prevents mosquito penetration.

Box 38-2. Manufacturers of Protective Clothing, Protective Shelters, and Insect Nets

PROTECTIVE CLOTHING*

Bug Baffler, Inc.
P.O. Box 444
Goffstown, NH 03045
(800) 662-8411
www.bugbaffler.com
Insect Out
P.O. Box 49643
Colorado Springs, CO 80949
(888) 488-0285
www.insectout.com
BugOut Outdoor Wear, Inc.
P.O. Box 185
Centerville, IA 52544
(877) 928-4688
www.bug-out-outdoorwear.com
Buzz Off Insect Repellent Apparel
(Nonmesh clothing impregnated with permethrin)
701 Green Valley Rd, Suite 302
Greensboro, NC 27408
(336) 272-4157
www.buzzoff.com
The Original Bug Shirt Company
908 Niagara Falls Blvd, #467
North Tonawanda, NY 14120
(800) 998-9096
www.bugshirt.com
Shannon Outdoor's Bug Tamer
1210-A Peachtree St
Louisville, GA 30434
(800) 852-8058
www.bugtamer.com

Continued

▌ Box 38-2. Manufacturers of Protective Clothing, Protective Shelters, and Insect Nets—cont'd

PROTECTIVE SHELTER AND INSECT NETS
Long Road Travel Supplies
111 Avenida Dr
Berkeley, CA 94708
(800) 359-6040
www.longroad.com
Travel Medicine, Inc.
369 Pleasant St
Northampton, MA 01060
(800) 872-8633
www.travmed.com
Wisconsin Pharmacal Co.
1 Repel Rd
Jackson, WI 53037
(800) 558-6614
www.pharmacalway.com

---

*Clothing includes hooded jackets, pants, head nets, ankle guards, gaiters, and mittens.

    e. Although mesh garments are effective barriers against insects, some people may find them uncomfortable during vigorous activity or in hot weather.

9. Lightweight insect nets and mesh shelters are available to protect travelers sleeping indoors or in the wilderness (see Box 38-2).

    a. Their effectiveness may be enhanced by treating them with a permethrin-based contact insecticide, which can provide weeks of efficacy after a single application (Fig. 38-1).

▶ REPELLENTS

For many people, applying an insect repellent may be the most effective and easiest way to prevent arthropod bites.

1. Development of the perfect insect repellent has been a scientific goal for years and has yet to be achieved.

2. The ideal agent would repel multiple species of biting arthropods, remain effective for at least 8 hours, cause no irritation to skin or mucous membranes, and possess no systemic toxicity, and it would be resistant to abrasion, greaseless, odorless, and not easily washed off.

3. No presently available insect repellent meets all of these criteria.

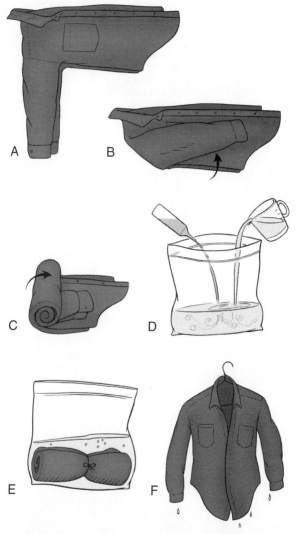

Figure 38-1. Technique for impregnating clothing or mosquito netting with permethrin solution. **A** to **C,** Lay jacket flat and fold it shoulder to shoulder. Fold sleeves to inside, roll tightly, and tie middle with string. For mosquito net, roll tightly and tie. **D,** Pour 2 oz (60 mL) of permethrin into plastic bag. Add 1 quart (1 L) water. Mix. Solution will turn milky white. **E,** Place garment or mosquito netting in bag. Shut or tie tightly. Let rest 10 minutes. **F,** Hang garment or netting for 2 to 3 hours to dry. Fabric can also be laid on a clean surface to dry. (Redrawn from Rose S: International Travel Health Guide. Northampton, MA, Travel Medicine, 1993, with permission.)

TABLE 38-1. DEET-Containing Insect Repellents

MANUFACTURER	PRODUCT NAME	FORM	DEET (%)
Sawyer Products Tampa, FL (800) 940-4664	Sawyer Controlled Release Sawyer Broad Spectrum Insect Repellent (with R-326 fly and gnat repellent)	Lotion Aerosol and pump spray	20 25
	Sawyer Maxi DEET	Pump spray	100
S.C. Johnson Wax Racine, WI (800) 558-5566	OFF! Skintastic	Pump spray	5
	OFF! Skintastic	Pump spray	7
	OFF! Skintastic with Sunscreen (SPF 30)	Pump spray	10
	OFF! Fresh Scent	Pump spray	25
	Deep Woods OFF!	Aerosol and pump spray	25
	Deep Woods OFF! Sportsman	Aerosol spray	30
	DEEP Woods OFF! Sportsman	Pump spray	100
Tender Corp. Littleton, NH (800) 258-4696	Ben's Tick and Insect Repellent	Aerosol, pump spray, roll-on	30
	Ben's 100 Tick and Insect Repellent	Pump spray	95
Spectrum Brands St. Louis, MO (800) 874-8892	Cutter All Family Insect Repellent	Aerosol, pump spray, wipes	7
	Cutter Skinsations Insect Repellent	Pump spray	7
	Cutter Unscented	Aerosol spray	10
	Cutter Backwoods	Aerosol and pump spray	23
	Cutter Backwoods	Wipes	30
	Cutter Outdoorsman	Pump	23
	Cutter Outdoorsman	Aerosol	28.5

TABLE 38-1. DEET-Containing Insect Repellents—cont'd

MANUFACTURER	PRODUCT NAME	FORM	DEET (%)
	Cutter Outdoorsman	Stick and lotion	30
	Cutter Tick Defense (with MGK 264 and 326)	Aerosol spray	25
	Cutter Max	Pump	100
	Repel Camp Lotion for Families	Lotion	10
	Repel Sun and Bug Stuff (SPF 15)	Lotion	20
	Repel Family Formula	Aerosol spray	23
	Repel Sportsman Formula	Lotion	20
	Repel Sportsman Formula	Pump spray	25
	Repel Sportsman Formula	Aerosol spray	29
	Repel Sportsman Formula	Wipes	30
	Repel Sportsman Max Formula	Aerosol spray	40
	Repel Hunter's Repellent with Earth Scent	Pump spray	55
	Repel 100% Insect Repellent	Pump spray	100
3M St. Paul, MN (888) 364-3577	Ultrathon	Aerosol	25
	Ultrathon	Lotion	35

4. Efforts to find such a compound have been hampered by the many variables that affect the inherent repellency of any chemical.

5. Repellents do not all share a single mode of action, and different species of insects may react differently to the same repellent.

6. To be effective as an insect repellent, a chemical must be volatile enough to maintain an effective repellent vapor concentration at the skin surface, but it must not evaporate so rapidly that it quickly loses its effectiveness.

7. Multiple factors play a role in effectiveness including concentration, frequency and uniformity of application, the user's activity level and overall attractiveness to blood-sucking arthropods, and the number and species of the organisms trying to bite.

8. The effectiveness of any repellent is reduced by abrasion from clothing; by evaporation from and absorption into the skin surface; by its tendency to be washed off via sweat, rain, or water; and by a windy environment.

9. Each 18° F (10° C) increase in ambient temperature can lead to as much as a 50% reduction in protection time.

10. Insect repellents do not cloak the user in a chemical veil of protection; any untreated exposed skin can be readily bitten by hungry arthropods.

Chemical Repellents (see Table 38-1)
DEET

1. *N,N*-diethyl-3-methylbenzamide (previously called *N, N*-diethyl-*m*-toluamide), or DEET, remains the gold standard of presently available insect repellents.

2. DEET has been registered for use by the general public since 1957. It is a broad-spectrum repellent, effective against many species of crawling and flying insects including mosquitoes, biting flies, midges, chiggers, fleas, and ticks.

3. The U.S. Environmental Protection Agency (EPA) estimates that about 30% of the U.S. population uses a DEET-based product every year; worldwide use exceeds 200 million people annually.

4. Decades of empirical testing of more than 20,000 other compounds has not yet led to the release of a superior repellent.

5. DEET may be applied directly to skin, clothing, mesh insect nets or shelters, window screens, tents, or sleeping bags.

6. Care should be taken to avoid inadvertent contact with plastics (e.g., watch crystals, eyeglass frames), rayon, spandex, leather, or painted and varnished surfaces because DEET may damage these. DEET does not damage natural fibers like wool and cotton.

7. In the United States, DEET is sold in concentrations from 5% to 100%, in multiple formulations including lotions,

solutions, gels, sprays, roll-ons, and impregnated towelettes (see Table 38-1).

8. As a general rule, higher concentrations of DEET provide longer-lasting protection. For most uses, however, there is no need to use the highest concentrations of DEET.

9. Products with 10% to 35% DEET provide adequate protection under most conditions. In fact, most manufacturers, responding to consumer demand, have recently begun to offer a greater variety of low-concentration DEET products and the vast majority of products now contain DEET concentrations of 40% or less.

10. Persons averse to applying DEET directly to their skin may get long-lasting repellency by applying it only to their clothing.

11. DEET-treated garments, stored in a plastic bag between wearings, maintain their repellency for several weeks.

12. Products with a DEET concentration higher than 35% are probably best reserved for circumstances in which the wearer will be in an environment with a high density of insects (e.g., a rain forest), where there is a high risk of disease transmission from insect bites, or when there may be rapid loss of repellent from the skin surface such as under conditions of high temperature and humidity or rain. Under these circumstances, reapplication of the repellent will most likely be necessary to maintain its effectiveness.

13. Sequential application of a DEET-based repellent and a sunscreen can reduce the efficacy of the sunscreen. In a study of 14 patients who applied a 33% DEET repellent followed by a sunscreen with a sun protection factor (SPF) of 15, the sunscreen's SPF was decreased by a mean of 33%, although the repellent maintained its potency.

14. Some products contain a combination of sunscreen and DEET and will deliver the SPF stated on the label. However, these products are generally not the best choice because it is rare that the need for reapplication of sunscreen and repellent is exactly the same.

15. Two companies (3M, Minneapolis, MN, and Sawyer Products, Tampa, FL) currently manufacture extended-release formulations of DEET that make it possible to deliver long-lasting protection without relying on high concentrations.

   a. The 3M product Ultrathon was originally developed for the U.S. military but is also available to the general public. This acrylate polymer formulation containing 35% DEET, when tested under many different environmental and climatic field conditions, was as effective as 75% DEET, providing up to 12 hours of greater than 95% protection against mosquito bites.

b. Sawyer Products' controlled-release 20% DEET lotion traps the chemical in a protein particle that slowly releases it to the skin surface, providing repellency equivalent to a standard 50% DEET preparation and lasting about 5 hours. Compared with a 20% ethanol-based preparation of DEET, 60% less of this encapsulated DEET is absorbed.

16. Case reports of potential DEET toxicity exist in the medical literature and have been extensively reviewed.

a. Fewer than 50 cases of significant toxicity from DEET exposure have been documented in the medical literature over the past 4 decades; more than three quarters of these resolved without sequelae.

b. Many of these cases involved long-term, excessive, or inappropriate use of DEET repellents; the details of exposure were frequently poorly documented, making causal relationships difficult to establish.

c. These cases have not shown a correlation between the concentration of the DEET product used and the risk of toxicity.

d. The reports of DEET toxicity that raise the greatest concern involve 18 cases of encephalopathy, 14 in children younger than 8 years of age. The EPA's analysis concluded that these cases "do not support a direct link between exposure to DEET and seizure incidence."

e. Animal studies in rats and mice show that DEET is not a selective neurotoxin.

f. Multiple studies have confirmed that children are not at greater risk for developing adverse effects from DEET when compared with older individuals.

g. Limited studies have been done investigating the safety of DEET use during pregnancy.

h. In these limited studies, no differences in survival, growth, or neurologic development have been detected in infants born to mothers who used DEET.

i. The EPA has issued guidelines to ensure safe use of DEET-based repellents (Box 38-3). Careful product choice and common-sense application greatly reduce the possibility of toxicity.

j. The current recommendation of the American Academy of Pediatrics is that children older than the age of 2 months can safely use up to 30% DEET. When required, reapplication of a low-strength repellent can

---

Box 38-3. Guidelines for Safe and Effective Use of Insect Repellents

- For casual use, choose a repellent with 10% to 35% DEET. Repellents with 10% DEET or less are most appropriate for use on children.
- Use just enough repellent to lightly cover the exposed skin; do not saturate the skin.
- Repellents should be applied only to exposed skin and clothing. Do not use under clothing.
- To apply to the face, dispense into palms, rub hands together, and then apply a thin layer to face.
- Young children should not apply repellents themselves.
- Avoid contact with eyes and mouth. Do not apply to children's hands, to prevent possible subsequent contact with mucous membranes.
- After applying, wipe repellent from the palmar surfaces to prevent inadvertent contact with eyes, mouth, and genitals.
- Never use repellents over cuts; wounds; or inflamed, irritated, or eczematous skin.
- Do not inhale aerosol formulations or get them in eyes. Do not apply when near food.
- Frequent reapplication is rarely necessary, unless the repellent seems to have lost its effectiveness. Reapplication may be necessary in hot, wet environments because of rapid loss of repellent from the skin surface.
- Once inside, wash treated areas with soap and water. Washing the repellent from the skin surface is particularly important when a repellent is likely to be applied for several consecutive days.
- If you suspect you are having a reaction to an insect repellent, discontinue its use, wash the treated skin, and consult a physician.

Modified from U.S. Environmental Protection Agency, Office of Pesticide Programs, Prevention, Pesticides, and Toxic Substances Division: Reregistration Eligibility Decision (RED): DEET (EPA-738-F-95-010). Washington, DC, EPA, 1998.

compensate for the inherent shorter duration of protection.

k. Questions about the safety of DEET may be addressed to the EPA-sponsored National Pesticide Information Center, available daily from 6:30 AM to 4:30 PM PST at 800-858-7378, or via their website at http://npic.orst.edu.

IR3535 (Ethyl-Butylacetylaminoproprionate)
1. IR3535 is an analog of the amino acid beta-alanine and has been sold in Europe as an insect repellent for 20 years.

2. In the United States this compound is classified by the EPA as a biopesticide, effective against mosquitoes, ticks, and flies.

3. IR3535 was brought to the U.S. market in 1999, sold exclusively by the Avon Corporation as Skin-So-Soft Bug Guard Plus, with 7.5% IR3535.

4. Depending on the species of mosquito and the testing method, this repellent has demonstrated widely variable effectiveness, with complete protection times ranging from 23 to 360 minutes.

5. In general, IR3535 provides longer-lasting repellency than the botanical citronella-based repellents, but it does not match the overall efficacy of DEET.

6. In 2006 Avon also released a 15% IR3535 spray to the market.

7. Avon's Skin-So-Soft Bath Oil was tested under laboratory conditions against *Aedes aegypti* mosquitoes. The effective half-life was found to be 0.51 hours.

8. In another study against *Aedes albopictus,* Skin-So-Soft oil provided 0.64 hours of protection from bites, and it was 10 times less effective than was 12.5% DEET.

9. Skin-So-Soft oil has been found to be somewhat effective against biting midges, but this effect is felt to be a result of its trapping the insects in an oily film on the skin surface.

10. It has been proposed that the limited mosquito repellent effect of Skin-So-Soft oil could result from its fragrance or from the presence of diisopropyl adipate and benzophenone in the formulation, both of which have some repellent activity.

Picaridin

1. The piperidine derivative picaridin (also known as KBR2023) is the newest insect repellent to become available in the United States.

2. Picaridin-based insect repellents have been sold in Europe since 1998 under the brand name Bayrepel.

3. In 2005 the first picaridin-based repellent was brought to the market in the United States, as Cutter Advanced, containing 7% of the active ingredient.

4. This nearly odorless, nongreasy repellent is effective against mosquitoes, biting flies, and ticks.

5. The 7% repellent should provide protection for up to 4 hours.

6. Studies have shown that, when used at higher concentrations of up to 20%, picaridin repellents can offer an efficacy comparable to that of DEET, giving up to 8 hours of protection.

7. The chemical is aesthetically pleasant and, unlike DEET, shows no detrimental effects on contact with plastics.
8. The EPA found picaridin to have a low toxicity risk.
9. In April 2005 the Centers for Disease Control and Prevention (CDC) released a statement adding picaridin to the list of approved repellents that could be used effectively to prevent mosquito-borne diseases (see Box 38-3).

Botanical Repellents

1. Thousands of plants have been tested as sources of insect repellents.
2. Although none of the plant-derived chemicals tested to date demonstrates the broad effectiveness and duration of DEET, a few show repellent activity.
3. Plants with essential oils that have been reported to possess repellent activity include citronella, neem, cedar, verbena, pennyroyal, geranium, catnip, lavender, pine, cajeput, cinnamon, vanilla, rosemary, basil, thyme, allspice, garlic, and peppermint.
4. Unlike DEET-based repellents, botanical repellents have been relatively poorly studied.
5. When tested, most of these essential oils tended to show short-lasting protection, lasting minutes to 2 hours.
6. A summary of readily available plant-derived insect repellents is shown in Table 38-2.

Citronella

1. It is the most common active ingredient found in "natural" or "herbal" insect repellents presently marketed in the United States.
2. Conflicting data exist on the efficacy of citronella-based products, varying greatly depending on the study methodology, location, and species of biting insect tested.
3. All Terrain Company (www.allterrainco.com) produces a citronella-based lotion in which the essential oil has been encapsulated into a beeswax matrix that slowly releases it to the skin surface, prolonging its efficacy.
4. In general, studies show that citronella-based repellents are less effective than are DEET repellents.
5. Citronella provides a shorter protection time, which may be partially overcome by frequent reapplication of the repellent.
6. In 1997, after analyzing available data on the repellent effect of citronella, the EPA concluded that citronella-based insect repellents must contain the following statement on their labels: "For maximum repellent effectiveness of this product, repeat applications at 1-hour intervals."

TABLE 38-2. Botanical Insect Repellents

MANUFACTURER	PRODUCT NAME	FORM	ACTIVE INGREDIENTS
HOMS, LLC Clayton, NC (800) 805-2483	Bite Blocker	Lotion, pump spray	Soybean oil 2%
Tender Corp. Littleton, NH (800) 258-4696	Natrapel	Lotion, pump spray, roll-on, wipes	Citronella oil 10%
All Terrain Co.	Herbal Armor	Pump spray and lotion	Citronella oil 12%, peppermint oil 2.5%, cedar oil 2%, lemongrass oil
	Herbal Armor	Lotion	1%, geranium oil 0.05%, in a slow-release encapsulated formula
	Bug & Sun SPF 15 Kids Herbal Armor	Pump spray	
	Kids Herbal Armor SPF 15	Lotion	
Green Ban Norway, IA (319) 446-7495	Green Ban for People: Regular	Oil	Citronella oil 5%, peppermint oil 1%
	Double Strength	Oil	Citronella oil 10%, peppermint oil 2%
Quantum Inc. Eugene, OR (800) 448-1448	Buzz Away	Towelettes, pump spray	Citronella oil 5%; oils of cedarwood, peppermint, eucalyptus, lemongrass
	Buzz Away, SPF 15	Lotion	

TABLE 38-2. Botanical Insect Repellents—cont'd

MANUFACTURER	PRODUCT NAME	FORM	ACTIVE INGREDIENTS
Kiss My Face Gardiner, NY (800) 262-5477	SunSwat SPF 15	Lotion	Citronella oil, bay, cedarwood, lavender, vetivert, patchouli, juniper, tea tree, lemon peel, pennyroyal, pansy, goldenseal oils
Lakon Herbals, Inc. Montpelier, VT (800) 865-2566	Bygone Bugzz	Lotion	Eucalyptus, rosemary, birch, peppermint, and geranium oils

7. Citronella candles have been promoted as an effective way to repel mosquitoes from one's local environment.
   a. One study compared the efficacy of commercially available 3% citronella candles, 5% citronella incense, and plain candles to prevent bites by *Aedes* species mosquitoes under field conditions.
   b. Subjects near the citronella candles had 42% less bites than controls that had no protection (a statistically significant difference). However, burning ordinary candles reduced the number of bites by 23%.
   c. No difference in efficacy between citronella incense and plain candles was found.
   d. The ability of plain candles to decrease biting may be due to their serving as a decoy source of warmth, moisture, and carbon dioxide.
8. The citrosa plant (*Pelargonium citrosum,* "Van Leenii") has been marketed as being able to repel mosquitoes through the continuous release of citronella oils. Unfortunately, when tested, these plants offer no protection against bites.

Bite Blocker
1. Bite Blocker is a "natural" repellent that was released to the U.S. market in 1997.
2. It combines soybean oil, geranium oil, and coconut oil in a formulation that has been available in Europe for several years.

3. Studies conducted at the University of Guelph showed that this product was capable of providing more than 97% protection against *Aedes* species mosquitoes under field conditions, even after 3.5 hours of application. During the same period, a 6.65% DEET-based spray afforded 86% protection, whereas Avon's Skin-So-Soft citronella-based repellent gave only 40% protection.

4. A second study showed that Bite Blocker provided a mean of 200 ± 30 (SD) minutes of complete protection from mosquito bites.

5. A laboratory study using three different species of mosquitoes showed that Bite Blocker provided an average protection time of about 7 hours.

6. Another study showed that it could give about 10 hours of protection against biting black flies; in the same test, 20% DEET protected for only about 6.5 hours.

Eucalyptus

1. A eucalyptus derivative (*p*-menthane-3,8-diol, or PMD) isolated from oil of the lemon eucalyptus plant has a strong lemony scent and has shown promise as an effective "natural" repellent.

2. This repellent has been popular in China for years and is currently sold in Europe as Mosi-Guard and in the United States as Repel Lemon Eucalyptus Repellent (Wisconsin Pharmacal Co., Inc., Jackson, WI) and as FiteBite Plant-Based Insect Repellent (Travel Medicine, Inc., Northampton, MA).

3. Field tests of this repellent have shown mean complete protection times ranging from 4 to 7.5 hours, depending on the mosquito species.

4. PMD-based repellents can cause significant ocular irritation, so care must be taken to keep them away from the eyes.

5. In 2005 the CDC added this repellent to the approved list of products that can be effectively used to prevent mosquito-borne diseases.

Efficacy of DEET versus Botanical Repellents

1. Limited data are available from studies that directly compare plant-derived repellents to DEET-based products.

2. Available data proving the efficacy of "natural" repellents are often sparse, and there is no uniformly accepted standard for testing these products. As a result, different studies often yield varied results, depending on how and where the tests were conducted.

3. Studies comparing "natural" repellents to low-strength DEET products, conducted under carefully controlled lab-

oratory conditions with caged mosquitoes, typically demonstrate dramatic differences in effectiveness between currently marketed insect repellents.

4. Citronella-based insect repellents usually provide the shortest-duration protection, often lasting only a few minutes.

5. Low-concentration DEET lotions (<7%) typically prove to be more effective than citronella-based repellents in their ability to prevent mosquito bites and can generally be expected to provide about 1.5 to 2 hours of complete protection.

6. Reapplication of these low-concentration DEET products can compensate for their shorter duration of action.

7. Because DEET repellents show a clear dose-response relationship, higher concentrations of DEET can be used to provide proportionately longer complete protection times— up to 6 to 8 hours after a single application.

8. Bite Blocker and oil of eucalyptus repellents appear to be the best of the botanical repellents.

9. Because of its pleasant aesthetic qualities, picaridin repellents may eventually replace DEET as the consumer's preferred repellent.

Alternative Repellents

Finding an oral insect repellent has always been of great interest. Oral repellents would be convenient and would eliminate the need to apply creams to the skin or put on protective clothing. Unfortunately, no effective oral repellent has been discovered.

1. For decades, lay literature has made the claim that vitamin B_1 (thiamine) works as a systemic mosquito repellent. When subjected to scientific scrutiny, however, thiamine has not been found to have any repellent effect on mosquitoes.

2. Additionally, ingested garlic has also never proven to be an effective deterrent.

Table 38-2 lists botanical repellents on the market.

▶ INSECTICIDES

Permethrin

1. Pyrethrum is a powerful, rapidly acting insecticide, originally derived from crushed dried flowers of the daisy *Chrysanthemum cinerariifolium*.

2. It does not repel insects but works as a contact insecticide, causing nervous system toxicity, leading to death, or "knockdown," of the insect.

3. The chemical is effective against mosquitoes, flies, ticks, fleas, lice, and chiggers.

4. Permethrin has low mammalian toxicity, is poorly absorbed by the skin, and is rapidly metabolized by skin and blood esterases.
5. Permethrin should be applied directly to clothing or to other fabrics (tent walls or mosquito nets), not to skin.
6. Permethrins are nonstaining, are nearly odorless, are resistant to degradation by heat or sun, and maintain their effectiveness for at least 2 weeks and through several launderings.
7. The combination of permethrin-treated clothing and skin application of a DEET-based repellent creates a formidable barrier against biting insects.
8. Permethrin-sprayed clothing also proved effective against ticks.
9. Permethrin-based insecticides available in the United States are listed in Table 38-3.
10. To apply to clothing do the following:
   a. Spray each side of the fabric (outdoors) for 30 to 45 seconds, just enough to moisten it.
   b. Allow it to dry for 2 to 4 hours before wearing it.

TABLE 38-3. Permethrin Insecticides

MANUFACTURER	PRODUCT NAME	FORM	ACTIVE INGREDIENT
Coulston Products Easton, PA (610) 253-0167	Duranon Odorless	Aerosol spray	Permethrin 0.5%
	Perma-Kill	Liquid concentrate	Permethrin 13.3%
Sawyer Products Tampa, FL (800) 940-4464	Permethrin Clothing Insect Repellent	Aerosol and pump sprays	Permethrin 0.5%
Spectrum Brands St. Louis, MO (800) 874-8892	Repel Permanone Clothing and Gear Insect Repellent	Aerosol spray	Permethrin 0.5%
3M St. Paul, MN (888) 364-3577	Clothing and Gear Insect Repellent	Aerosol spray	Permethrin 0.5%

11. Permethrin solution is also available for soak-treating large items such as mesh bed nets or for treating multiple garments simultaneously.
12. Permethrin-pretreated shirts, pants, socks, and hats can also be purchased.
    a. The manufacturer (Buzz Off Insect Shield, Greensboro, NC) claims that its product will maintain insecticidal effect through 25 machine washings.

▶ REDUCING LOCAL MOSQUITO POPULATIONS

Consumers may still find advertisements for small ultrasonic electronic devices that are meant to be carried on the body and claim to repulse mosquitoes by emitting "repellent" sounds such as that of a dragonfly (claimed to be the natural enemy of the mosquito), male mosquito, or bat.

1. Multiple studies, conducted in the field and in the laboratory, show that these devices do not work.
2. Mass-marketed backyard bug zappers, which use ultraviolet light to lure and electrocute insects, are also ineffective: Mosquitoes continue to be more attracted to humans than to the devices.
3. An estimated 71 to 350 billion beneficial insects may be killed annually in the United States by these devices.
4. Newer technology, using more specific bait such as a warm, moist plume of carbon dioxide, as well as other known chemical attractants (e.g., octenol), may prove to be a more successful way to lure and selectively kill biting insects.
5. Pyrethrin-containing yard foggers set off before an outdoor event can temporarily reduce the number of biting arthropods in a local environment.
    a. These products should be applied before any food is brought outside and should be kept away from animals or fishponds.
6. Burning coils that contain natural pyrethrins or synthetic pyrethroids (such as d-allethrin or d-*trans*-allethrin) can also temporarily reduce local populations of biting insects.
    a. Some concerns have been raised about the cumulative safety of long-term use of these coils in an indoor environment.
7. Wood smoke from campfires can also reduce the likelihood of being bitten by mosquitoes. The smoke's ability to repel insects may vary depending on the type of wood or vegetation burned.

▶ **INTEGRATED APPROACH TO PERSONAL PROTECTION**

An integrated approach to personal protection is the most effective way to prevent arthropod bites, regardless of where one is in the world and which species of insects may be attacking.

1. Maximal protection is best achieved through avoiding infested habitats and using protective clothing, topical insect repellents, and permethrin-treated garments.
2. When appropriate, mesh bed nets or tents should be used to prevent nocturnal insect bites.
3. DEET-containing insect repellents are the most effective products currently on the U.S. market, providing broad-spectrum, long-lasting repellency against multiple arthropod species.
4. Insect repellents alone, however, should not be relied on to provide complete protection.
   a. Mosquitoes, for example, can find and bite any untreated skin and may even bite through thin clothing.
   b. Deerflies, biting midges, and some blackflies prefer to bite around the head and readily crawl into the hair to bite where there is no protection.
5. Wearing protective clothing including a hat reduces the chances of being bitten.
6. Treating clothes including the hat with permethrin maximizes their effectiveness by causing knockdown of any insect that crawls or lands on the treated clothing.
7. To prevent chiggers or ticks from crawling up the legs, pants should be tucked into the boots or stockings.
8. Persons traveling to parts of the world where insect-borne disease is a potential threat can protect themselves best if they learn about indigenous insects and the diseases they might transmit.
9. Protective clothing, mesh insect tents or bedding, insect repellent, and permethrin spray should be carried.
10. Travelers would be wise to check the most current CDC recommendations.

Toxic Plant Ingestions

GENERAL CONSIDERATIONS

1. Supportive care
2. History should include the following:
   a. Time of ingestion
   b. Amount and part of plants ingested
   c. Initial symptoms
   d. Time between ingestion and onset of symptoms
   e. Method of preparation (e.g., drying, cooking, boiling)
   f. Number of persons who ate the same plant, and their symptoms

ORGAN SYSTEM PRINCIPLES

Toxic effects of certain plants can be grouped into categories designated by major effects on the central nervous, cardiovascular, gastrointestinal, renal, endocrine-metabolic, hematopoietic, and reproductive systems.

▶ CENTRAL NERVOUS SYSTEM

Anticholinergic Plants (Tropane Alkaloids)
Plants causing human toxicity include *Atropa belladonna* (deadly nightshade), *Mandragora* spp. (mandrake), *Hyoscyamus niger* (black henbane), *Datura* spp. (jimsonweed), and *Brugmansia* spp. (angel's trumpet).

Anticholinergic Syndrome
1. Hyperthermia—hot as a hare (or hot as Hades)
2. Visual disturbances including blurred and decreased vision
3. Dry skin, decreased or absent sweating
4. Skin erythema (flushing)
5. Altered mental status including delirium

Jimsonweed (Fig. 39-1)
Young, thin, tender stems of jimsonweed contain the highest concentration of tropane alkaloids. However, the seeds also contain high concentrations of the alkaloids, and as little as one-half teaspoonful of seeds may cause death from cardiopulmonary arrest.

Symptoms may appear within minutes and may last for days. These include the following:
1. Tachycardia
2. Dry mouth

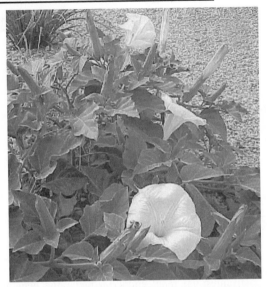

Figure 39-1. Jimsonweed (*Datura* species) is a bush with trumpet-like flowers.

3. Agitation
4. Nausea and vomiting
5. Incoherence
6. Disorientation
7. Auditory and visual hallucinations
8. Mydriasis (blurred vision and photophobia are sequelae); anisocoria if one eye has topical contact
9. Decreased bowel sounds
10. Slurred speech
11. Hyperthermia
12. Flushed skin
13. Urinary retention
14. Hypertension
15. Seizures, flaccid paralysis, and coma

Deadly Nightshade

All parts of deadly nightshade contain tropane alkaloids, but the highest concentrations are in the ripe fruit and green leaves; each berry may contain up to 2 mg of atropine. The berries may be mistaken for bilberries (hurtleberries). The most severely poisoned victims have anticholinergic symptoms, with hypertonia, hyperthermia, respiratory failure, and coma. Other common symptoms include meaningless speech, lethargy, tachycardia, mydriasis, and flushing.

Treatment
1. Decontamination and supportive care including oral administration of activated charcoal, airway protection, intravenous (IV) fluids, and vasopressors for hypotension resistant to IV fluids
2. Treat hyperthermia
3. Agitation can be treated with administration of benzodiazepines. Haloperidol and phenothiazines should not be used because these agents may enhance toxicity.
4. Foley catheterization and nasogastric tube placement may be necessary if bladder distention and decreased gut motility develop, respectively.

Nicotinic Plants
(Pyridine-Piperidine Alkaloids)
Nicotine alkaloids are found mainly in the Solanaceae family of plants. Other families containing nicotine alkaloids include Hippocastanaceae (horse chestnut) and Asclepiadaceae (milkweed).

Tobacco Plants
Nicotiana tabacum is the major source of commercial tobacco. One to two cigarettes, ingested and absorbed, could be lethal to a child.

Nicotinic Syndrome
Hypertension, tachycardia, vomiting, diarrhea, abdominal pain, salivation, bronchorrhea, muscle fasciculations, spasms, confusion, agitation, tremor, and convulsions (stimulation) are followed by hypotension, bradyarrhythmias (occasionally asystole), paralysis, coma, and respiratory failure (blockade). When death occurs, it is generally because of respiratory paralysis.

Poison Hemlock
Conium maculatum (poison hemlock) (Fig. 39-2) is also known as spotted hemlock, California or Nebraska fern, stinkweed, fool's parsley, and carrot weed. It has a mousy odor and unpleasant bitter taste and burns the mouth and throat. All plant parts are poisonous; the roots are especially toxic. Poisoning may also occur after eating birds that have consumed poison hemlock.
   Initially, stimulation causes:
1. Sialorrhea
2. Nausea and vomiting
3. Diarrhea
4. Abdominal cramping
5. Tremor
6. Tachycardia

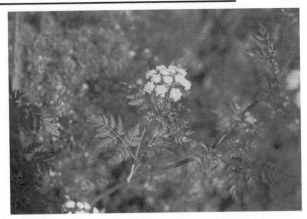

Figure 39-2. Poison hemlock *(Conium maculatum).*

followed by:
1. Dry mucosae
2. Gastrointestinal hypotonia
3. Diminished cardiac contraction
4. Bradycardia
5. Muscle swelling and stiffness

Betel Nut

Areca catechu (areca palm) produces betel nut.

Clinical effects resemble nicotinic syndrome and cholinergic toxicity:
1. Central nervous system (CNS) effects (dizziness, euphoria, subjective arousal, altered mental status, hallucinations, psychosis, convulsions)
2. Cardiac effects (tachycardia, hypertension, palpitations, arrhythmias, bradycardia, hypotension, chest discomfort, and acute myocardial infarction in susceptible individuals)
3. Pulmonary effects (bronchospasm, tachypnea, dyspnea), gastrointestinal (GI) effects (salivation, vomiting, diarrhea)
4. Urogenic effects (urinary incontinence) and musculoskeletal effects (weakness and paralysis)
5. Other: flushing, diaphoresis, warm sensations, red- or orange-stained oral mucosa and saliva, and dark brown- or black-stained teeth

Quinolizidine Alkaloids

Common toxic plants in this group include golden chain tree *(Laburnum anagyroides),* Kentucky coffee tree *(Gymnocladus dioica),* necklace pod sophora *(Sophora tomentosa),* and mescal bean bush *(Sophora secundiflora).*

Treatment

1. Supportive care with particular attention to airway protection and ventilation is necessary.
2. Benzodiazepines and barbiturates are given for seizures.
3. Adequate urine output is maintained, with consideration of urine alkalinization.
4. Treating initial excessive adrenergic stimulation with phentolamine is ill advised because this complicates the nicotinic blockade that follows.
5. Symptomatic bradycardia can be treated with atropine, and hypotension with IV fluids and inotropic agents (e.g., dopamine) if needed.

Hallucinogenic Plants

Chemical relationships exist among serotonin, psilocybin (*Psilocybe* spp.), and D-lysergic acid diethylamide (LSD).

Morning Glory *(Ipomoea violacea)*

About 300 seeds, or enough to fill a cupped hand, are equivalent to 200 to 300 mg of LSD, with similar systemic and hallucinatory effects. Ingestion of Hawaiian baby woodrose seeds *(Argyrlia nervosa)* presents similarly.

Nutmeg *(Myristica fragrans)*

Nutmeg contains myristicin, which is metabolized to amphetamine-like compounds.

Cannabis *(Cannabis sativa)*

The primary psychoactive component is most concentrated in the flowering tops.

Effects include mild mood-altering qualities, euphoria, alteration in perceptions, time distortion, intensification of ordinary sensory experiences, impairment of short-term memory and attention, impairment of motor skills and reaction times, anxiety, psychosis symptoms, and tachycardia.

Peyote Cactus *(Lophophora williamsii)*

Effects include slight rise in blood pressure and heart rate, tachypnea, hyperreflexia, mydriasis, ataxia, perspiration, flushing, salivation, and urination.

Mescal Bean Bush or Texas Mountain Laurel *(Sophora secundiflora)*

The beans contain the toxic alkaloid cytisine, which causes nausea, numbing sensations, hallucinations, unconsciousness, convulsions, and death through respiratory failure.

Khat or Evergreen Khat Tree *(Catha edulis)*

Khat is also known as chat, qat, eschat, mirra, qaad, and jaad. Khat leaves and bark are chewed, with the juice of the masticated plant being swallowed for stimulatory effects. Khat contains cathinone, cathine (norpseudoephedrine), and norephedrine.

Effects include increased energy and alertness, feelings of increased endurance and self-esteem, enhanced imaginative ability, higher capacity to associate ideas, euphoria, tachycardia, increased blood pressure, tachypnea, mydriasis, anorexia, hypomania, insomnia, delusions, paranoid psychosis, aggression, depression, anxiety, hyperthermia, and endocrine disturbances.

Anticholinergic Plants

Henbane *(Hyoscyamus niger)*, jimsonweed *(Datura stramonium)*, and mandrake *(Mandragora officinarum)* contain tropane alkaloids and can produce hallucinations.

Treatment

Treatment of patients exposed to hallucinogenic plants is supportive. First-line treatment for agitation is generally benzodiazepines.

Sedating Plants (Isoquinoline Alkaloids)
Poppy

Papaver somniferum flowers yield opium.

Neuromuscular Blocking Plants (Indole Alkaloids)
Yellow or Carolina Jasmine (*Gelsemium sempervirens*)

Convulsant Plants (Indoles, Resins)
Strychnine

Strychnine, found in seeds of the tree *Strychnos nux-vomica*, is a powerful CNS stimulant.

Symptoms include hyperreflexia, hypersensitivity to stimuli, migratory rippling movements of the muscles, twitching, severe muscle spasm, rigidity, and spinal convulsions (generally, flexor spasm of the upper limbs, extensor spasm of the lower limbs, opisthotonic posturing, and spasms of the jaw muscles, all without loss of consciousness or postictal states). In between the spasms, which last from 30 seconds to 2 minutes, the muscles become completely relaxed. Respiratory and secondary cardiac failure may ensue during severe convulsions.

Treatment

1. Decontamination and support including activated charcoal, benzodiazepines, and barbiturates.
2. Chemical paralysis with a nondepolarizing agent, endotracheal intubation, and mechanical ventilation may be required for severely poisoned patients.

Water Hemlock

Water hemlock *(Cicuta maculata)* and chinaberry *(Melia azedarach)* are two of the most toxic resin-containing plants. Chinaberry produces primarily GI symptoms (see later). The resin of *C. maculata*, an unsaturated aliphatic alcohol called cicutoxin, possesses convulsive properties.

Symptoms
1. Early symptoms are primarily GI including abdominal pain, vomiting, and diarrhea
2. Profuse perspiration, salivation, and respiratory distress
3. Tachycardia and hypertension or bradycardia and hypotension
4. Epileptiform seizure activity or spastic and tonic movements including opisthotonus without seizure activity
5. Pupils may be any size
6. Rhabdomyolysis and renal failure
7. Death associated with persistent seizures, cerebral edema, ventricular fibrillation, pulmonary edema, cardiopulmonary arrest, and disseminated intravascular coagulation

Treatment
1. Symptomatic and supportive with particular attention to the airway
2. Activated charcoal
3. Benzodiazepine and barbiturate administration for seizure control
4. Adequate urine output maintenance and alkalinization of urine to treat rhabdomyolysis

Purine Alkaloids

Cardiotoxins That Inhibit Na⁺ K⁺ ATPase (Cardiac Glycosides)

Cardiotoxins That Inhibit $Na^+ K^+$ ATPase (Cardiac Glycosides)

Cardiac glycosides are found in *Digitalis purpurea* (foxglove, Fig 39-3), *Digitalis lanata, Nerium oleander* (common oleander, Fig. 39-3), (Fig. 39-4), *Thevetia peruviana* (yellow oleander), *Convallaria majalis* (lily of the valley), *Urginea maritima* (squill or sea onion), *Urginea indica, Strophanthus gratus* (ouabain), *Asclepias* species (balloon cotton, red-headed cotton-bush, milkweeds), *Calotropis procera* (king's crown), *Carissa spectabilis* (wintersweet), *C. acokanthera* (bushman's poison), *Cerbera manghas* (sea mango), *Plumeria rubra* (frangipani), *Cryptostegia grandiflora* (rubber vine), *Euonymus europaeus* (spindle tree), *Cheiranthus, Erysimum* (wallflower), and *Helleborus niger* (henbane).

Clinical Presentation
1. Nausea and vomiting
2. Visual changes (yellow and green colors, "halos," geometric shapes, scintillations, photophobia)
3. Mental status changes (disorientation, psychosis, lethargy, stupor, dysarthria, weakness, dizziness, seizures)
4. Cardiac disturbances (palpitations, bradycardia, atrioventricular block, sinus node block, extrasystoles, ventricular arrhythmias, syncope)

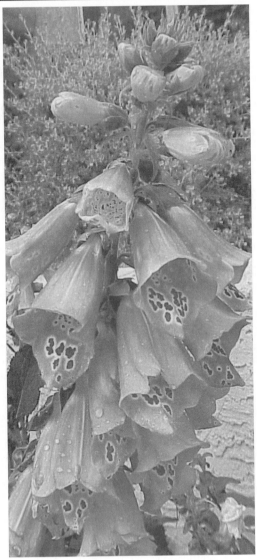

Figure 39-3. *Digitalis purpurea* (foxglove). (Courtesy Kimberlie Graeme, MD.)

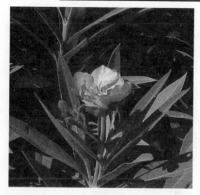

Figure 39-4. *Nerium oleander* (common oleander) plants have white or pink flowers. (Courtesy Kimberlie Graeme, MD.)

5. Hyperkalemia
6. When death occurs, it is generally caused by cardiotoxicity

Treatment
Cardiac glycoside toxicity from plant ingestions has been successfully treated with:
1. Activated charcoal to limit enterohepatic circulation
2. Cardiac pacing
3. Antiarrhythmic agents
4. Digoxin-specific Fab fragments (e.g., Digibind)
5. Maintenance of fluid and electrolyte balance
6. Theoretically, administration of exogenous calcium could be harmful

Cardiotoxins That Open Sodium Channels (Steroid Alkaloids, Resins)
Steroid alkaloids form principal toxic components of several common cardiotoxic plants: monkshood (*Aconitum* spp.) (Fig. 39-5), American hellebore *(Veratrum viride),* and death camas (*Zigadenus* spp.).

Symptoms
1. Begin within 3 minutes to 6 hours of ingestion and may persist for several days
2. Nausea and vomiting
3. Salivation
4. Diaphoresis
5. Dyspnea
6. Restlessness

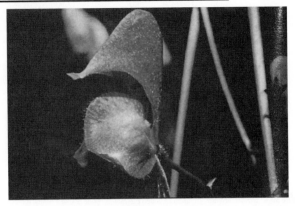

Figure 39-5. Monkshood (*Aconitum* species).

7. Cardiac effects are clinically similar to cardiac glycoside toxicity, with enhanced vagal tone, bradycardia, heart block, ectopic beats, supraventricular tachycardia, bundle branch block, junctional escape rhythms, ventricular tachycardia, bifascicular ventricular tachycardia, polymorphic ventricular tachycardia, torsades de pointes, ventricular fibrillation, asystole, and hypotension.
8. Occasionally, death ensues, generally from ventricular arrhythmias such as refractory ventricular fibrillation.

Veratrum Alkaloids
Veratrum and *Zigadenus* species belong to the lily family.

Symptoms
1. Generally occur within 30 minutes to 3 hours and resolve within 24 to 48 hours
2. Diaphoresis, nausea, vomiting, diarrhea, abdominal pain, hypotension, bradycardia, arrhythmias, and shock
3. Syncope, respiratory depression, scotomata, paresthesias, fasciculations, muscle spasticity, hyperreflexia, vertigo, ataxia, dizziness, coma, seizures, and death may also occur

Treatment
1. Treatment of cardiotoxic steroid alkaloid poisoning is supportive and includes atropine, crystalloid fluids, and vasopressors
2. Victims may require mechanical ventilation and cardiopulmonary resuscitation
3. Magnesium may suppress ventricular tachycardia
4. Lidocaine, amiodarone and hemoperfusion have been also been used to treat ventricular arrhythmias

Grayanotoxins

Resins called grayanotoxins are found in rhododendrons, mountain laurels, and azaleas. Grayanotoxins produce toxicity similar to the steroid alkaloids, veratrum and aconite, by binding to myocardial sodium channels and increasing their permeability. Symptoms include salivation, emesis, hypotension, bradycardia, arrhythmias, hypotension, chest pain, dizziness, circumoral and extremity paresthesias, incoordination, and muscular weakness.

▶ OTHER CARDIOTOXINS

Taxine Alkaloids

Taxus species include *Taxus baccata* (English yew) and *Taxus brevifolia* (Western yew).

Although GI toxicity is most common, dizziness, pupil dilation, muscle weakness and convulsions have also been reported. Severe toxicity is characterized by bradycardia, heart block, ventricular tachycardia, ventricular fibrillation, widened QRS complexes, and cardiac arrest.

Lidocaine administration and cardiac pacing have also been reportedly beneficial in the treatment of humans poisoned with yew.

▶ ORAL AND GASTROINTESTINAL SYSTEM

Gastrointestinal Irritants

Chinaberry Trees
Melia azedarach plants contain toxins that induce gastroenteritis. Immature berries are green but turn yellow and wrinkle with age. After ingestion of as little as one berry, severe gastroenteritis and often bloody diarrhea ensue. Symptoms may be rapid or delayed for several hours after ingestion.

Treatment is supportive, with replacement of fluids and electrolytes and administration of activated charcoal. If hypotension ensues, it generally responds to IV fluids.

Solanum

The *Solanum* species include *Solanum tuberosum* (potato), *Solanum gracile* (wild tomato), *Solanum carolinense* (horse nettle), *Solanum pseudocapsicum* (Jerusalem cherry), *Solanum dulcamara* (woody nightshade), *Solanum nigrum* L. var. *americanum* (black nightshade), and other nightshade plants.

Solanine generally produces gastroenteritis, but bradycardia, weakness, and CNS and respiratory depression may be seen. Treatment is supportive, with replacement of fluids and electrolytes and administration of activated charcoal. If hypotension ensues, it generally responds to IV fluids. Atropine may be beneficial if bradycardia develops.

Saponin Glycosides (Pokeweed)

Phytolacca americana, or *Phytolacca decandra*, is most commonly known as pokeweed but is also known as Virginia poke, inkberry, pocan, pigeonberry, American cancer-root, garget, red ink, American nightshade, scoke, jalap, and redwood. The root is the most toxic part of the plant.

Symptoms
1. Fulminant gastroenteritis with vomiting and diarrhea 2 to 4 hours after ingestion.
2. Diarrhea may appear foamy from the sudsing effect of saponin glycosides.
3. Hypotension may follow significant GI fluid losses.
4. Severe ingestions may result in weakness, loss of consciousness, seizures, and respiratory depression.

Treatment
1. Administration of activated charcoal
2. Fluid replacement for dehydration secondary to GI losses
3. Airway support
4. Seizures should be treated with benzodiazepines. Hematologic changes generally resolve within weeks

Anthraquinone Glycosides

Herbal teas that contain leaves, flowers, or bark of senna *(Cassia senna)*, leaves of aloe *(Aloe barbadensis)*, and bark of buckthorn *(Rhamnus frangula)* can cause severe diarrhea. Treatment is supportive, emphasizing adequate volume and electrolyte replacement.

Toxins That Inhibit Protein Synthesis (Phytotoxins)

Phytotoxins (Ricin, Abrin)

Phytotoxins are found in the families Fabaceae including *Abrus precatorius* (jequirity bean, rosary pea, prayer bead), which contains abrin, and Euphorbiaceae including the *Ricinus communis* (castor bean), which contains ricin (Fig. 39-6).

Symptoms
1. The oral lethal dose is estimated to be 1 mg/kg, theoretically as little as 1 castor bean in a child and 8 to 10 in an adult.
2. Latent period of 1 to 6 hours, followed by nausea, vomiting, diarrhea, hemorrhagic gastritis, abdominal pain, thirst, dehydration, hypotension, and shock.
3. Death may occur from dehydration and electrolyte imbalances; convulsions may precede death. Death usually

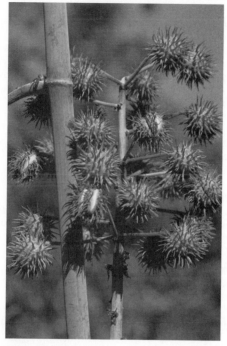

Figure 39-6. Guatemalan castor bean plant. (Photo courtesy Paul Auerbach, MD.)

occurs on the third day or later because of multi-organ failure.

Treatment
Treatment is supportive including fluid and electrolyte replacement and activated charcoal administration.

Toxins That Inhibit Cell Division
Colchicine
Colchicine toxicity can occur after ingestion of *Sandersonia aurantiaca* (Christmas-bells, Chinese lantern lily); *Gloriosa superba* (glory lily); and, more commonly, *Colchicum autumnale,* all of the lily family.

Symptoms
1. Acute poisoning may occur after a latent period of several hours.

2. Initial GI effects are severe abdominal pain, nausea, vomiting, diarrhea, and hemorrhagic gastroenteritis.
3. Electrolyte abnormalities, volume depletion, acidosis, shock, arrhythmias, and multi-organ failure occur.
4. Muscular weakness and ascending paralysis may cause respiratory arrest, which may occur with a clear sensorium.

Treatment
1. Symptomatic and supportive
2. Assisted ventilation as needed
3. Parenteral analgesics cautiously to relieve severe abdominal pain because colchicine sensitizes victims to CNS depressants
4. Fluid and electrolyte replacement

Podophyllum
Podophyllum peltatum is most commonly known as the mayapple, but it has also been called American mandrake. Treatment is similar to that for colchicine.

Hepatotoxic Agents
Pyrrolizidine Alkaloids
Plants containing pyrrolizidine alkaloids include *Senecio vulgaris* (groundsel), *Senecio longilobus* (gordolobo), *Senecio jacobaea* (tansy ragwort), *Senecio latifolius* (Dan's cabbage or "muti"), *Symphytum officinale* (comfrey), *Gynura segetum, Ilex paraguayensis* (mate), *Heliotropium* spp., *Crotalaria* spp. (rattlebox), *Amsinckia intermedia* (fiddle neck or tar weed), *Baccharis pteronoides, Astragalus lentiginosus, Gnaphalium, Cynoglossum, Echium, Tussilago farfara,* and *Adenotyles alliariae* (alpendost). These plants are consumed in herbal preparations, in breads made with grains that are contaminated with pyrrolizidine-containing weeds ("bread poisoning"), and in teas. Toxicity is associated with hepatic veno-occlusive disease; hepatomegaly; cirrhosis; and Budd-Chiari syndrome, which is characterized by obstruction of the trunk or large branches of the hepatic vein. Treatment is supportive.

Oral Irritants (Glycosides, Oxalates)
Daphne
Daphne *(Daphne mezereum)*, with its fragrant succulent berries, represents a significant risk to curious children, in whom only a few ingested berries may be lethal. The fruits contain a coumarin glycoside and a diterpene that irritate mucous membranes, with swelling of the tongue and lips. Blisters form if berries are rubbed on the skin. Severe gastroenteritis with GI bleeding may

occur after ingestion. In addition, progressive weakness, paralysis, seizures, and coma may develop. Treatment is supportive.

Insoluble Oxalates
Philodendron, Dieffenbachia (dumb cane), *Spathiphyllum* species (peace lily), and *Colocasia* species (elephant's ear, common cala) contain insoluble oxalates arranged in numerous needles of calcium oxalate (raphides).

Symptoms
1. Painful edematous swelling including angioedema
2. Dysphagia
3. Vesicle, bullae, or ulcer formation of the oral mucous membranes
4. Esophageal erosions
5. Respiratory obstruction caused by edema
   Treatment is supportive, with special attention to maintaining a patent airway.

Plants That Induce Hypoglycemia
Ackee Fruit
Unripe ackee fruit, *Blighia sapida*, contains hypoglycemic compounds.

Symptoms
1. Vomiting, abdominal pain, hypotonia, convulsions, and coma
2. Severe hypoglycemia
   Treatment is largely supportive and consists of securing an airway and administering activated charcoal, glucose, and IV fluids.

▶ PLANTS THAT INHIBIT CELLULAR RESPIRATION
Cyanogenic Plants
Amygdalin is the cyanogenic glycoside found in the seeds of apples and pits of cherries, peaches, plums, and apricots. Black or wild cherries *(Prunus serotina)* are considered the most dangerous. Linseeds *(Linum usitatissimum)* and cycad seeds *(Cycas* spp.) are also cyanogenic.

Symptoms
1. GI distress, bitter almond breath
2. CNS (agitation, anxiety, excitement, weakness, numbness, hypotonia, spasticity, coma, seizures)
3. Respiratory (hyperpnea, dyspnea, apnea, cyanosis)
4. Cardiovascular (tachycardia and hypertension followed by bradycardia and hypotension, heart block, ventricular arrhythmias, asystole)

5. Metabolic acidosis
6. Skin color may be pink or cyanotic

Treatment
1. 100% oxygen
2. Cyanide antidote kit, which includes amyl nitrite, sodium nitrite (3% solution given intravenously based on hemoglobin and weight; generally 300 mg in a nonanemic adult), and sodium thiosulfate (12.5 g)
3. Not available in the United States, hydroxocobalamin is used as antidotal therapy in some countries
4. Supportive care including mechanical ventilation, intravenous fluids, and vasopressors

Mushroom Toxicity

40

The four major types of mushroom toxins are gastrointestinal toxins, disulfiram-like toxins, neurotoxins, and protoplasmic toxins.

▶ DISORDERS CAUSED BY GASTROINTESTINAL TOXINS (Table 40-1)

Signs and Symptoms
1. Nausea, vomiting, intestinal cramping, and diarrhea within 1 to 2 hours of ingestion
2. Stools usually watery and occasionally bloody with fecal leukocytes
3. Chills, headaches, and myalgias possible
4. Spontaneous remission of symptoms in 6 to 12 hours

Treatment
1. Initiate supportive treatment including intravenous or oral fluid and electrolyte replacement.
2. For a severe case, administer an antiemetic such as prochlorperazine (Compazine), 2.5 to 10 mg IV or a 25-mg suppository, or ondansetron (Zofran), 4 mg oral dissolving tablet or IV.
3. Treat diarrhea with loperamide (Imodium, 4 mg initially, followed by 2 mg after each loose stool, up to 8 mg/day).

▶ DISORDERS CAUSED BY DISULFIRAM-LIKE TOXINS (Table 40-2)

Signs and Symptoms
1. If a person ingests these mushrooms and subsequently ingests alcohol, symptoms similar to those of an alcohol-disulfiram (Antabuse) reaction
   a. Severe headache, flushing, and tachycardia within 15 to 30 minutes of alcohol ingestion
   b. Hyperventilation, shortness of breath, palpitations
   c. Chest pain and orthostatic hypotension in severe cases; may be confused with an allergic reaction or acute myocardial infarction
2. Sensitivity to alcohol ingestion 2 to 6 hours after ingestion and lasting for up to 72 hours

Treatment
1. Initiate supportive treatment. Propranolol may be used for supraventricular tachycardia.

TABLE 40-1. Gastrointestinal Disorders: Causative Mushrooms and Identification

NAME	DESCRIPTION
Chlorophyllum molybdites (green-spored parasol) (see Plate 18)	This summer mushroom has a large, whitish cap (often 10 to 40 cm [4 to 16 inches] in diameter) that is initially smooth and becomes convex with maturity. Tan or brown warts may be present. The gills are free from the stalk, initially white to yellow and becoming green with maturity. The stalk is 5 to 25 cm (2 to 10 inches) long, smooth, and white. The ring is generally brown on the underside.
Omphalotus olearius (jack-o'-lantern) (see Plate 19)	This bright-orange to yellow mushroom has sharp-edged gills. It often grows in clusters at the base of stumps or on buried roots of deciduous trees. The cap is 4 to 16 cm (1½ to 6½ inches) in diameter on a stalk that is 4 to 20 cm (1½ to 8 inches) long. Gills are olive to orange, with white to yellow spores.
Amanita flavor-ubescens and *Amanita brun-nescens*	Both have broad caps (3 to 15 cm [1¼ to 6 inches] in diameter) with loosely attached warts. The caps are yellowish to brown. The stalks are 3 to 18 cm (1¼ to 7 inches) long, enlarging toward the base with a superior ring.

TABLE 40-2. Disulfiram-like Disorders: Causative Mushroom and Identification

NAME	DESCRIPTION
Coprinus atramentarius (inky cap) (see Plate 20)	This mushroom has a 2- to 8-cm (1- to 3-inch) cylindric cap on a 4- to 5-cm (1½- to 2-inch) thin stalk. The cap is white, occasionally orange or yellow at the top, with a surface that is characteristically shaggy. The mature cap often develops cracks at its margins, which turn up. The cap blackens as it matures and then liquefies.

2. Note that symptoms resolve spontaneously within 3 to 6 hours.
3. Be aware that activated charcoal is not beneficial.

▶ DISORDERS CAUSED BY NEUROLOGIC TOXINS (MUSCARINE) (Table 40-3)

Signs and Symptoms
1. Symptoms developing within 15 to 30 minutes of ingesting muscarine-containing mushrooms
2. Salivation, lacrimation, urination, diaphoresis, and emesis (SLUDGE); diarrhea; abdominal pain
3. Bradycardia and bronchospasm
4. Constricted pupils
5. Copious bronchial secretions that may cause respiratory failure, requiring mechanical ventilation

Treatment
1. Treatment consists of supportive care with oxygen, suctioning, and intravenous fluid replacement if available.
2. Administer atropine, 0.01 mg/kg IV or IM for children and 1 mg for adults, to manage profound secretions or bradycardia. Repeat the dose prn until secretions are manageable.
3. Symptoms resolve spontaneously within 6 to 24 hours.

TABLE 40-3. Muscarine Disorders: Causative Mushrooms and Identification

NAME	DESCRIPTION
Amanita muscaria (see Plate 21)	This mushroom has a cap 5 to 30 cm (2 to 12 inches) in diameter that is scarlet red with white warts. The stalk is white, often hollow, and grows 15 to 20 cm (6 to 8 inches) long, tapering upward. It has a prominent cup and volva and numerous rings. Gills are free and white.
Inocybe patouillardii (see Plate 22)	The *Inocybe* family contains small brown mushrooms with conical caps up to 6 cm (2½ inches) in diameter. Stalks are 2 to 10 cm (¾ to 4 inches) long, covered with fine brown to white hairs. Gills are brown and notched.
Clitocybe dealbata	*Clitocybe* mushrooms are whitish tan to gray, with 15- to 33-mm (¾- to 1½-inch) caps on hairless stalks 1 to 5 cm (½ to 2 inches) long. Gills run down the stalk.

▶ **ISOXAZOLE REACTIONS** (Table 40-4)

Signs and Symptoms
1. Begin within 30 minutes of ingestion and last 2 hours
2. With mild ingestion (10 mg), dizziness and ataxia
3. With ingestion of 15 mg or more:
   a. Pronounced ataxia, visual disturbances
   b. Delirium or manic behavior
   c. Visual hallucinations, seizures, muscle twitching, hyper-activity

Treatment
1. Treatment is primarily supportive.
2. Provide appropriate sedation with phenobarbital (30 mg IV qh) or diazepam (5 mg IV q15–20 min prn in an adult or 0.1 to 0.3 mg/kg in a child) if necessary, but use with caution in the wilderness.
3. Atropine may worsen the central nervous system symptoms associated with isoxazole derivatives. Therefore withhold it unless the muscarinic effects are serious.

▶ **DISORDERS CAUSED BY HALLUCINOGENIC MUSHROOMS** (Table 40-5)

Signs and Symptoms
1. With ingestion of 10 mg of the mushroom, moderate euphoria
2. With ingestion of 20 mg, hallucinations and a loss of time sensation
   a. Heightened imagination developing within 15 to 30 minutes of ingestion
   b. Hallucinations lasting 4 to 6 hours
3. Fever and seizures in children

TABLE 40-4. Isoxazole Reactions: Causative Mushrooms and Identification

NAME	DESCRIPTION
Amanita muscaria *Amanita pantherina* (see Plate 23)	See Table 40-3. This mushroom is 5 to 15 cm (2 to 6 inches) long with a cap 5 to 15 cm in diameter. The cap is white to pink early and becomes reddish-brown or brown with maturity. The stalk has a distinct ring, with a volva or cup at the bottom. When the flesh is cut or injured, it develops a pinkish tinge. Gills are free and produce white spores.

TABLE 40-5. Hallucinogenic Disorders: Causative Mushrooms and Identification

NAME	DESCRIPTION
Members of the *Psilocybe* family (see Plate 24)	These are little brown mushrooms with 0.5- to 4-cm (¼- to 1½-inch) broad caps that are smooth and become sticky or slippery when wet. The stalks are slender and 4 to 15 cm (1½ to 6 inches) long. Gills are gray to purple-gray. The flesh of these mushrooms turns blue or greenish when bruised or cut.
Members of the *Panaeolus* family	These little brown mushrooms are about the same size as *Psilocybe*. Gills are dark gray or black with black spores. Unlike *Psilocybe*, the caps are not sticky or slippery when wet.

Treatment
1. Place the victim in a quiet, supportive environment.
2. Reserve activated charcoal administration for the victim of a large ingestion.
3. When necessary, accomplish sedation with benzodiazepines (diazepam, 5 mg q15–20 min prn in an adult or 0.1 to 0.3 mg/kg in a child), phenobarbital (30 mg qh), or haloperidol (3 to 5 mg q8h in an adult or 0.10 mg/kg/day in equally divided doses q8h in a child). No evidence exists for use of newer antipsychotic medications.

▶ DISORDERS CAUSED BY PROTOPLASMIC POISONS
(Table 40-6)

Gyromitra Toxin
Signs and Symptoms
1. Symptoms delayed for 4 to 50 hours (average, 5 to 12 hours) after ingestion
2. Initially, nausea, vomiting, severe diarrhea
3. In some victims: dizziness, weakness, muscle cramps, loss of coordination
4. With severe ingestion: delirium, seizures, coma
5. Hepatic failure developing over several days after ingestion, although hepatic damage is generally mild
6. Severe hepatic failure and death possible

TABLE 40-6. Protoplasmic Disorders: Causative Mushrooms and Identification

NAME	DESCRIPTION
Gyromitra Toxin *Gyromitra esculenta* (false morel) (see Plate 25)	This mushroom grows in the spring near pines and in sandy soil. It is 5 to 16 cm (2 to 6½ inches) in height with a reddish-brown to dark brown, irregularly shaped cap. The cap's surface is curved and folded, resembling a human brain. The stalk is often as thick as the cap. The inside of the cap and the stalk are hollow.
Amatoxin *Amanita phalloides* (death cap) (see Plate 26)	This mushroom grows under deciduous trees in the fall and has a white to greenish cap 4 to 16 cm (1½ to 6½ inches) in diameter, often with remnants of the veil (warts). The stalk is thick, 5 to 18 cm (2 to 7 inches) long, with a large bulb at the base, often with a volva or cup. A thin ring is usually present on the stalk. Gills are generally free and white to green.
Amanita virosa (see Plate 27)	This mushroom resembles *Amanita phalloides,* but the cap is more yellowish or white.

Treatment
1. Administer activated charcoal, although it is of little proven value.
2. For a victim who develops significant neurologic symptoms, give pyridoxine, 25 mg/kg IV up to 25 g per day.
3. Be aware that no specific antidote or treatment is available for fulminant hepatic failure.

Amatoxin (see Table 40-6)
Signs and Symptoms
1. After a latent period of 4 to 16 hours: severe nausea, vomiting, abdominal cramps, diarrhea; gastrointestinal symptoms abating over the next 12 to 24 hours
2. Hepatic failure between 48 and 72 hours after ingestion in most victims

3. Endocrinopathies possible including severe hypoglycemia, hypocalcemia, and decreased thyroid function
4. Greater toxicity and higher mortality in children

Treatment
1. Administer activated charcoal, 1 g/kg PO q4–6h.
2. Administer normal saline solution intravenously to correct dehydration.
3. Give silibinin (milk thistle, also called silymarin), if available, IV 20 to 40 mg/kg/day in divided doses. If IV preparation is not available, give oral preparation in dose of 1.4 to 4.2 g/day.
4. Administer benzyl penicillin (penicillin G), 300,000 to 1 million U/kg/day IV in divided doses if silibinin is not available.
5. Administer cimetidine, 4 to 10 g IV in an adult for 3 days.
6. Experimental: hyperbaric oxygen treatment (dives to 2 atmospheres for 30 minutes once or twice a day).

Animal Attacks

41

Recommended oral antibiotics for prophylaxis of domestic animal and human bite wounds are listed in Appendix H.

▶ WOUND CARE

Evaluate for potential blunt trauma and injury to deeper and vital structures by penetrating teeth, claws, or horns. When you are in the proper setting for immunization, ensure appropriate coverage against tetanus.

1. Irrigate the wound using, in order of preference, normal saline (NS) solution, boiled or otherwise disinfected drinking water, tap water, or filtered fresh (stream) water.
   a. Do not use seawater or brackish water.
   b. Do not soak the wound.
2. If possible, add a germicidal agent to the irrigating solution. In order of preference, use 1% povidone-iodine solution (not "scrub"), 1% benzalkonium chloride, or ordinary hand (camping) soap. In a heavily contaminated wound, a 5% to 10% povidone-iodine solution may be used.
3. Complete the irrigation with a germicide-free solution (e.g., plain water) to rinse all irritating chemicals from the wound. Use 2% benzalkonium chloride to cleanse wounds inflicted by animals suspected of being rabid (see Chapter 42). For rabies-prone wounds, they may also be infiltrated with 1% procaine hydrochloride.
   a. Perform the irrigation technique at approximately 10 psi. This can be achieved by attaching a 19-gauge needle or plastic IV catheter to a 35-mL syringe; a pressure of 20 psi, to dislodge adherent debris, can be achieved by attaching a 19-gauge needle or plastic IV catheter to a 12-mL syringe.
   b. Use 100 to 200 mL of irrigating solution for a wound a few inches long.
4. Clean the wound, if necessary, by swabbing with a soft, clean cloth or sterile gauze. Follow with a repeat irrigation.
5. If the wound edges are macerated, crushed, or extremely contaminated, perform sharp débridement.
6. If the wound must be closed to control bleeding, to allow dressing, or to facilitate evacuation, do so in a manner that allows drainage. Use tape, surgical adhesive strips, or loose approximating sutures or staples in preference to a tight closure. It is not necessary and may be harmful to shave the skin around the wound.

    a. Do not suture bite wounds of the hand. These should be irrigated, débrided, and initially left open. Do not suture bite wounds older than 6 to 12 hours (limbs) or 12 to 24 hours (face).

    b. Immobilize the hand with a bulky mitten dressing in an elevated position, and start the victim promptly on an antibiotic (see Appendix F). If the wound is a human bite, choose amoxicillin/clavulanate, cephalexin, or penicillin and dicloxacillin.

7. Cover the wound with a sterile dressing or a clean, dry cloth. You can use a topical antiseptic ointment such as mupirocin for abrasions and shallow wounds. Do not plug deep puncture wounds with antiseptic so that they cannot drain.

8. Apply a splint if appropriate to restrict motion.

9. If the wound is of the high-risk type (see following features) or treatment is hours away, administer a prophylactic antibiotic (e.g., azithromycin, amoxicillin/ clavulanate, ciprofloxacin, trimethoprim-sulfamethoxazole [co-trimoxazole]). Dicloxacillin, tetracycline, and erythromycin cannot be relied on to offer coverage against *Pasteurella multocida*. High-risk wounds have the following features:

    a. Location: hand, wrist, or foot; scalp or face in infants; over a major joint (possible perforation); through-and-through wound of cheek

    b. Type of wound: puncture; tissue crush; carnivore bite over a vital structure (artery, nerve, or joint)

    c. Victim risk factor: older than age 50 years; asplenic; chronic alcoholic; immunosuppressed; diabetic; has peripheral vascular insufficiency; receiving chronic corticosteroid therapy; has prosthetic or diseased cardiac valve; has prosthetic or seriously diseased joint

    d. Animal species: domestic cat; large cat; human bite wound to hand; primate; pig

▶ WOUND INFECTION

The causative organisms in a wound infection after animal attack are most often *Staphylococcus* or *Streptococcus*, but you must consider signs and symptoms consistent with an anaerobic infection. Less common pathogens such as *Pasteurella* or *Eikenella* are usually sensitive to and effectively treated with most common antibiotics such as amoxicillin/clavulanate, 500 mg PO bid, azithromycin (perhaps less effective), 250 mg PO qd, cefuroxime, 500 mg PO bid, ciprofloxacin, 500 mg PO bid, and co-trimoxazole, DS tablet bid. For a human bite of the hand, a reasonable approach is dicloxacillin, 500 mg PO qid, plus ampicillin, 500 mg PO qid, or cefuroxime, 500 mg PO bid. Erythromycin is a poor choice for *Pasteurella*.

▶ SPECIFIC ANIMAL CONSIDERATIONS

Dog

1. If a dog's large teeth cause facial or scalp wounds in a small child, particularly an infant, be alert for the possibility of an underlying skull or facial bone fracture.
2. For a bite made by a large dog or any other animal with large teeth, when the bite is close to a major vessel, examine the wound for absent or diminished pulse, sensory or motor deficit, large or expanding hematoma, or extremely active bleeding. Any of these may indicate an arterial injury.

Cat

1. Do not suture a cat bite puncture because it has a high likelihood of becoming infected.
2. *P. multocida* causes an infection that may follow a cat bite. The appropriate prophylactic antibiotic is cefuroxime, amoxicillin/clavulanate, cefixime, trimethoprim-sulfamethoxazole, or ciprofloxacin.
3. With bites from large cats, suspect deep penetration, even with a seemingly trivial surface wound.

Ferret

Ferrets are classified in the same category as cats and dogs regarding rabies pathogenesis and viral shedding patterns. They may be confined and observed for 10 days rather than being routinely euthanized after biting.

Porcupine

1. Be aware that porcupine quills not only penetrate human skin but also can migrate up to 25 cm (10 inches). The quills are barbed, and their cores are spongy, allowing them to absorb body fluid and expand, which makes removal even more difficult.
2. Pull the quill straight out. In a deep penetration, you may need to make a small nick in the skin to allow egress of the entrapped barb.

Skunk

1. The skunk sprays its victim with musk from anal sacs. The musk causes skin irritation, keratoconjunctivitis, temporary blindness, nausea, and occasionally seizures and loss of consciousness. The chief component of the musk is butylmercaptan.

2. Neutralize the butylmercaptan with a strong oxidizing agent such as sodium hypochlorite in a 5.25% solution (household bleach), further diluted 1:5 or 1:10 in water. Then cleanse the area with tincture of green soap, followed by a dilute bleach rinse. Tomato juice as a shampoo has been advocated for deodorizing hair, which should then be washed and can be mildly bleached or cropped short.

Herbivores

Bites from horses, donkeys, cattle, sheep, camels, deer, and most other herbivores are treated with the same antibiotics as bites from dogs, cats, and humans.

Pigs

Bites from domestic pigs may be at risk for infections from bacteria that are resistant to amoxicillin-clavulanate, so the addition of ciprofloxacin is recommended as prophylaxis.

▶ AVOIDING AND MITIGATING ANIMAL ATTACKS

To avoid animal attacks and bites do the following:
1. Do not leave young children alone with biting animals.
2. Never pet an unfamiliar dog, especially if it is tied up or confined.
3. Do not pet, nuzzle, or kiss animals. Do not pet them on the head.
3. Avoid sudden movements around animals.
4. Do not try to take food or favored objects away from animals.
5. Never try to separate fighting animals unless you are well protected; use a bucket of water or a hose.
6. Do not invade the territory of nursing animals or animals with young offspring.
7. Do not corner or threaten animals, unless in a purposeful defensive gesture (such as when under attack by a cougar).
8. Know the likely animals you might encounter and their likely behaviors when frightened, hungry, irritated, and threatened, and how they will respond to your behaviors for the purposes of pacification, intimidation, and defense.
9. Do not reach into the cages of animals.
10. After handling food, wash hands before touching a hungry animal.

▶ BEAR ATTACK PREVENTION AND RISK REDUCTION

Prevent Predatory Behavior

1. Avoid camping along bear travel corridors or at feeding sites.
2. Use proper food storage to render human food unavailable to bears.
3. Avoid campsites littered with human refuse.
4. Reduce food odors by cooking and eating at a site away from the sleeping area. Do not sleep in clothes worn while cooking or eating.
5. Do not leave garbage or food buried or poured into the ground at the campsite.
6. Keep sleeping bags at least partially unzipped to facilitate a quick exit.
7. Sleep in a tent. Equip each tent with a flashlight. Consider equipping with pepper spray or, in knowledgeable hands, a firearm.

Avoiding an Encounter

1. Make noise so that the bear knows a person is present. Bear bells may not be sufficiently loud.
2. Remain alert to the terrain and environment in bear country. An "upwind bear" is more likely to be surprised by you, as is one in heavy forestation, near loud rushing water, in the rain, or in fog.
3. Avoid ripened berry patches, streams with spawning fish, and elk calving grounds. A collection of ravens may indicate carrion and the presence of feeding bears.
4. If you see bear signs (e.g., tracks, scratchings, droppings, or a prey carcass), consider that a bear is in the vicinity.
5. Do not approach bears or any wild animals too closely for a better view or photograph.

Avoiding an Attack

1. Allow the bear to know that you are human and not a prey species. Once the bear sees you, step out away from any visual obstruction and make it clear that you are a human. If you attempt to hide, you may confuse the bear. Speak in a calm voice to allow the bear to identify you.
2. Do not make sudden movements or yell out.
3. Do not stare directly at the bear. Look to the side or stand sideways to the bear.
4. Do not climb a tree or run away.

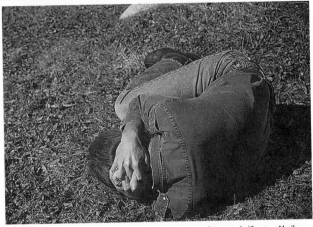

Figure 41-1. Curling into the fetal position to defend against a bear attack. (Courtesy Marilynn G. French.)

If a Bear Attacks

1. Do not run, try to climb a tree, fight, or scream.
2. Drop to the ground and protect the head and neck by interlocking the hands behind the head (ear level) and flexing the head forward, either in the fetal position or flat on the ground face down (Fig. 41-1). Use elbows to cover the face if the bear turns you over.
3. Do not hold out an arm to ward off the attack.
4. Never try to look at the bear during an attack.
5. After the attack, stay down until you are sure the bear has left the area.
6. When you believe the bear has left the area, peek around while moving as little as possible, try to determine which way the bear went, and then pick the best option for leaving the area.

Zoonoses

42

▶ **DEFINITION**

Zoonoses are diseases of animals that may be transmitted to humans under natural conditions.

▶ **DISORDERS**

Rabies

In the United States the most common rabid animals are skunks, raccoons, bats, and foxes. Overseas, additional animals that can become rabid are wolves, jackals, mongooses, weasels, and dogs. Woodchucks and cattle may be rabid. In the United States, rodents, urban cats and dogs, domestic ferrets, rabbits, and hares are currently considered at low risk. No case of rabies has been reported or documented in either wild or captive bears. Rabies virus is transmitted in saliva or by aerosols of saliva, secretions, and excretions (bats). Transmission by bat is especially worrisome because bat teeth, the size of 27- to 30-gauge needles, inflict wounds that are difficult to detect. Because the virus is sensitive to desiccation and ultraviolet light, once contaminated materials are dry or exposed to sunlight, they rapidly become noninfectious.

Signs and Symptoms
1. Incubation period: 9 days to more than 1 year, usually (in humans) 2 to 16 weeks
2. Initial symptoms are nonspecific
   a. Malaise, fatigue, anxiety, agitation, irritability, insomnia, depression, fever, headache, nausea, vomiting, sore throat, abdominal pain, anorexia
   b. Early pain, pruritus, or paresthesias at the site of the bite in approximately half of victims
3. Neurologic symptoms after prodromal period, which lasts 2 to 10 days; may be in the form of furious or paralytic (dumb) rabies
4. Furious rabies: increasing agitation, hyperactivity, seizures, and episodes in which the victim may thrash about, bite, and become aggressive, alternating with periods of relative calm
   a. Hallucinations possible
   b. Severe laryngeal spasm or spasm of respiratory muscles possible when the victim attempts to drink, or even looks at, water (hydrophobia)

    c. Pharyngeal spasm possible when air is blown on the victim's face (aerophobia)

5. Paralytic (dumb) rabies: progressive lethargy, incoordination, ascending paralysis, coma

Postexposure Treatment

1. Capture the offending animal.
   a. If not obviously diseased or acting abnormally, the domestic cat or dog should be quarantined for a 10-day period.
   b. Rabies prophylaxis can be started and discontinued if the animal remains well for 10 days.
   c. If the animal dies or develops neurologic symptoms within 10 days, the animal's brain should be examined. The brain should be double bagged in plastic and kept refrigerated or on ice (not frozen or chemically fixed) in a leakproof container.
   d. Any wild animal that bites a person should be killed immediately, and the brain sent for diagnostic laboratory studies.

2. Swab the wound thoroughly with 2% benzalkonium chloride or 20% soap solution. Simple flushing is not sufficient; the wound should be physically swabbed. After a few minutes' contact time, irrigate the chemical agent from the wound (see Chapter 20). If nothing else is available, scrub the wound vigorously with soap and water.

3. Infiltrate the wound edges with procaine hydrochloride 1%.

4. Administer rabies antiserum.
   a. The drug of choice is human rabies immune globulin (HRIG, 150 IU of neutralizing antibody per milliliter), administered as a single dose of 20 IU/kg. Theoretically, HRIG may be effective at any time before development of symptoms and should be given regardless of the time since the biting accident.
   b. Infiltrate the full dose around the bite wound. If the wound is in a small site, such as the finger, inject as much as feasible in that area. Inject the remainder intramuscularly at a site distant from the vaccine administration, such as in the upper outer quadrant of the buttocks in an adult or the anterolateral aspect of the thigh in a small child.
   c. Give the antiserum at the same time that active immunization (vaccine) is started, as described next. Be certain to use a different syringe and different anatomic site for the vaccine and HRIG administration. If HRIG is not administered when active immunization is started, it can be given up to 7 days after the first vaccine dose.

5. Administer human diploid cell vaccine (HDCV). The vaccine is given as a 1-mL dose regardless of the victim's age on days 0, 3, 7, 14, and 28. Inject it intramuscularly into the deltoid in an adult and into the thigh muscles in an infant or small child. Do not give the vaccine in the same syringe or site as human rabies immune globulin, and do not give it into the buttock (in order to avoid a poorly immunogenic deposition into fat).
6. A person who has undergone pre-exposure immunization with HDCV or purified chick embryo cell vaccine (PCEC) should receive booster doses of the same vaccine on days 0 and 3.
7. After immunization, antirabies titers 2 to 4 weeks after the immunization series is completed should show complete virus neutralization at a 1:5 serum dilution in the rapid fluorescent focus inhibition test (RFFIT) or a titer of at least 0.5 IU. If the response is inadequate, an additional booster dose of rabies vaccine can be given each week until a satisfactory response is obtained.

Prevention
1. Obtain pre-exposure immunization in humans by administering either HDVC or PCEC in three 1-mL intramuscular (deltoid muscle in adults and anterior thigh in children) injections on days 0, 7, and 21 or 28.
2. Check the antirabies titer, and give a booster dose of vaccine if the titer drops below complete virus neutralization at a 1:5 serum dilution in the rapid fluorescent focus inhibition test (RFFIT) or a titer of at least 0.5 IU.

Cat-Scratch Disease
Cat-scratch disease has been linked to the organism *Bartonella* (formerly *Rochalimaea*) *henselae.* Most cases are caused by scratches from cats, but dog and monkey bites, as well as thorns and splinters, have been implicated. Most cases occur in children, with an average incubation period of 3 to 10 days.

Signs and Symptoms
1. Characteristic feature: regional lymphadenitis, usually involving lymph nodes of the arm or leg
   a. May affect only one lymph node
   b. Nodes often painful and tender, and about 25% suppurate
2. Raised, red, slightly tender, and nonpruritic papule with a small central vesicle or eschar that resembles an insect bite at the site of primary inoculation
3. Mild systemic symptoms including fever (usually <39° C [102.2° F]), chills, malaise, anorexia, and nausea

4. Evanescent morbilliform and pleomorphic rashes lasting up to 48 hours
5. Parinaud's oculoglandular syndrome: conjunctivitis and ipsilateral, enlarged, tender preauricular lymph node
6. Rarely, encephalopathy, seizures, transverse myelitis, arthritis, splenic abscess, optic neuritis, or thrombocytopenic purpura

Treatment
1. Cat-scratch disease usually resolves spontaneously in weeks to months. In approximately 2% of victims (usually adults) the course is prolonged and involves systemic complications.
2. Antibiotics that may help shorten the course of illness include trimethoprim-sulfamethoxazole, rifampin, gentamicin, and ciprofloxacin. Antibiotics not thought to be of benefit include amoxicillin/clavulanate, erythromycin, dicloxacillin, cephalexin, ceftriaxone, cefaclor, and tetracycline.

Leptospirosis

Leptospirosis is caused by *Leptospira interrogans,* which infects many wild and domestic animals. Dogs are the most common vectors. The organism is shed in the urine. Humans contract the disease when they come in contact with contaminated water or soil. Doxycycline 100 mg PO once weekly may be used to prevent illness when traveling in endemic countries and participating in high-risk activities such as rafting, kayaking, or swimming in fresh water.

Signs and Symptoms
1. After incubation period (average 7 to 12 days, range 1 to 26 days), initial phase (4 to 7 days) of abrupt high fever, chills, headache, malaise, prostration, myalgias, lymph node enlargement, nonproductive cough, and prominent conjunctival suffusion without exudate; nausea, vomiting, and abdominal pain possible
2. Apparent recovery for a few days, followed by return of less dramatic fever associated with relentless headache with meningeal signs; severe cases initially interpreted as aseptic meningitis, infectious hepatitis, or fever of unknown origin (FUO)
3. Maculopapular, petechial, or purpuric rash; uveitis (iridocyclitis); arrhythmias; splenic enlargement
4. Weil's syndrome (icteric form): jaundice, petechial hemorrhages, renal insufficiency

Treatment
1. The treatment of choice is doxycycline, 100 mg PO bid for 7 days. Tetracycline, 2 g PO in four divided doses for

7 to 14 days, is an alternative. Another choice is procaine penicillin G, 3 million U/day IM in four divided doses for 7 to 10 days.
2. A Jarisch-Herxheimer reaction may be seen within a few hours of initial treatment.

Rat-Bite Fever

Rat-bite fever is an acute illness caused by *Streptobacillus moniliformis* or *Spirillum minus,* which are part of the oral flora of rodents including squirrels. It may also result from bites by weasels, dogs, cats, and pigs.

Signs and Symptoms
1. Streptobacillary rat-bite (Haverhill) fever:
   a. Incubation period of 1 to several weeks; disease transmitted by contaminated food, milk, or water or by simply playing with pet rats, without a history of bite or injury
   b. Initial symptoms: fever; chills; cough; malaise; headache; and, less frequently, lymphadenitis; followed by a nonpruritic morbilliform or petechial rash, which frequently involves the palms and soles
   c. Migratory polyarthritis in 50% of victims
   d. Centralized lymphadenitis; absence of meningeal signs
2. Spirillar rat-bite fever:
   a. Incubation period 7 to 21 days, during which the bite lesion heals
   b. Onset heralded by chills, fever, lymphadenitis, and dark-red macular rash
   c. Myalgias common, but arthritis absent, which helps in the differentiation from streptobacillary rat-bite fever
   d. Disease episodic and relapsing, with a 24- to 72-hour cycle

Treatment
1. Administer procaine penicillin, 600,000 units IM bid for 7 to 10 days. Alternative drugs for penicillin-allergic persons are tetracycline, 30 mg/kg/day PO in four divided doses, or streptomycin, 15 mg/kg/day IM in two divided doses.
2. Erythromycin is not effective.

Tularemia

Tularemia represents a variety of syndromes caused by *Francisella tularensis.* This bacterium is a common parasite of rabbits, rodents, hares, moles, beavers, muskrats, squirrels, rats, and mice. The primary mode of transmission to humans is via a bloodsucking arthropod such as a tick or by skin or eye inoculation resulting from skinning, dressing, or handling a diseased animal.

Signs and Symptoms

1. Abrupt onset of fever, often with chills and temperature up to 41.5° C (106° F)
2. Headache, which may mimic meningitis in severity
3. Hepatomegaly, splenomegaly
4. Six clinical presentations
   a. Ulceroglandular form (most common)
      - Typical skin lesion beginning as red papule or nodule that indurates and ulcerates
      - Frequently painful and tender
      - Ulcers associated with handling infected animals usually located on the hand, with associated lymphadenopathy in the epitrochlear or axillary area
      - Infection transmitted by tick bite, usually initiated on the lower extremity and associated with inguinal or femoral lymphadenopathy
      - Possible exudative pharyngitis
   b. Oculoglandular form
      - Unilateral conjunctivitis in and around a nodular lesion on the conjunctiva, extreme ocular pain, photophobia, itching, lacrimation, mucopurulent eye discharge
      - Enlargement of the ipsilateral preauricular lymph node
   c. Glandular form: enlarged, tender lymph nodes without an associated skin lesion
   d. Typhoidal form: fever, chills, debility, possible exudative pharyngitis
   e. Oropharyngeal form
      - Exudative pharyngitis associated with cervical lymphadenitis
      - Also may be seen with typhoidal or oculoglandular form
   f. Pneumonic form: pneumonia, with cough, chest pain, shortness of breath, sputum production, and hemoptysis

Treatment

Streptomycin is the drug of choice; administer in a dose of 30 to 40 mg/kg/day IM in two divided doses for 3 days, followed by half the dose for another 4 to 7 days. Alternative antibiotics include intravenous gentamicin or oral tetracycline or chloramphenicol. The latter two drugs are given as 50 to 60 mg/kg/day in four divided doses for 14 days. Relapse may occur with the oral drugs. If no other antibiotic is available, give ciprofloxacin or norfloxacin. Ceftriaxone does not appear to be effective.

Brucellosis

Brucella organisms are carried chiefly by swine, cattle, goats, and sheep. They are usually transmitted to humans by direct skin contact or from the ingestion of contaminated milk products. The incubation period in humans is 1 to 15 weeks.

Signs and Symptoms

1. No specific symptoms or signs; thus the nickname "mimic" disease
2. Most characteristic clinical manifestation: undulating fever
3. Acute form: headache, weakness, diaphoresis, myalgias, arthralgias; anorexia, constipation, and weight loss in the first 3 to 4 weeks; hepatomegaly and splenomegaly
4. Subacute or "undulant" form: similar to acute, but milder symptoms, with addition of arthritis and orchitis
5. Chronic form: symptoms persist for more than 1 year; arthralgias and extra-articular rheumatism; mimics chronic fatigue syndrome

Treatment

1. Administer tetracycline, 50 mg/kg/day PO in four divided doses for 21 days. Doxycycline is an alternative. In severe cases, add streptomycin, 20 to 40 mg/kg IM qd for 1 week. In the next week, continue streptomycin at a dose of 15 mg/kg. Alternatively, rifampin can be added to doxycycline.

Trichinosis

Trichinosis is an infection caused by nematodes of the genus *Trichinella*. The infection is acquired by ingesting larvae encysted in skeletal muscle, usually raw or undercooked pork. It can also be acquired from wild game such as bear, raccoon, horse, walrus, cougar, and wild swine.

Signs and Symptoms

1. Nausea, vomiting, and abdominal pain approximately 5 days after ingestion of infective meat; diarrhea or fever possible; gastrointestinal symptoms persisting for 4 to 6 weeks
2. Larvae invade skeletal muscle as early 7 days after ingestion
   a. Capillary damage during larval migration, which appears as facial (especially periorbital) edema, photophobia, blurred vision, diplopia, and complaints of pain associated with eye movements
   b. Splinter hemorrhages in the nail beds, along with cutaneous petechiae and hemorrhagic lesions in the conjunctivae
   c. Fever up to 41° C (105° F)

3. After 2 weeks: cough, dyspnea, pleuritic chest pain, hemoptysis, meningitis symptoms, headache
4. After 3 weeks: myalgias, muscle stiffness

Treatment
1. Be aware that no satisfactory, safe, and effective drug is available for the elimination of larvae.
2. Thiabendazole, 25 mg/kg bid for 5 days (maximum 3 g/day), is effective against adult worms in the intestine, but its efficacy against larvae is questionable. Mebendazole (200 to 400 mg tid for 3 days, then 400 to 500 mg tid for 10 days) is better tolerated, but poor intestinal absorption reduces its use in extraintestinal trichinosis. Albendazole and flubendazole are well absorbed and may be more effective, but supporting data are scarce.
3. Use prednisone, 30 to 60 mg/day PO, for 10 to 30 days for relief from severe inflammatory manifestations.

Prevention
1. Cook meat to an internal temperature of 65.6° C to 77° C (150° F to 170° F).
2. Most *Trichinella* larvae are killed by freezing. Holding the meat at −15° C (5° C) for 20 days, −23.3° C (−10° F) for 10 days, or −28.9° C (−20° F) for 6 days is recommended.
3. Salting, drying, and smoking are not always effective. *Trichinella nativa* found in Arctic mammals is resistant to freezing.

Hantavirus Pulmonary Syndrome
Hantavirus pulmonary syndrome is a severe viral respiratory illness predominantly transmitted through a rodent vector such as the deer mouse. Other small mammals such as brush mice and western chipmunks may be infected. The animals shed virus in saliva, urine, and feces for weeks.

Signs and Symptoms
1. Prodrome of fever, myalgia, and variable respiratory symptoms, which may include cough and shortness of breath with minimal bronchospasm; then rapid onset of acute respiratory distress
2. Headache, chills, abdominal pain, nausea, vomiting; possible hemorrhage related to thrombocytopenia
3. Rapid deterioration including respiratory failure and hypotension

Treatment
Note that therapy is supportive and based on symptoms. Ribavirin is being used on protocol as an investigational agent. The protocol calls for administration of a 2-g loading

dose of intravenous ribavirin, followed by 15 mg/kg q6h for 4 days, then 7.5 mg/kg q8h for another 4 days.

Prevention

1. Eliminate rodents, and reduce the availability of food sources and nesting sites used by rodents inside the home. Maintain snap traps and use rodenticides; in areas where plague occurs, control fleas with insecticides.
2. Keep food and water covered and stored in rodent-proof metal or thick, plastic containers. Keep cooking areas clean.
3. Dispose of clutter. Contain and elevate garbage.
4. Remove food sources that might attract rodents. Avoid feeding or handling rodents.
5. Spray dead rodents, nests, and droppings with a general-purpose household disinfectant or 10% bleach solution before handling. Dispose of all excreta and nesting materials in sealed bags. Always wear rubber or plastic gloves.
6. Avoid contact with rodents and rodent burrows. Do not disturb dens.
7. Do not use cabins or other enclosed shelters that are rodent infested until they have been appropriately cleaned and disinfected. Seal holes and cracks in dwellings to prevent entrance by rodents. Avoid sweeping, vacuuming, or stirring dust until the area is thoroughly wet with disinfectant.
8. Do not pitch tents or place sleeping bags in areas close to rodent feces or burrows or near possible rodent shelters (garbage dumps, wood piles).
9. If possible, do not sleep on bare ground.
10. Burn or bury all garbage promptly. Clear brush and trash from around homes and outbuildings.
11. Use only bottled water or water that has been disinfected for oral consumption, cooking, washing dishes, and brushing teeth.

Plague

Plague is a bacterial illness caused by *Yersinia pestis*. Plague is carried by various rodent reservoirs and transmitted by fleas. Carnivorous mammals can acquire plague by ingesting infected rodents or by being bitten by their fleas. Plague in cats is a serious problem.

Signs and Symptoms
Bubonic Plague

1. Incubation period of 2 to 6 days, then appearance of enlarged, tender lymph nodes (buboes) proximal to the point of percutaneous entry

2. Inguinal nodes most often involved because fleas usually bite humans on the legs; axillary buboes from skinning an animal as the mode of transmission
3. High fever, chills, malaise, headache, myalgias
4. Cardiovascular collapse with shock and hemorrhagic phenomena possible, with blackened, hemorrhagic skin lesions

Septicemic Plague
1. Fever, chills, malaise, headache, abdominal pain, nausea, vomiting, diarrhea
2. Eventual cardiovascular collapse with disseminated intravascular coagulation (DIC)

Pneumonic Plague
1. Incubation period of 2 to 3 days, then acute, fulminant disease
2. Characterized by symptoms of pneumonia including fever, cough, shaking chills, headache, tachypnea, and bloody sputum

Treatment for All Types of Plague
1. Initiate treatment if there is any suspicion that the disease may be present.
2. The drug of choice is streptomycin, 30 mg/kg/day IM in four divided doses for 5 days. A less preferred alternative is gentamicin, 5 mg/kg/day IV in four divided doses, reduced to 3 mg/kg/day after clinical improvement. Tetracycline is often used concurrently with streptomycin. The loading dose is 15 mg/kg PO up to 1 g total dose. Follow this with 40 to 50 mg/kg in six divided doses on the first day. Thereafter, administer 30 mg/kg PO in four divided doses for 10 to 14 days. An alternative to tetracycline is chloramphenicol, administered in a loading dose of 25 mg/kg PO up to 3 g total, followed by 50 to 75 mg/kg PO in four divided doses for 10 to 14 days. Sulfadiazine is a less satisfactory alternative. A loading dose of 25 mg/kg is given orally, followed by 75 mg/kg orally in four divided doses for 10 to 14 days. If none of these drugs is available, give co-trimoxazole (320 mg trimethoprim and 1600 mg sulfamethoxazole) PO bid or tid for 14 days. Ciprofloxacin (400 mg IV q12h for adults; 15 mg/kg IV q12h for children) is another alternative.

Prevention
1. The greatest risk of contagion is by aerosol transmission from victims with pneumonic plague. Therefore keep them in strict quarantine and isolation for a minimum of 48 hours after antibiotic therapy is begun (suspected case)

or 4 days after beginning antibiotic therapy (obvious case). Contact personnel should wear gloves, gowns, masks, and eye protection.
2. Treat individuals directly exposed to pneumonic plague prophylactically with tetracycline, 500 mg PO q6h for 6 days, for adults, or co-trimoxazole (otitis media dose) for children.

Anthrax

Anthrax is a bacterial illness caused by *Bacillus anthracis*. Naturally occurring anthrax is acquired from contact with infected animals (usually herbivores) or contaminated animal products but has recently become an agent of bioterrorism. It can be transmitted by inhalation, inoculation, or ingestion. The spore form of anthrax is highly resistant to physical and chemical agents and can persist in the environment for years. Anthrax is not transmitted from person to person.

Signs and Symptoms
The incubation period is 1 to 5 (range up to 60) days. Cutaneous anthrax is the most common form.

Inhalation Anthrax
1. First stage is a few hours to a few days of a flu-like illness: nonspecific symptoms of fever, dyspnea, cough, headache, vomiting, chills, weakness, abdominal pain
2. Second stage is abrupt onset of acute hemorrhagic mediastinitis, characterized by fever, dyspnea, diaphoresis, and hypotension
3. Mortality rate approaches 90%, even with treatment; hemorrhagic meningitis with meningismus, delirium, and obtundation; shock and death within 24 to 36 hours

Cutaneous Anthrax
1. Variable local edema, followed by pruritic macule or papule by second day, with or without tiny vesicles
2. Blackened, painless, and depressed eschar, often with extensive local edema; eschar dries and falls off in 7 to 14 days
3. Lymphangitis, painful lymphadenopathy

Gastrointestinal (Ingestion) Anthrax
1. Germination of spores in the upper gastrointestinal tract leads to oral or esophageal ulcer(s), with regional lymphadenopathy, edema, and sepsis.
2. Germination of spores in terminal ilium or cecum leads to local lesions, nausea, vomiting, and malaise progressing to bloody diarrhea, peritonitis, and sepsis.
   a. Ascites, acute abdomen

Treatment of Anthrax

1. Ciprofloxacin, 500 mg IV (preferred) or PO q12h for adults and 10 to 15 mg/kg/day divided every 12 hours for children not to exceed the adult dose, is the treatment of choice for penicillin-resistant inhalation anthrax, for gastrointestinal anthrax with severe symptoms, and for empirical therapy while awaiting susceptibility testing results. Alternative agents based on in vitro data are ofloxacin, 400 mg IV q12h, or levofloxacin, 500 mg q12h. If the strain is proven susceptible, administer penicillin G, 4 million U IV q4h, or doxycycline, 100 mg IV q12h. Treatment is continued for 60 days.

2. All victims should be vaccinated with three doses of anthrax vaccine (days 0, 14, and 28). Continue antibiotic prophylaxis until three doses of vaccine have been administered. If vaccine is not available, antibiotics should be continued for 60 days (to treat delayed germination of spores in the event of inhalation).

Prevention

1. If vaccine is available, all exposed persons should be vaccinated with three doses of anthrax vaccine (days 0, 14, and 28).

2. Begin antibiotic prophylaxis immediately after exposure with ciprofloxacin (500 mg PO q12h) or doxycycline (100 mg PO q12h). If it is determined that the strain of anthrax is penicillin susceptible, therapy can be changed to penicillin or amoxicillin (500 mg PO q8h for adults; 40 mg/kg in three divided doses q8h for children weighing less than 20 kg).

3. Continue antibiotic prophylaxis until three doses of vaccine have been administered. If vaccine is not available, antibiotics should be continued for 60 days (to treat delayed germination of spores in the event of inhalation).

Glanders

Glanders occurs in a few Asian and African countries such as India, China, Mongolia, and Egypt and is primarily a disease of horses. Occasionally, infections occur in dogs, cats, sheep, and goats. Humans are infected by exposure to sick horses. Infection can occur by inhalation of respiratory droplets or by contact with infected discharges.

Signs and Symptoms

1. Incubation period of 1 to 5 days
2. Pustular cutaneous eruptions
3. Thick indurated lymphatics that may ulcerate

4. Mucopurulent discharge from the eyes or nose
5. Pneumonia
6. Depending on the severity, the patient may have anorexia, fever, weight loss, headache, nausea, diarrhea, or septicemic shock

Treatment
1. Administer sulfadiazine, 100 mg/kg/day in three divided dosed for 3 weeks.
2. Treatment with tetracyclines and streptomycin is also recommended.

Prevention
Glanders can be transmitted from one person to another, so strict infection control should be exercised with suspected patients.

Avian Influenza

The highly pathogenic H5N1 avian influenza virus has been reported mainly in Vietnam, Indonesia, Hong Kong, Thailand, China, Egypt, and Eastern Europe. Most infections in humans result from contact with infected birds or their contaminated feces.

Signs and Symptoms
1. Sudden onset of high fever, headache, malaise, cough, sore throat, and myalgias
2. Gastrointestinal manifestations such as diarrhea may also occur.

Treatment
Administer oseltamivir (Tamiflu) 75 mg bid (adult dose and adolescents 13 years and older) for 5 days. Treatment should begin within 48 hours of symptom onset. The recommended dose of oseltamivir for pediatric patients 1 year and older is shown in Table 42-1. Oseltamivir capsules may be opened and mixed with sweetened liquids. Oseltamivir is not recommended for pediatric patients younger than 1 year old.

TABLE 42-1. Pediatric Dose of Oseltamivir for Treatment of Influenza

>1 yr:
<15 kg: 2 mg/kg PO bid for 5 days; not to exceed 30 mg PO bid
15-23 kg: 45 mg PO bid
24-40 kg: 60 mg PO bid
>40 kg: Administer as in adults

TABLE 42-2. Pediatric Dose of Oseltamivir for Prophylaxis of Influenza

>1 yr:
<15 kg: 30 mg PO qd for 10 days
>15-23 kg: 45 mg PO qd for 10 days
24-40 kg: 60 mg PO qd for 10 days
>40 kg: Administer as in adults

Prevention
The recommended dose of oseltamivir for prophylaxis of influenza in adults and adolescents 13 years and older following close contact with an infected individual is 75 mg once daily for 10 days. The recommended dose for pediatric patients 1 year and older is shown in Table 42-2.

Diarrhea and Constipation

43

▶ TRAVELERS' DIARRHEA

Travelers' diarrhea (TD) is the most important travel-related illness in terms of frequency and economic impact.

Definition

TD refers to an illness contracted while traveling, although in about 15% of sufferers, symptoms begin after the return home.

Most clinical studies define TD as the passage of three or more unformed stools in a 24-hour period in association with one or more enteric symptoms including the following:
Abdominal cramps
Fever
Fecal urgency
Tenesmus
Passage of bloody, mucoid stools
Nausea and vomiting

Transmission

1. The enteric pathogens that cause TD are usually spread by fecal-oral contamination. Water and food are the most common vehicles.
2. The risk of TD is high among short-stay travelers in the developing tropical regions of Latin America, southern Asia, and Africa.
3. TD is a syndrome and not a specific disease. Although a large percentage of cases is caused by strains of *Escherichia coli,* TD can be caused by any number of water-borne or food-borne enteric pathogens including the following (Table 43-1):
   a. Viruses such as rotavirus and Norwalk virus
   b. Enteric bacteria such as enterotoxigenic *E. coli, Shigella, Campylobacter, Aeromonas, Salmonella,* and *Vibrio*
   c. Intestinal protozoa including *Giardia lamblia, Entamoeba histolytica,* and *Cryptosporidium*
   d. *Cyclospora* (a recently described cyanobacterium-like microorganism)

Signs and Symptoms
1. Acute diarrhea, possibly accompanied by nausea, loss of appetite, abdominal cramps, low-grade fever, and malaise (Table 43-2)
2. Symptoms beginning as early as 8 to 12 hours after contaminated food or water has been ingested

TABLE 43-1. Major Pathogens in Travelers' Diarrhea (Travel to Developing Tropical Regions)

AGENT	FREQUENCY (%)
Bacteria	**50-80**
Enterotoxigenic	
Escherichia coli	5-50
Enteroaggregative *E. coli*	5-30
Salmonella species	1-15
Shigella species	1-15
Campylobacter jejuni	1-30
Aeromonas species	0-10
Plesiomonas shigelloides	0-5
Other	0-5
Viruses	**0-20**
Rotavirus	0-20
Norovirus	1-20
Protozoa	**1-5**
Giardia lamblia	0-5
Entamoeba histolytica	0-5
Cryptosporidium parvum	0-5
Unknown	**10-40**

TABLE 43-2. Pathophysiologic Syndromes in Diarrheal Disease

SYNDROME	AGENT
Acute watery diarrhea	Any agent, especially with toxin-mediated diseases (e.g., enterotoxigenic *Escherichia coli*, *Vibrio cholerae*)
Febrile dysentery	*Shigella*, *Campylobacter jejuni*, *Salmonella*, enteroinvasive *E. coli*, *Aeromonas* species, *Vibrio* species, *Yersinia enterocolitica*, *Entamoeba histolytica*, inflammatory bowel disease
Vomiting (as predominant symptom)	Viral agents, preformed toxins of *Staphylococcus aureus* or *Bacillus cereus*
Persistent diarrhea (>14 days)	Protozoa, small bowel bacterial overgrowth, inflammatory or invasive enteropathogens (*Shigella*, enteroaggregative *E. coli*)
Chronic diarrhea (>30 days)	Small bowel injury, inflammatory bowel disease, irritable bowel syndrome (postinfectious), Brainerd diarrhea

3. Watery diarrheal stools
4. Dysentery (i.e., invasive disease) in 10% to 15% of cases, particularly with *Shigella, Campylobacter jejuni* or *Salmonella* as cause
   a. Passage of bloody stools occurs.
   b. Fever up to 40° C (104° F). Fever is a reaction to an intestinal inflammatory process. High fever suggests that a pathogen has invaded the intestinal mucosa, and classically this has meant bacterial enteropathogens.
   c. Dysentery is often associated with abdominal colic, tenderness, and tenesmus.
5. Dehydration. An important part of the initial assessment is to measure the level of hydration, which includes a determination of vital signs, orthostatic pulse and blood pressure, mental status, skin turgor, hydration of mucous membranes, and urine output. Dehydration is most common in pediatric and elder populations.
6. Vomiting as the predominant symptom suggests food intoxication secondary to enterotoxin produced by *Staphylococcus aureus, Bacillus cereus,* or *Clostridium perfringens* or gastroenteritis secondary to viruses such as rotavirus in infants or norovirus in any age group.
7. An abdominal examination of persons with TD often shows mild tenderness, but there should not be signs of peritoneal irritation.
8. With persistent diarrhea (longer than 14 days' duration), consider possible infection with intestinal parasites such as *G. lamblia, E. histolytica, Cryptosporidium* (see later discussions), *Isospora, Cyclospora,* or less common entities including the following:
   a. Pseudomembranous enterocolitis *(Clostridium difficile)* after recent antibiotic use
   b. Lactase deficiency induced by small-bowel pathogens
   c. Viral enteropathogens such as rotavirus or Norwalk virus
   d. Small-bowel bacterial overgrowth syndrome
   e. Other less common enteric parasites such as *Strongyloides stercoralis* or *Trichuris trichiura*
   f. Postinfective malabsorption syndrome
   g. Tropical sprue
   h. Brainerd diarrhea
   i. Inflammatory bowel disease
   j. Others (see Table 43-2)

Treatment (Table 43-3)
1. TD typically runs a self-limited course of less than 1 week. Recovery without antimicrobial treatment is the norm in healthy adults. However, most travelers choose to avoid

TABLE 43-3. Nonspecific Drugs for Therapy in Adults

AGENT	THERAPEUTIC DOSAGE
Attapulgite	Initially 3 g, then 3 g after each loose stool or every 2 hours (not to exceed 9 g/day); should be safe during pregnancy and childhood (available in 600-mg tabs, or liquid 600 mg/tsp)
Loperamide	Initially 4 mg, then 2 mg after each loose stool (not to exceed 8 to 16 mg/day); do not use in dysenteric diarrhea
Bismuth sub- salicylate	30 mL or two 262-mg tablets every 30 min for 8 doses; may repeat on day 2

the inconvenience and discomfort of diarrhea by seeking medical treatment.

2. Severe, watery TD can cause life-threatening fluid loss. Treating serious dehydration is an urgent priority, especially in elderly persons, young children, and infants.

3. Fluid replacement is the cornerstone of therapy.

   a. Treating dehydration often significantly decreases malaise.

   b. Urine frequency, color, and volume can serve as markers of adequate rehydration and should be monitored qualitatively.

   c. Make sure the victim drinks oral fluids to approximate fluid losses in the stools.

   (1) Generally, any fruit juice alternated with bottled or disinfected water can be used for oral rehydration in mild to moderate diarrhea.

   (2) Packets of oral rehydration salts produced according to World Health Organization (WHO) guidelines can be reconstituted to make oral rehydration solution (see following discussion). These packets are increasingly available in pharmacies throughout the world.

   (3) Sports electrolyte solutions also provide adequate fluid replacement if diluted to about half their strength. Full-strength sports drinks are often hypertonic and may delay gastric absorption.

   (4) Maximum gastrointestinal absorption of water occurs when the consumed drink has a glucose concentration of 2.5%. Highly sweetened drinks such as undiluted apple juice, soft drinks, and undiluted Gatorade have glucose concentrations of 6% or higher.

4. To make an oral rehydration solution (ORS), one of the following methods is generally used:
   a. Method 1: 1 tsp salt, 2 to 3 tbsp sugar or honey, 1 L clean or disinfected water (This formula lacks bicarbonate and potassium.)
   b. Method 2: 8-oz cup orange, apple, or other fruit drink, 3 cups clean or disinfected water, 1 tsp salt (This formula lacks potassium.)
   c. Method 3: half-strength athletic drink such as Gatorade
   d. Method 4: Starch-based ORS solutions such as Ricelyte or Cera-Lyte. These are excellent; they contain rice starch, which decreases osmotic load and enhances absorption, and electrolytes. Unfortunately, these solutions are not always available.
   e. Method 5: Use a WHO formula ORS packet (usually available and inexpensive in most developing countries). Add the packet to 1 L clean or disinfected water. WHO ORS is equivalent to the following:

Sodium chloride 3.5 g
Potassium chloride 1.5 g
Sodium bicarbonate 2.5 g
Glucose 20 g

   f. Method 6—Make a WHO-ORS solution: ½ tsp salt, ¼ tsp salt substitute (potassium chloride), ½ tsp baking soda (bicarbonate), 2 to 3 tbsp table sugar or 2 tbsp honey or Karo syrup, 1 L clean or disinfected water

5. Treatment with intravenous (IV) fluids is indicated for the following:
   a. Patients with hemodynamic decompensation (hypotension)
   b. Inability to retain oral fluids
   c. Systemic compromise (high fever and toxicity)
   d. Moderate toxicity or dehydration and a severe underlying disease
   e. Patients at extremes of age

Nonspecific Therapy

Symptomatic medications are useful for treatment of mild to moderate diarrhea because they decrease symptoms and allow patients to return more quickly to normal activities (see Table 43-3).

Probiotics

Lactobacillus preparations and yogurt are safe, but evidence is insufficient to establish their value in the therapy of acute diarrhea.

Adsorbents

1. Adsorbent agents bind nonspecifically to water and other intraluminal material including bacteria and toxins and potentially to other medications such as antibiotics.
2. The most common medication in this group is attapulgite (see Table 43-3). Attapulgite is a nonabsorbable magnesium aluminum silicate that is more active than the combination of kaolin and pectin (Kaopectate).
3. By adsorbing water, these agents give stools more form or consistency but do not decrease stool frequency, cramps, or duration of illness.

Antimotility Drugs

Narcotic analogs related to opiates are the major antimotility drugs. In addition to slowing intestinal motility, these drugs alter water and electrolyte transport, probably affecting both secretion and absorption.

Use an antiperistaltic drug such as the over-the-counter agents loperamide (Imodium) or diphenoxylate plus atropine (Lomotil) to offer relief to victims with watery diarrhea and cramps.

a. Of the two drugs, loperamide is better tolerated and has fewer central opiate effects than diphenoxylate plus atropine.
b. Avoid antiperistaltic drugs alone (i.e., without antibiotics) if blood or mucus is present in the stool or if victim has signs of serious illness (high fever, recurrent vomiting, severe abdominal pain) because the inhibition of gut motility may facilitate intestinal infection by invasive bacterial enteropathogens. This theoretically deleterious effect does not appear to be an issue when loperamide is used concurrently with an effective antimicrobial agent.
c. Be aware that these drugs can be valuable for long bus rides or summit bids where social constraints make frequent rest stops impractical.
d. Antiperistaltic drugs can be important for controlling fluid balance in a victim with profuse diarrhea who is unable to tolerate sufficient oral fluids to maintain a positive fluid balance.
e. The dose for loperamide is 4 mg for the initial dose and 2 mg after every loose stool, up to a total dose of 8 mg/day.
f. Antiperistaltic drugs should only be used up to a maximum of 48 hours in acute diarrhea.
g. The combination of loperamide plus an antibiotic is a potentially effective single-dose treatment for TD (e.g., ciprofloxacin 750 to 1000 mg single dose, plus loperamide 4 mg).

Antisecretory Drugs

1. Because increased secretion of water and electrolytes is the major physiologic derangement in acute watery diarrhea, therapy aimed at this effect is appealing.
2. Give bismuth subsalicylate (BSS, Pepto-Bismol).
   a. 30 mL BSS liquid or 2 BSS tablets PO q 30 min, maximum eight doses in 24 hours
3. BSS often improves both diarrhea and cramps.
4. This is a reasonable alternative to starting antibiotic therapy in a patient with mild diarrhea.

Antimicrobial Therapy

1. Empiric antimicrobial therapy is indicated in acute TD and febrile, dysenteric illness because of the high frequency of bacteria as an etiologic agent.
2. Travelers with acute diarrhea and mild symptomatology usually do not need empiric antimicrobial therapy and can be treated with oral fluids and electrolytes.
3. Those travelers with acute diarrhea and moderate symptoms (serious enough to change their itinerary) can be treated with antimicrobial empiric therapy or symptomatic therapy with loperamide or bismuth subsalicylate.
4. Travelers with severe and incapacitating symptoms, or with dysentery, should be treated with empiric antimicrobial therapy immediately after the first passage of unformed stool (Table 43-4).
5. Additional considerations follow:
   a. Azithromycin has been found to be a reasonable alternative for the treatment of acute TD. Although it remains to be tested in adequate clinical trials, 500 mg of azithromycin daily for 1 to 3 days appears to be safe and effective.
   b. Resistance to quinolone antibiotics can develop during the treatment of *C. jejuni* infections. Azithromycin (Zithromax) 500 mg tablets, 1 tablet qd for 3 days, may be used for quinolone-resistant *Campylobacter* infections.
   c. Loperamide 4 mg plus ciprofloxacin (Cipro) 750 to 1000 mg may be sufficient as a single-dose treatment for TD but is not commonly recommended.
   d. An individual with a more severe diarrheal syndrome (frequent profuse stools) will often experience relief within hours of beginning empiric antibiotic therapy. Despite the drug's rapid effect, the individual should continue to take the antibiotic for a total of 3 days to prevent relapse.
   e. If the patient has begun initial treatment of diarrhea with BSS therapy, at least 8 hours must elapse before optimum antibiotic therapy can occur because BSS impairs the absorption of oral antimicrobial agents.

TABLE 43-4. Antimicrobial Therapy for Diarrhea in Adults

DIAGNOSIS	RECOMMENDATION
Empiric Therapy in Bacteriologically Unconfirmed Disease	
Travelers' diarrhea	Rifaximin 200 mg tid or 400 mg bid for 3 days; norfloxacin 400 mg bid, ciprofloxacin 500 mg bid or levofloxacin 500 mg qd for 1 to 3 days; or azithromycin 500-1000 mg single dose
Febrile and/or dysenteric disease	Norfloxacin 400 mg bid, ciprofloxacin 500 mg bid, levofloxacin 500 mg qd for 3 days; or azithromycin 500-1000 mg qd for 3 days
Persistent diarrhea	Consider a trial with metronidazole 250 mg qid for 7 days
Organism-Specific Therapy in Laboratory-Confirmed Diarrhea	
Enterotoxigenic and enteroaggregative *Escherichia coli* diarrhea	Rifaximin 200 mg tid or 400 mg bid for 3 days; ciprofloxacin 1000 mg single dose or 500 mg bid for 1 to 3 days; norfloxacin 400 mg bid or levofloxacin 500 mg qd for 1 to 3 days; or azithromycin 500-1000 mg single dose
Cholera	Ciprofloxacin 1000 mg single dose or 500 mg bid for 3 days; norfloxacin 400 mg bid or levofloxacin 500 mg qd for 3 days or doxycycline 300-mg single dose
Salmonellosis (typhoid fever or systemic infection)	Norfloxacin 400 mg bid, ciprofloxacin 500 mg bid, or levofloxacin 500 mg qd for 7 to 10 days; in patients with underlying disease or immunocompromised persons
Salmonellosis (intestinal nontyphoid salmonellosis without systemic infection)	Antimicrobial therapy controversial (see text)
Shigellosis	Norfloxacin 400 mg bid, ciprofloxacin 500 mg bid, levofloxacin 500 mg qd for 3 days
Campylobacteriosis	Erythromycin 500 mg qid for 5 days; azithromycin 500-1000 mg qd, norfloxacin 400 mg bid, ciprofloxacin 500 mg bid or levofloxacin 500 mg qd for 3 days
Enteropathogenic *E. coli* diarrhea	Unclear if antimicrobial therapy is necessary
Clostridium difficile colitis	Metronidazole 250 mg qid to 500 mg tid; or vancomycin 125 mg qid for 7 to 14 days

bid, twice daily; qd, daily; qid, four times daily; tid, three times daily.

   f. If blood or mucus is present in the stool, advise the victim to take an antibiotic as described earlier but to refrain from using antiperistaltic medications alone (i.e., without an antibiotic).

   g. If the patient is ill with what appears to be a resistant bacterial pathogen, a viral or parasitic infection, or a toxin-induced gastroenteritis (food poisoning), be aware that antibiotic therapy will not alter the course of the diarrhea.

   h. Advise any victim who does not respond to empiric antibiotic treatment or who has diarrhea for more than 1 week to obtain clinical follow-up that includes a complete workup for bacterial and parasitic pathogens.

   i. Because fluoroquinolones are not yet approved for use in children, TMP/SMX plus a macrolide, nalidixic acid, or azithromycin may be given.

   j. Rifaximin is a new antibacterial rifamycin derivative indicated for the treatment of infectious diarrhea and other conditions of the gastrointestinal tract. It is virtually unabsorbed by the oral route, leading to fewer systemic adverse reactions. Rifaximin may prove to be the ideal drug for TD. Large clinical studies are pending.

Prevention

1. Take dietary precautions. The risk of illness is lowest when most of a traveler's meals are self-prepared and eaten in a private home, highest when food is obtained from street vendors, and intermediate when food is consumed at public restaurants. Unfortunately, many studies evaluating risk have found little correlation between routine precautions and illness.

   a. Dietary recommendations to decrease the potential for transmission of fecal pathogens through food and water are as follows:

      (1) Avoid tap water and ice made from untreated water (most enteric organisms can survive freezing).

      (2) Low-quality bottled water may be contaminated; inquire about the best brands.

      (3) Bottled and carbonated drinks, beer, and wine are probably safe.

      (4) Boiled or disinfected water is safe.

      (5) Alcohol in mixed drinks does not disinfect.

      (6) Homemade beverages cannot be guaranteed.

      (7) Ice in block form is often handled with unsanitary methods.

      (8) Avoid unpasteurized cheese and dairy products.

(9) Avoid raw vegetables and salads, which may be contaminated by fertilization with human waste or washing with contaminated water.

(10) Anything that can be peeled or have the surface removed is generally safe.

(11) Fruits and hearty vegetables can be disinfected by immersion and washing in iodinated water or by exposure to boiling water for 30 seconds.

(12) Avoid raw seafood and fish.

(13) Avoid raw meat because adequate cooking kills all microorganisms and parasites. If the meat is left at room temperature and recontaminated, cooked food can incubate pathogenic bacteria.

b. Safe foods usually include the following:

(1) Well-cooked foods served steaming hot

(2) Baked foods (e.g., bread)

(3) Foods with high sugar content (e.g., syrups, jellies)

(4) Peeled fruits (if you are the peeler)

2. Use of prophylactic medications to prevent TD.

a. Of the nonantibiotic drugs, only BSS (Pepto-Bismol) has been shown by controlled studies to offer reasonable protection and safety. The current recommended dose of BSS (for prevention) is 2 tablets 4 times per day. Mild side effects include constipation, nausea, and blackened tongue or stools. BSS taken concurrently with antibiotics should be avoided because of the potential binding of BSS to the antibiotic, which prevents absorption.

b. Do not give BSS to someone with a history of aspirin allergy.

c. Give BSS with caution to small children; people with gout or renal insufficiency; and those taking probenecid, methotrexate, anticoagulants, or products containing aspirin.

3. Antimicrobial prophylaxis for TD.

a. A broad-spectrum antibiotic taken during travel can effectively prevent illness, but resolution of TD within a few hours can usually be obtained after oral antibiotic therapy with an oral quinolone antibiotic. It is probably unnecessary for the average traveler to ingest an antibiotic for the full duration of a trip. Travelers wanting to avoid illness can initiate empiric antibiotic therapy immediately after the onset of symptoms.

b. Antimicrobial prophylaxis of TD might be a reasonable strategy for residents of a low-risk country going to a high-risk area for fewer than 5 weeks with one or more of the following:

(1) Underlying illness such as acquired immunodeficiency syndrome (AIDS); inflammatory bowel disease; or a cardiac, renal, or central nervous system disorder

(2) An itinerary that is so rigid and critical that a person cannot tolerate any inconvenience caused by signs and symptoms; such travelers include competitive athletes, politicians, sales representatives, and people going to special events.

c. For specific antibiotic therapy recommended to prevent TD see Table 43-5.

d. Despite its dramatic protection against diarrhea, the routine use of antimicrobial prophylaxis by travelers is not recommended because of the following:

(1) Potential for adverse side effects

(2) Alteration of normal bacterial flora

TABLE 43-5. Prophylactic Medications for Prevention of Traveler's Diarrhea*

AGENT	PROTECTIVE EFFICACY	PROPHYLAC-TIC DOSE	COMMENT
Bismuth sub-salicylate	65%	Two 262-mg tablets before meals and at bedtime	Safe; temporary darkening of stools and tongue
Fluoroqui-nolones	90%	Norfloxacin 400 mg, ciprofloxacin 500 mg, or levofloxacin 500 mg once a day	Side effects, increased resistance
Rifaximin	70%-80%	Rifaximin 200 mg once or twice a day with meals	Safe, nonabsorbable, no increased resistance; should be considered the standard agent for prophylaxis during high-risk travel

*Not generally recommended for travelers; used only in special situations (see text) and for no longer than 3 weeks.

(3) Tendency to "lower one's guard." Travelers taking prophylactic antibiotics may relax their vigilance, which can increase their risk of acquiring other nonbacterial infections.

▶ FOOD POISONING

Food poisoning results when toxins produced by bacteria are found in foods in concentrations sufficient to produce symptoms. This is not an infection, but a true poisoning. Most food poisoning is caused by *S. aureus* or *B. cereus*.

Signs and Symptoms
1. Diarrhea that develops within 6 to 12 hours after a suspicious meal, most likely caused by ingesting a preformed toxin
2. Often a common source is found to have affected multiple persons
3. Usually preceded by severe nausea and vomiting
4. Symptoms usually limited to 24 hours
5. Physical examination nonspecific

Treatment
1. Treatment is directed toward fluid and electrolyte replacement and the control of nausea.
2. No specific antibiotic therapy exists.

▶ INFECTION CAUSED BY INTESTINAL PROTOZOA

All intestinal protozoa are transmitted by the fecal-oral route. Protozoa typically cause subacute or chronic gastrointestinal symptoms but may also invade the bowel wall and cause severe dysentery with an acute presentation.

Giardia lamblia
G. lamblia is a flagellate protozoan with a life cycle that involves two forms. Trophozoites are responsible for symptomatic illness. They are rarely infective because they die quickly outside of the body. Some trophozoites encyst and are passed in the stools of infected hosts. Cysts are typically the form passed through fecal-oral contact and cause infection. Cysts are hardy in the external environment and retain viability in cold water for as long as 2 or 3 months. The infective dose of *Giardia* for humans is 10 to 25 cysts.

Giardiasis is a zoonosis with cross-infectivity from animals to humans. Animals that have been implicated as carriers include beavers, cattle, dogs, cats, rodents, sheep, and deer. In North America, *Giardia* is transmitted primarily through drinking water. Worldwide, person-to-person transmission may be more common.

Signs and Symptoms

1. Average incubation period 1 to 3 weeks
2. Sometimes abrupt onset of explosive, watery diarrhea accompanied by abdominal cramps, foul flatus, vomiting, fever, and malaise; typically lasts 3 to 4 days before transition to more common subacute syndrome
3. Onset usually insidious, with symptoms that wax and wane
4. Stools becoming mushy and malodorous
5. Watery diarrhea alternating with soft stools and even constipation
6. Middle and upper abdominal cramping, substantial burning acid indigestion, sulfurous belching, nausea, bowel distention, early satiety, foul flatus
7. Dysenteric symptoms (blood and pus in the stool) not features of giardiasis; fever and vomiting infrequent except during initial onset
8. May develop into a chronic process associated with malabsorption and weight loss

Treatment

1. Treatment in the wilderness is typically initiated empirically.
2. Note that a cure can be achieved with one of several drugs. However, no drug is effective in all cases. In resistant cases, longer courses of two drugs taken concurrently may be effective.
3. Relapse may occur up to several weeks after treatment, which requires a second course of the same medication or an alternative drug.
4. Three groups of drugs are currently being used (Table 43-6):
   a. Nitroimidazoles (metronidazole, tinidazole, albendazole, ornidazole, nimorazole)
   b. Nitrofuran derivatives (furazolidone)
   c. Acridine compounds (mepacrine, quinacrine)
5. Metronidazole (Flagyl, 250 mg three times a day for 5 to 7 days for adults) is often used in the United States. Cure rates of 85% to 90% are comparable with those with quinacrine but with better tolerance.
6. Tinidazole (Fasigyn, 2000 mg in a single dose) has the same success rate with better compliance and is now approved for use in the United States. Nitazoxanide (Alinia) has comparable efficacy to metronidazole and is available in suspension for children as young as 1 year of age (100 mg twice a day for 3 days for younger than 4 years, 200 mg twice a day for 3 days for ages 4 to 11 years, 500 mg twice a day for adults).
7. Quinacrine (Atabrine, 100 mg three times a day for 5 days for adults and 7mg/kg/day in three divided doses for 5 days

TABLE 43-6. Antiparasitic Therapy for Infectious Diarrhea in Adults

DIAGNOSIS	RECOMMENDATION
Giardiasis	Metronidazole 250 mg tid (15 mg/kg/day for children), albendazole* 400 mg qd, or quinacrine† 100 mg tid for 7 days; or tinidazole* 2000-mg single dose; or nitazoxanide 500 mg bid for 3 days (100 mg bid for 3 days for children 1 to 4 yr of age; 200 mg bid for 3 days for children 4 to 11 yr of age)
Entamoeba histolytica excretion (asymptomatic)	Iodoquinol 650 mg tid for 20 days or paromomycin 500 mg tid for 7 days
Entamoeba histolytica diarrhea	Metronidazole 750 mg tid for 5 to 10 days or tinidazole* 1000 mg bid for 3 days, followed by iodoquinol 650 mg tid for 20 days or paromomycin 500 mg tid for 7 days
Cryptosporidiosis	Nitazoxanide 500 mg bid for 3 days; in severe cases or patients with AIDS, consider nitazoxanide 500 mg bid for 2 wk, paromomycin 500-750 mg tid or qid for 2 wk; or azithromycin 1200 mg qd for 4 wk
Cyclosporidiosis	TMP/SMX 160 mg/800 mg bid for 7 days, followed by 160 mg/800 mg 3 times/wk in patients with AIDS
Isosporiasis	TMP/SMX 160 mg/800 mg qid for 10 days, followed by 160 mg/800 mg bid for 3 wk, or pyrimethamine 75 mg qd with folinic acid 10 mg qd for 2 wk
Microsporidiosis	Albendazole* 400 mg bid for 2 to 4 wk, followed by chronic suppression in patients with AIDS

*Albendazole and tinidazole were recently approved and are available in the United States.
†Quinacrine is not commercially available in the United States.
bid, twice daily; qd, daily; qid, four times daily; tid, three times daily; TMP/SMX, trimethoprim and sulfamethoxazole.

for children) achieves cure rates of about 95%. Unfortunately, it is no longer available in the United States because it produces more frequent side effects, especially in children. No pediatric liquid form is available.

8. For use in severely symptomatic individuals or pregnant women, the nonabsorbable drug paromomycin (Humatin, 25 to 30 mg/kg in three divided doses for 5 to 10 days) has been effective. When considering treatment during pregnancy, when possible, withhold treatment until after discussing with an obstetrician because none of the treatment options is considered completely safe (see Table 43-6).

Entamoeba histolytica

Entamoeba histolytica is found worldwide. Approximately 10% of the world's population carries the parasite. The prevalence in tropical countries is 30% to 50%. Despite its high prevalence, amebiasis accounts for less than 1% of cases of TD.

As with *Giardia*, the life cycle of *E. histolytica* involves two forms and one host. When a cyst is ingested through fecal contamination of food or water or via person-to-person contact, it divides and produces trophozoites. The trophozoites are the reproductive form, residing in the host and causing illness. The trophozoite cannot survive the external environment and is unlikely to transmit infection. Encystment occurs in the gut, and cysts pass in the stool. The cysts are typically infectious when they are passed. Extraintestinal disease sometimes occurs by hematogenous spread. Abscesses develop primarily in the liver but may also involve the brain and lungs.

▶ NONDYSENTERIC DISEASE

Signs and Symptoms
80% to 99% of infections result in an asymptomatic carrier state. In individuals who develop illness, the following may be noted:
1. Most often, colonic inflammation without dysentery, causing lower abdominal cramping and altered stools
2. Weight loss, anorexia, nausea
3. Subacute infection developing into a nondysenteric bowel syndrome with symptoms of intermittent diarrhea, abdominal pain, weight loss, and flatulence

▶ DYSENTERIC (INVASIVE) DISEASE

Signs and Symptoms
1. Dysentery developing suddenly or after a period of mild symptoms
2. Symptoms developing in as few as 8 to 10 days, but more often after weeks to months
3. Ill appearance, with frequent bloody stools, tenesmus, moderate to severe abdominal pain and tenderness, and fever (considerable variation in severity)
4. Rarely, significant fever
5. Complications in 1% to 4% of victims: bowel perforation, toxic megacolon, strictures, or an ameboma (inflammatory lesion containing trophozoites that develops in the colon)
6. Amoebic liver abscess acutely or years after infection
7. In the wilderness, diagnosis considered in any victim with dysentery who is not responding to an appropriate antibiotic
8. Asymptomatic cyst shedding and active gastrointestinal illness that persist for years if amebiasis is not treated

Treatment (see Table 43-6)
1. In general, treatment is effective for invasive infections but disappointing for luminal infections (no regimen is completely effective in eradicating intestinal infection).
2. Treatment is based on the location of the infection and the degree of symptoms.
3. Medications are divided as follows:
   a. Tissue amebicides, which are well absorbed and combat invasive amebiasis in the bowel and liver
   b. Luminal drugs, which are poorly absorbed and act primarily within the gut
4. Treat invasive disease with a tissue-active drug followed by a luminal agent.
5. For oral therapy, note that high-dose metronidazole (Flagyl) is the drug of choice (750 mg tid for 5 to 10 days).
6. Give the luminal-acting drug iodoquinol (diiodohydroxyquin, Yodoxin) 650 mg tid for 20 days.
7. Tinidazole (Tiniba, Fasgyn), which was recently approved and is now available in the United States, can be given 1000 mg bid for 3 days followed by iodoquinol 650 mg tid for 20 days or paromomycin 500 mg tid for 7 days.
8. Emetine and dehydroemetine (1 mg/kg/day, maximum 90 mg/day) are used parenterally in severe cases of amebiasis, primarily extraintestinal, followed by iodoquinol for 20 days. These two drugs have frequent systemic side effects including the development of cardiac arrhythmias requiring hospitalization for cardiac monitoring. Because this class of drugs is related to ipecac, the drugs also cause vomiting.

▶ CRYPTOSPORIDIUM

Cryptosporidium is a coccidian parasite that belongs to the phyla Sporozoa. It is a re-emergent enteric pathogen in humans. The infection has been described in those who have contact with animals such as veterinarians and farmers; infants in day care centers; travelers to endemic areas; and AIDS or other immunocompromised patients. It may infect large numbers of individuals in community-wide waterborne outbreaks. *Cryptosporidium* has attracted renewed interest recently because of an increase in reported cases. Ingestion of untreated surface water, well water, or raw milk has been implicated as methods of transmission. Foodborne transmission is also suspected.

Signs and Symptoms
1. Syndrome generally mild and self-limited (typical duration of 5 to 6 days, range 2 to 26 days)
2. Asymptomatic infection may occur

3. Definitive diagnosis by stool examination or serologic techniques

4. Watery diarrhea (without blood or pus); abdominal cramps; nausea; flatulence; and, at times, vomiting and low-grade fever

5. Immunocompromised hosts experience more frequent and prolonged infections, with profuse chronic watery diarrhea, malabsorption, and weight loss lasting months to years

Treatment
1. No clearly effective treatment has been found.
2. The disease is usually mild and self-limited in immunocompetent hosts; therefore only supportive care is necessary.
3. Anticryptosporidial agents such as paromomycin (500 to 750 mg 3 or 4 times a day for 2 weeks) and azithromycin (1200 mg daily for 4 weeks) may be used in immunocompetent persons with persistent infection and in immuno-compromised patients.

▶ CYCLOSPORA CAYETANENSIS

Cyclospora is a protozoan parasite found in the ground water of developing countries. It was first discovered as a cause of diarrhea among travelers visiting Nepal. The organism has shown to be an important cause of acute and protracted diarrhea. *Cyclospora* is endemic in many developing countries in all continents, with the highest rates occurring in Nepal, Haiti, and Peru. In the United States most of the native outbreaks have been from areas east of the Rocky Mountains, usually associated with ingestion of contaminated imported raspberries.

Signs and Symptoms
1. The onset of diarrhea is usually abrupt.
2. *Cyclospora* causes a protracted watery diarrhea that can persist for weeks.
3. Definitive diagnosis is made by finding the microorganism in a stool sample treated with a modified acid-fast stain.

Treatment
1. Unfortunately, *Cyclospora* is resistant to halogen-based water disinfection methods (e.g., iodine and chlorine).
2. It is best killed by bringing drinking water to a boil.
3. The treatment of choice is TMP/SMX (160/800 mg 4 times a day for 10 days)

▶ CONSTIPATION

Constipation is a common malady on many wilderness sojourns. The most common cause for constipation on backcountry trips is dehydration. Additionally, lack of roughage from eating foods often void of natural fiber may contribute. On certain trips, psychologic factors including apprehension about using primitive toilet facilities and simple inconvenience may be a factor.

Treatment
1. Increase fluid intake.
2. Patients should be advised to drink eight glasses of water daily.
3. Patients should try to drink an extra glass of water for every drink of coffee, tea, or alcohol (i.e., diuretics).
4. Increase dietary fiber.
   a. It is helpful to bring along bran or psyllium seed (e.g., Metamucil) or methylcellulose (Citrucel) for this purpose.
   b. Patients should ingest plenty of water or taking fiber can be counterproductive.
   c. Fiber is not a laxative and will not typically induce an immediate bowel movement.
   d. Fiber products such as psyllium or methylcellulose may cause gas or bloating.
   e. If fruits and vegetables are available, the patient should eat plenty of them.
5. Stool softeners such as docusate sodium (Colace 50 to 500 mg/day PO in 1 to 4 divided doses) enhance the absorption of water and fat into stool, causing stool to soften. These drugs can be helpful, but they often lose their effectiveness over time.
6. At times a stronger stimulant medication may be indicated. Dozens of products are on the market.
7. Bisacodyl (Dulcolax) is generally safe and effective.
   a. Bisacodyl should be taken with a full glass of water.
   b. The patient should swallow the tablets or capsules whole (i.e., do not chew or crush them).
8. Bisacodyl is also available as a rectal suppository. To use a rectal suppository follow these steps:
   a. If it is warm and the suppository is soft, insert it (in its wrapping) into cold water for 1 or 2 minutes before use.
   b. After removing the wrapper, moisten the suppository with water or petroleum jelly.
   c. The patient should lie on his or her side.
   d. With the pointed end first, push the suppository into the rectum.
   e. The suppository should be retained for 15 to 20 minutes.

Field Water Disinfection

44

▶ RISK AND ETIOLOGY

Infectious agents in contaminated drinking water with the potential for waterborne transmission include bacteria, viruses, protozoa, and parasites. Risk of waterborne illness depends on the number of organisms consumed, which is determined by the volume of water, concentration of organisms, and treatment system efficiency (Boxes 44-1 to 44-3).

▶ DEFINITIONS

1. Disinfection, the desired result of field water treatment, means the removal or destruction of harmful microorganisms.
2. Pasteurization is similar to disinfection but specifically refers to the use of heat, usually at temperatures below 100° C (212° F), to kill most pathogenic organisms.
3. Disinfection and pasteurization should not be confused with sterilization, which is the destruction or removal of all life forms.
4. The goal of disinfection is to achieve potable water, indicating only that a water source, on average over a period of time, contains a "minimal microbial hazard" so that the statistical likelihood of illness is acceptable.
5. Water sterilization is not necessary because not all organisms are enteric human pathogens.
6. Purification is the removal of organic or inorganic chemicals and particulate matter to remove offensive color, taste, and odor. The term is frequently used interchangeably with "disinfection," but purification may not remove or kill enough microorganisms to ensure microbiologic safety (Box 44-4).

▶ HEAT

1. The boiling time required is important when fuel is limited.
2. Enteric pathogens including cysts, bacteria, viruses, and parasites can be killed at a temperature well below boiling.
3. Thermal death is a function of both time and temperature; therefore lower temperatures are effective with longer contact times
4. Microorganisms have varying sensitivity to heat; however, all common enteric pathogens are readily inactivated by heat (Table 44-1).

Box 44-1. Waterborne Enteric Pathogens

BACTERIAL
Escherichia coli
Shigella
Campylobacter
Vibrio cholerae
Salmonella
Yersinia enterocolitica
Aeromonas

VIRAL
Hepatitis A
Hepatitis E
Norovirus
Poliovirus
Miscellaneous enterics (>100 types: e.g., adenovirus, enterovirus, calicivirus, ECHO viruses, astrovirus, coronavirus)
Giardia lamblia
Entamoeba histolytica
Cryptosporidium
Blastocystis hominis
Isospora belli
Balantidium coli
Acanthamoeba
Cyclospora

PARASITIC
Ascaris lumbricoides
Ancylostoma duodenale (hookworm)
Taenia spp. (tapeworm)
Fasciola hepatica (sheep liver fluke)
Dracunculus medinensis
Strongyloides stercoralis
Trichuris trichiura (whipworm)
Clonorchis sinensis (oriental liver fluke)
Paragonimus westermani (lung fluke)
Diphyllobothrium latum (fish tapeworm)
Echinococcus granulosus (hydatid disease)

ECHO, enteropathic cytopathogenic human orphan.

5. Given its environmental stability and clinical virulence, hepatitis A virus is a special concern. It should respond to heat as do other enteric viruses, but data indicate that it has greater thermal resistance.
6. The boiling point decreases with the lower atmospheric pressure present at high elevations (Table 44-2). Because heat inactivation occurs below typical boiling temperatures,

---

Box 44-2.   Enteric Pathogens in U.S. Wilderness or Recreational Water

COMMONLY REPORTED
Giardia
Cryptosporidium

OCCASIONALLY REPORTED WITH FIRM EIDENCE FOR WATERBORNE
Campylobacter
Hepatitis A
Hepatitis E
Enterotoxigenic *Escherichia coli*
E. coli 0157:H7
Shigella
Enteric viruses

UNUSUAL OCCURRENCES, WATERBORNE SUSPECTED
Yersinia enterocolitica
Aeromonas hydrophila
Cyanobacterium (blue-green algae)

Box 44-3.   Water Quality: Key Points

- In wilderness water, most sediment is inorganic and clarity is not an indication of microbiologic purity.
- In general, cloudiness indicates higher risk of contamination.
- A major factor determining the amount of microbe pollution in surface water is human and animal activity in the watershed.
- Streams do not purify themselves.
- Settling effect of lakes may make them safer than streams, but care should be taken not to disturb bottom sediments when obtaining water.
- Groundwater is generally cleaner than surface water because of the filtration action of overlying sediments.

---

elevation should not make a large difference (unless hepatitis A is of concern).

7. The 10-minute boiling rule is for the sterilization of water including the destruction of heat-resistant bacterial spores, which are generally not enteric pathogens. Disinfection of water requires less than 10 minutes. Pasteurization of food and beverages is accomplished at 65° C (150° F) for 30 minutes or at 71° C (160° F) for 1 to 5 minutes. Enteric

---

Box 44-4. Heat

ADVANTAGES
- Does not impart additional taste or color to water
- Single-step process that inactivates all enteric pathogens
- Efficacy is *not* compromised by contaminants or particles in the water, as happens with halogenation and filtration
- Can pasteurize water without sustained boiling

DISADVANTAGES
- Does not improve the taste, smell, or appearance of poor-quality water
- Fuel sources may be scarce, expensive, or unavailable
- Does not prevent recontamination during storage

Relative susceptibility of microorganisms to heat: protozoa > bacteria > viruses.

pathogens are killed within seconds by boiling water and rapidly at temperatures above 60° C (140° F). The majority of the time required raising the temperature of water to the boiling point works toward disinfection, so water is safe to drink by the time it has reached a full boil. For an extra margin of safety (e.g., hepatitis A), keep the water covered and hot for several minutes after boiling or boil for 1 full minute (up to 3 minutes at high altitude).

8. A pressure cooker saves time and fuel at all elevations.
9. Pasteurization has been successfully achieved using solar heating. A solar cooker constructed from a foil-lined cardboard box with a glass window in the lid can be used for disinfecting large amounts of water by pasteurization. This could be a low-cost method for improving water quality, especially in refugee camps and disaster areas (see "Ultraviolet Light" later; Tables 44-1 to Table 44-2; Box 44-5).

▶ FILTRATION AND CLARIFICATION

Filtration

1. Field filters that rely solely on the mechanical removal of microorganisms may be adequate for cysts and bacteria but may not reliably remove viruses, which are a major concern in water where high levels of fecal contamination are present (e.g., in developing countries).
2. They have the advantages of being simple and requiring no holding time.

TABLE 44-1. Data on Heat Inactivation of Microorganisms as Reported in the Literature

ORGANISM	LETHAL TEMPERATURE/TIME
Giardia	55° C (131° F) for 5 min
	100° C (212° F) immediately
	50° C (122° F) for 10 min (95% inactivation)
	60° C (140° F) for 10 min (98% inactivation)
	70° C (158° F) for 10 min (100% inactivation)
	55° C (131° F)
Entamoeba histolytica	Similar to *Giardia*
Nematode cysts, helminth eggs, larvae, cercariae	50-55° C (122-131° F)
Cryptosporidium	45-55° C (113-131° F) for 20 min
	55° C (131° F) warmed over 20 min
	64.2° C (148° F) within 2 min
	72° C (162° F) heated up over 1 min
Escherichia coli	55° C (131° F) for 30 min
	60-62° C (140-144° F) for 10 min
Salmonella and *Shigella*	65° C (149° F) for <1 min
Vibrio cholerae	60-62° C (140-144° F) for 10 min
	100° C (212° F) for 30 sec
E. coli, Salmonella, Shigella, Campylobacter	60° C (140° F) for 3 min (3-log reduction)
	65° C (149° F) for 3 min (all but few *Campylobacter*)
	75° C (167° F) for 3 min (100% kill)
E. coli	50° C (122° F) for 10 min ineffective
	60° C (140° F) for 5 min
	70° C (158° F) for 1 min
Viruses	55-60° C (131-140° F) within 20-40 min
	70° C (158° F) for >1 min
Hepatitis A	98° C (208° F) for 1 min
	85° C (185° F) for 1 min
	61° C (142° F) for 10 min (50% disintegrated)
	60° C (140° F) for 19 min (in shellfish)
Hepatitis E	60° C (140° F) for 30 min
Bacterial spores	>100° C (212° F)

TABLE 44-2. Boiling Temperatures at Various Altitudes

ALTITUDE (ft)	ALTITUDE (m)	BOILING POINT
5000	1524	95° C (203° F)
10,000	3048	90° C (194° F)
14,000	4267	86° C (187° F)
19,000	5791	81° C (179° F)

Box 44-5. Summary of Clarification Techniques

TECHNIQUE	PROCESS USES	ADVANTAGES
Sedimentation	Settling by gravity of large particulates	Requires long time Greatly improves water aesthetics
Coagulation-flocculation	Removes suspended particles, most microorganisms, some dissolved substances	Simple process, easily applied in field Greatly improves water quality Improves efficacy of filtration and chemical disinfection
Activated charcoal	Removes organic and some inorganic chemicals	Removes toxins such as pesticides and removes chemical disinfectants Improves taste of water
Filtration	Physical and chemical process	Removes microorganisms If charcoal stage, may improve taste and remove chemicals

3. They do not add any unpleasant taste and may improve taste and appearance of water.
4. Most viruses adhere to larger particles or clump together into larger aggregates that may be removed by a filter. However, filtration is not an adequate method to eliminate viruses because the infectious dose of an enteric virus may be quite small. Filters are often expensive and can add considerable weight and bulk to a backpack.

5. Some devices are designed as purely mechanical filters, whereas others combine filtration with granular activated carbon (GAC). Most of the filters containing iodine resins have been withdrawn from the market. Currently only one drink-through bottle uses an iodine resin.

6. The filter pore size required to remove microorganisms effectively is difficult to determine. Microorganisms possess elasticity and deform under pressure, making it possible for them to squeeze through filter pores. Most field filters are depth filters with maze-like passageways that trap particles and organisms smaller than the average diameter of a passage.

7. Being familiar with the functional removal rate of certain organisms rather than with the rated pore size of the filter is more useful and important. Good testing data are necessary to back claims; however, objective comparative data are not generally available.

8. The size of a microorganism is the primary determinant of its susceptibility to filtration. Filters are rated by their ability to retain particles of a certain size, which is described by two terms. Absolute rating means that 100% of a certain size of particle is retained. Nominal rating indicates that more than 90% of a given particle size will be retained.

9. All filters eventually clog from suspended particulate matter, present even in clear streams, requiring cleaning or replacement of the filter. The ability to easily service a unit in the field is an advantage.

10. As a filter clogs, it requires increasing pressure to drive water through it, which can force microorganisms through the filter.

Reverse Osmosis

1. A reverse-osmosis filter uses high pressure (100 to 800 psi) to force water through a semipermeable membrane that filters out dissolved ions, molecules, and solids.

2. Reverse osmosis is generally used for desalinating water.

3. It may also be used to remove biologic contaminants.

4. Small hand-pumped reverse osmosis units have been developed. High price and slow output currently limit their use by land-based wilderness travelers.

5. Essential survival item for ocean travelers (Box 44-6; Table 44-3).

Clarification of cloudy water can be achieved by sedimentation, coagulation-flocculation (C-F), or adsorption.

1. Large particles settle by gravity over 1 to 2 hours in sedimentation. Although filters remove particulate debris, thus

Box 44-6. Filtration

ADVANTAGES

- Simple to operate
- Mechanical filters require no holding time for treatment (water is treated as it comes out of the filter)
- Large choice of commercial products
- Adds no unpleasant taste and often improves taste and appearance of water
- Rationally combined with halogens for removal or destruction of all pathogenic waterborne microbes

DISADVANTAGES

- Adds bulk and weight to baggage
- Most filters not reliable for removal of viruses
- Expensive relative to chemical treatment
- Channeling of water or high pressure can force microorganisms through the filter
- Eventually clogs from suspended particulate matter; may require some maintenance or repair in field

Susceptibility of microorganisms to filtration: protozoa > bacteria > viruses.

TABLE 44-3. Microorganism Susceptibility to Filtration

ORGANISM	AVERAGE SIZE (mm)	MAXIMUM RECOMMENDED FILTER RATING (mm)
Viruses	0.03	N/S
Escherichia coli	0.5 × 3-8	0.2-0.4
Campylobacter	0.2-0.4 × 1.5-3.5	Same as above
Microsporidia	1-2	N/S
Cryptosporidium oocyst	2-6	1
Giardia cyst	6-10 × 8-15	3-5
Entamoeba histolytica cyst	5-30 (average 10)	Same as *Giardia*
Cyclospora	8-10	Same as *Giardia*
Nematode eggs	30-40 × 50-80	20
Schistosome cercariae	50 × 100	Coffee filter or fine cloth
Dracunculus larvae	20 × 500	Coffee filter or fine cloth

N/S, Not specified.

improving the appearance and taste of "dirty" water, they clog quickly if the water contains large particles.

2. Smaller suspended particles can be removed by coagulation-flocculation (C-F). This is accomplished in the field by adding alum (aluminum potassium sulfate) (Box 44-7). Alum is used in the food industry as a pickling powder and is nontoxic. C-F will remove contaminants that cause an unpleasant color and taste, some dissolved metals, and some microorganisms (Table 44-4).

Halogens

Halogens (chlorine and iodine) are effective disinfectants that are active against bacteria, viruses, *Giardia*, and cysts of amebae, excluding *Cryptosporidium*. They are readily available and inexpensive.

Box 44-7. Water Clarification Using Alum

1. Add a pinch of alum to each gallon of water.
2. Mix well, stir occasionally for 30 minutes, and then allow 30 to 60 minutes for settling.
3. The water should clear; if it does not, add another pinch of alum.
4. Decant or pour the water through a paper filter to remove clumps of flocculate.
5. Granular activated charcoal (GAC) removes organic pollutants, chemicals, and radioactive particles by adsorption. This improves the color, taste, and smell of the water. Although some microorganisms adhere to GAC or become trapped in charcoal filters, GAC does not remove all microorganisms, so it does not disinfect.
6. GAC can be used to remove halogens (iodine, chlorine) after disinfection.
7. If GAC is used to remove iodine or chlorine, wait until after the required contact time for disinfection before running water through charcoal or adding charcoal to the water.
8. Filters that use iodine resins, followed by GAC, rely on a different dynamic for disinfection.
9. Although residual-free iodine is largely removed by GAC, iodine is thought to remain bound to microorganisms following the resin pass-through and GAC pass-through phases.
10. The necessary contact time for iodine resins is not absolutely determined, but it is clearly less than that required with standard iodine solutions.

TABLE 44-4. Factors Affecting Halogen Disinfection

	EFFECT	COMPENSATION
Primary Factors		
Concentration	Measured in milligrams per liter (mg/L) or the equivalent, parts per million (ppm); higher concentration increases rate and proportion of microorganisms killed.	Higher concentration allows shorter contact time for equivalent results. Lower concentration requires increased contact time.
Contact time	Usually measured in minutes; longer contact time assures higher proportion of organisms killed.	Contact time is inversely related to concentration; longer time allows lower concentration.
Secondary Factors		
Temperature	Cold slows reaction time.	Some treatment protocols recommend doubling the dose (concentration) of halogen in cold water, but if time allows, exposure time can be increased instead, or the temperature of the water can be increased.
Water contaminants, cloudy water (turbidity)	Halogen reacts with organic nitrogen compounds from decomposition of organisms and their wastes to form compounds with little or no disinfecting ability, effectively decreasing the concentration of available halogen. In general, turbidity increases halogen demand.	Doubling the dose of halogen for cloudy water is a crude means of compensation that often results in a strong halogen taste on top of the taste of the contaminants. A more rational approach is to first clarify water to reduce halogen demand.
pH	The optimal pH for halogen disinfection is 6.5 to 7.5. As water becomes more alkaline, approaching pH 8.0, much higher doses of halogens are required.	Most surface water is neutral to slightly acidic, so compensating for pH is not necessary. Tablet formulations of halogen have the advantage of some buffering capacity.

Concentration and Demand

1. Disinfection with halogens depends on both the concentration of halogen and the amount of time the halogen is in contact with the water (contact time). An increase in one allows a decrease in the other.
2. Minor factors affecting this method include the water temperature (cold slows reaction time) and presence of organic contaminants in the water, which react with halogen and decrease its disinfectant action.
3. Use 4 parts per million (ppm) as a target concentration for surface water and allow extra contact time, especially if the water is cold.
4. In cold water, the contact time or dose should be increased; in polluted water, the dose must be increased.
5. In cloudy water that will not settle out by sedimentation, the halogen dose should be at least 8 ppm to account for the greater halogen demand that results from the presence of organic material. Ideally, use C-F to clarify the water before halogenation and then use a smaller amount of halogen.

Pathogen Sensitivity

1. Bacteria are extremely sensitive to halogens.
2. Viruses and *Giardia* require higher concentrations or longer contact times.
3. Certain parasite eggs such as *Ascaris* are resistant but are not usually spread by water. These types of resistant cysts and eggs are susceptible to heat or filtration.
4. *Cryptosporidium* cysts are extremely resistant to halogens.
5. Although *Cryptosporidium* oocysts have been found in surface water and have been identified as the etiologic agent in cases of travelers' diarrhea and municipal water-borne outbreaks, it is unclear how much risk they pose in pristine wilderness waters.
6. The resistance of *Cryptosporidium* will require an alternative to halogens or a combination of methods to ensure removal and inactivation of all pathogens.

Chlorine versus Iodine

1. Compared with chlorine, iodine is less affected by pH or nitrogenous wastes, and it tastes better.
2. Chlorine (Table 44-5) and iodine (Table 44-6) are available in either liquid or tablet form.
3. Concern surrounds the physiologic activity of iodine.
   a. At levels used for water disinfection, iodine is safe for most people.
   b. Despite iodine's relative safety, some alteration in thyroid function can be measured and some persons experience magnification of existing thyroid problem.

TABLE 44-5. Experimental Data for 99.9% Kill with Chlorine

CONCENTRATION	TIME	pH	TEMPERATURE
Giardia lamblia (consistent with *Entamoeba histolytica*)			
0.5 mg/L	6-24 hr	6-8	3-5° C (37-41° F)
4.0 mg/L	60 min	6-8	3-5° C (37-41° F)
8.0 mg/L	30 min	6-8	3-5° C (37-41° F)
3.0 mg/L	10 min	6-8	15° C (59° F)
1.5 mg/L	10 min	6-8	25° C (77° F)
Enteric Viruses			
0.5 mg/L	40 min	7.8	2° C (35.6° F)
0.3 mg/L	30 min	7.8	25° C (77° F)
Escherichia coli			
0.03 mg/L	5 min	7.0	2-5° C (35.6-41° F)

TABLE 44-6. Experimental Data for 99.9% Kill with Iodine

CONCENTRATION	TIME	pH	TEMPERATURE
Giardia and *Amebae* Cysts			
3.0 mg/L	15 min	7.0	20° C (68° F)
7.0 mg/L	30 min	7.4	3° C (37.4° F)
Poliovirus			
0.3 mg/L	1.5 min	7.0	25° C (77° F)
Escherichia coli			
1.0 mg/L	1 min	6.5-8.5	2-5° C (35.6- 41° F)

    c. Hypersensitivity reactions to iodine can occur.
    d. Iodine use is not recommended for persons with unstable thyroid disease or a known iodine allergy.
    e. Iodine should not be used during pregnancy for more than several weeks because of the risk of neonatal goiter.

   f. Caution dictates limiting exposure (daily iodination of all drinking water) to periods of 1 month or less.
4. Iodine resins may reduce toxicity concerns because they leave low concentrations of dissolved iodine in the water. They also allow for the complete removal of iodine residual with GAC. Iodine resins have been incorporated into many different filter designs now available for field use.
   a. Most designs incorporate two stages in addition to the iodine resin. A microfilter, generally 1 micron (μm), effectively removes *Cryptosporidium*, *Giardia*, and other halogen-resistant parasitic eggs or larva. Because iodine resins kill bacteria and viruses rapidly, no significant contact time is required for most water.
   b. The addition of a third stage of activated charcoal removes dissolved residual; however, the importance of iodine residual for disinfection has not been established.
5. Halogens can be applied with equal ease to large and small quantities of water (Tables 44-7 to 44-9).

Problems
1. The taste of the water can be unpleasant when the halogen concentration exceeds 4 to 5 mg/L.
2. The potency of some products (tablets, solutions) decreases with time and is affected by prolonged exposure to moisture or heat (tablets) and air (e.g., iodine crystals).
3. Liquids are corrosive and can stain clothes and equipment.
4. The actual concentration (after halogen demand) is not known.
5. *Cryptosporidium* is highly resistant.

TABLE 44-7. Iodine Solutions

PREPARATION	IODINE (%)	IODIDE (%)	TYPE OF SOLUTION
Iodine topical solution	2.0	2.4 (sodium)	Aqueous
Lugol's solution	5.0	10.0 (potassium)	Aqueous
Iodine tincture	2.0	2.4 (sodium)	Aqueous-ethanol
Strong iodine solution	7.0	9.0 (potassium)	Ethanol (85%)

TABLE 44-8. Water Disinfection Techniques and Halogen Doses

	ADDED TO 1 L OR QUART OF WATER	
IODINATION TECHNIQUES	AMOUNT FOR 4 ppm	AMOUNT FOR 8 ppm
Iodine tabs Tetraglycine hydroperiodide EDWGT Potable Aqua Globaline	½ tab	1 tab
2% Iodine solution (tincture)*	0.2 mL or 5 gtts	0.4 mL or 10 gtts
10% Povidone-iodine solution*†	0.35 mL or 8 gtts	0.70 mL or 16 gtts
Saturated solution: iodine crystals in water	13 mL	26 mL
Saturated solution: iodine crystals in alcohol	0.1 mL	0.2 mL
CHLORINATION TECHNIQUES	AMOUNT FOR 5 ppm	AMOUNT FOR 10 ppm
Sodium hypochlorite (household bleach 5%)†	0.1 mL or 2 gtts	0.2 mL or 4 gtts
Calcium hypochlorite (Redi Chlor [¹⁄₁₀ g tab])		¼ tab/2 quarts
Sodium dichloroisocyanurate (AquaClear)		1 tab (8.5 mg NaDCC)
Chlorine plus flocculating agent (Chlor-Floc)		1 tab

*Measure with dropper (1 drop = 0.05 mL) or tuberculin syringe.
†Povidone-iodine solutions release free iodine in levels adequate for disinfection, but scant data are available.
EDWGT, emergency drinking water germicidal tablet; gtts, drops; ppm, parts per million.

Improving the Taste of Water Disinfected with Halogens

1. Add flavoring to the water only after adequate contact time. Iodine will react with sugar additives, thereby reducing the free iodine available for disinfection.
2. Use charcoal (GAC) to remove halogen after contact time.
3. Reduce the concentration and increase the contact time in clean water. For a small group of people, use a collapsible plastic container to disinfect water with low doses of iodine during the day or overnight.
4. Iodine and chlorine taste and iodine color can be removed by chemical reduction. In addition, a much higher halogen dose (shorter contact time) can be used if followed by chemical reduction. To remove iodine and chlorine taste and iodine color by chemical reduction:
   a. Add a few granules per liter of ascorbic acid (vitamin C, available in powder or crystal form) or sodium thiosulfate (nontoxic) after the required contact time.
   b. These chemicals reduce iodine or chlorine to iodide or chloride, which has no taste or color.
   c. Ascorbic acid leaves behind a slightly tart taste.
   d. Iodide still has physiologic activity, which means that a person with unstable thyroid disease or known iodine allergy or a pregnant woman should continue to exercise caution.

Superchlorination-Dechlorination

1. High doses of chlorine are added to the water in the form of calcium hypochlorite crystals to achieve concentrations of 30 to 200 ppm of free chlorine.
2. These extremely high levels are above the margin of safety for field conditions and rapidly kill all bacteria, viruses, and protozoa and could kill *Cryptosporidium* with overnight contact times.
3. After at least 10 to 15 minutes, several drops of 30% hydrogen peroxide solution are added. This reduces hypochlorite to chloride, forming calcium chloride and oxygen.
4. The minor disadvantage of a two-step process is offset by excellent taste.
5. This is a good technique for highly polluted or cloudy water and for disinfecting large quantities. It is the best technique for storing water on boats or for emergency use. Water is then dechlorinated in needed quantities when ready to use.
6. The ingredients can be easily obtained and packaged in small Nalgene bottles (Box 44-8; see Table 44-9).

Box 44-8. Improving the Taste of Halogens

- Decreased dose; increased contact time
- Clarification of cloudy water, which decreases amount of halogen needed
- Removal of halogen
- Use of granular activated carbon (GAC)
- Chemical reduction
- Ascorbic acid
- Sodium thiosulfate
- Superchlorination/dechlorination
- Use of KDF (zinc-copper) brush or media
- Alternative techniques:
  - Heat
  - Filtration
  - Chlorine dioxide or mixed species (Miox)

TABLE 44-9. Recommendations for Contact Time with Halogenations in the Field

CONCEN-TRATION OF HALOGEN	CONTACT TIME IN MINUTES AT VARIOUS WATER TEMPERATURES		
	5° C (41° F)	15° C (59° F)	30° C (86° F)
2 ppm	240	180	60
4 ppm	180	60	45
8 ppm	60	30	15

NOTE: Data indicate that very cold water requires prolonged contact time with iodine or chlorine to kill *Giardia* cysts. These contact times have been extended from the usual recommendations in cold water to account for this and for the uncertainty of residual concentration.

▶ **MISCELLANEOUS DISINFECTANTS**

Mixed Species Disinfection (Miox Purifier)

1. Passing a current through a simple brine salt solution generates free available chlorine, as well as other "mixed species" disinfectants that have been demonstrated effective against bacteria, viruses, and bacterial spores.
2. The exact composition of the solution is not well delineated because many of the compounds are relatively unstable; however, the resulting solution has greater disinfectant ability than a simple solution of sodium hypochlorite.

3. It has even been demonstrated to inactivate *Cryptosporidium,* suggesting that chlorine dioxide is among the chemicals generated.
4. Plan for prolonged contact time, if *Cryptosporidium* is a strong concern.
5. High technology approach will appeal to some.
6. Potential for malfunction and battery depletion.
7. A new point-of-use commercial product is Miox, marketed by Mountain Safety Research (Seattle, WA) (Box 44-9).

Chlorine Dioxide

1. Chlorine dioxide is capable of inactivating most waterborne pathogens including *Cryptosporidium parvum* oocysts at practical doses and contact times.
2. It is as least as effective a bactericide as chlorine, and in many cases superior.
3. It is far superior as a virucide.
4. New technology enables cost-effective and portable chlorine dioxide generation in the field. Current products include MicroPUR MP-1, Aquamira, and Miox (Box 44-10).

Ultraviolet Light

1. In sufficient doses, all waterborne enteric pathogens are inactivated by ultraviolet (UV) radiation.
2. Bacteria and protozoan parasites require lower doses than enteric viruses and bacterial spores.

Box 44-9. Chlorine Dioxide

ADVANTAGES
- Effective against all microorganisms including *Cryptosporidium*
- Low doses have no taste or color
- Portable device now available for individual and small group field use; simple to use
- More potent than equivalent doses of chlorine
- Less affected by nitrogenous wastes

DISADVANTAGES
- Volatile, so do not expose tablets to air and use generated solutions rapidly
- No persistent residual, so does not prevent recontamination during storage
- Sensitive to sunlight; keep bottle shaded or in pack during treatment

---

Relative susceptibility of microorganisms to chlorine dioxide: bacteria > viruses > protozoa.

Box 44-10. Ultraviolet Irradiation

ADVANTAGES
- Effective against all microorganisms
- Imparts no taste
- Portable device now available for individual and small group field use; simple to use
- Available from sunlight

DISADVANTAGES
- Requires clear water
- Does not improve water aesthetics
- Does not prevent recontamination during storage
- Expensive
- Require power source
- Requires direct sunlight, prolonged exposure; dose low and uncontrolled

---

Relative susceptibility of microorganisms to ultraviolet: protozoa > bacteria > viruses.

3. *Giardia* and *Cryptosporidium* are susceptible to practical doses of UV and may be more sensitive because of their relatively large size.
4. UV treatment does not require chemicals and does not affect the taste of the water.
5. UV works rapidly, and an overdose to the water presents no danger.
6. UV light has no residual disinfection power; water may become recontaminated, or regrowth of bacteria may occur.
7. Particulate matter can shield microorganisms from UV rays.
8. A portable field unit is now available, the SteriPEN. These units require a power source and have great potential.
9. Another approach uses simple solar disinfection ("SODIS") technique (see http://www.sodis.ch/).
    a. Transparent bottles (e.g., clear plastic beverage bottles), preferably lying on a dark surface, are exposed to sunlight for a minimum of 4 hours.
    b. Oxygenation induces greater reductions of bacteria, so agitation is recommended before solar treatment in bottles.
    c. Where strong sunshine is available, solar disinfection of drinking water is an effective, low-cost method for improving water quality and may be of particular use in refugee camps and disaster areas (Tables 44-10 to 44-12).

TABLE 44-10. Summary of Field Water Disinfection Techniques

	BACTERIA	VIRUSES	GIARDIA/ AMEBAE	CRYPTOSPORIDIUM	NEMATODES/ CERCARIAE
Heat	+	+	+	+	+
Filtration	+	+/−*	+	+	+
Halogens	+	+	+	−	+/−†
Chlorine dioxide	+	+	+	+	+/−†

*Most filters make no claims for viruses. Reverse osmosis is effective. The General Ecology filtration system claims virus removal.
†Eggs are not very susceptible to halogens but have very low risk of waterborne transmission.

TABLE 44-11. Advantages and Disadvantages of Disinfection Techniques

	HEAT	FILTRATION	HALOGENS	CHLORINE DIOXIDE	2-STEP PRCCESS	UV
Availability	Wood can be scarce	Many commercial choices	Many common and specific products	Several new products generate ClO_2	Filtration plus halogen, or clarification plus second stage	New portable commercial device; sunlight
Cost	Fuel and stove costs	Moderate expense	Cheap	Depends on method, generally inexpensive	Depends on choice of stages	Commercial device relatively expensive
Effectiveness	Can sterilize or pasteurize	Most filters not reliable for viruses	*Cryptosporidium* cysts are resistant	All organisms and some parasitic eggs are resistant	Highly effective, should cover all organisms	All organisms
Optimal application	Clear water	Clear or slightly cloudy; turbid water clogs filters rapidly	Clear; need increased dose if cloudy	Clear water, but ClO_2 less affected by nitrogenous compounds	May be adapted to any source water	Requires clear water, small volumes
Taste	Does not change taste	Can improve taste, especially if charcoal stage	Tastes worse unless halogen is removed or "neutralized"	Unchanged, may leave some chlorine taste	Depends on sequence and choice of stages; generally improves	Unchanged

	HEAT	FILTRATION	HALOGENS	CHLORINE DIOXIDE	2-STEP PROCESS	UV
Time	Boiling time (minutes)	Filtration time (minutes)	Contact time (minutes to hours)	Prolonged, if need to ensure *Cryptosporidium*	Combination of time for each stage disinfection	Minutes
Other considerations	Fuel is heavy and bulky	Adds weight and space; requires maintenance to keep adequate flow	Works well for large quantities and for water storage. Some understanding of principles is optimal; damaging if spills or container breaks	More experience and testing would be reassuring; likely to replace iodine for field use	More rational to use halogens first if filter has charcoal stage; C-F is best means of cleaning very turbid water, then followed by halogen, filtration or heat	Sunlight currently for emergency situations or no other methods available; commercial product good for high-quality source water, small group use

C-F, Coagulation-flocculation; UV, ultraviolet.

TABLE 44-12. Choice of Method for Various Types of Source Water

	"PRISTINE" WILDERNESS	DEVELOPED OR DEVELOPING COUNTRY		
	WATER WITH LITTLE HUMAN OR DOMESTIC ANIMAL ACTIVITY	TAP WATER IN DEVELOPING COUNTRY	CLEAR SURFACE WATER NEAR HUMAN AND ANIMAL ACTIVITY*	CLOUDY WATER
Primary concern	*Giardia*, enteric bacteria	Bacteria, *Giardia*, small numbers of viruses	All enteric pathogens, including *Cryptosporidium*	All enteric pathogens plus micro-organisms
Effective methods	Any single-step method†	Any single-step method†	1. Heat 2. Filtration plus halogen (can be done in either order); iodine resin filters (see text) 3. Chlorine dioxide 4. Ultraviolet (commercial product, not sunlight)	C-F followed by second step (heat, filtration or halogen)

*Includes agricultural runoff with cattle grazing or sewage treatment effluent from upstream villages or towns.
†Includes heat, filtration, halogens and chlorine dioxide, ultraviolet.
C-F, Coagulation-flocculation.

► CHOOSING THE PREFERRED TECHNIQUE

1. The best technique for disinfection for either an individual or a group depends on the number of persons, space and weight available, quality of source water, personal taste preferences, and availability of fuel.
2. Unfortunately, optimal protection for all situations may require a two-step process of filtration or C-F and halogenation because halogens do not kill *Cryptosporidium* and filtration misses some viruses.
3. Heat works as a one-step process, but it will not improve the taste and look of water if it is cloudy or tastes poor initially.
4. An iodine resin, combined with microfiltration to remove resistant cysts, is also a viable one-step process for all situations.

Alpine Camping

1. For alpine camping where a high-quality water source is available, heat, mechanical or iodine resin filtration, or a low-dose halogen can be used.
2. The only limitation for halogens is *Cryptosporidium* cysts, but in high-quality pristine surface water the cysts are generally found in insufficient numbers to pose significant risk.
3. Heat is limited by fuel supply.
4. Filtration has the advantage of imparting no taste and requiring no contact time.

Agricultural Runoff and Discharge from Upstream Towns

1. Treat water with agricultural runoff or sewage plant discharge from an upstream town or city with heat or a two-step process of filtration to remove *Cryptosporidium,* then with a halogen to ensure destruction of all viruses.
2. You can also use an iodine resin filter with microfiltration. A filter containing a charcoal element has the added advantage of removing many chemicals such as pesticides.

Surface Water in Undeveloped Countries

1. View all surface water in undeveloped countries, even if visually clear, as highly contaminated with enteric pathogens.
2. Heat is effective for disinfection, but simple mechanical filtration is not adequate because of the potential for enteric viruses.
3. A halogen is reasonable but will miss *Cryptosporidium* and parasite eggs.
4. A two-stage process offers added protection.

Cloudy Water in Developed or Undeveloped Countries

1. Pretreat cloudy water in developed or undeveloped countries that does not clear with sedimentation with co-agulation-flocculation, and then disinfect with heat or a halogen.
2. Note that filters can clog rapidly with silted or cloudy water.

Systems Where Water Will Be Stored

1. Halogens have a distinct advantage in locations where the water will be stored for a time such as on a boat or in a home without running water.
2. Iodine works for short-term but not prolonged storage because it is a poor algicide.
3. Note that when only heat or filtration is used before storage, the water can become recontaminated and bacterial regrowth can occur. Superchlorination-dechlorination is particularly useful in this situation because a high level of chlorination can be maintained for a long period.
    a. When ready to use the water, pour it into a smaller container and dechlorinate it.
    b. If another means of chlorination is used, maintain a minimum residual of 3 to 5 mg/L in the water.
4. Silver has been approved by the EPA for preservation of stored water.
5. On oceangoing vessels where water must be desalinated during the voyage, only reverse-osmosis membrane filters are adequate. Halogens should then be added to the water in the storage tanks (see Tables 44-10 to 44-12).

Hydration and Dehydration

45

HYDRATION AND DEHYDRATION ASSESSMENT AND TREATMENT

Water accounts for 50% to 70% of the body's weight. Because sweating involves loss of body mass, measuring changes in body weight (BW) is the simplest way to rapidly assess hydration status. Daily BW tends to be stable, so changes can be attributed to water loss. Body weight measurement, before, during and after endurance activity, corrected for fluid intake and urine output, is a simple, practical, and reliable method of measuring sweat rate and thus hydration status (Table 45-1).

▶ URINE MARKERS

Urine Color
In the backcountry, the color of urine can be used as a rough guide to monitor hydration status.
1. Strongly yellow-colored urine is indicative of hypohydration.
2. Pale urine indicates adequate hydration.

Dark yellow or orange urine can also be caused by recent use of laxatives or consumption of B complex vitamins or carotene. Orange urine is often caused by phenazopyridine (Pyridium) (used in the treatment of urinary tract infections), rifampin, and warfarin.

Urine Specific Gravity
Urine dipsticks that measure specific gravity can be carried on backcountry trips and used as a marker of hydration. A urine specific gravity of more than 1.02 indicates a state of hypohydration.

Treatment
1. Administer oral rehydration fluids to victims who are conscious and coherent.
2. Administer intravenous fluids (2 L normal saline over 4 hours for adults and 20 mL/kg for children) to victims who are severely dehydrated or unable to ingest oral fluids.

▶ HYDRATION STRATEGIES

1. Drink 500 mL of fluid about 2 hours before endurance or strenuous activity to promote adequate hydration and allow time for excretion of excess water.
2. Replace water losses caused by sweating at a rate equal to the sweat rate (Table 45-2).

TABLE 45-1. Signs and Symptoms of Dehydration

SIGNS/ SYMPTOMS	MILD DEHYDRA-TION	MODERATE DEHYDRATION	SEVERE DEHYDRA-TION
Level of consciousness	Alert	Lethargic	Obtunded
Capillary refill	2 sec	2-4 sec	>4 sec, cool limbs
Mucous membranes	Normal	Dry	Parched, cracked
Tears	Normal	Decreased	Absent
Heart rate	Slight increase	Increased	Very increased
Respiratory rate	Normal	Increased	Increased and hyperpnea
Blood pressure	Normal	Normal, but orthostasis	Decreased
Pulse	Normal	Thready	Faint or impalpable
Skin turgor	Normal	Slow	Tenting
Eyes	Normal	Sunken	Very sunken
Urine output	Decreased	Oliguria	Oliguria/ anuria

    a. Sweat losses range from 0.3 to 1.2 L/hour for an individual doing mild work while wearing cotton clothes.

    b. Sweat losses range from 1 to 2 L/hour for an individual doing mild work and wearing nonpermeable clothing.

    c. Sweat losses range from 1 to 2.5 L/hour for an individual doing strenuous work or during high exercise intensity in a hot climate.

3. The perception of thirst is a poor indicator of hydration. Individuals can be 2% to 8% dehydrated before feeling thirsty.

4. Beverages containing electrolytes and carbohydrates offer little advantage over water in maintaining hydration or electrolyte concentration or in improving intestinal absorption.

5. Fluid-replacement beverages that are sweetened (with carbohydrates or artificial sweeteners) and cooled (to between 15° and 21° C) stimulate ingestion of more fluid.

6. Meals should be consumed regularly to return normal electrolyte losses.

7. During prolonged exercise, frequent (every 15 to 20 minutes) consumption of moderate (150-mL) to large (350-mL) volumes of low-osmolarity fluid may improve the gastric emptying rate.

TABLE 45-2. Fluid Replacement Guidelines for Warm-Weather Training (Applies to Average Acclimated Soldier Wearing BDU in Hot Weather)*

HEAT CATEGORY	WBGT INDEX (°F)	EASY WORK		MODERATE WORK		HARD WORK	
		WORK/REST CYCLE	WATER INTAKE (q/hr)	WORK/REST CYCLE	WATER INTAKE (q/hr)	WORK/REST CYCLE	WATER INTAKE (q/hr)
1	78-81.9 (26-28° C)	NL	½	NL	¾	40/20 min	¾
2 (green)	82-84.9 (28-29.4° C)	NL	½	50/10 min	¾	30/30 min	1
3 (yellow)	85-87.9 (29.4-31° C)	NL	¾	40/20 min	¾	30/30 min	1
4 (red)	88-89.9 (31-32.2° C)	NL	¾	30/30 min	¾	20/40 min	1
5 (black)	>90	50/10 min	1	20/40 min	1	10/50 min	1

*The work/rest times and fluid replacement volumes will sustain performance and hydration for at least 4 hours of work in the specified heat category. Individual water needs will vary ± ¼ quart per hour.

Rest means minimal physical activity (sitting or standing), accomplished in shade if possible.

CAUTION: Hourly fluid intake should not exceed 1½ quarts. Daily fluid intake should not exceed 12 quarts.

Wearing body armor: Add 5° F to WBGT index. Wearing mission-oriented protective posture (MOPP, chemical protection) overgarment, add 10° F to WBGT index.

EASY WORK: Weapon maintenance; walking hard surface at 2.5 mph, ≤30-lb load; manual handling of arms; marksmanship training; drill and ceremony.

MODERATE WORK: Walking in loose sand at 2.5 mph, no load; walking hard surface at 3.5 mph, ≤40-lb load; calisthenics; patrolling; individual movement techniques (e.g., low crawl, high crawl); defensive position construction; field assaults.

HARD WORK: Walking on hard surface at 3.5 mph, ≥40-lb load; walking in loose sand at 2.5 mph with load.

1 quart = 946 mL.

BDU, battle dress uniform; NL, no limit to work time per hour; WBGT, wet bulb global temperature.

From Montain SJ, Latzka WA, Sawka MN: Fluid replacement recommendations for training in hot weather. Mil Med 164:502, 1999.

8. Optimal performance is attainable only with sufficient drinking during exercise to minimize dehydration. Even low levels of dehydration (1% loss of body mass) impair cardiovascular and thermoregulatory responses and reduce capacity for exercise.

9. To restore hydration status after exercise, a person should consume 1 L (4 cups) of fluid for every kilogram of weight lost during the activity.

Malaria

46

Malaria is a mosquito-transmitted, blood-borne, parasitic infection present throughout tropical and developing areas of the world. Parasites are transmitted by 30 to 40 (out of 430) species of the female *Anopheles* mosquito, which tends to bite between dusk and dawn. Estimated worldwide incidence is 300 to 500 million cases per year. Malaria infection causes a severe febrile illness that is potentially fatal.

Four species of malaria typically cause disease in humans:
1. *Plasmodium vivax* (worldwide distribution, but uncommon in sub-Saharan Africa)
2. *Plasmodium falciparum* (worldwide distribution)
3. *Plasmodium ovale* (West Africa)
4. *Plasmodium malariae* (worldwide distribution)

▶ CLINICAL MANIFESTATIONS AND COMPLICATIONS
(Table 46-1)

1. Clinical manifestations first evident 1 to 2 weeks after entry into endemic area (sooner if infected blood obtained through transfusion or shared needles)
2. No pathognomonic signs, but common symptoms (Table 46-2)
3. Paroxysms of chills followed by high fever and sweating
   a. May last several hours and occur every 2 to 3 days
   b. Classic periodic attacks often not observed in severe *P. falciparum* malaria; fever possibly constant
4. Abdominal cramps, diarrhea
5. Cerebral malaria (associated with high levels of *P. falciparum* parasitemia), characterized by high fevers, confusion, and eventually coma and death
6. Acute renal failure, pulmonary edema
7. Definitive diagnosis only by the presence of parasite-containing red blood cells (detected on thick and thin blood smears)
8. Clinical attacks during the first 4 to 8 weeks after return from the area of exposure
9. Prolonged latent incubation times (up to 3 years) reported
10. Complications are more common with *P. falciparum* infection than with other species of malaria.
11. Factors indicating a poor prognosis for persons with severe malaria include clinical, biochemical, and hematologic features (Table 46-3).

TABLE 46-1. Clinical Manifestations and Complications of Human *Plasmodium* Infection

PLASMODIUM SPECIES	MANIFESTATIONS AND COMPLICATIONS
All species	Fever, chills, rigors, sweats, headache Weakness Myalgias Vomiting Diarrhea Hepatomegaly Splenomegaly Jaundice Anemia Thrombocytopenia
P. falciparum	Hyperparasitemia Cerebral malaria: seizures, obtundation, coma Severe anemia Hypoglycemia Acidosis Renal failure Pulmonary edema (noncardiogenic) Vascular collapse
P. vivax and *P. ovale*	Splenic rupture Relapse months to years after primary infection because of latent hepatic stages
P. malariae	Low-grade fever, fatigue Chronic asymptomatic parasitemia Immune complex glomerulonephritis

TABLE 46-2. Common Symptoms and Their Incidence in Malaria

SYMPTOM	INCIDENCE (%)
Fever	97
Chills	97
Headaches	94
Nausea/vomiting	62
Abdominal pain	56
Myalgia	50
Backache	9
Dark urine	3

TABLE 46-3. Indicators of a Poor Prognosis in Severe Malaria

INDICATOR	FACTOR	COMMENTS
Clinical	Age <3	
	Impaired consciousness	
	Seizures ≥3 in 24 hr	
	Absent corneal reflexes	
	Papilledema	
	Decerebrate/decorticate rigidity	
	Opisthotonus	
	Respiratory distress	
	Shock	
Biochemical	Hypoglycemia	Glucose <40 mg/dL
	Acidosis	Plasma bicarbonate <15 mmol/L
	Hyperlactatemia	Lactate >45 mg/dL
	Renal impairment	Serum creatinine >3 mg/dL; BUN >60 mg/dL
	Elevated aminotransferases	>3 times normal
	Hyperbilirubinemia	Serum total bilirubin >2.5 mg/dL
Hematologic	Hyperparasitemia	>500,000 parasites/mL or >10,000 mature trophozoites and schizonts/mL
	Anemia	Hemoglobin <5 g/dL; packed cell volume <15%
	Visible malarial pigment	>5% neutrophils with malarial pigment

BUN, blood urea nitrogen.

▶ **PRESUMPTIVE SELF-TREATMENT**

If treatment is required, this implies failure of malaria chemo-prophylaxis. Taking prophylactic medications does not exclude the possibility of becoming infected because no current drug or drug regimen can be considered to provide 100% protection against malaria. Presumptive self-treatment should be used only as an interim measure, and travelers should be advised to seek medical evaluation as soon as possible so that thick and thin blood smears can be obtained for precise diagnosis. Presumptive self-treatment should be taken immediately if the traveler develops an influenza-like illness with fevers and chills and professional medical care is not available within 24 hours.

Note the drugs used for stand-by therapy (Table 46-4). Have the victim take a treatment dose of one of the antimalarial agents when signs and symptoms suggest an acute attack and prompt medical attention is not available.

Treatment
Malaria treatment consists of rapid and appropriate antimalarial therapy (Table 46-5), as well as supportive care.

Prevention
Chemoprophylaxis:
General Principles
1. Determine the risk of malaria infection for a geographic location.
   a. Use the Centers for Disease Control Internet site for up-to-date changes in malaria risk worldwide: www.cdc.gov/travel/
2. Chemoprophylaxis (Table 46-6) should be prescribed for nonimmune individuals including children traveling to malaria-endemic areas. The health care provider must consider several factors when choosing an appropriate chemoprophylactic regimen for the traveler. These include destination-specific malaria risk and resistance patterns, age, underlying medical conditions, allergies, tolerability, and length of stay. Pediatric dosages are based on weight and should never exceed adult dosages.
   a. Be aware that resistance to multiple antimalarial drugs has made prevention and treatment of *P. falciparum* malaria a major problem in some endemic areas.
3. Start administration of the antimalarial drug 1 to 2 weeks (chloroquine or mefloquine) or 1 to 2 days (doxycycline or atovaquone/proguanil) before departure to allow time to accomplish the following:
   a. Become familiar with any drug side effects.
   b. Switch to an alternative drug if necessary.
   c. Habituate to the timing of doses.
   d. Build up to steady-state drug levels.
4. Maintain the antimalarial drug-dosing schedule during exposure.
5. Continue the antimalarial drug regimen for 4 weeks (chloroquine, mefloquine, and doxycycline) or 7 days (atovaquone/proguanil) after leaving the area of malaria infection.

TABLE 46-4. Medications for Presumptive Self-Treatment* of Malaria†

DRUG	ADULT DOSAGE	PEDIATRIC DOSAGE‡	ADVERSE EFFECTS	COMMENTS
Atovaquone-proguanil (Malarone)	4 adult tablets‡ (each dose contains 1000 mg atovaquone and 400 mg proguanil) orally as a single daily dose for 3 consecutive days	Single daily dose to be taken for 3 consecutive days <5 kg: not indicated 5-8 kg: 2 pediatric tablets‡ 9-10 kg: 3 pediatric tablets 11-20 kg: 1 adult tablet 21-30 kg: 2 adult tablets 31-40 kg: 3 adult tablets ≥41 kg: 4 adult tablets	Nausea, vomiting, abdominal pain, diarrhea, increased transaminase levels, seizures	Approved for once-a-day dose, but dose can be divided in half to reduce nausea and vomiting; take with food or milk. Contraindicated in persons with severe renal impairment (creatinine clearance <30 mL/min). Adult tablet not recommended for children <5 kg, pregnant women, women breastfeeding infants <5 kg, and persons on atovaquone-proguanil prophylaxis.
Or: Mefloquine	750 mg salt PO followed 12 hr later by 500 mg salt. Total dose = 1250 mg salt	15 mg/kg (13.7 mg base) followed 12 hr later by 10 mg/kg (9.1 mg base) Total dose = 25 mg salt/kg		See mefloquine comments in Table 46-60.

Continued

TABLE 46-4. Medications for Presumptive Self-Treatment* of Malaria†—cont'd

DRUG	ADULT DOSAGE	PEDIATRIC DOSAGE‡	ADVERSE EFFECTS	COMMENTS
Or: Quinine sulfate	650 mg PO q8h × 3-7 days	30 mg/kg/day in 3 doses × 3-7 days		See quinine comments in Table 46-6.
Plus: Doxycycline	100 mg PO bid	4 mg/kg/day in 2 doses × 7 days		See doxycycline comments in Table 46-6.

*Self-treatment drug is to be used for febrile illness if professional medical care is not available within 24 hr. Medical care should be sought immediately after treatment.

†Caused by *Plasmodium falciparum*, *Plasmodium ovale*, *Plasmodium vivax*, and *Plasmodium malariae*.

‡Each adult tablet contains 250 mg atovaquone and 100 mg proguanil; each pediatric tablet contains 62.5 mg atovaquone and 25 mg proguanil. Pediatric dosages should never exceed adult dosages.

TABLE 46-5. Medications for the Treatment of Malaria*

DRUG	ADULT DOSAGE	PEDIATRIC DOSAGE†	ADVERSE EFFECTS	COMMENTS
Chloroquine-Sensitive *Plasmodium falciparum, Plasmodium vivax, Plasmodium ovale, Plasmodium malariae*				
Drug of Choice:				
Chloroquine phosphate (Aralen)‡	1 g salt (600 mg base) PO immediately, followed by 500 mg salt (300 mg base) PO at 6, 24, and 48 hr. Total dosage: 2500 mg salt (1500 mg base)	10 mg base/kg (max. 600 mg base) PO immediately, followed by 5 mg/kg (base) PO at 6, 24, and 48 hr. Total dosage: 25 mg/kg (base)	Pruritus, nausea, headache, skin eruptions, dizziness, blurred vision, insomnia. May exacerbate psoriasis	Has been used extensively and safely in pregnancy.

Continued

TABLE 46-5. Medications for the Treatment of Malaria*—cont'd

DRUG	ADULT DOSAGE	PEDIATRIC DOSAGE†	ADVERSE EFECTS	COMMENTS
Chloroquine-Resistant *P. falciparum* Oral Drugs of Choice:				
Atovaquone-proguanil (Malarone)	2 adult tablets§ (500 mg atova-quone/ 200 mg proguanil) bid × 3 days daily OR 4 adult tablets§ (1 g atovaquone/ 400 mg proguanil) qd × 3 days	<5 kg: not indicated 5-8 kg: 2 pediatric tablets/day§ × 3 days. 9-10 kg: 3 pediatric tablets/day§ × 3 days. 11-20 kg: 1 adult tablets§/day × 3 days. 21-30 kg: 2 adult tablets§/day × 3 days. 31-40 kg: 3 adult tablets§/day × 3 days. >40 kg: 2 adult tab-lets§ bid × 3 days OR 4 adult tablets§ qd × 3 days.	Headache, nausea, vomiting, abdominal pain, diarrhea, increased transaminase levels, seizures	Approved for once-a-day dosing but dose can be divided in half to reduce nausea and vomiting. Take with food or milk. Contraindicated in persons with severe renal impairment (creatinine clearance <30 mL/min). Adult tablet not recommended for children <5 kg, pregnant women, women breastfeeding infants <5 kg.

DRUG	ADULT DOSAGE	PEDIATRIC DOSAGE†	ADVERSE EFFECTS	COMMENTS
Quinine sulfate	650 mg salt (542 mg base) q8h × 3-7 days	30 mg salt/kg/ day in 3 doses × 3-7 days	—	In Southeast Asia, continue treatment for 7 days because of increased relative resistance to quinine.
Plus: Doxycycline (Vibramycin, Vibra-Tabs, Doryx, Periostat and others, generic)	100 mg bid × 7 days	>8 yr: 4 mg/kg/day in 2 doses × 7 days	Gastrointestinal upset, vaginal candidiasis, photosensitivity, allergic reactions, blood dyscrasias, azotemia in renal diseases, hepatitis	Contraindicated in children ≤8 yr and pregnant women.

Continued

TABLE 46-5. Medications for the Treatment of Malaria*—cont'd

DRUG	ADULT DOSAGE	PEDIATRIC DOSAGE†	ADVERSE EFECTS	COMMENTS
Or Plus: Tetracycline (Achromycin, Sumycin, Panmycin, and others)	250 mg qid × 7 days	25 mg/kg/day in 4 doses × 7 days	Gastrointestinal upset, vaginal candidiasis, photosensitivity, allergic reactions, blood dyscrasias, azotemia in renal diseases, hepatitis	Contraindicated in children ≤8 yr and pregnant women.
Or Plus: Clindamycin (Cleocin and others)	20 mg/kg/day divided in 3 doses × 7 days	20 mg/kg/day in 3 doses × 7 days	—	For use in pregnancy.

DRUG	ADULT DOSAGE	PEDIATRIC DOSAGE†	ADVERSE EFFECTS	COMMENTS
Alternatives: Mefloquine (Lariam, Mephaquine, generic)	750 mg salt followed by 500 mg 6-12 hr later. Total dose = 1250 mg salt	<45 kg: 15 mg/kg (13.7 mg base) followed by 10 mg/kg (9.1 mg base) 6-12 hr later. Total dose = 25 mg salt/kg	Gastrointestinal disturbance, headache, insomnia, vivid dreams, visual disturbances, depression, anxiety disorder, dizziness	Contraindicated in persons with active depression or a previous history of depression, generalized anxiety disorder, psychosis, schizophrenia, other major psychiatric disorders, or seizures. Contraindicated for treatment in pregnancy. Not recommended for persons with cardiac conduction abnormalities. Use with caution in travelers involved in tasks requiring fine motor coordination and spatial discrimination. In the U.S., a 250-mg tablet of mefloquine contains a 228-mg mefloquine base. Outside the U.S., a 275-mg mefloquine tablet contains a 250-mg mefloquine base. Do not give with quinine, quinidine, or halofantrine. In areas of reported resistance (e.g., the Thailand-Myanmar and Thailand-Cambodia borders and the Amazon basin), 25 mg/kg should be used.

Continued

TABLE 46-5. Medications for the Treatment of Malaria*—cont'd

DRUG	ADULT DOSAGE	PEDIATRIC DOSAGE†	ADVERSE EFECTS	COMMENTS
Or: Artesunate	4 mg/kg/day × 3 days	4 mg/kg/day × 3 days	—	Available in U.S. only from the manufacturer.
Plus: Mefloquine (Lariam, Mephaquin, generic)	750 mg salt followed by 500 mg 6-12 hr later. Total dose = 1250 mg salt	<45 kg: 15 mg/kg followed by 10 mg/kg (9.1 mg base) 6-12 hr later. Total dose = 25 mg salt/kg	Gastrointestinal disturbance, headache, insomnia, vivid dreams, visual disturbances, depression, anxiety disorder, dizziness	Contraindicated in persons with active depression or a previous history of depression, generalized anxiety disorder, psychosis, schizophrenia, other major psychiatric disorders, or seizures. Contraindicated for treatment in pregnancy. Not recommended for persons with cardiac conduction abnormalities. Use with caution in travelers involved in tasks requiring fine motor coordination and spatial discrimination. In the U.S., a 250-mg tablet of mefloquine contains a 228-mg mefloquine base. Outside the U.S., a 275-mg mefloquine tablet contains a 250-mg mefloquine base. Do not give with quinine, quinidine, or halofantrine. In areas of reported resistance (e.g., the Thailand-Myanmar and Thailand-Cambodia borders and the Amazon basin), 25 mg/kg should be used.

DRUG	ADULT DOSAGE	PEDIATRIC DOSAGE†	ADVERSE EFECTS	COMMENTS
Chloroquine-Resistant _P. vivax_ (Oral)				
Drug of Choice:				
Quinine sulfate	650 mg q8h × 3-7 days	30 mg/kg/day in 3 doses × 3-7 days	—	In Southeast Asia, continue treatment for 7 days because of increased relative resistance to quinine.
Plus:				
Doxycycline (Vibramycin, Vibra-Tabs, Doryx, Periostat and others, generic)	100 mg bid × 7 days	>8 yr: 4 mg/kg/day in 2 doses × 7 days	Gastrointestinal upset, vaginal candidiasis, photosensitivity, allergic reactions, blood dyscrasias, azotemia in renal diseases, hepatitis	Contraindicated in children ≤8 yr and pregnant women.

Continued

TABLE 46-5. Medications for the Treatment of Malaria*—cont'd

DRUG	ADULT DOSAGE	PEDIATRIC DOSAGE†	ADVERSE EFECTS	COMMENTS
Or: Mefloquine (Lariam, Mephaquin, generic)	750 mg salt followed by 500 mg salt 6-12 hr later. Total dose = 1250 mg salt	<45 kg: 15 mg/kg (13.7 mg base) followed by 10 mg/kg (9.1 mg base) 6-12 hr later. Total dose = 25 mg/kg salt	Gastrointestinal disturbance, headache, insomnia, vivid dreams, visual disturbances, depression, anxiety disorder, dizziness	Contraindicated in persons with active depression or a previous history of depression, generalized anxiety disorder, psychosis, schizophrenia, other major psychiatric disorders, or seizures. Contraindicated for treatment in pregnancy. Not recommended for persons with cardiac conduction abnormalities. Use with caution in travelers involved in tasks requiring fine motor coordination and spatial discrimination. In the U.S., a 250-mg tablet of mefloquine contains a 228-mg mefloquine base. Outside the U.S., a 275-mg mefloquine tablet contains a 250-mg mefloquine base. Do not give with quinine, quinidine, or halofantrine. In areas of reported resistance (e.g., the Thailand-Myanmar and Thailand-Cambodia borders and the Amazon basin), 25 mg/kg should be used.

DRUG	ADULT DOSAGE	PEDIATRIC DOSAGE†	ADVERSE EFECTS	COMMENTS
Alternatives: Chloroquine phosphate (Aralen)	25 mg base/kg in 3 doses over 48 hr	Same as adult dosage	Pruritus, nausea, headache, skin eruptions, dizziness, blurred vision, insomnia. May exacerbate psoriasis	Has been used extensively and safely in pregnancy. If chloroquine phosphate is not available, hydroxychloroquine sulfate is effective (400 mg of hydroxychloroquine sulfate = 500 mg of chloroquine sulfate).
Plus: Primaquine phosphate	30 mg base/day × 14 days	0.6 mg/kg/day × 14 days	—	Take with food. Contraindicated in persons with G6PD deficiency, and during pregnancy and breastfeeding unless the infant being breastfed has a documented normal G6PD level.

Continued

TABLE 46-5. Medications for the Treatment of Malaria*—cont'd

DRUG	ADULT DOSAGE	PEDIATRIC DOSAGE†	ADVERSE EFECTS	COMMENTS
All Plasmodium (Parenteral) **Drugs of Choice:** Quinidine gluconate	10 mg salt 6.25 mg base)/kg loading dose (max. 600 mg salt) in normal saline slowly over 1-2 hr, followed by continuous infusion of 0.02 mg salt (0.0125 mg base)/kg/min until oral therapy can be started or parasitemia is >1%. Treat for 7 days in multidrug-resistant areas, 3 days in nonmultidrug-resistant areas	Same as adult dosage	—	In patients with severe malaria, use with one of the following: doxycycline, tetracycline, or clindamycin. Continuous ECG, blood pressure, and glucose monitoring are recommended, especially in pregnant women and children. The loading dose should be decreased or omitted in patients who have received quinine or mefloquine. For problems with quinidine availability, call the manufacturer (Eli Lilly, 800-821-0538) or the CDC Malaria Hotline (770-488-7788). If >48 hr of parenteral therapy is required, the quinine or quinidine dosage should be decreased by ⅓ to ½.

DRUG	ADULT DOSAGE	PEDIATRIC DOSAGE†	ADVERSE EFECTS	COMMENTS
Quinine dihydrochloride (IV)	20 mg/kg loading dose IV in 5% dextrose over 4 hr, followed by 10 mg/kg over 2-4 hr q8h (max. 1800 mg/day) until oral therapy can be started or parasitemia is >1%. Treat for 7 days in multidrug-resistant areas, 3 days in non-multidrug-resistant areas	Same as adult dosage	—	In patients with severe malaria, use with one of the following: doxycycline, tetracycline, or clindamycin. Not available in the U.S. Continuous ECG, blood pressure, and glucose monitoring are recommended, especially in pregnant women and children. The loading dose should be decreased or omitted in patients who have received quinine or mefloquine. If >48 hr of parenteral therapy is required, the quinine or quinidine dosage should be decreased by 1/3 to 1/2.
Alternative: Artemether	3.2 mg/kg IM, then 1.6 mg/kg daily × 5-7 days	Same as adult dosage	—	Available in the U.S. only from the manufacturer.

Continued

TABLE 46-5. Medications for the Treatment of Malaria*—cont'd

DRUG	ADULT DOSAGE	PEDIATRIC DOSAGE†	ADVERSE EFECTS	COMMENTS
Prevention of Relapses: *Plasmodium vivax* and *Plasmodium ovale*				
Only Drug of Choice:				
Primaquine phosphate	30 mg base (52.6 mg salt)	0.6 mg base/kg/day × 14 days	—	For individuals who have had prolonged exposure to *P. vivax* or *P. ovale*. Take with food. Contraindicated in persons with G6PD deficiency, and during pregnancy and breastfeeding unless the infant being breastfed has a documented normal G6PD level. Relapses have been reported with this regimen and should be treated with a second 14-day course of 30 mg base/day. In Southeast Asia and Somalia, the higher dosage (30 mg base/day) should be used initially.

*Caused by *Plasmodium falciparum*, *Plasmodium ovale*, *Plasmodium vivax*, and *Plasmodium malariae*.
†Should never exceed adult dosage.
‡Hydroxychloroquine sulfate can be used if chloroquine phosphate is not available. 400 mg of hydroxychloroquine sulfate = 500 mg of chloroquine phosphate.
§Adult tablet contains 250 mg atovaquone and 100 mg proguanil hydrochloride. Pediatric tablet contains 62.5 mg atovaquone and 2.5 mg proguanil.
ECG, electrocardiography; G6PD, glucose-6-phosphate dehydrogenase; IM, intramuscularly; IV, intravenously; U.S., United States.

TABLE 46-6. Medications Used for Prevention of Malaria*

DRUG	TRADE NAME	ADULT DOSAGE	PEDIATRIC DOSAGE	WHEN TO START BEFORE TRAVEL	HOW LONG TO CONTINUE AFTER RETURN	ADVERSE EFFECTS	COMMENTS
Chloroquine-Sensitive Areas **Drug of choice:**							
Chloro-quine phosphate	Aralen, generic	300 mg base (500 mg salt) orally, once/wk	Base: 5 mg/kg (salt: 8.3 mg/kg) orally, once/wk, up to maximum adult dose of 300 mg base	1-2 wk	4 wk	Pruritus, nausea, headache, skin eruptions, dizziness, blurred vision, insomnia. May exacerbate psoriasis	Has been used extensively and safely in pregnancy. Where *P. vivax* and *P. ovale* are found, some recommend prima-quine phosphate 52.6 mg (30 mg base)/day (for children, 0.6 mg base/kg/ day) during the last 2 weeks of prophylaxis. Others prefer to avoid the risk of toxicity and rely on surveillance to detect cases.

Continued

TABLE 46-6. Medications Used for Prevention of Malaria*—cont'd

DRUG	TRADE NAME	ADULT DOSAGE	PEDIATRIC DOSAGE	WHEN TO START BEFORE TRAVEL	HOW LONG TO CONTINUE AFTER RETURN	ADVERSE EFFECTS	COMMENTS
Alternative: Hydroxy-chloro-quine sulfate	Plaque-nil	310 mg base (400 mg salt) orally, once/wk	Base: 5 mg/kg (salt: 6.5 mg/kg) orally, once/wk up to maximum adult dose of 310 mg base	1-2 wk	4 wk	Pruritus, nausea, headache, skin eruptions, dizziness, blurred vision, and insomnia	Has been used extensively and safely in pregnancy. Where *P. vivax* and *P. ovale* are found, some recommend primaquine phosphate 52.6 mg (30mg base)/day (for children, 0.6 mg base/kg/day) during the last 2 weeks of prophylaxis. Others prefer to avoid the risk of toxicity and rely on surveillance to detect cases.

DRUG	TRADE NAME	ADULT DOSAGE	PEDIATRIC DOSAGE	WHEN TO START BEFORE TRAVEL	HOW LONG TO CONTINUE AFTER RETURN	ADVERSE EFFECTS	COMMENTS
Chloroquine-Resistant Areas							
Drug of choice:							
Atova-quone-proguanil	Malar-one	1 adult tablet orally, daily	11-20 kg: 1 pediatric tablet† daily. 21-30 kg: 2 pediatric tablets‡ daily. 31-40 kg: 3 pediatric tablets‡ daily. ≥40 kg: 1 adult tablet† daily.	1 to 2 days	7 days	Headaches, nausea, vomiting, abdominal pain, diarrhea, increased transaminase levels, seizures	Approved for once-a-day dose but dose can be divided in two to reduce nausea and vomiting; take with food or milk. Contraindicated in persons with severe renal impairment (creatinine clearance <30 mL/min). Not recommended for children <11 kg, pregnant women, and women breast feeding infants <11 kg. Where *P. vivax* and *P. ovale* are found, some recommend primaquine phosphate 52.6 mg (30mg base)/day (for children, 0.6 mg base/kg/day) during the last 2 weeks of prophylaxis. Others prefer to avoid the risk of toxicity and rely on surveillance to detect cases.

Continued

TABLE 46-6. Medications Used for Prevention of Malaria*—cont'd

DRUG	TRADE NAME	ADULT DOSAGE	PEDIATRIC DOSAGE	WHEN TO START BEFORE TRAVEL	HOW LONG TO CONTINUE AFTER RETURN	ADVERSE EFFECTS	COMMENTS
Or: Doxycy-cline	Vibramy-cin, Vi-bra-Tabs, Doryx, Periostat, and others, generic	100 mg orally daily	>8 years: 2 mg/kg/day up to adult dosage of 100 mg/day	1-2 days	4 wk	Gastroin-testinal up-set, vaginal candidia-sis, photo-sensitivity, allergic reactions, blood dyscrasias, azotemia in renal diseases, hepatitis	Contraindicated in children ≤8 years and pregnant women. Where P. vivax and P. ovale are found, some recommend prima-quine phosphate 52.6 mg (30 mg base)/day (for children, 0.6 mg base/kg/day) during the last 2 weeks of prophylaxis. Others prefer to avoid the risk of toxicity and rely on surveillance to detect cases.

DRUG	TRADE NAME	ADULT DOSAGE	PEDIATRIC DOSAGE	WHEN TO START BEFORE TRAVEL	HOW LONG TO CONTINUE AFTER RETURN	ADVERSE EFFECTS	COMMENTS
Or: Mefloquine	Lariam, Mephaquine, generic	228-mg base (250 mg salt) orally, once/wk	≤9 kg: 4.6 mg/kg base (5 mg/kg salt). 10-20 kg: ¼ tablet§ once/wk. 21-30 kg: ½ tablet§ once/wk. 31-45 kg: ¾ tablet§ once/wk. >45 kg: 1 tablet once/wk	1-2 wk	4 wk	Gastrointestinal disturbance, headache, insomnia, vivid dreams, visual disturbances, depression, anxiety disorder, dizziness	Contraindicated in persons with active depression or a previous history of depression, generalized anxiety disorder, psychosis, schizophrenia, other major psychiatric disorders, or seizures. Not recommended for persons with cardiac conduction abnormalities. Use with caution in travelers involved in tasks requiring fine motor coordination and spatial discrimination. In the US, a 250-mg tablet of mefloquine contains a 228-mg mefloquine base. Outside the US, a 275-mg mefloquine tablet contains a 250-mg mefloquine base.

Continued

TABLE 46-6. Medications Used for Prevention of Malaria*—cont'd

DRUG	TRADE NAME	ADULT DOSAGE	PEDIATRIC DOSAGE	WHEN TO START BEFORE TRAVEL	HOW LONG TO CONTINUE AFTER RETURN	ADVERSE EFFECTS	COMMENTS
Mefloquine—cont'd							Where *P. vivax* and *P. ovale* are found, some experts recommend primaquine phosphate 52.6 mg (30 mg base)/day (for children, 0.6 mg base/kg/day) during the last 2 weeks of prophylaxis. Others prefer to avoid the risk of toxicity and rely on surveillance to detect cases.

DRUG	TRADE NAME	ADULT DOSAGE	PEDIATRIC DOSAGE	WHEN TO START BEFORE TRAVEL	HOW LONG TO CONTINUE AFTER RETURN	ADVERSE EFFECTS	COMMENTS
Or: Prima- quine	—	30 mg base (52.6 mg salt) orally, daily	0.6 mg/kg base (1 mg/kg salt) up to adult dosage, orally, daily	1-2 days	3-7 days	—	An option for primary prophylaxis in special circumstances and in consultation with malaria experts. Take with food. Contraindicated in persons with G6PD deficiency, during pregnancy and breastfeeding (unless the infant being breastfed has a documented normal G6PD level).

*Caused by *Plasmodium falciparum*, *P. ovale*, *P. vivax*, and *P. malariae*.

†Adult tablets contain 250 mg atovaquone and 100 mg proguanil hydrochloride.

‡Pediatric tablets contain 62.5 mg atovaquone and 25 mg proguanil hydrochloride.

§Approximate tablet fraction is based on a recommended dosage of 5 mg/kg body weight once weekly. A pharmacist should prepare exact doses for children weighing 10 kg.

¶Should never exceed adult dosage.

G6PD, glucose-6-phosphate dehydrogenase; US, United States.

Other Malaria Prevention Strategies

1. Apply behavioral modification strategies.
    a. Limit exposure to mosquitoes (i.e., time spent outdoors, particularly at dusk and during nighttime).
    b. Use physical barriers such as screens, doors, nets, and curtains.
    c. Wear protective clothing (long sleeves and long pants when possible, sprayed or impregnated with insecticide).
    d. Use mosquito bed nets (sprayed or impregnated with insecticide).
    e. Use mosquito coils and candles.
2. Insect repellents and insecticides are highly recommended as adjuncts to malaria chemoprophylaxis. They provide additional protection from insect-transmitted infections that have no vaccines or chemoprophylaxis. The most effective insect repellent for skin application contains diethyltoluamide (DEET). Examples include the following:
    a. Ultrathon Insect Repellent: 35% DEET in polymer formulation; provides up to 12-hour protection against mosquitoes; also effective against ticks, biting flies, chiggers, fleas, and gnats (3M, Minneapolis, MN)
    b. DEET plus Insect Repellent: 17.5% DEET with 2.5% R 326; apply q4h for mosquitoes, q8h for biting flies (Sawyer Products, Safety Harbor, FL)
    c. Skedaddle Insect Protection for Children: 10% DEET using molecular entrapment technology (Little Point Corp., Cambridge, MA)
3. Permethrin-containing spray insecticide is effective for external clothing and mosquito nets. Examples include the following:
    a. Permanone Tick Repellent (Coulston International Corp., Easton, PA)
    b. Duranon Tick Repellent: permethrin in a formula lasting up to 2 weeks; repels ticks, chiggers, and mosquitoes (Coulston International Corp., Easton, PA)
    c. Peripel: permethrin liquid for soaking bed nets (Burroughs Wellcome, Great Britain)
4. Partial immunity can be stimulated by repeated infections in residents of malaria-endemic areas; however, this immunity is gained at the expense of chronic anemia and is lost when residents go abroad for work or study.
5. Malaria vaccines are being investigated and may become available in the future.

Travel-Acquired Illnesses

47

SOURCES OF INFORMATION

The Centers for Disease Control and Prevention (CDC) publishes several authoritative sources of information on travel medicine. Health Information for International Travel (the "yellow book") is updated annually. Two other periodicals, the weekly *Morbidity and Mortality Weekly Report* (MMWR) and *Summary of Health Information for International Travel* (the "blue sheet," published biweekly), provide updated information on the status of immunization recommendations, worldwide disease outbreaks, and changes in health conditions. A reliable way to obtain current travel health information including vaccine requirements, malaria chemoprophylaxis, and disease outbreaks for various regions of the world is to consult the CDC Database of Health Information for International Travel website at www.cdc.gov/travel/contentyellowbook.aspx. For nonmedical information of interest to the traveler, the U.S. State Department can be accessed at http://travel.state.gov/. Additional resources for travel medicine information are listed at the end of the chapter.

Aside from the diarrheal diseases, the major travel-acquired illnesses are as follows:

- Yellow fever
- Dengue fever
- Hepatitis
- Typhoid and paratyphoid fevers
- Meningococcal disease
- Japanese B encephalitis
- Malaria (see Chapter 46)

These disorders are often preventable if the traveler takes specific precautions or prophylactic agents.

MAJOR VIRAL INFECTIONS

▶ YELLOW FEVER

Yellow fever is one of the viral hemorrhagic fevers. It is caused by a single-stranded ribonucleic acid (RNA) flavivirus that is transmitted by mosquitoes. The liver is the principal target organ. All recent cases of American yellow fever were acquired in the jungle environment; however, urban transmission continues to occur in Africa.

Signs and Symptoms
1. May appear as an undifferentiated viral syndrome
2. Specific diagnosis in the wilderness is extremely difficult; clinical suspicion is based on immune status, geographic distribution of the disease, travel history, and characteristic triphasic fever, as follows:
   a. Headache, fever, and malaise, often accompanied by bradycardia and conjunctival suffusion
   b. After 3 to 4 days, brief remission
   c. Within 24 hours, intoxication phase: jaundice; fever; prostration; and, in severe cases, hypotension, shock, oliguria, and obtundation; hemorrhage usually manifested as hematemesis, but bleeding from multiple sites possible
   d. Signs of a poor prognosis include early onset of the intoxication phase, hypotension, severe hemorrhage with disseminated intravascular coagulation (DIC), renal failure, shock, and coma

Treatment
1. Perform a careful physical examination. Be aware that the laboratory evaluation includes thick and thin blood smears to rule out malaria and blood cultures for bacterial pathogens; both of these necessitate evacuation to a qualified medical facility. If the victim's condition progresses to the intoxication phase, arrange for immediate evacuation to an intensive care unit (ICU).
2. Note that no effective antiviral treatment is available for yellow fever.
3. Supportive care in the field includes the following:
   a. Control fever with acetaminophen (do not use salicylates).
   b. Give IV fluids and oral rehydration fluids.
   c. Transfer the victim to a hospital as quickly as possible.

Prevention
1. Give yellow fever vaccine (>95% of those vaccinated achieve significant antibody levels). Be aware that booster doses of vaccine are recommended every 10 years.
2. Avoid the causative organism through mosquito protection measures in endemic areas including repellent and proper netting.

▶ DENGUE

Dengue virus is a single-stranded RNA flavivirus that is transmitted by the day-biting urban mosquito *Aedes aegypti* or the jungle mosquito *Aedes albopictus*. *A. aegypti* is the principal vector for dengue viruses worldwide. Viral transmission is maintained through a mosquito-human cycle without a major animal reservoir.

Signs and Symptoms (compare dengue with malaria in Table 47-1)

1. Clinically, may range from undifferentiated viral symptoms with fever and mild respiratory/gastrointestinal symptoms to dengue hemorrhage fever (see later)
2. Incubation period: 5 to 8 days
3. Early prodromal symptoms of nausea and vomiting common, followed by high fever lasting for days (mean, 5 days)
4. Headache and lymphadenopathy common, as well as myalgias ("breakbone fever")
5. After several days, often maculopapular or morbilliform rash spreading outward from chest
6. Dengue can progress to severe forms, referred to as *dengue hemorrhage fever* (DHF) or *dengue shock syndrome* (DSS). Severe DHF/DSS may progress to circulatory failure with shock and spontaneous bleeding from almost any site.
7. After infection, patients often develop extreme fatigue persisting for weeks or months.
8. DHF/DSS is unlikely in travelers not previously infected with dengue.
9. Awareness of the local epidemiology of DHF/DSS is important in establishing the diagnosis. Definitive diagnosis of all forms requires serology (antibody identification) or viral isolation from serum.

TABLE 47-1. Clinical Illness in Malaria and Dengue Fever

SIGNS AND SYMPTOMS	MALARIA	DENGUE FEVER
Fever	+++	+++
Chills	+++	++
Headache	+++	+++
Malaise		++
Anorexia		++
Nausea, vomiting	++	++
Abdominal pain	++	
Myalgia	++	++
Arthralgia		++
Backache	+	
Dark urine	+	

+++, >90% of patients; ++, >50% of patients; +, <10% of patients.

Treatment
1. Treatment is symptomatic.
2. In DHF/DSS, administer acetaminophen for fever and myalgias (do not use salicylates).
3. Vigorously maintain hydration.
4. Be aware that severe DHF or any DSS is a medical emergency and requires immediate evacuation and hospitalization.
5. No specific therapy exists for any form of dengue.

▶ HEPATITIS VIRUSES

The causes of hepatitis may be divided into two groups. First, the so-called *named,* or more accurately, *lettered* viruses now include hepatitis A to G. These are associated with defined clinical syndromes and elevated liver function tests. Second, other organisms that cause hepatitis as part of a more systemic infection include Epstein-Barr virus, cytomegalovirus, toxoplasmosis, and leptospirosis.

Hepatitis A

Hepatitis A virus (HAV) is transmitted mainly through the fecal-oral route, either by person-to-person contact or by ingestion of contaminated food or water. Occasional cases are associated with exposure to nonhuman primates. HAV is endemic worldwide, but underdeveloped regions have a significantly higher prevalence. In most instances, resolution of the acute disease is permanent, but rare cases of relapse have been noted. Death from HAV is rare. After natural infection, HAV antibodies confer immunity. HAV patients are infectious for approximately 2 weeks before the onset of symptoms. Viral shedding declines with the onset of jaundice. The victim is typically not infectious 1 to 2 weeks after the onset of clinical disease.

Signs and Symptoms
1. Incubation period ranging from 2 to 7 weeks
2. Infection is often asymptomatic or mild, especially in children
3. Classic syndrome: early onset of anorexia, followed by nausea, vomiting, fever, and abdominal pain
4. Symptoms possibly accompanied by hepatosplenomegaly
5. Jaundice after gastrointestinal syndrome by several days to a few weeks; resolution of jaundice lasting another 3 to 4 weeks
6. Although rare, HAV sometimes (0.5% to 1%) follows a fulminant course, resulting in hepatic necrosis, hepatic

encephalopathy, and death. The incidence of fulminant hepatitis increases with age.

7. Clinical presentation is often milder than with other types of viral hepatitis, but not distinctive enough to allow clinical differentiation.
8. A number of clinical tests are available to confirm the diagnosis, but diagnosis in the field is empiric.

Treatment
1. No specific therapy exists for HAV infection.
2. Instruct affected persons to adhere to enteric precautions to avoid transmission to others (compulsive hand washing).
3. Although infectivity drops sharply soon after the onset of jaundice. To be safe, continue enteric and blood-drawing precautions for 2 weeks.

Prevention
1. See discussion of HAV vaccine in Chapter 48.
2. See discussion of dietary precautions in Chapter 43.

Hepatitis B

Hepatitis B virus (HBV) is transmitted through the exchange of blood; semen; or, rarely, saliva from infected people. Although spread is possible from persons with acute disease, in most cases chronic carriers spread the disease. In many areas of the developing world, chronic carriers are 10% to 20% of the total population. The risk is much higher among persons regularly exposed to body fluids including medical personnel and those who engage in sexual contact abroad. Victims with HBV infection may be infectious within 1 to 2 weeks after inoculation, well before any clinical symptoms develop.

Signs and Symptoms
1. Range of incubation period 7 to 22 weeks
2. Manifestations similar to those of HAV: fever, anorexia, nausea, vomiting, abdominal pain
3. Additional prodrome of rash, arthralgias, or arthritis and fever in up to 20% of HBV patients (rare in HAV)
4. Jaundice developing a short time after gastrointestinal symptoms
5. With self-limited disease, recovery complete by 6 months
6. With fulminant (1% to 3%) course, hepatic necrosis, hepatic encephalopathy, often death
7. Other possibilities:
   a. Asymptomatic chronic carrier state
   b. Chronic active hepatitis
   c. Chronic progressive hepatitis
8. Definitive diagnosis requires antigen and antibody tests

Treatment
1. No specific field therapy exists for HBV.
2. Note that prolonged and sometimes persistent viremia makes blood and body fluid precautions necessary until antigen and antibody testing show noninfectivity.
3. Note: for patients with chronic infection, therapy with interferon-alfa is sometimes recommended.

Prevention
Prophylaxis is indicated for travelers at high risk, specifically, medical workers or those anticipating sexual contact with local inhabitants in endemic areas (see Chapter 48).

▶ OTHER FORMS OF HEPATITIS

Hepatitis C
1. Previously "non-A, non-B hepatitis," hepatitis C is similar to HBV in both transmission and clinical course.
2. Unlike hepatitis B, protective antibody responses have not been demonstrated.
3. Treatment of acute hepatitis C is supportive.
4. Treatment of chronic infection is with interferon-alpha, though the overall results are disappointing and side effects are significant.

Hepatitis D
1. Formerly the "delta agent," active hepatitis D is found only in individuals who are positive for hepatitis B surface antigen (HbsAg).
2. Precautions against transmission are the same as for hepatitis B.
3. No specific vaccine or immune globulin for the delta agent exists.
4. The best preventive measure is to be vaccinated for hepatitis B because delta agent infection cannot occur in the absence of the former virus.

Hepatitis E
1. Hepatitis E was formerly called "enterically transmitted non-A, non-B hepatitis."
2. Hepatitis E is similar to HAV in both transmission and clinical course.
3. It is the second most common cause of viral hepatitis transmitted via the enteric route.
4. Diagnosis in travelers from endemic areas can be made on the basis of IgM antibody to hepatitis E in serum or testing of stool for viral antigen.

5. Vaccines are not available.
6. Prophylaxis is appropriate advice for travelers and involves counseling with respect to precautions regarding ingestion of food and water in endemic areas.

Hepatitis F and G

1. Hepatitis F is a poorly defined hepatitis virus of uncertain significance.
2. Hepatitis G is a member of the flavivirus family with limited homology to hepatitis C. Its significance as a cause of hepatitis is also unclear.

Hepatitis C-G Treatment

No specific vaccine exists for these forms. Immunity to hepatitis D is conferred with immunity to HBV. As with other types of hepatitis, the best method of prevention is avoidance of infected body fluids and adherence to safe sexual practices. Additional blood-borne precautions include avoiding potentially infected needles, tattooing, and body piercing.

▶ JAPANESE B ENCEPHALITIS

1. Japanese encephalitis is a viral infection transmitted by *Culex* mosquitoes. Transmission takes place year-round in tropical and subtropical areas and during the late spring, summer, and early fall in temperate climates. This disease occurs primarily in rural areas, often associated with pig farming.
2. Encephalitis is caused by a neurotropic flavivirus.
3. After initial replication near the mosquito bite, viremia occurs and, if prolonged, may seed infection to the brain.
4. The virus causes central nervous system nerve cell destruction and necrosis.
5. Most infections in endemic areas involve children, but this disease may occur in any age group.
6. At present, Japanese B encephalitis transmission is most likely in India, Southeast Asia, China, Korea, Indonesia, the far western Pacific region, eastern Russia, and Japan.
7. Recent outbreaks and case reports of Japanese B encephalitis in islands of the Torres Strait that runs between Northern Australia and Papua New Guinea indicate that the virus has spread south from Asia.

Signs and Symptoms

1. No clinical illness in most infections
2. Encephalitis (about 1 in 300 infections)
3. Mild, undifferentiated febrile illness (encephalitis victims often with a similar prodrome)
4. Headache, lethargy, fever, confusion; possible tremors or seizures

5. Reported mortality with clinical encephalitis: 10% to 50%
6. Encephalitis syndrome not easily distinguished from other arboviral encephalitis
7. Definitive diagnosis: serologic testing

Treatment
1. Be aware that no specific therapy exists for this disease.
2. Provide supportive care and hydration.
3. Note that supportive care often requires an ICU.
4. Practice blood and body fluid precautions.

Prevention
1. The main interventions are prophylactic: vaccination and reduced arthropod exposure.
2. An effective inactivated vaccine is recommended for travelers to endemic areas in the transmission season who will be staying for longer than 1 month.
3. See discussion of Japanese encephalitis vaccine in Chapter 48.

MAJOR BACTERIAL INFECTIONS

▶ TYPHOID AND PARATYPHOID FEVER (ENTERIC FEVERS)

Typhoid fever occurs worldwide, but its prevalence and attack rates are much higher in undeveloped countries. Humans are the only host for *Salmonella typhi*, the most common cause of the typhoid fever syndrome. Nearly all cases are contracted through the ingestion of contaminated food and water. The risk of transmission is relatively high in Mexico, Peru, India, Pakistan, Chile, sub-Saharan Africa, and Southeast Asia.

Salmonella species are gram-negative enteric bacilli. *Salmonella typhi* is the prime cause of typhoid fever, but other species may cause a typhoid fever-like syndrome. The term *enteric fever* is used to describe a severe systemic infection with *Salmonella paratyphi* (paratyphoid fever). The clinical appearance of *S. paratyphi* infection is similar to that seen with typhoid (see next), but typically, *S. paratyphi* infection runs a shorter course.

Signs and Symptoms
1. Onset of illness is usually 10 to 14 days after exposure to the pathogen.
2. Gastroenteritis is possible early in the course of the disease with associated abdominal pain and constipation. Diarrhea is more common in younger children.
3. Fever
   a. Usually the first sign of disease
   b. May be accompanied by bradycardia

    c. Increases slowly over several days and remains constant for 2 to 3 weeks, after which defervescence begins
4. Headaches, malaise, anorexia
5. "Rose spots" (2- to 4-mm maculopapular blanching lesions) classically described on the trunk, although not seen in most victims
6. Hepatomegaly, splenomegaly in many patients
7. Uncomplicated, untreated typhoid fever usually resolves spontaneously in 3 to 4 weeks
8. Life-threatening complications:
    a. Intestinal perforation leading to peritonitis
    b. Gastrointestinal hemorrhage
    c. Pneumonia
    d. Multisystem failure with myocardial involvement
9. Definitive diagnosis possible by bacterial culture
10. Possible for victims to remain asymptomatic carriers and continue to shed organisms for years

Treatment
1. Give antibiotics:
    a. Ciprofloxacin, 500 mg bid for 2 weeks (or other quinolone)
    b. In cases of quinolone resistance (either laboratory or clinical unresponsiveness), ceftriaxone or other third-generation cephalosporins are indicated.
    c. In the absence of the previously mentioned antibiotics, use one of the following, but remember that resistance has been noted:
        1. Ampicillin, 100 mg/kg/day in four divided doses for at least 2 weeks
        2. Co-trimoxazole: 80 mg trimethoprim plus 400 mg sulfamethoxazole/day in two divided doses for at least 2 weeks
        3. Chloramphenicol, 50 mg/kg/day in four divided doses for 2 weeks
2. Make certain that the patient has adequate nutrition and food support.
3. High-dose steroids are not recommended for those with less severe disease but may be used cautiously in those with severe disease.
4. Be aware that relapse can occur after 2 weeks of therapy and necessitates retreatment with the same regimen.

Prevention
1. Because typhoid vaccine does not ensure protection, tell vaccinated persons to avoid potentially contaminated food and drink (see Chapter 43).
2. See discussion of typhoid fever vaccine in Chapter 48.

▶ MENINGOCOCCAL DISEASE

Meningococcal disease is caused by *Neisseria meningitidis,* a gram-negative diplococcus. Meningococcal meningitis classically attacks children and young adults and is often seen in epidemic form. Despite effective antibiotic therapy and immunization, this disease remains problematic in many parts of the world.

Epidemic situations pose the greatest health problem to both travelers and resident populations. Since 1970, large outbreaks have occurred in Brazil; China; the Sahel region of sub-Saharan Africa; New Delhi, India; and Nepal.

Transmission of the organism occurs through respiratory secretions, so close contact is believed to be important in the spread of the disease.

Signs and Symptoms
1. Variety of forms, including but not limited to the following:
   a. Bacteremia with septic shock
   b. Meningitis, often with bacteremia
   c. Pneumonia
2. Sustained meningococcemia may lead to severe toxemia with hypotension, fever, and disseminated intravascular coagulation.
3. Meningitis caused by *N. meningitidis* is marked by the classic triad of fever, headache, and stiff neck and possibly accompanied by bacteremia and any of several skin manifestations including petechiae, pustules, or maculopapular rash.
4. Severe meningitis may progress to mental status deterioration, hypotension, congestive heart failure, disseminated intravascular coagulation, and death.
5. During an epidemic, a presumptive diagnosis can be made on the basis of clinical presentation.
6. Definitive diagnosis requires culture of the organism from cerebrospinal fluid or blood.
7. Several commercial kits for measuring meningococcal antigen are now available for use on cerebral spinal fluid or blood samples.

Treatment
1. Be aware that meningococcal meningitis, or sepsis, is a medical emergency, with suspected victims requiring immediate evacuation to an appropriate medical facility.
2. Note that, fortunately, the organism remains sensitive to many antibiotics such as the following:
   a. Penicillin G, 300,000 U/kg/day (up to 24 million U/day) IV in divided doses q2h for 7 to 10 days for serious disease

   b. Ceftriaxone, 2 g q12h IV

   c. Chloramphenicol, 12.5 mg/kg q6h IV (note that there has been emergence of chloramphenicol-resistant strains of *N. meningitidis*)

3. Give supportive care including close monitoring for hypotension and cardiac failure (will necessitate ICU technology) and IV fluid support.
4. Be aware that dexamethasone may be of value for victims in a coma or with evidence of increased intracranial pressure.
5. Make sure that close contacts receive prophylaxis to eradicate the organism (ciprofloxacin, 500 mg PO as a single dose, or rifampin, 600 mg PO q12h for four doses).

Prevention
See discussion of meningococcal vaccine in Chapter 48.

MALARIA

See Chapter 46.

TRAVEL MEDICINE INFORMATION RESOURCES

▶ TELEPHONE INFORMATION

- Centers for Disease Control and Prevention (CDC) Travelers' Health Hotline: 877-FYI-TRIP
- United States Department of State Overseas Citizens' Services: 888-407-4747

▶ OFFICIAL REFERENCES

- Centers for Disease Control: *Health Information for International Travel, 2004–5*, Washington, DC, USA
- Government Printing Office (revised annually) Telephone: 202-738-3238
- World Health Organization: *International Travel and Health, Vaccination Requirements and Health Advice*, 1999, World Health Organization Publications Center USA, 49 Sheridan Avenue, Albany, NY 12210 (revised annually)
- *Morbidity and Mortality Weekly Report*, Centers for Disease Control and Prevention, Atlanta, GA 30333; Subscriptions available at the website www.cdc.gov

▶ PRETRAVEL CLINIC DIRECTORIES

- International Society of Travel Medicine, website www.istm.org
- American Society of Tropical Medicine and Hygiene, website www.astmh.org

▶ TRAVELERS' CLINIC DIRECTORY

English-Speaking Physicians: International Association for
Medical Assistance to Travelers (IAMAT), 1623 Military Rd.
#279, Niagara Falls, NY 14304-1745
Telephone: 716-754-4883

▶ REFERENCE TABLES FOR PEDIATRIC TRAVEL

- Access www.istm.org, then at the left-hand column click on
  "Education and Training," then "Education and Scientific
  Information," then "Drugs and Vaccines for Pediatric Trav-
  elers: an Integrated Table."

Immunizations for Travel   48

▶ ROUTINE IMMUNIZATIONS

The vaccines currently recommended in childhood include those against tetanus, diphtheria, pertussis, varicella, rotavirus, measles mumps rubella, poliovirus, *Haemophilus influenzae* type b (Hib), hepatitis A, and hepatitis B. The recommended immunization schedules for persons aged 0 to 6 years (Table 48-1) and 7 to 18 years (Table 48-2) are published each year as approved by the Advisory Committee on Immunization Practices (www.cdc.gov/vaccines/recs/acip), the American Academy of Pediatrics (www.aap.org), and the American Academy of Family Physicians (www.aafp.org). Recommendations for immunization against influenza, meningococcal disease, and pneumococcal pneumonia are based on underlying health and age. A catch-up immunization schedule is available for persons aged 4 months to 18 years who start late or who are more than 1 month behind schedule with any particular immunization.

Travelers should record all immunizations in The International Certificates of Vaccination (the "little yellow booklet") as approved by the World Health Organization (WHO). Routine immunizations are those customarily given in childhood and updated in adult life including the following:

1. *Tetanus and diphtheria.* Booster doses of tetanus/diphtheria (Td) vaccine given at 10-year intervals throughout life are recommended to maintain immunity. If the person has no record or recollection of immunization, it is advisable to obtain this vaccine before traveling. The diphtheria and tetanus toxoids and acellular pertussis vaccine (DTaP) is used for primary immunization of children younger than 7 years of age. Tetanus and diphtheria toxoids and acellular pertussis vaccine (Tdap) is recommended beginning at age 11 to 12 years for persons who have completed the recommended DTP/DTaP vaccination series and have not received a tetanus and diphtheria toxoids (TD) booster dose.

2. *Pertussis.* Immunization is given in childhood as DTaP, and was formerly given as diphtheria-pertussis-tetanus (DPT) vaccine. Tetanus and diphtheria toxoids and acellular pertussis vaccine (Tdap) is recommended beginning at age 11 to 12 years for persons who have completed the recommended DTP/DTaP vaccination series and have not received a tetanus and diphtheria toxoids (TD) booster dose.

3. *Measles, mumps, and rubella.* A single dose of measles, mumps, and rubella (MMR) vaccine is recommended for all

601

TABLE 48-1. Recommended Immunization Schedule for Persons Aged 0–6 Years—UNITED STATES

VACCINE ▼ AGE ▶	BIRTH	1 MO	2 MO	4 MO	6 MO	12 MO	15 MO	18 MO	19–23 MO	2–3 YR	4–6 YR
Hepatitis B[1]	HepB	HepB			HepB						
Rotavirus[2]			see footnote 1 / Rota	Rota	Rota						
Diphtheria, Tetanus, Pertussis[3]			DTaP	DTaP	DTaP		DTaP	DTaP			DTaP
Haemophilus influenzae type b[4]			Hib	Hib	Hib[4]	see footnote 3 / Hib	Hib				
Pneumococcal[5]			PCV	PCV	PCV	PCV	PCV			PPV	
Inactivated Poliovirus			IPV	IPV		IPV	IPV				IPV
Influenza[6]					Influenza (Yearly)						
Measles, Mumps, Rubella[7]						MMR	MMR				MMR
Varicella[8]						Varicella	Varicella				Varicella
Hepatitis A[9]						HepA (2 doses)				HepA Series	
Meningococcal[10]										MCV4	MCV4

☐ Range of recommended ages   ☐ Certain high-risk groups

This schedule indicates the recommended ages for routine administration of currently licensed childhood vaccines, as of December 1, 2007, for children aged 0 through 6 years. Additional information is available at www.cdc.gov/vaccines/recs/schedules. Any dose not administered at the recommended age should be administered at any subsequent visit, when indicated and feasible. Additional vaccines may be licensed and recommended during the year. Licensed combination vaccines may be used whenever any components of the combination are indicated and other components of the vaccine are not contraindicated and if approved by the Food and Drug Administration for that dose of the series. **Providers should consult the respective Advisory Committee on Immunization Practices statement for detailed recommendations, including for high risk conditions: http:www.cdc.gov/vaccines/pubs/ACIP-list.htm.**

Clinically significant adverse events that follow immunization should be reported to the Vaccine Adverse Event Reporting System (VAERS). Guidance about how to obtain and complete VAERS form is available at www.vaers.hhs.gov or by telephone, 800-822-7967.

1. **Hepatitis B vaccine (HepB).** *(Minimum age: birth)* **At birth:** • Administer monovalent HepB to all newborns prior to hospital discharge. • If mother is hepatitis surface antigen (HBsAg)-positive, administer HepB and 0.5 mL of hepatitis B immune globulin (HBIG) within 12 hours of birth. • If mother's HBsAg status is unknown, administer HepB within 12 hours of birth. Determine the HBsAg status as soon as possible and if HBsAg-positive, administer HBIG (no later than age 1 week). • If mother is HBsAg-negative, the birth dose can be delayed, **in rare cases,** with a provider's order and a **copy of the mother's negative HBsAg** laboratory report in the infant's medical record. **After the birth dose:** • The HepB series should be completed with either monovalent HepB or a combination vaccine containing HepB. The second dose should be administered at age 1–2 months. The final dose should be administered no earlier than age 24 weeks. Infants born to HBsAg-positive mothers should be tested for HBsAg and antibody to HBsAg after completion of at least 3 doses of a licensed HepB series, at age 9–18 months (generally at the next well-child visit). **4-month dose:** • It is permissible to administer 4 doses of HepB when combination vaccines are administered after the birth dose. If monovalent HepB is used for doses after the birth dose, a dose at age 4 months is not needed.

2. **Rotavirus vaccine (Rota).** *(Minimum age: 6 weeks)* • Administer the first dose at age 6-12 weeks. • Do not start the series later than age 12 weeks. • Administer the final dose in the series by age 32 weeks. Do not administer any dose later than age 32 weeks. • Data on safety and efficacy outside of these age ranges are insufficient.

3. **Diphtheria and tetanus toxoids and acellular pertussis vaccine (DTaP).** *(Minimum age: 6 weeks)* • The fourth dose of DTaP may be administered as early as age 12 months, provided 6 months have elapsed since the third dose. • Administer the final dose in the series at age 4–6 years.

4. **Haemophilus influenzae type b conjugate vaccine (Hib).** *(Minimum age: 6 weeks)* • If PRP-OMP (PedvaxHIB® or ComVax® [Merck]) is administered at ages 2 and 4 months, a dose at age 6 months is not required. • TriHIBit® (DTaP/Hib) combination products should not be used for primary immunization but can be used as boosters following any Hib vaccine in children age 12 months or older.

5. **Pneumococcal vaccine.** *(Minimum age: 6 weeks for pneumococcal conjugate vaccine [PCV]; 2 years for pneumococcal polysaccharide vaccine [PPV])* • Administer one dose of PCV to all healthy children aged 24–59 months having any incomplete schedule. • Administer PPV to children aged 2 years and older with underlying medical conditions.

6. **Influenza vaccine.** *(Minimum age: 6 months for trivalent inactivated influenza vaccine [TIV]; 2 years for live, attenuated influenza vaccine [LAIV])* • Administer annually to children aged 6–59 months and to all close contacts of children aged 0–59 months. • Administer annually to children 5 years of age and older with certain risk factors, to other persons (including household members) in close contact with persons in groups at higher risk, and to any child whose parents request vaccination. • For healthy nonpregnant persons (those who do not have underlying medical conditions that predispose them to influenza complications) ages 2–49 years, either LAIV or TIV may be used. • Children receiving TIV should receive 0.25 mL if age 6-35 mos or 0.5 mL if age 3 years or older. • Administer 2 doses (separated by 4 weeks or longer) to children younger than 9 years who are receiving influenza vaccine for the first time or who were vaccinated for the first time last season, but only received one dose.

Continued

TABLE 48-1. Recommended Immunization Schedule for Persons Aged 0–6 Years—UNITED STATES—cont'd

7. **Measles, mumps, and rubella vaccine (MMR).** *(Minimum age: 12 months)* • Administer the second dose of MMR at age 4–6 years. MMR may be administered before age 4–6 years, provided more than 4 weeks have elapsed since the first dose and both doses are administered at age 12 months or older.

8. **Varicella vaccine.** *(Minimum age: 12 months)* • Administer second dose at age 4–6 years; may be administered 3 months or more after first dose.
   • Don't repeat second dose if administered 28 days or more after first dose.

9. **Hepatitis A vaccine (HepA).** *(Minimum age: 12 months)* • HepA is recommended for all children aged 1 yr (i.e., aged 12–23 months). The 2 doses in the series should be administered at least 6 months apart. • Children not fully vaccinated by age 2 years can be vaccinated at subsequent visits. • HepA is recommended for certain other groups of children, including in areas where vaccination programs target older children.

10. **Meningococcal vaccine.** *(Minimum age: 2 years for meningococcal conjugate vaccine (MCV4) and for meningococcal polysaccharide vaccine (MPSV4)* • MCV4 is recommended for children aged 2–10 years with terminal complement deficiencies or anatomic or functional asplenia and certain other high-risk groups. Use of MPSV4 is also acceptable. • Persons who received MPSV4 3 or more years prior and remain at increased risk for meningococcal disease should be vaccinated with MCV4.

TABLE 48-2. Recommended Immunization Schedule for Persons Aged 7–18 Years—UNITED STATES

VACCINE ▼ AGE ▶	7–10 YR	11–12 YR	13–18 YR
Diphtheria, Tetanus, Pertussis[1]	see footnote 1	Tdap	Tdap
Human Papillomavirus[2]	see footnote 2	HPV (3 doses)	HPV Series
Meningococcal[3]	MCV4	MCV4	MCV4
Pneumococcal[4]		PPV	
Influenza[5]		Influenza (Yearly)	
Hepatitis A[6]		HepA Series	
Hepatitis B[7]		HepB Series	
Inactivated Poliovirus[8]		IPV Series	
Measles, Mumps, Rubella[9]		MMR Series	
Varicella[10]		Varicella Series	

☐ Range of recommended ages   ☐ Catch-up immunization   ☐ Certain high-risk groups

This schedule indicates the recommended ages for routine administration of currently licensed childhood vaccines, as of December 1, 2007, for children aged 7–18 years. Additional information is available at www.cdc.gov/vaccines/recs/schedules. Any dose not administered at the recommended age should be administered at any subsequent visit, when indicated and feasible. Additional vaccines may be licensed and recommended during the year. Licensed combination vaccines may be used whenever any components of the combination are indicated and other components of the vaccine are not contraindicated and if approved by the Food and Drug Administration for that dose of the series. Providers should consult the respective Advisory Committee on Immunization Practices statement for detailed recommendations, including for high risk conditions: http:www.cdc.gov/vaccines/pubs/ACIP-list.htm. Clinically significant adverse events that follow immunization should be reported to the Vaccine Adverse Event Reporting System (VAERS). Guidance about how to obtain and complete VAERS form is available at www.vaers.hhs.gov or by telephone, 800-822-7967.

Continued

TABLE 48-2. Recommended Immunization Schedule for Persons Aged 7–18 Years—UNITED STATES—cont'd

1. **Tetanus and diphtheria toxoids and acellular pertussis vaccine (Tdap).** *(Minimum age: 10 years for BOOSTRIX® and 11 years for ADACEL™)* • Administer at age 11–12 years for those who have completed the recommended childhood DTP/DTaP vaccination series and have not received a tetanus and diphtheria toxoids (Td) booster dose. • 13–18 year olds who missed the 11–12 year Tdap or received Td only, are encouraged to receive one dose of Tdap 5 years after the last Td/DTaP dose.

2. **Human papillomavirus vaccine (HPV).** *(Minimum age: 9 years)* • Administer the first dose of the HPV vaccine series to females at age 11–12 years. • Administer the second dose 2 months after the first dose and the third dose 6 months after the first dose. • Administer the HPV vaccine series to females at age 13–18 years if not previously vaccinated.

3. **Meningococcal vaccine.** • Administer MCV4 at age 11–12 years and at age 13–18 years if not previously vaccinated. MPSV4 is an acceptable alternative. • Administer MCV4 to previously unvaccinated college freshmen living in dormitories. • MCV4 is recommended for children aged 2–10 years with terminal complement deficiencies or anatomic or functional asplenia and certain other high-risk groups. • Persons who received MPSV4 3 or more years prior and remain at increased risk for meningococcal disease should be vaccinated with MCV4.

4. **Pneumococcal polysaccharide vaccine (PPV).** • Administer PPV to certain high-risk groups.

5. **Influenza vaccine.** • Administer annually to all close contacts of children aged 0–59 months. • Administer annually to persons with certain risk factors, health-care workers, and other persons (including household members) in close contact with persons in groups at higher risk. • Administer 2 doses (separated by 4 weeks or longer) to children younger than 9 years who are receiving influenza vaccine for the first time or who were vaccinated for the first time last season, but only received one dose. • For healthy nonpregnant persons (those who do not have underlying medical conditions that predispose them to influenza complications) ages 2–49 years, either LAIV or TIV may be used.

6. **Hepatitis A vaccine (HepA).** • The 2 doses in the series should be administered at least 6 months apart. • HepA is recommended for certain other groups of children, including in areas where vaccination programs target older children.

7. **Hepatitis B vaccine (HepB).** • Administer the 3-dose series to those who were not previously vaccinated. • A 2-dose series of Recombivax HB® is licensed for children aged 11–15 years.

8. **Inactivated poliovirus vaccine (IPV).** • For children who received an all-IPV or all-oral poliovirus (OPV) series, a fourth dose is not necessary if the third dose was administered at age 4 years or older. • If both OPV and IPV were administered as part of a series, a total of 4 doses should be administered, regardless of the child's current age.

9. **Measles, mumps, and rubella vaccine (MMR).** • If not previously vaccinated, administer 2 doses of MMR during any visit, with 4 or more weeks between the doses.

10. **Varicella vaccine.** • Administer 2 doses of varicella vaccine to persons younger than 13 years at least 3 months apart. Do not repeat the second dose, if administered 28 or more days following the first dose. • Administer 2 doses of varicella vaccine to persons aged 13 years or older at least 4 weeks apart. • Administer 2 doses of vaccine minimum 4 weeks apart to persons younger than 13 years without evidence of immunity.

infants at 15 months of age. The Immunization Practices Advisory Committee recommends a second dose of measles vaccine in childhood on entry into grade school, middle school, or high school; this is required by law in many states. Also, persons born after 1957 are assumed to be susceptible and should receive a second dose of measles vaccine. The second dose of measles vaccine is usually administered as MMR vaccine. MMR vaccine is a live attenuated virus preparation that is contraindicated in pregnancy and in persons with compromised immunity. Transmission of naturally occurring measles is higher among populations in developing countries than in the United States, so travelers are at higher risk of exposure.

4. *Poliovirus.* Poliomyelitis vaccine is usually not boosted after childhood in the United States except for anticipated high-risk exposure through work or travel to areas where polio is endemic. An inactivated (killed) virus polio vaccine (IPV) regimen is recommended for a primary immunization series given before 18 years of age. IPV is also recommended for booster doses in people 18 years of age and older because of a higher risk of complications associated with the live oral vaccine (OPV) in older patients. Polio has been nearly eradicated worldwide, except for India. All traveling adults should have received a primary course of the polio vaccine.

5. *H. influenzae type B (Hib).* Immunization is acquired in childhood. The risk for invasive *H. influenzae* disease including meningitis is greatest in children younger than 7 years old, and the infection is common among children in the developing world. Primary immunization is recommended at 2 months of age or as soon as possible thereafter. Three different conjugate vaccines are commercially available against *H. influenzae* type B. Two doses of PRP-OMP vaccine, or three doses of HbOC vaccine given 2 months apart, are recommended for all children younger than 12 months of age. After 12 months of age, a single dose of either vaccine is sufficient for immunization. The third Hib conjugate vaccine, PRP-D, is approved for use only in children 15 months or older and is given as a single dose. Immunization against Hib is not recommended for adults.

6. Influenza vaccine is recommended for all health care workers and for international travelers because prolonged air travel and exposure to crowded or extreme environments create a predisposition to infection. Other considerations are based on conventional recommendations regarding underlying health and age (e.g., all people older than

65 years of age and those with chronic lung, heart, or kidney disease or with impaired immunity).

7. The 23-valent polysaccharide vaccine against pneumococcal pneumonia consists of a single dose and is recommended for all persons older than 65 years of age and those with chronic lung, heart, or kidney disease or with impaired immunity. A revaccination dose at 3 to 5 years after the initial dose is recommended for certain risk groups.

8. Pneumococcal congregate vaccine is routinely recommended for infants younger than 2 years of age to prevent pneumococcal disease including meningitis and septicemia.

▶ COMMONLY RECOMMENDED TRAVELERS' VACCINES
(Table 48-3)

Specific recommendations are based on the following risk factors:
- Geographic destination(s)
- Duration of trip
- Style of travel
- Purpose of trip
- Underlying health of traveler
- Access to medical care during trip

Cholera
Cholera vaccine is not highly efficacious and is no longer endorsed by the WHO as a requirement for entry into any country. It is no longer available in the United States. Some countries still require cholera vaccine for travelers arriving from a cholera-endemic area. The primary series consists of two doses given a week or more apart. However, a single cholera dose should meet entry requirements. Travelers going to cholera-endemic or cholera-epidemic areas should follow food and water precautions to prevent all forms of travelers' diarrhea. Persons with underlying gastric conditions such as achlorhydria or partial gastric resection may benefit from immunization in view of the increased susceptibility to infection.

An oral live cholera vaccine is now available in Europe and Canada. This vaccine is moderately effective as a single dose and confers immunity for 3 years. Adverse reactions are uncommon.

Typhoid Fever
An oral typhoid fever vaccine is available. Even if a typhoid fever vaccine is administered before travel, it is essential to follow routine precautions related to the ingestion of food and water because efficacy of vaccination is only 40% to 80%.

TABLE 48-3. Vaccines and Immunoglobulin for Adult Travelers Who Completed Childhood Immunizations

VACCINE	ROUTE (DOSE)	SCHEDULE	SIDE EFFECTS, PRECAUTIONS, AND CONTRAINDICATIONS*	COMMENTS
Hepatitis A (Havrix and Vaqta)	IM (1 mL)	Primary: single dose Booster dose at 6-12 mo for long-lasting protection. Additional booster doses: not recommended	Local reactions: <56% Fever: <5% Headache: 16%	Prevaccine hepatitis A serology may be cost effective for some travelers (see text).
Hepatitis B (Recombivax and Engerix-B)	IM (adult and pediatric formulations)	Primary: 1 dose at 0, 1, and 6 mo Booster: not routinely recommended Accelerated schedules: see text	Local reaction: 3%-29% Fever: 1%-6%	
Hepatitis A and B antigens combined (Twinrix)	IM (1 mL)	Primary: 1 dose at 0, 1, and 6 mo booster: not routinely recommended Accelerated schedules: see text	Local reactions: approximately 56% Systemic reactions: similar to single antigen products	Give at least 2 doses of vaccine before departure to provide protection against hepatitis A.

Continued

TABLE 48-3. Vaccines and Immunoglobulin for Adult Travelers Who Completed Childhood Immunizations—cont'd

VACCINE	ROUTE (DOSE)	SCHEDULE	SIDE EFFECTS, PRECAUTIONS, AND CONTRAINDICATIONS*	COMMENTS
Immunoglobulin (Ig)	IM (buttocks)	Travel of <3 mo duration: 0.02 mL/kg Travel <3 mo: 0.06 mL/kg every 4-6 mo	Local discomfort: common Systemic allergy: rare	Should not be given <2 wk after or 3 mo before MMR, or varicella vaccines. Hepatitis A vaccine is preferred.
Influenza	IM (0.5 mL)	1 dose of current vaccine annually	Local reactions: <33% Systemic reactions: occasional Allergic reaction: rare Avoid in persons with history of anaphylaxis to eggs	
Influenza (Flumist)	Intranasal (0.5 mL)	Primary: 1 dose per season	Mild upper respiratory symptoms: occasional Avoid in persons with history of anaphylaxis to eggs, Guillain-Barré syndrome, or immunosuppression	Approved for persons 5-49 yr.

VACCINE	ROUTE (DOSE)	SCHEDULE	SIDE EFFECTS, PRECAUTIONS, AND CONTRAINDICATIONS*	COMMENTS
Japanese B encephalitis	SC (1 mL)	Primary: 1 dose at 0, 7, and 30 days Booster: 1 dose at 24-mo intervals	Local reactions: 20% Mild systemic reactions: 10% Allergic reactions (urticaria, rash, angioedema, or respiratory distress): approximately 0.6% Sudden death or encephalomyelitis: rare Avoid in pregnancy or in persons with multiple allergies	Observe recipients for delayed allergic reactions for 30 min after each dose. Complete series ≥10 days before departure.

Continued

TABLE 48-3. Vaccines and Immunoglobulin for Adult Travelers Who Completed Childhood Immunizations—cont'd

VACCINE	ROUTE (DOSE)	SCHEDULE	SIDE EFFECTS, PRECAUTIONS, AND CONTRAINDICATIONS*	COMMENTS
Measles (monovalent or combined with rubella and mumps [MMR])	SC (0.5 mL)	Primary: 2 doses separated by at least 1 yr Booster: none	Fever, 5-21 days after vaccination: 5%-15% Transient rash: 5% Local reaction among persons who received killed vaccine (1963-1967): 4%-55% Severe allergic reactions, CNS complications, thrombocytopenia (MMR): rare Avoid in pregnancy, immunocompromised hosts, and persons with history of anaphylaxis to eggs or neomycin	Do not give Ig within 3 mo of vaccine dose. If MMR and yellow fever vaccine are not given simultaneously, separate by ≥28 days.
Meningococcal polysaccharide-protein conjugate tetravalent vaccine (Menactra)	IM (0.5 mL)	Primary: Single dose Booster: Not determined	Local reactions: 10%-60% Systemic reactions: occasional fever, headache, and malaise	Replaces tetravalent polysaccharide vaccine (Menamune).

VACCINE	ROUTE (DOSE)	SCHEDULE	SIDE EFFECTS, PRECAUTIONS, AND CONTRAINDICATIONS*	COMMENTS
Mumps	SC (0.5 mL)	Primary: 1 dose (usually as MMR) Booster: none	Mild allergic reactions: uncommon Parotitis: rare Avoid in pregnancy, immunocompromised hosts, and persons with history of anaphylaxis to eggs or neomycin	Do not give Ig within 3 mo of vaccine dose. If MMR and yellow fever vaccine are not given simultaneously, separate by ≥28 days.
Pneumococcal polysaccharide	SC or IM (0.5 mL)	Primary: single dose at age 65 or age 60 if high risk. Booster: high-risk patients after 5 yr	Mild local reactions: approximately 50% Systemic symptoms: <1% Arthus-like reaction with booster doses may occur Avoid in persons with moderate to severe acute illness	Opportunity to update routine vaccination in older travelers.
Poliomyelitis	SC or IM (0.5 mL)	Booster: 1 adult dose	Local reactions: occasional	Additional boosters not recommended. Access CDC or WHO databases for current regions with polio transmission.

Continued

TABLE 48-3. Vaccines and Immunoglobulin for Adult Travelers Who Completed Childhood Immunizations—cont'd

VACCINE	ROUTE (DOSE)	SCHEDULE	SIDE EFFECTS, PRECAUTIONS, AND CONTRAINDICATIONS*	COMMENTS
Rabies: human diploid cell vaccine (HDCV); purified chick embryo cell (PCEC); rabies vaccine adsorbed (RVA)	IM (1 mL)	Pre-exposure: 1 dose at 0, 7, and 21 or 28 days. Booster doses depend on ongoing risk and results of serology (see text)	Mild local or systemic reactions: occasional immune complex–like reactions after booster dose of HDCV (2-21 days after vaccination): 6%	Target children in endemic areas who might not tell parents about bites.
Rubella	SC (0.5 mL)	Primary: 1 dose (usually as MMR) Booster: none	Transient arthralgias in adult women beginning 3-25 days after vaccination: up to 25% Arthritis: <2% Avoid in pregnancy, immunocompromised hosts, and persons with history of anaphylaxis to neomycin	Do not give Ig within 3 mo of vaccine dose. If MMR and yellow fever vaccine are not given simultaneously, separate by ≥28 days.

VACCINE	ROUTE (DOSE)	SCHEDULE	SIDE EFFECTS, PRECAUTIONS, AND CONTRAINDICATIONS*	COMMENTS
Tetanus-diphtheria (Td)	IM (0.5 mL)	Booster dose every 10 yr	Local reactions: common Systemic symptoms: occasional Anaphylaxis: rare Arthus-like reactions possible after multiple previous boosters Avoid if Guillain-Barré syndrome occurs ≤6wk after previous dose	Consider booster at 5 yr for travelers to remote areas or regions without adequate health care facilities when sustaining punctures or other significant wounds is possible. After one dose DTaP give Td every 10 yr
Tetanus-diphtheria acellular pertussis (TDaP)	IM (0.5 mL)	1 dose to replace a Td dose	See Td	
Typhoid Ty21a	Oral capsules	Primary: 1 capsule every other day for 4 doses Booster: every 5 yr	Gastrointestinal upset or rash: infrequent Avoid in pregnancy and in persons with febrile illness, taking antibiotics, or immunocompromised state.	Refrigerate capsules. If already taking mefloquine, separate doses by 24 hr.
Typhoid Vi polysaccharide	IM (0.5 mL)	Primary: single dose Booster: every 2 yr	Local reaction: 7% Headache: 16% Fever: <1%	

Continued

TABLE 48-3. Vaccines and Immunoglobulin for Adult Travelers Who Completed Childhood Immunizations—cont'd

VACCINE	ROUTE (DOSE)	SCHEDULE	SIDE EFFECTS, PRECAUTIONS, AND CONTRAINDICATIONS*	COMMENTS
Varicella	SC (0.5 mL)	Primary: 2 doses at ≥4-wk interval No booster	Local reactions: 20% Fever: 15% Localized or mild systemic varicella rash: 6% Avoid in pregnancy and immunocompromised hosts, if severe allergic reactions to gelatin or neomycin or if serum immune globulin within 5 mo	Rare transmission of vaccine strain to susceptible hosts; therefore avoid if close contacts are immunosuppressed.
VZV vaccine (Oka/Merck)	SC (0.65 mL)	1 dose	Local reactions: 33% Fever: 1.8% See Varicella for contraindications	Consider for all adults ≥60 yr of age to lower the burden of herpes zoster and decrease the incidence of postherpetic neuralgia.

VACCINE	ROUTE (DOSE)	SCHEDULE	SIDE EFFECTS, PRECAUTIONS, AND CONTRAINDICATIONS*	COMMENTS
Yellow fever	SC (0.5 mL)	Primary: single dose Booster: every 10 yr	Mild headache, myalgia, fever (5-10 days after vaccination): 25% Immediate hypersensitivity: rare Viscerotropic syndrome or neurotropic disease: rare (see text) Avoid if allergic to eggs	If subject can eat eggs without a reaction, he or she can take vaccine.

VACCINE	PRIMARY SERIES	BOOSTER
Cholera (parenteral)	2 doses 1 wk or more apart (0.5 mL SC or IM)	6 mo pediatric dose 0.3 mL for 5-10 yr of age, 0.2 mL for 6 mo to 4 yr of age
Plague	1st dose (1 mL IM); 2nd dose (0.2 mL IM) 4 wk later; dose 3 (0.2 mL IM) 3-6 mo after dose 2	Boost if risk of exposure persists: give first 2 booster doses (0.1-0.2 mL) 6 mo apart, then give 1 booster dose at 1- to 2-yr intervals as needed

Continued

TABLE 48-3. Vaccines and Immunoglobulin for Adult Travelers Who Completed Childhood Immunizations—cont'd

VACCINE	PRIMARY SERIES	BOOSTER
Tick-borne encephalitis	3 doses given SC on days 0, 30, and 180 days	Boost at 3- to 5-yr intervals
Tuberculosis (BCG vaccine)†	1 dose percutaneously with multiple-puncture disk; half strength for infants <1 mo old	Revaccination after 2-3 mo in those who remain tuberculin negative to 5 TU skin test

*Moderate or severe acute illness with or without fever or a serious reaction to a previous dose is a contraindication to all vaccines.
†Caution may be contraindicated in patients with any of the following conditions: pregnancy, leukemia, lymphoma, generalized malignancy, immunosuppression from HIV infection or treatment with corticosteroids, alkylating drugs, antimetabolites, or radiation therapy.
ID, intradermally; IM, intramuscularly; PO, orally; SC, subcutaneously.
Modified from information in *Health Information for International Travel 2004-5* (www.cdc.gov/travel/contentYellowBook.aspx) and Hill DR, Ericsson CD, Pearson RD, et al: The practice of travel medicine: Guidelines by the Infectious Diseases Society of America. Clin Infect Dis 43:1499-1539, 2006.

Oral Vaccine
1. Licensed in the United States since 1989
2. Contains live attenuated *Salmonella typhi*
3. Given as a series, taken every other day for four doses
4. Booster interval of 5 years
5. Better tolerated than the older injectable form; minimal side effects including gastrointestinal upset, fever, or headache
6. Not recommended for children younger than 6 years of age
7. Liquid formulation taken with a buffer more effective than capsules; also easily administered to young children but not yet licensed in the United States

Hepatitis A
1. Hepatitis A is the leading vaccine-preventable disease among international travelers to the developing world.
2. Hepatitis A is a serious viral infection with a transmission similar to polio, cholera, typhoid, and travelers' diarrhea (i.e., fecal contamination of food and water).
3. Adventure travelers who venture off usual tourist routes may be at increased risk compared with other groups of travelers.
4. Two hepatitis A inactivated viral vaccines are approved in the United States:
   a. Havrix (SmithKline Beecham)
   b. VAQTA (Merck)
5. Both vaccines are safe, efficacious, and produce long-lasting immunity. Each vaccine is given by intramuscular injection into the deltoid muscle.
6. Within 7 to 10 days after the first monovalent hepatitis A vaccine dose, most vaccine recipients develop protective levels of antibodies.
7. A second dose, constituting a booster dose, is given 6 to 18 months after the first dose. Immunity is likely lifelong, so booster does are not recommended in immunocompetent travelers.
8. Hepatitis A vaccine products are thought to be interchangeable. Travelers who fail to receive their second dose of vaccine within 6 to 12 months should receive one full dose of monovalent vaccine with the anticipation of lifelong immunity.

Immune Globulin (Human Ig)
Protection against hepatitis A can be obtained from immune globulin ("gamma globulin") containing preformed antibodies against hepatitis A.
1. No longer recommended unless you do not have time to wait 2 weeks after the first hepatitis A vaccine dose before initiating exposure to hepatitis A

2. Pre-exposure—recommended dose: 0.02 mL/kg IM if the stay is less than 3 months; for longer periods, 0.06 mL/kg IM
3. Postexposure: for a person having intimate contact (household or sexual) with an infected individual, use 0.02 mL/kg IM if the dose can be given within 2 weeks of exposure

Hepatitis B

Hepatitis B vaccine is now recommended as a routine immunization for children in the United States. Only adults at high risk need to receive immunization, but consideration should be given to immunizing all U.S. adults regardless of travel.

Immunization should be considered for travelers staying 6 or more months in Asia, Africa, or other endemic areas. In addition, immunization is recommended for travelers at high risk such as medical workers or those anticipating sexual contact with locals in endemic areas. Two vaccines are available: Recombivax and Engerix B. Both are recombinant vaccines containing killed virus and are felt to be interchangeable.

Vaccine Summary
1. Recombivax
   a. Standard adult dose at 0, 1, and 6 months
   b. Approved for an accelerated dosage schedule of 0, 1, and 2 months
2. Engerix B
   a. Standard adult dose at 0, 1, and 6 months
   b. Approved for an accelerated dosage schedule of 0, 1, and 2 months
3. Literature supports a highly accelerated 3-week schedule with dosing at 0, 7, and 21 days with a 12-month booster.
4. A combined hepatitis A and hepatitis B vaccine (Twinrix, SmithKline Beecham) is available. It is dosed at 0, 1, and 6 months. Because a smaller dose of Hepatitis A antigen is used in this preparation, travelers must receive their second dose before traveling for reliable protection. Literature also supports a highly accelerated 3-week dosing schedule (see previous instruction).

Meningococcus

Meningococcal vaccine is recommended for people traveling to countries or regions where outbreaks have been reported. The vaccine is also recommended for people traveling to live and work in certain areas of Africa (sub-Saharan) and South America (Brazil), where outbreaks of the disease are frequent among the residents. The vaccine is required for travel to Saudi Arabia in the late spring. It is prudent to check with local and federal health officials to determine current recommendations for vaccination because epidemic areas are not geographically fixed and previously uninvolved areas may experience epidemics.

Vaccine Summary
1. Meningococcal polysaccharide vaccine (Menomune, Aventis) is a quadrivalent vaccine inducing immunity against serogroups A, C, Y, and W-135.
2. Clinical efficacy is reduced because vaccine only covers four serotypes (five primary serotypes exist).
3. Duration of immunity is not established; revaccination is recommended for adults every 3 years if high risk continues.
4. Vaccine efficacy is variable in young children, so a second dose of vaccine after 2 to 3 years is recommended for children living in high-risk areas who received the first vaccine dose when younger than 4 years of age.
5. The vaccine is contraindicated in children younger than 2 years of age.
6. A new quadrivalent meningococcal polysaccharide-protein conjugate vaccine has been released for use in persons 11 to 55 years of age. Check to see if approval has been obtained for use in 2- to 10-year-olds. Compared with the polysaccharide vaccine, the conjugate vaccine promises longer-lasting immunity. Travelers who had been previously immunized with polysaccharide vaccine and need revaccination should receive conjugate vaccine.

Japanese Encephalitis Virus

Japanese encephalitis is a viral infection transmitted by *Culex* mosquitoes in mainland Asia and Southeast Asia. Pigs and some species of birds are natural reservoirs for the virus. Transmission is year-round in tropical and subtropical areas and during the late spring, summer, and early fall in temperate climates. Japanese encephalitis is not considered a risk for short-term travelers visiting tourist destinations in urban and developed resort areas.

The risk of infection can be greatly decreased by personal measures that prevent mosquito bites (e.g., protective clothing, insect repellents, bed nets). Vaccine should be offered to the following groups:
- Travelers who anticipate prolonged stays in rural endemic areas, especially areas of pig farming
- Travelers (e.g., expatriate workers, students) planning to live in an endemic area

Vaccine Summary
1. Recommended doses are given at 0, 7, and 30 days, with the third dose given on day 14 if required.
2. A booster is recommended every 2 to 3 years.
3. Expected efficacy is greater than 90%.

4. Adverse reactions to Japanese encephalitis virus vaccine include local pain and swelling at the injection site in about 20% of recipients, systemic symptoms (fever, headache, malaise, rash) in about 10% of recipients, and hypersensitivity reactions (mainly urticaria, angioedema, or both).
5. The Centers for Disease Control and Prevention (CDC) recommends that vaccine recipients do the following:
   a. Be directly observed for 30 minutes after injection of Japanese encephalitis virus vaccine
   b. Not depart on their journey until 10 days after the last dose because of the possibility of delayed adverse reactions

Rabies
See Chapter 42.

Plague
Plague is a bacterial disease caused by *Yersinia pestis*. It is transmitted to humans by fleas or direct contact with infected animals. Person-to-person spread is common through respiratory secretions. International travelers on standard tourist itineraries to countries where plague is reported are unlikely to be at high risk. Persons at risk of exposure include field biologists and persons who will reside or work in rural areas, where avoidance of rodents and fleas is difficult. It is recommended that travelers at risk avoid flea bites by using topical insect repellents containing DEET and permethrin insecticides on clothing and bed nets (see Chapter 37).

Vaccine Summary
1. A killed bacterial vaccine, it has poorly documented protective efficacy.
2. Primary series of three injections is recommended, with the first two doses given 4 or more weeks apart and the third dose given 3 to 6 months later.
3. Boosters are given every 6 months to 2 years for as long as exposure is present.
4. Both local and systemic side effects are possible including mild pain, redness, and induration at the injection site; with repeated doses, malaise, fever, and headache with increasing severity are possible.
5. An alternative to plague vaccine is the use of prophylactic oral tetracycline (500 mg/day) or doxycycline (100 mg bid) during periods of active exposure to plague-infected animals or humans (unproved as yet by controlled clinical studies).

Tick-Borne Encephalitis

Tick-borne encephalitis (TBE) is a viral disease spread by ticks in parts of Europe and the Commonwealth of Independent States (the former Soviet Union). It is transmitted to humans by bites from infected ticks, primarily *Ixodes ricinus,* usually found in forested areas of endemic regions from April through August. A similar TBE is caused by *Ixodes persulcatus.* This TBE results in systemic infection after ingestion of unpasteurized dairy products from infected cows, goats, or sheep.

The infection rate for TBE is very low, even in endemic areas. Vaccination against TBE is not available in the United States. Travelers planning outdoor activities in endemic areas need to rely on personal measures (DEET on exposed areas of skin and permethrin-based insecticide on clothing) to avoid tick attachment and bites. All travelers to endemic areas should avoid ingestion of unpasteurized dairy products.

Vaccine Summary
1. A three-dose injection series of inactivated vaccine (Encepur: Novartis or FSME-Immun: Baxter AG) given over 12 months is available in Europe; it is not routinely recommended by the CDC for travelers to endemic Western Europe.
2. A booster is given at 3- to 5-year intervals.
3. No vaccine is generally obtained by most travelers from North America to endemic areas because of lack of availability and long immunization schedule.

Tuberculosis (BCG Vaccine)

BCG (bacille Calmette-Guérin) vaccine is widely used worldwide for childhood immunization against tuberculosis. In the United States the CDC does not routinely recommend BCG. No consensus exists on the efficacy of BCG vaccine, but the vaccine is approved for use in children who will live where tuberculosis is prevalent or where exposure to adults with active or recently arrested tuberculosis is likely. It is also recommended for children of infected mothers. Vaccination may be appropriate for health care personnel who have negative results of purified protein derivative (PPD) skin tests and who are going to work in areas of high endemic prevalence and have limited access to medical diagnosis and treatment.

Vaccine Summary
1. Like other live attenuated vaccines, BCG vaccine is contraindicated in persons with immunosuppression caused by congenital conditions, chemotherapy, radiation therapy, HIV infection, or another condition resulting in impaired immune response. Pregnancy is considered a relative contraindication.

2. Epidemiologic data suggest that the vaccine may be more useful in protecting children from disseminated extrapulmonary complications of tuberculosis than in protecting adults from primary pulmonary infection.
3. Occasionally, children in families going abroad for extended residence are requested by the receiving country to provide proof of BCG vaccination to qualify for a visa.
4. A BCG vaccine is commercially available in the United States and is approved by the American Academy of Pediatrics Committee on the Control of Infectious Diseases for use in children traveling to live in areas in which tuberculosis is prevalent or there is a likelihood of exposure to adults with active or recently arrested tuberculosis.
5. Persons immunized with BCG vaccine test positive on PPD skin tests for many years afterward, regardless of the degree of protection conferred by the vaccine.

Yellow Fever

Yellow fever is a viral infection transmitted by *Aedes aegypti* mosquitoes in equatorial South America and Africa. The vaccine for yellow fever is highly immunoprotective.

Vaccine Summary
1. Vaccine strain is an attenuated live virus and well tolerated.
2. It is administered as a single injection.
3. Significant antibody levels are achieved in more than 95% of persons vaccinated.
4. Booster interval is every 10 years, although persistent antibody titers have been detected 30 to 40 years after vaccination.
5. The vaccine is not recommended for infants younger than 9 months of age because of postvaccination encephalitis.
6. It is also not recommended during pregnancy unless risk of yellow fever is thought to be greater than risk of adverse effects from vaccine.
7. Other contraindications are immunosuppression or history of severe allergy to eggs.
8. Vaccine-associated viscerotropic disease has been reported in a small number of first-time recipients of yellow fever vaccine. This may be associated with thymic dysfunction and/or age older than 60 years.
9. Another method for reducing the risk of yellow fever (or any mosquito-borne disease) is liberal use of mosquito repellent and netting in endemic areas.

Cold Water Immersion and Near Drowning

49

▶ COLD WATER IMMERSION

Cold Shock Response

Cold water immersion precipitates drowning by several mechanisms. Sudden cold water immersion produces profound cardiovascular and respiratory responses. Reflex sympathetic output can markedly increase blood pressure and heart rate, resulting in lethal arrhythmias.

An immediate and involuntary gasp occurs after cold water immersion. This is followed by hyperventilation. Pulmonary ventilation increases up to fivefold because of increased tidal volume and respiratory rate. The initial gasp can result in aspiration of water and laryngospasm. Hyperventilation produces respiratory alkalosis with resultant muscle tetany and cerebral hypoperfusion. This response can increase the risk of drowning in a person struggling to maintain an airway freeboard in rough water.

The respiratory stimulation produced by cold water immersion significantly decreases breath-holding duration. This fact has enormous implications for survivors who must maintain an airway freeboard in rough water.

Peripheral cold water–induced vasoconstriction exacerbates rapid cooling of muscles and nerves in the extremities, resulting in loss of strength and coordination. The ability to swim, maintain freeboard, avoid obstacles, and climb from the water may be greatly impaired.

The combination of hyperventilation and muscle dysfunction can be lethal for a swimmer in rough water. A personal floatation device (PFD) helps but does not prevent even small waves from submerging a swimmer's head.

If cold water immersion occurs, the following is recommended:

1. Try to enter the water without submersing the head.
2. Pull oneself out of the water as quickly as possible.
3. Minimize exposure (i.e., get as much of one's body as possible out of the water and onto a floating object).
4. Ensure flotation if one must remain in the water.
5. Minimize heat loss by remaining as still as possible in the heat escape lessening position (HELP), in which arms are pressed against the chest and legs are pressed together, or by huddling with other survivors.
6. Drawstrings should be tightened in clothing to decrease the flow of cold water within clothing layers.

Rescue and Treatment

1. Attempt to maintain hypothermic patients in a horizontal position during retrieval from water and aboard the rescue vehicle.
2. Conscious victims should not be required to assist in their own rescue or to ambulate once out of the water because physical activity increases afterdrop and may induce ventricular fibrillation.
3. After recovery from the water, immediately begin to rewarm the victim (see Chapter 3).

▶ NEAR DROWNING

General Evaluation

1. Assume an underlying cause for the event. Anticipate cervical spine fracture or a significant head injury. Other common causes include hypoglycemia (with or without diabetes), seizure disorder, and acute myocardial infarction.
2. Initiate resuscitation whenever possible until a reliable core temperature can be measured.

▶ NEAR DROWNING AND DROWNING CLASSIFICATIONS AND GENERAL TREATMENT

Grade 0—No Cough or Difficulty Breathing

1. Warm, dry, and release at scene.

Grade 1—Normal Lung Auscultation with Cough

1. Rest, dry, warm, reassure, and release. Consider observation for a few hours to identify shortness of breath. If the victim continues to cough or becomes short of breath, administer oxygen, 4 to 6 L/min, by facemask; increase the flow to 8 to 10 L/min if the victim continues to be short of breath.
2. Examine for signs of distress:
   a. Tachypnea
   b. Dyspnea
   c. Persistent cough
   d. Tachycardia or unexplained hypertension
   e. Increasing anxiety
   f. Pallor or cyanosis, first acral, then central
3. Anticipate vomiting.
4. Anticipate that the victim's condition will deteriorate. Begin to plan transport or evacuation.

Grade 2—Rales, Small Amount of Frothy Sputum ("Foam"), Strong Radial Pulses

1. Administer oxygen, 4 to 6 L/min, by facemask; increase the flow to 8 to 10 L/min if the victim continues to be short of breath.
2. Observe for 6 hours minimum.

Grade 3—Acute Pulmonary Edema with Strong Radial Pulses

1. High-flow oxygen by nonrebreather mask (12 to 15 L/min), advanced cardiac life support (ACLS), and rapid evacuation

Grade 4—Acute Pulmonary Edema with Hypotension

1. High-flow (12 to 15 L/min) oxygen by nonrebreather mask, ACLS, prepare for endotracheal intubation and pressors, rapid evacuation

Grade 5—Respiratory Arrest

1. ACLS, respiratory support including endotracheal intubation (see Grade 6 later), rapid evacuation

Grade 6—Cardiopulmonary Arrest

1. ACLS, CPR, rapid evacuation
2. Manage the airway. Perform endotracheal intubation or administer high-flow oxygen by bag-valve-mask.
3. Position the victim on the side to allow water to drain from the mouth. Proper positioning must be balanced with consideration given to an obvious or occult cervical or thoracic spine injury.
4. Do not perform the Heimlich maneuver unless the airway is obstructed or the abdomen is rigidly distended (presumably with water) and mechanical ventilation is deemed to be otherwise impossible. Forced emesis achieved with this maneuver may cause the victim to aspirate and worsen the pulmonary injury.
5. Note any trauma, and deploy cervical spine precautions if indicated.
6. After cold water (<10° C [50° F]) submersion, victims have been revived even after one hour of submersion. These remarkable saves are presumably due to the protective effects of profound hypothermia. If possible, perform CPR on cold water drowning victims until they reach the hospital.

Termination of Resuscitation

1. The victim has sustained an obviously fatal injury (e.g., limb loss with severe hemorrhage).
2. The victim displays normal body temperature and absent vital signs with or without postmortem lividity after 30 minutes of resuscitative efforts.
3. The victim displays rigor mortis.
4. The victim is hypothermic and has no signs of life after rewarming.
5. The victim is hypothermic, and the rescue effort must be discontinued because of rescuer fatigue.

Scuba Diving–Related Disorders

50

The disorders related to scuba diving include those caused by dysbarism, nitrogen narcosis, contaminated breathing gas, and decompression sickness (DCS).

▶ DYSBARISM

Dysbarism encompasses all the pathologic changes caused by altered environmental pressure. At sea level, atmospheric pressure is 14.7 lb/sq in. Each 10-m (33-foot) descent under water increases the pressure by 1 atmosphere. Gas in enclosed spaces obeys Boyle's law, which states that the pressure of a given quantity of gas when its temperature remains unchanged varies inversely with its volume.

Mask Squeeze

An air space is present between the face and the glass of a scuba (self-contained underwater breathing apparatus) diving mask. If nasal exhalations do not maintain air pressure within this space during descent, the volume of air contracts, creating negative pressure. This leads to capillary rupture, which is potentially dangerous after keratotomy because of the slow healing rate of corneal incisions.

Signs and Symptoms
1. Skin ecchymoses in mask pattern
2. Conjunctival hemorrhage similar to strangulation injury

Treatment
1. No treatment is necessary because the manifestations are self-limited.
2. Orbital hemorrhage is a rare complication and is associated with diplopia, proptosis, and visual loss. Prompt referral should be made for MRI and ophthalmologic care. Recompression therapy is not indicated.

Ear Canal Squeeze

A tight-fitting wet suit hood, ear plugs, exostoses, or cerumen impaction can trap air in the external auditory canal. On descent, this air contracts in the enclosed space between the tympanic membrane and the (occluded) external opening of the ear.

Signs and Symptoms
1. Pain, swelling, erythema, and petechiae or hemorrhagic blebs (bullae) of external ear canal wall
2. Hemorrhage possible
3. In severe cases, tympanic membrane rupturing outward

Treatment
1. If a remediable occlusion exists, correct it.
2. If inflammation of the external canal occurs without tympanic membrane rupture, instill ear drops suitable for the treatment of otitis externa (a fluoroquinolone combined with a steroid component) as directed for 2 to 3 days.
3. If the tympanic membrane is perforated, seek otolaryngologic evaluation. Do not allow further diving until the membrane has healed. Instill fluoroquinolone otic drops.
4. Do not incise bullae.

Middle Ear Squeeze (Barotitis Media)

If air cannot enter the middle ear via the (contracted or blocked) eustachian tube during an underwater descent, the existing air in the middle ear space contracts, creating a relative vacuum and pulling the tympanic membrane inward (Fig. 50-1).

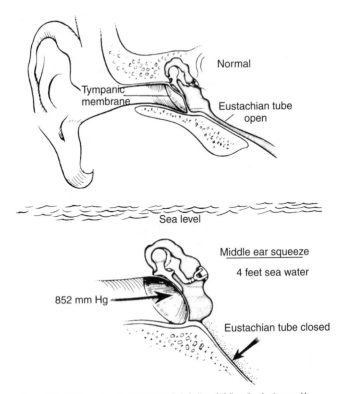

Figure 50-1. Middle ear trauma. Symptoms include feeling of "fullness" and pain caused by stretching of tympanic membrane.

Signs and Symptoms
1. Initially, slight pain that progresses to severe pain with further underwater descent
2. Hemorrhage in the tympanic membrane revealed on otoscopy; ranges from erythema over the malleus to gross blood throughout the tympanic membrane; blood around the mouth and nose and hearing loss also possible
3. If the tympanic membrane ruptures:
   a. Sudden severe pain, accompanied by vertigo as water rushes into the middle ear
   b. Total hearing loss in the affected ear

Treatment
1. Before tympanic membrane rupture, administer an oral decongestant and a long-acting topical decongestant nasal spray such as oxymetazoline. In a severe case, if the tympanic membrane is intact, a short course of prednisone (50 mg PO, tapered over 7 days) may be helpful. An antihistamine may be administered if there is an allergic component.
2. Repeated gentle autoinflation of the middle ear by use of the Frenzel maneuver may help to displace any collection of middle ear fluid through the eustachian tube.
3. For tympanic membrane rupture, administer an antibiotic such as amoxicillin/clavulanate for 7 days. In addition, administer fluoroquinolone otic drops. Suspend all diving activities until the tympanic membrane is fully healed or has been surgically repaired and eustachian tube function allows easy autoinflation.

Barosinusitis

Barosinusitis, or "sinus squeeze," results from an inability to inflate a paranasal sinus during descent, at which time contraction of the trapped air creates a relative vacuum. This damages the sinus wall mucosa, which ultimately hemorrhages. Less often, a "reverse sinus squeeze" can occur on ascent in the water because the expanding air cannot be vented from the sinus.

Signs and Symptoms
1. Pain in and over the affected sinus, with radiation similar to that seen with sinusitis (e.g., into the upper teeth with maxillary involvement)
2. May be accompanied by epistaxis

Treatment
1. Give oral and topical decongestants (mucosal vasoconstrictors) such as pseudoephedrine and oxymetazoline.
2. Administer an analgesic as appropriate.

3. If an episode of sinus squeeze has occurred, particularly with epistaxis, and the victim subsequently develops symptoms of sinusitis (pain, fever, tenderness over the affected sinus, nasal discharge), administer an appropriate antibiotic such as amoxicillin/clavulanate or azithromycin.

Barodontalgia

Barodontalgia, or "tooth squeeze," is caused by entrapped gas in the interior of a tooth or in the structures surrounding a tooth. The confined gas develops either positive or negative pressure relative to the ambient pressure, which places force on the surrounding sensitive dental structures.

Signs and Symptoms
1. Tooth pain, with normal referral pathways
2. Expulsion of a filling or crown; "exploding" or cracked tooth
3. Imploded tooth

Treatment
1. Supply symptomatic and supportive therapy for the specific type of dental trauma.
2. Administer an analgesic.

Labyrinthine Window Rupture (Inner Ear Barotrauma)

Labyrinthine window rupture affects the inner ear, with possible injury to the cochleovestibular system. This may lead to permanent deafness or vestibular dysfunction.

Signs and Symptoms
1. Roaring tinnitus, vertigo, hearing loss
2. Feeling of "fullness" in or blockage of the affected ear
3. Nausea, vomiting, nystagmus, pallor, diaphoresis, disorientation, ataxia
4. Symptoms of inner ear barotrauma developing immediately or delayed for hours

Treatment
1. Allow the victim to rest in bed, with the head elevated 30 degrees.
2. Make sure the victim avoids strenuous activities.
3. Suspend all diving activities until the victim is cleared by an otolaryngologist.

Alternobaric Vertigo

Alternobaric vertigo usually occurs with ascent and is caused by the sudden development of unequal middle ear pressure.

Signs and Symptoms
1. Asymmetric vestibular stimulation and resultant pronounced vertigo
2. Vertigo usually transient but may last for several hours or days

Treatment
1. Allow the victim to rest in a supine position, with the head elevated 30 degrees.
2. Make sure the victim avoids strenuous activities.
3. If labyrinthine window rupture is suspected, suspend all diving activities until the victim is cleared by an otolaryngologist.

Lung Squeeze

Lung squeeze is observed in a breath-holding diver who descends to a depth at which total lung volume is reduced to less than residual volume, which causes transpulmonic pressure to exceed intraalveolar pressure. This produces the transudation of fluid or blood (from rupture of pulmonary capillaries) into the alveoli.

Signs and Symptoms
1. Shortness of breath, cough, hemoptysis
2. In severe cases, pulmonary edema

Treatment
1. Administer oxygen, 5 L/min, by nonrebreather facemask.
2. Suspend all diving activities.

Pulmonary Barotrauma of Ascent (Pulmonary Overpressurization Syndrome)

Pulmonary barotrauma of ascent results from expansion of gas trapped in the lungs, which ruptures alveoli or is forced across the pulmonary capillary membrane.

Signs and Symptoms
1. History of rapid and uncontrolled ascent to the surface before onset of symptoms
2. Pneumomediastinum: gradually increasing hoarseness or "brassy" voice, neck fullness, substernal chest pain several hours after diving
3. Subcutaneous emphysema (crepitus) possible
4. In severe cases, possible chest pain, dyspnea, bloody sputum, dysphagia
5. Syncope possible
6. Pneumothorax
   a. Pleuritic chest pain, breathlessness, dyspnea
   b. With tension pneumothorax, progressive respiratory difficulty, cyanosis, distended neck veins, hyper-resonant

chest percussion, tracheal shift, absent or diminished breath sounds

Treatment
1. For pneumomediastinum, administer supplemental oxygen, 5 L/min, by nonrebreather mask. Have the victim rest.
2. For pneumothorax, administer supplemental oxygen, 5 L/min, by nonrebreather mask.
   a. Observe the victim closely for worsening condition.
   b. Be prepared to insert a thoracostomy (chest) tube or a decompression flutter valve.

Arterial Gas Embolism

Arterial gas embolism results from air bubbles entering the pulmonary venous circulation from ruptured alveoli. Gas bubbles are showered into the heart, from which they may be distributed to the coronary and carotid arteries. Arterial gas embolism typically develops immediately after a diver surfaces.

Signs and Symptoms
Sudden loss of consciousness on surfacing from a dive should be considered to indicate air embolism until proved otherwise.
1. Cardiac: chest pain related to myocardial ischemia, arrhythmias, or cardiac arrest
2. Neurologic
   a. Possibly confusing pattern, as showers of bubbles randomly embolize cerebral circulation
   b. Manifestations often typical of acute stroke (cerebrovascular accident), although hemiplegia infrequent
   c. Most often observed signs: loss of consciousness, monoplegia or asymmetric multiplegia, focal paralysis, paresthesias or other sensory disturbances, convulsions, aphasia, confusion, blindness or other visual field defects, vertigo, dizziness, headache
   d. Rare signs: sharply circumscribed areas of glossal pallor

Treatment
1. Transport the victim for recompression treatment in a hyperbaric (oxygen) chamber.
   a. If an aircraft is used, do not expose the victim to significant cabin altitude. Ideally, the aircraft will be pressurized to sea level.
   b. In an unpressurized aircraft, maintain the flying altitude as low as possible, not to exceed 300 m (1000 feet) above sea level.
2. Maintain the victim in a supine position.

3. Administer oxygen, 5 to 10 L/min, by nonrebreather facemask.
4. Begin an intravenous infusion of isotonic solution to maintain urine output at 1 to 2 mL/kg/hr.
5. Obtain help with the treatment of dive-related incidents 24 hours a day by calling the Divers Alert Network at Duke University (919-684-8111).
6. If it is available, administer IV lidocaine per protocol as an adjunct to recompression therapy.

Nitrogen Narcosis

Nitrogen narcosis is the increasing development of anesthesia or intoxication as the partial pressure of nitrogen in inspired compressed air increases at depth.

Signs and Symptoms
1. Usually becomes apparent at depths between 21 and 30 m (70 and 100 feet)
2. Lightheadedness, loss of fine sensory discrimination, giddiness, euphoria
3. Progressively worsening symptoms at deeper depths
   a. When deeper than 45 m (150 feet): severe intoxication, manifested by increasingly poor judgment and impaired reasoning, overconfidence, and slowed reflexes
   b. At depths of 75 to 90 m (250 to 300 feet): auditory and visual hallucinations, feeling of impending blackout
   c. By 120 m (400 feet): loss of consciousness

Treatment
Have the victim ascend to a shallower depth for symptoms to resolve.

Contaminated Breathing Gas

The pressurized air within a scuba tank may be contaminated with oil or carbon monoxide.

Signs and Symptoms
1. With oil contamination: cough, shortness of breath, oily taste in mouth
2. With carbon monoxide contamination: headache, nausea, dizziness during the dive
   a. Examination at the surface: lethargy, mental dullness, nonspecific neurologic deficits
   b. May be confused with those accompanying DCS (see next) or air embolism (see earlier)

Treatment
Administer oxygen, 5 to 10 L/min, by nonrebreather facemask.

Decompression Sickness

DCS is caused by the formation of bubbles of inert gas (e.g., nitrogen) within the intravascular and extravascular spaces after a reduction in ambient pressure.

Signs and Symptoms

1. Symptoms developing in the first hour after surfacing from a dive, with some victims noticing symptoms within 6 hours after diving; rarely, symptoms not noted until 24 to 48 hours after diving
2. Musculoskeletal DCS or "limb bends": periarticular joint pain most common symptom
   a. Shoulders and elbows most often affected
   b. Pain usually described as dull ache deep within the affected joint, but also characterized as sharp or throbbing
   c. Pain worse with joint movement, or "grating" sensation
   d. Vague area of numbness surrounding the affected joint
   e. Palpable tenderness
   f. Variably present diagnostic feature: pain temporarily relieved by inflation to 150 to 250 mm Hg of sphygmomanometer cuff placed around the joint
3. Neurologic DCS: back pain, girdling abdominal pain, extremity heaviness or weakness, paresthesias of extremities, anal sphincter weakness or fecal incontinence, loss of bulbocavernosus reflex, bladder distention and urinary retention, paralysis, hyperesthesia or hypoesthesia, paresis, scotomata, headache, dysphagia, confusion, visual field deficit, spotty motor or sensory deficits, disorientation, mental dullness
4. Fatigue
5. Cutaneous: pruritus, mottling, local or generalized hyperemia, marbled skin
6. "Chokes": dyspnea, substernal pain made worse on deep inhalation, nonproductive cough, cyanosis, tachypnea, tachycardia
7. Vasomotor DCS: weakness, sweating, unconsciousness, hypotension, tachycardia, pallor, mottling, decreased urine output

Treatment

1. Transport the victim for recompression treatment in a hyperbaric (oxygen) chamber.
2. If an aircraft is used, do not expose the victim to significant cabin altitude. Ideally, the aircraft will be pressurized to sea level.
3. In an unpressurized aircraft, maintain the flying altitude as low as possible, not to exceed 300 m (1000 feet) above sea level.

4. Maintain the victim in a supine position.
5. Administer oxygen, 5 to 10 L/min, by nonrebreather face-mask.
6. Begin an intravenous infusion of isotonic solution to maintain urine output at 1 to 2 mL/kg/hr.
7. Obtain help with the treatment of dive-related incidents 24 hours a day by calling the Divers Alert Network at Duke University (919-684-8111).

Although experimental proof of their efficacy is lacking, high-dose parenteral corticosteroids have been widely recommended as an adjunct to recompression treatment. They are used much less often than in the past. If you elect to use these, administer hydrocortisone hemisuccinate, 1 g, or methylprednisolone sodium succinate, 125 mg, followed by dexamethasone, 4 to 6 mg q6h for 72 hours.

Flying after Diving

Flying too soon after diving can seriously jeopardize decompression safety, leading to development of DCS during or after the flight because of the reduced atmospheric pressure present in most commercial aircraft.

1. Observe a minimum surface interval of 12 hours between the last dive and flying in a commercial jet.
2. Divers who make daily, multiple dives for several days or who make dives that require decompression stops are advised to attempt to attain an interval of at least 18 hours between diving and flying. However, it would seem prudent to extend the interval to 24 hours or longer to minimize the risk of DCS.

Absolute Contraindications for Diving

The following conditions are felt to be absolute contraindications for diving:

1. Spontaneous pneumothorax
2. Acute asthma with abnormal pulmonary function
3. Cystic or cavitary disease of the lungs
4. Obstructive or restrictive lung disease
5. Epilepsy or seizure disorder
6. Atrial septal defect (ASD)
7. Symptomatic coronary artery disease
8. Chronic perforated tympanic membrane
9. Chronic inability to equalize sinus and/or middle ear
10. Intraorbital gas
11. Pregnancy
12. Sickle cell disease
13. Meniere's disease

Injuries from Nonvenomous Aquatic Animals

51

Sharks, barracuda, moray eels, needlefish, and coral present dangers to those venturing into the ocean. The injuries inflicted range from bites or stings to cuts and abrasions.

▶ **GENERAL TREATMENT**

Wound Management

1. Irrigate all wounds with a sterile diluent, preferably normal saline (NS) solution. Seawater is not recommended because it carries a hypothetical risk of infection. Use disinfected tap water if NS solution is not available.
   a. Note that proper irrigation technique involves using a 19-gauge needle or 18-gauge plastic IV catheter attached to a syringe to deliver a pressure of 10 to 20 psi.
   b. Flush a minimum of 100 to 250 mL of irrigant through each wound.
   c. If the wound was caused by a stingray, warm the irrigant to 45° C (113° F) (see Chapter 52).
2. Add an antiseptic to the irrigation fluid. Use povidone-iodine in a concentration of 1% to 5% with a contact time of 1 to 5 minutes. After antiseptic irrigation, thoroughly irrigate the wound with NS solution.
3. With a coral cut or abrasion, scrub the area to remove debris that cannot be irrigated from the wound.
4. Remove any crushed or devitalized tissue using sharp dissection.
5. In the field, perform wound closure using the technique that is least constrictive and therefore less prone to trap bacteria, which could initiate a wound infection. Unless a wound preparation equivalent to that achieved in a hospital is undertaken, it is often better to approximate the wound edges with adhesive strips or loosely placed sutures than to perform a tight approximation of the margins.
6. At the earliest sign of wound infection, release sufficient fasteners to allow prompt and thorough drainage from the wound. Initiate antibiotic therapy.
7. Administer appropriate antitetanus prophylaxis.

Antibiotic Therapy

The following recommendations are based on the malignant potential of soft tissue infections caused by *Vibrio* (sea water) or *Aeromonas* (natural freshwater) species.

1. Be aware that minor abrasions or lacerations (e.g., coral cuts, superficial sea urchin puncture wounds) do not require prophylactic antibiotics in the normal host. However, for persons who are chronically ill (e.g., diabetes, hemophilia, thalassemia), are immunologically impaired (e.g., leukemia, AIDS, chemotherapy, prolonged corticosteroid therapy), or have serious liver disease (e.g., hepatitis, cirrhosis, hemochromatosis), particularly those with elevated serum iron levels, immediately begin a regimen of oral ciprofloxacin, trimethoprim/sulfamethoxazole (co-trimoxazole), or tetracycline/doxycycline. Note that penicillin, ampicillin, amoxicillin, and erythromycin are not acceptable alternatives. Although other quinolones have not been extensively tested against *Vibrio* species, they may be useful alternatives.

2. Note that the appearance of an infection indicates the need for prompt débridement and antibiotic therapy. If an infection develops, choose antibiotic coverage that will also be efficacious against *Staphylococcus* and *Streptococcus* species. Vancomycin is recommended in the event of methicillin resistance.

3. From an infection perspective, consider the following as serious injuries: large lacerations, extensive or deep burns, deep puncture wounds, and a retained foreign body.

   a. These injuries may be caused by shark or barracuda bites, stingray spine wounds, any spine puncture that enters a joint space, and full-thickness coral cuts.

   b. If the victim will require hospitalization for any of these serious injuries and intravenous antibiotics are accessible, the recommended drugs for prophylaxis include gentamicin, tobramycin, amikacin, co-trimoxazole, cefoperazone, cefotaxime, and ceftazidime.

4. Manage infected wounds with antibiotics as noted earlier, with consideration of adding imipenem-cilastatin or meropenem for severe, progressive infections and sepsis.

5. If a wound infection is minor and has the appearance of a classic erysipeloid reaction *(Erysipelothrix rhusiopathiae)* (see Plate 28), penicillin, cephalexin, or ciprofloxacin should be administered.

▶ INJURIES CAUSED BY SHARKS AND BARRACUDA

Treatment

1. Manage abrasions caused by contact with sharkskin as if they were second-degree burns. Cleanse the wound thoroughly; then apply a thin layer of mupirocin (Bactroban) ointment or silver sulfadiazine cream under a sterile dressing.

2. Control active hemorrhage with pressure if possible. If necessary, ligate large disrupted vessels.

3. Insert at least two large-bore intravenous lines.
4. Keep the victim well oxygenated and warm.
5. Transport the victim to a proper emergency facility equipped to handle major trauma and appropriate surgical management of the wounds.
6. If the wound is more than minor, administer a prophylactic antibiotic (see earlier).

Prevention of Shark Attacks
1. Avoid shark-inhabited water, particularly at dusk and at night.
2. Do not swim through schools of bait fish in the presence of sharks.
3. Do not enter waters posted with shark warnings.
4. Do not wander too far from shore.
5. Do not swim with animals (e.g., dogs or horses) in shark waters.
6. Photograph hazardous sharks from within the confines of a protective cage.
7. Swimmers should remain in groups.
8. Avoid turbid water, drop-offs, deep channels, inlets, mouths of rivers, and sanitation waste outlets.
9. Do not swim in waters frequented by recreational or commercial fishers.
10. Do not swim in water that has been recently churned up by a storm.
11. Be alert when crossing sandbars.
12. Do not enter the water with an open wound, particularly if it is bleeding.
13. Do not wear flashy metal objects.
14. Do not carry captured fish.
15. Be alert when schools of fish behave in an erratic manner or when pods of porpoises cluster more tightly or head toward shore.
16. Do not tease or corner a shark.
17. Do not splash on the surface or create a commotion in the water.

▶ MORAY EEL INJURY

Morays are forceful and vicious biters that can inflict severe puncture wounds with their narrow and vise-like jaws, which are equipped with long, sharp, retrorse, and fang-like teeth.

Treatment
1. Explore each wound to locate any retained teeth.
2. Irrigate each wound copiously.
3. Because the risk for infection is high, do not suture any puncture wounds unless it is necessary temporarily to control hemorrhage.

4. If the wound is extensive and more linear in configuration (resembling a dog bite), débride the wound edges and loosely approximate them with nonabsorbable sutures or staples.
5. Administer a prophylactic antibiotic (see earlier).

▶ SEA LION BITE

"Seal finger" follows a bite wound from a seal or sea lion or from contact of even a minor skin wound with the animal's mouth or pelt. The signs and symptoms include an incubation period of 1 to 15 (typically, 4) days, followed by painful swelling of the digit, with or without joint involvement. Severe pain may precede the appearance of the initial furuncle, swelling, or stiffness. As the lesion worsens, the skin becomes taut and shiny and the entire hand may swell and take on a brownish-violet hue (see Plate 40). *Mycoplasma* species may be the inciting pathogens. The treatment is tetracycline 1.5 gm PO initially, followed by 500 mg PO qid for 4 to 6 weeks. Fluoroquinolone or macrolide antibiotics may be useful if tetracycline is not available.

▶ NEEDLEFISH INJURY

The pointed snout (teeth) of a needlefish that leaps from the water can penetrate into a human victim, creating a stab wound with a residual foreign body (the fish). Other fishes, such as sailfish and marlin, may also impale human victims.

Signs and Symptoms
Stab wound that may contain a foreign body

Treatment
1. Be aware that the major risk is wound infection caused by the retained organic material. Another risk is vascular injury.
2. Cleanse the wound thoroughly, then débride and dress it.
3. If the wound is more than superficial, administer a prophylactic antibiotic (see earlier). If the distal circulation is impeded, undertake immediate evacuation.

▶ CORAL CUTS AND ABRASIONS

Signs and Symptoms
1. Initial reactions: stinging pain, erythema, pruritus
2. Break in skin surrounded within minutes by erythematous wheal, which fades over 1 to 2 hours
3. Red, raised welts and local pruritus accompanied by low-grade fever and malaise, known as "coral poisoning"

4. Progresses to cellulitis with ulceration and tissue sloughing
5. Healing over 3 to 6 weeks, with prolonged morbidity
6. Lymphangitis and reactive bursitis also seen

Treatment

1. Promptly and vigorously scrub the wound with soap and water, and then irrigate copiously to remove all foreign material.
2. Use hydrogen peroxide to bubble out tiny particles of organic material deposited from the surface of the coral.
3. If a stinging sensation is prominent, be aware that envenomation may have occurred. Briefly rinse the area with diluted (half-strength or 2.5%) household vinegar to diminish discomfort. Follow with a thorough NS solution or tap water irrigation.
4. If a coral-induced laceration is severe, close it with adhesive strips rather than sutures, if possible, because the margins of the wound are likely to become inflamed and necrotic. Be aware that serial débridement may become necessary.
5. To achieve a bed of healing tissue, apply twice-daily, sterile, wet-to-dry dressings using NS solution or a dilute antiseptic (e.g., povidone-iodine 1% to 5%). Alternatively, use a nontoxic topical antiseptic ointment (e.g., bacitracin, mupirocin, polymyxin B-bacitracin-neomycin) sparingly and cover the wound with a nonadherent dressing.
6. Be aware that despite the best efforts at primary irrigation and decontamination, the wound may heal slowly, with moderate to severe soft tissue inflammation and ulcer formation. Débride all devitalized tissue regularly using sharp dissection. Continue this regimen until healthy granulation tissue is formed.
7. Treat any wound that appears infected with an antibiotic (see earlier).

Envenomation by Marine Life

52

Interactions with various forms of marine life can result in anaphylactic reactions or envenomation.

▶ ANAPHYLAXIS

Signs and Symptoms
For signs and symptoms typical of anaphylactic reactions, see Chapter 26.

Treatment
1. Maintain the airway and administer oxygen.
2. Obtain intravenous access. Administer lactated Ringer's (LR) or normal saline (NS) solution to support the blood pressure to a minimum of 90 mm Hg systolic.
3. Administer epinephrine.
   a. Begin with aqueous epinephrine 1:1000 SC in the deltoid region.
   b. The dose for adults is 0.3 to 0.5 mL and for children 0.01 mL/kg.
   c. An alternative is to inject the contents of an EpiPen or EpiPen Jr. intramuscularly into the lateral thigh region. Repeat in 20 minutes if relief is partial.
   d. If the reaction is limited to pruritus and urticaria, there is no wheezing or facial swelling, and the victim is older than 45 years, administer an antihistamine and reserve epinephrine for a worsened condition.
4. If the reaction is life threatening and there is no response to subcutaneous or intramuscular epinephrine, administer intravenous epinephrine.
   a. Give an adult a 0.1-mg bolus of 1:1000 aqueous epinephrine (0.1 mL) diluted in 10 mL of NS solution (final dilution 1:100,000) infused over 10 minutes.
   b. Prepare a mixture for continuous infusion by adding 1 mg 1:1000 aqueous epinephrine (1 mL) to 250 mL of NS solution, to create a concentration of 4 µg/mL. This infusion should be started at 1 µg/minute (15 minidrops/minute) and increased to 4 to 5 µg/minute if the clinical response is inadequate.
   c. In infants and children, starting dose is 0.1 µg/kg/minute up to a maximum of 1.5 µg/kg/minute, noting that infusion rates in excess of 0.5 µg/kg/minute may be associated with cardiac ischemia and arrhythmias.
5. Relieve bronchospasm by administering micronized albuterol or metaproterenol by hand-held metered-dose inhaler (MDI).

6. Administer antihistamines.
   a. For a mild reaction, give diphenhydramine, 50 to 75 mg IV, IM, or PO. The dose for children is 1 mg/kg.
   b. Nonsedating antihistamines such as fexofenadine, 60 mg, or cimetidine, 300 mg, are adjuncts.
7. Administer corticosteroids.
   a. If the reaction is severe or prolonged, or if the victim is regularly medicated with corticosteroids, administer hydrocortisone, 200 mg, methylprednisolone, 50 mg, or dexamethasone, 15 mg IV with a 10-day oral taper to follow. The parenteral dose of hydrocortisone for children is 2.5 mg/kg.
   b. With oral therapy, administer prednisone, 60 to 100 mg for adults and 1 mg/kg for children.

▶ REACTION TO SPONGES

Sponges are stationary animals that attach to the sea floor or coral beds. Embedded in their connective tissue matrices are spicules of silicon dioxide or calcium carbonate. Other chemical toxins and secondary coelenterate (stinging) inhabitants contribute to the skin irritation and systemic manifestations that result from dermal contact.

Signs and Symptoms
1. Within a few hours after contact: burning and itching of the skin, possibly progressing to local joint swelling and stiffness, soft tissue edema, and blistering
   a. Skin becoming mottled or purpuric
   b. If untreated, subsidence of minor reaction in 3 to 7 days
2. With involvement of large areas of skin: fever, chills, malaise, dizziness, nausea, muscle cramps, and formication
   a. Bullae becoming purulent
   b. Surface skin desquamation after 10 days

Treatment
1. Gently dry the skin.
2. To remove embedded microscopic spicules, apply sticky adhesive tape, a commercial facial peel, or a thin layer of rubber cement; then peel away the adherent spicules.
3. Apply a 5% acetic acid (vinegar) soak for 10 to 30 minutes three or four times a day. If vinegar is not available, use isopropyl alcohol 40%. Do not use a topical steroid preparation as the primary (initial) decontaminant because this may worsen the reaction.
4. After decontamination and at least two vinegar applications, use a mild emollient cream to soothe the skin.

5. If the allergic component is mild, apply a topical steroid preparation. If the allergic component is severe, as manifested by weeping, crusting, and vesiculation, administer a systemic corticosteroid (e.g., prednisone, 60 to 100 mg, tapered over 14 days).

6. Perform frequent follow-up wound checks because significant infections sometimes develop. Culture infected wounds and administer antibiotics (see Chapter 51).

Prevention
1. Ensure that all divers and net handlers wear proper gloves.
2. Do not allow sponges to be broken, crumbled, or crushed with bare hands.
3. Be aware that dried sponges may remain toxic.

▶ JELLYFISH STINGS (ALSO FIRE CORAL, HYDROIDS, AND ANEMONES)

These creatures sting with a variation of the microscopic stinging cell, the nematocyst, which is stimulated to fire its venom-bearing injector into the victim by physical contact, hypotonicity, or chemical stimulation. An encounter with a single long-tentacled creature can simultaneously trigger hundreds of thousands of stinging cells.

Signs and Symptoms
1. Skin irritation: stinging, pruritus, paresthesias, burning, throbbing, redness, tentacle prints, impression patterns (see Plate 29), blistering, local edema, petechial hemorrhages, skin ulceration, necrosis, and secondary infection
2. Neurologic: malaise, headache, aphonia, diminished touch and temperature sensation, vertigo, ataxia, spastic or flaccid paralysis, mononeuritis multiplex, parasympathetic dysautonomia, plexopathy, peripheral nerve palsy, delirium, loss of consciousness, and coma
3. Cardiovascular: anaphylaxis, hemolysis, hypotension, small artery spasm, bradycardia, tachycardia, congestive heart failure, and ventricular fibrillation
4. Respiratory: rhinitis, bronchospasm, laryngeal edema, dyspnea, cyanosis, pulmonary edema, and respiratory failure
5. Musculoskeletal: abdominal rigidity, myalgia, muscle cramp/spasm, arthralgia, and arthritis
6. Gastrointestinal: nausea, vomiting, diarrhea, dysphagia, hypersalivation, and thirst
7. Ocular: conjunctivitis, chemosis, corneal ulcer, iridocyclitis, elevated intraocular pressure, and lacrimation
8. Other: chills, fever, acute renal failure, and nightmares

Treatment
1. For systemic reactions:
    a. Maintain the airway and administer oxygen.
    b. Obtain intravenous access. Administer LR or NS solution to support the blood pressure to at least 90 mm Hg systolic.
    c. Treat anaphylaxis if present (see Chapter 37).
    d. If the sting is from the box jellyfish *(Chironex fleckeri)* (Fig. 52-1 and Plate 30) or severe and from the sea wasp *(Chiropsalmus quadrigatus)*, consider immediate administration of *C. fleckeri* antivenom. Administer this in a dose of 1 ampule (20,000 U/ampule) IV diluted 1:5 to 1:10 in isotonic crystalloid. A large sting in an adult may require the initial administration of two ampules. Alternatively, administer this in a dose of 3 ampules intramuscularly into the thigh. Antivenom administration may be repeated once or twice every 2 to 4 hours until there is no further worsening of the reaction (skin discoloration, pain, or systemic effects).

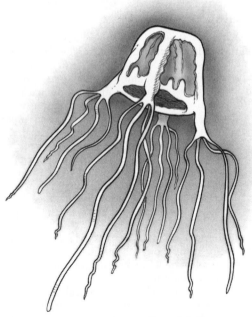

Figure 52-1. The dreaded Indo-Pacific box jellyfish *(Chironex fleckeri)*.

    e. If the sting is from the Irukandji *(Carukia barnesi)*, hypertension from catecholamine stimulation may be severe. If necessary, administer an alpha-adrenergic blocking agent (phentolamine, 5 mg IV initially, followed by an infusion of up to 10 mg/hour).

    f. Authorities NO LONGER recommend the pressure-immobilization technique to treat a box jellyfish sting or any other jellyfish sting.

2. For dermatitis:

    a. If possible, apply a topical decontaminant immediately (described in step d later). If more than 1 or 2 minutes will elapse before the application of the decontaminant, rinse the wound with sea water. Do not rinse gently with fresh water; if fresh water is to be used, the stream must be forceful (e.g., jet stream from a shower or hose).

    b. Hot packs or showers to tolerance (45° C [113° F]) may be more effective than dry, (nonmoist), cold (insulated ice) packs.

    c. Do not rub or abrade the wound.

    d. If these have been done, apply a topical decontaminant. The efficacy may vary depending on the stinging species.

- Acetic acid 5% (vinegar) is the decontaminant of choice with a box jellyfish *(C. fleckeri)* sting.
- For other stings, diminish the pain using vinegar, isopropyl (rubbing) alcohol 40%, sodium bicarbonate (baking soda), papain (papaya latex or nonseasoned meat tenderizer, the latter in a brief [<15 minutes] application), or dilute household ammonia. Other substances that may be effective include sugar or olive oil, or lemon or lime juice. Urinating on the sting is generally not helpful. A sting from the Australian *Physalia physalis,* a recently differentiated species, should not be doused with vinegar.
- Do not apply a solvent (e.g., formalin, ether, gasoline).
- Perfume, aftershave, or high-proof liquor may worsen the skin reaction.

    e. After decontamination, remove the adherent nematocysts. Apply shaving cream or a paste of soap or baking soda, flour, or talc, and shave the area with a razor or other sharp edge.

    f. Apply a local anesthetic ointment or mild steroid preparation to soothe the skin.

    g. If the reaction is severe, administer a systemic corticosteroid (e.g., prednisone, 60 to 100 mg, tapered over 14 days).

    h. Inspect the wound regularly for ulceration and the onset of infection.

Prevention
1. Give all jellyfish a wide berth when swimming or diving.
2. Wear a "stinger suit" when immersed in jellyfish-infested water.
3. When diving, scan for surface concentrations of stinging animals.
4. If "stinger enclosures" are present, do not venture beyond their confines.
5. Consider the use of a topical skin protective preparation such as Safe Sea (jellyfish-safe sunblock).

▶ SEA BATHER'S ERUPTION

Sea bather's eruption, commonly misnomered "sea lice," predominantly involves covered areas of the body and has been attributed to stings from the microscopic larvae of certain jellyfish and anemones.

Signs and Symptoms
1. Stinging of the skin while still in the water or immediately on exiting; may be intensified by the application of fresh water
2. Skin redness, papules (see Plate 31), urticaria, and blisters minutes to 12 hours after exposure
   a. Most common areas: buttocks, genitals, and under breasts (women)
   b. Individual lesions resembling insect bites
   c. Also seen under bathing caps and swim fins and along the edge of the cuffs of wet suits
3. Fever, chills, headache, fatigue, malaise, vomiting, conjunctivitis, and urethritis

Treatment
1. Apply a topical decontaminant. Acetic acid 5% (vinegar) seems to be less effective than papain. Otherwise, scrub thoroughly with soap and water.
2. After decontamination, apply calamine lotion with 1% menthol to control itching. A high-potency topical corticosteroid preparation may be of benefit.
3. If the reaction is severe, administer a systemic corticosteroid (e.g., prednisone, 60 to 100 mg, tapered over 14 days).

▶ STARFISH PUNCTURE

The most common venomous starfish (Fig. 52-2) have glandular tissue interspersed underneath the epidermis that covers the rigid spines, which may attain a length of 4 to 6 cm (1.5 to 2.5 inches). The envenomation occurs when a spine punctures the skin.

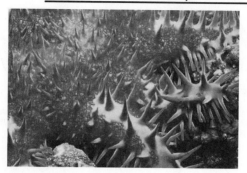

Figure 52-2. Spines of the crown-of-thorns starfish *(Acanthaster planci)*. (Photo by Paul Auerbach, MD.)

Signs and Symptoms
1. Intense pain, moderate bleeding, local soft tissue edema
2. With multiple stings: paresthesias, nausea, vomiting, lymph-adenopathy, muscular paralysis

Treatment
1. Immerse the wound into nonscalding, hot water to tolerance (45° C [113° F]) for 30 to 90 minutes or until there is significant pain relief.
2. Remove any obvious spine fragments. Do not attempt to crush remaining fragments.
3. Observe closely for subsequent wound infection.
4. Consider prophylactic antibiotics (see Chapter 51).

▶ SEA URCHIN SPINE PUNCTURE OR ENVENOMATION BY PEDICELLARIAE

Sea urchins envenom their victims in one of two ways: (1) puncture wound by sharp, venom-bearing spine(s) or (2) inoculation of venom via the venom gland in the base of flower-like, stalked pincer organs (globiferous pedicellariae) (Fig. 52-3).

Signs and Symptoms
1. Intense pain, burning, local muscle aching, erythema, soft tissue edema, and black or purple tattoos (see Plate 32) at sites of spine punctures
2. Malaise, weakness, arthralgias, aphonia, dizziness, syncope, generalized muscular paralysis, respiratory distress, and hypotension

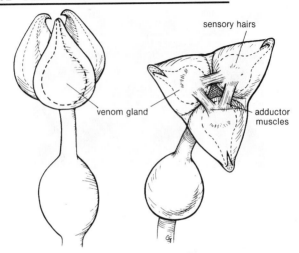

Figure 52-3. Globiferous pedicellaria of sea urchin used to hold and envenom prey.

Treatment
1. Immerse the wound into nonscalding, hot water to tolerance (45° C [113° F]) for 30 to 90 minutes or until significant pain relief.
2. Remove any obvious spine fragments. Do not attempt to crush remaining fragments. If spines are felt to remain within the victim near a joint, splint the affected limb.
3. If pedicellariae are attached, apply shaving foam and scrape them away with a razor.
4. Observe closely for subsequent wound infection.
5. Consider prophylactic antibiotics (see Chapter 51).

▶ SEA CUCUMBER IRRITATION

Sea cucumbers are worm- or sausage-shaped bottom feeders (Fig. 52-4). They produce in their body walls a visceral cantharidin-like toxin that is concentrated in tentacular organs that can be projected and extended anally when the animal mounts a defense.

Signs and Symptoms
1. Contact dermatitis when the tentacular organs contact the skin
2. Corneal and conjunctival irritation from contact with the tentacles or high concentrations of the toxin
3. Toxin is a potent cardiac glycoside and may cause severe illness or death on ingestion

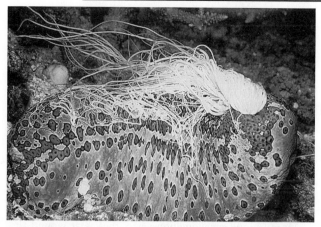

Figure 52-4. Extruded tentacular organs of Cuvier from within a sea cucumber. (Photo by Paul Auerbach, MD.)

Treatment
1. Wash the skin with soap and water.
2. Because sea cucumbers may dine on stinging cells of jellyfish, initial skin detoxication should include topical application of 5% acetic acid (vinegar), papain, or 40% to 70% isopropyl alcohol.
3. If the eye is involved, it should be anesthetized with proparacaine 0.5% and irrigated to 100 to 250 mL of normal saline to remove foreign matter. Slit lamp examination and fluorescein staining to identify corneal defects are recommended.

▶ BRISTLEWORM IRRITATION

Certain segmented marine worms have chitinous bristles arranged in soft rows around the body. These are dislodged into the human victim when a worm is handled.

Signs and Symptoms
Burning sensation, raised red urticarial rash, papular dermatitis, soft tissue edema, and pruritus

Treatment
1. Remove all large visible bristles using a forceps.
2. Dry the skin gently.
3. To remove embedded spines, apply sticky adhesive tape, a commercial facial peel, or a thin layer of rubber cement; then peel away the adherent spines.

4. Apply acetic acid 5% (vinegar), isopropyl alcohol 40%, dilute ammonia, or a paste of unseasoned meat tenderizer for 10 to 15 minutes to achieve pain relief.
5. Apply a thin layer of a topical corticosteroid preparation.
6. If the reaction is severe, administer a systemic corticosteroid (e.g., prednisone, 60 to 100 mg, tapered over 14 days).

▶ CONE SHELL (SNAIL) STING

These cone-shaped shelled mollusks intoxicate their victims by injecting rapid-acting venom by means of a detachable, dart-like radular tooth (Fig. 52-5).

Signs and Symptoms
1. Mild sting (puncture) that resembles bee or wasp sting
2. Alternative initial symptoms: localized ischemia, cyanosis, numbness in area around wound
3. More serious envenomations: paresthesias at wound site, which become perioral and then generalized
4. Dysphagia, nausea, syncope, weakness, areflexia, aphonia, diplopia, blurred vision, pruritus, disseminated intravascular coagulation, generalized muscular paralysis leading to respiratory failure, cardiac failure, and coma

Treatment
1. Apply the pressure immobilization technique for venom sequestration (see Chapter 36): If practical by virtue of the sting's location, place a cloth or gauze pad 6 to 8 cm (2.5 to 3 inches) by 2 cm (1-inch thickness) directly over the sting and hold it firmly in place using a circumferential

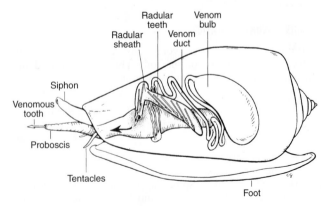

Figure 52-5. Venom apparatus of cone shell.

bandage 15 to 18 cm (6 to 7 inches) wide, applied at lymphatic-venous occlusive pressure. If the cloth or gauze pad is not available, a rolled bandage may be used alone.

   a. Do not occlude the arterial circulation, as determined by the detection of arterial pulsations and proper capillary refill.
   b. Splint the limb, and do not release the bandage until after the victim has been brought to proper medical attention and you are prepared to provide systemic support, or after 24 hours.
   c. Check frequently that swelling beneath the bandage has not compromised the arterial circulation.

▶ BLUE-RINGED OCTOPUS BITE

The blue-ringed octopus bite injects the victim with a venom containing tetrodotoxin, a paralytic agent that blocks peripheral nerve conduction.

Signs and Symptoms
1. Local reaction: one or two puncture wounds characterized by minimal discomfort, described as minor ache, slight stinging, or pulsating sensation
   a. Occasionally, initial numbness at the site, followed in 5 to 10 minutes by discomfort that may spread to involve the entire limb, persisting for up to 6 hours
   b. Within 30 minutes: redness, swelling, tenderness, heat, and pruritus
   c. Most common local tissue reaction: absence of symptoms, small spot of blood, or tiny blanched area
2. Within 10 to 15 minutes: oral and facial numbness, followed rapidly by diplopia, blurred vision, aphonia, dysphagia, ataxia, myoclonus, weakness, sense of detachment, nausea, vomiting, flaccid muscular paralysis, and respiratory failure

Treatment
1. Apply the pressure immobilization technique for venom sequestration (see Chapter 36 and earlier Treatment section for cone shell sting).
2. Be prepared to assist ventilations. Administer oxygen.

▶ STINGRAY SPINE PUNCTURE

The venom organ of stingrays consists of one to four venomous stingers on the dorsum of the whiplike caudal appendage. The cartilaginous spine(s) is covered with venom glands and an epidermal sheath. When the spine(s) enters the victim, the sheath is disrupted and venom extruded, so the wound is both a puncture/laceration and an envenomation.

Signs and Symptoms
1. Immediate local intense pain with central radiation, soft tissue edema, and dusky (ischemic) discoloration with surrounding erythema
2. Rapid (hours to days) fat and muscle hemorrhage and necrosis
3. Weakness, nausea, vomiting, diarrhea, diaphoresis, vertigo, tachycardia, headache, syncope, seizures, inguinal or axillary pain, muscle cramps, fasciculations, generalized edema (with truncal wounds), paralysis, hypotension, and arrhythmias

Treatment
1. Immerse the wound into nonscalding hot water to tolerance (45° C [113° F]) for 30 to 90 minutes or until significant pain relief. No reason exists to add ammonia, magnesium sulfate, potassium permanganate, or a solvent to the soaking solution. Do not immerse the wound into ice water.
2. Remove any obvious spine fragments. This may be done during the hot water soak. However, if the spine is seen to be lodged in the victim and has acted as a dagger deeply into the chest, abdomen, or neck and may have penetrated a critical blood vessel of the heart, it should be managed as would be a weapon of impalement (e.g., knife). In this case, the spine should be left in place (if possible) and secured from motion until the victim is brought to a controlled operating room environment where emergency surgery can be performed to guide its extraction and control bleeding that may occur on its removal.
3. Administer appropriate pain medications. Consider local or regional anesthetic administration.
4. Administer prophylactic antibiotics if the wound is more than minor or if the victim is immunocompromised (see Chapter 51).
5. Do not suture the wound closed unless bleeding cannot be controlled with pressure or this wound closure method is necessary for evacuation.

▶ SCORPIONFISH SPINE PUNCTURE

Scorpionfish (Fig. 52-6), lionfish (Fig. 52-7), and stonefish (Fig. 52-8) envenom their victims using dorsal, anal, and pelvic spines, which are erected as a defense mechanism (Fig. 52-9). Other venomous fish that sting in a manner similar to scorpionfish include the Atlantic toadfish, European ratfish, rabbitfishes, stargazers, and leatherbacks. Other marine fishes carry spines that envenom to a lesser degree.

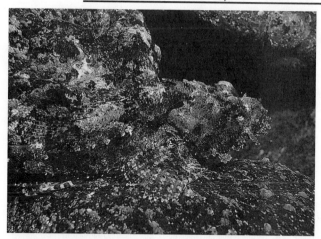

Figure 52-6. Scorpionfish assuming the coloration of its surroundings. (Photo by Paul Auerbach, MD.)

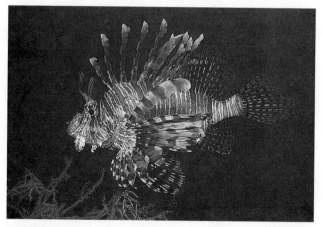

Figure 52-7. Adult lionfish. (Photo by Paul Auerbach, MD.)

Signs and Symptoms
The severity of the envenomation depends on the number and type of stings, species, amount of venom released, and age and underlying health of the victim. In general, the severity is considered to be stonefish > scorpionfish > lionfish.
1. Immediate, intense pain with central radiation
    a. If untreated, pain peaking at 60 to 90 minutes and persisting for 6 to 12 hours (stonefish)

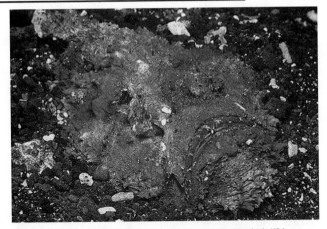

Figure 52-8. The deadly stonefish *(Synanceja horrida)*. (Photo by Paul Auerbach, MD.)

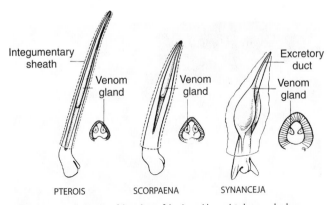

Figure 52-9. Lionfish, scorpionfish, and stonefish spines with associated venom glands.

    b. Stonefish pain possibly severe enough to cause delirium and persisting at high levels for days

2. Wound and surrounding area initially ischemic and then cyanotic, with more broadly surrounding areas of erythema, edema, and warmth

    a. Vesicles possible

    b. Tissue sloughing within 48 hours

3. Anxiety, headache, tremors, maculopapular rash, nausea, vomiting, diarrhea, abdominal pain, diaphoresis, pallor, restlessness, delirium, seizures, limb paralysis, peripheral

neuropathy, lymphangitis, arthritis, fever, hypertension, respiratory distress, pulmonary edema, bradycardia, tachycardia, atrioventricular block, ventricular fibrillation, congestive heart failure, syncope, and hypotension

Treatment
1. Immerse the wound into nonscalding hot water to tolerance (45° C [113° F]) for 30 to 90 minutes or until significant pain relief occurs. No reason exists to add ammonia, magnesium sulfate, potassium permanganate, or a solvent to the soaking solution. Do not immerse the wound into ice water.
2. Remove any obvious spine fragments. This may be done during the hot water soak.
3. Administer appropriate pain medications. Consider local or regional anesthetic administration.
4. Administer prophylactic antibiotics if the wound is more than minor or the victim is immunocompromised (see Chapter 51).
5. Give stonefish antivenin in cases of severe systemic reaction from stings of Synanceja species. The antivenom is supplied in ampules containing 2 mL (2000 units) of hyperimmune horse serum, with 1 vial neutralizing one or two significant punctures. Administer to the victim with all due anticipation of anaphylaxis associated with the administration of an antivenin product.

▶ CATFISH SPINE STING

The most frequent stinger is the freshwater catfish; the marine coral catfish has also been reported to sting humans. The venom apparatus consists of dorsal and pectoral fin spines. Some catfish generate skin secretions that are toxic.

Signs and Symptoms
1. Instantaneous stinging, throbbing, or scalding pain with central radiation; normally, pain subsiding within 30 to 60 minutes, but possibly lasting up to 48 hours
2. Area around the wound ischemic, with central pallor that grows cyanotic before onset of erythema and edema
3. Local muscle spasm, diaphoresis, fasciculations, weakness, syncope, hypotension, and respiratory distress

Treatment
1. Immerse the wound into nonscalding hot water to tolerance (45° C [113° F]) for 30 to 90 minutes or until significant pain relief occurs. No reason exists to add ammonia, magnesium sulfate, potassium permanganate, or a solvent to the soaking solution. Do not immerse the wound in ice water.

2. Remove any obvious spine fragments. This may be done during the hot water soak.
3. Administer appropriate pain medications. Consider local or regional anesthetic administration.
4. Administer prophylactic antibiotics if the wound is more than minor or the victim is immunocompromised (see Chapter 51).
5. Be aware that tiny Amazonian catfishes swim up the human urethra and are not easily dislodged. Ingestion of a large quantity of ascorbic acid, which is then excreted in the urine, may soften the spines and allow the fish to be "passed."

▶ WEEVERFISH SPINE STING

The weeverfish is the most venomous fish of the temperate zone. It is found in the Mediterranean Sea, Eastern Atlantic Ocean, and European coastal areas. The venom apparatus consists of dorsal and opercular spines associated with venom glands.

Signs and Symptoms
1. Instantaneous burning, scalding, or crushing pain with central radiation
   a. Peak of pain at 30 minutes with subsidence within 24 hours, but can last for days
   b. Possibly of an intensity sufficient to induce irrational behavior and syncope
2. Little bleeding at puncture wound site; often appears pale and edematous initially
   a. Over 6 to 12 hours, wound becoming red, ecchymotic, and warm
   b. Increasing edema for 7 to 10 days, causing the entire limb to become swollen
3. Headache, delirium, aphonia, fever, chills, dyspnea, diaphoresis, cyanosis, nausea, vomiting, seizures, syncope, hypotension, and cardiac arrhythmias

Treatment
1. Immerse the wound into nonscalding hot water to tolerance (45° C [113° F]) for 30 to 90 minutes or until significant pain relief occurs. No reason exists to add ammonia, magnesium sulfate, potassium permanganate, or a solvent to the soaking solution. Do not immerse the wound into ice water.
2. Remove any obvious spine fragments. This may be done during the hot water soak.
3. Administer appropriate pain medications. Consider local or regional anesthetic administration.

4. Administer prophylactic antibiotics if the wound is more than minor or the victim is immunocompromised (see Chapter 51).

▶ SEA SNAKE BITE

Sea snakes have a venom apparatus consisting of two to four maxillary fangs and a pair of associated venom glands. Most bites do not result in envenomation.

Signs and Symptoms
1. Onset potentially delayed by up to 8 hours
2. No appreciable local reaction to a sea snake bite other than the initial pricking sensation
3. Initially, euphoria, malaise, or anxiety
4. Over 30 to 60 minutes, classic muscle aching and stiffness (particularly of the bitten extremity and neck muscles), along with dysarthria and sialorrhea
5. Within 3 to 6 hours, moderate to severe pain with passive movements of the neck, trunk, and limbs
6. Ascending flaccid or spastic paralysis, beginning in lower extremities
7. Nausea, vomiting, myoclonus, muscle spasm, ophthalmoplegia, ptosis, dilated and poorly reactive pupils, facial paralysis, and trismus
8. In severe cases, skin cool and cyanotic, loss of vision, and possible coma

Treatment
1. Apply the pressure immobilization technique for venom sequestration (see Chapter 36).
2. Be prepared to assist ventilations. Administer oxygen.
3. With any evidence of envenomation, give polyvalent sea snake antivenom. The minimum effective adult dosage is 1 ampule (1000 units). The victim may require 3 to 10 ampules depending on the severity of the envenomation. Administer the antivenom with all due anticipation of anaphylaxis associated with the administration of an antivenom product. Tiger snake antivenom is no longer recommended for use if sea snake antivenom is unavailable.

Seafood Toxidromes

53

Toxidromes associated with seafood that may be encountered in the wilderness are ciguatera fish poisoning, clupeotoxin fish poisoning, scombroid fish poisoning, tetrodotoxin fish poisoning, paralytic shellfish poisoning, *Vibrio* fish poisoning, anisakiasis, domoic acid intoxication, gempylotoxication, botulism, and *Pfiesteria* syndrome.

▶ CIGUATERA FISH POISONING

Ciguatera fish toxins are carried by more than 400 species of bottom-feeding reef fishes. The most frequently affected fish are the jacks, snappers, triggerfishes, and barracudas. Others include mullet, moray eels, porgies, wrasses, parrotfishes, and surgeonfishes. All toxins to date have been unaffected by freeze-drying, heat, cold, and gastric acid, and none has any effect on the odor, color, or taste of the fish. The free algae dinoflagellate *Gambierdiscus toxicus* is responsible for producing ciguatoxins. Other dinoflagellates may generate toxins that play a role in ciguatera syndrome. The toxic fish is generally unremarkable in taste and smell.

Signs and Symptoms
1. Onset possible within 15 to 30 minutes of ingestion and generally within 1 to 3 hours; increasing severity over ensuing 4 to 6 hours; almost all victims develop symptoms by 24 hours
2. Abdominal pain, nausea, vomiting, and diarrhea usually occurring 3 to 6 hours after ingestion and possibly persisting for 48 hours
3. Headache, metallic taste, chills, paresthesias (particularly of the extremities and circumoral region), pruritus (particularly of the palms and soles after a delay of 2 to 5 days), tongue and throat numbness or burning, sensation of "carbonation" during swallowing, odontalgia or dental dysesthesias, dysphagia, dysuria, dyspnea, weakness, fatigue, tremor, fasciculations, athetosis, meningismus, aphonia, ataxia, vertigo, pain and weakness in the lower extremities, visual blurring, transient blindness, hyporeflexia, seizures, nasal congestion and dryness, conjunctivitis, maculopapular rash, skin vesiculations, dermatographia, sialorrhea, diaphoresis, arthralgias, myalgias (particularly in the lower back and thighs), painful ejaculation with urethritis, insomnia, bradycardia, hypotension, central respiratory failure, and coma
4. Tachycardia and hypertension possible

5. More severe reactions in persons previously stricken with the poisoning
6. Pathognomonic symptom: reversal of hot and cold tactile perception, which may result from generalized thermal hypersensitivity or paresthesias
7. Pruritus exacerbated by anything that increases skin temperature (blood flow), such as exercise or alcohol consumption
8. If parrotfish ingested, possible second phase, showing locomotor ataxia, dysmetria, and resting or kinetic tremor

Treatment
1. Be aware that therapy is supportive and based on symptoms.
2. Control nausea and vomiting with an antiemetic (prochlorperazine, 2.5 mg IV; ondansetron, 4 mg IV or PO dissolving tablet; or promethazine, 25 mg IM).
3. Control hypotension with intravenous crystalloid volume replacement or oral rehydration if tolerated.
4. For arrhythmias, heart block, hypotension, or severe neurologic symptoms, administer mannitol (20% solution), 1 g/kg IV over 45 to 60 minutes during the acute phase (days 1 to 5).
5. Bradyarrhythmias may respond to atropine (0.5 mg IV, up to 2 mg).
6. For pruritus, administer hydroxyzine, 25 mg PO q6–8h. Cool showers may help. Amitriptyline, 25 mg PO bid, may relieve pruritus and dysesthesias, as well as emotional depression.
7. In the recovery phase, avoid ingestion of fish, fish sauces, shellfish, shellfish sauces, alcoholic beverages, and nuts and nut oils.

▶ CLUPEOTOXIN FISH POISONING

Clupeotoxin fish poisoning involves plankton-feeding fish, which ingest planktonic blue-green algae and surface dinoflagellates. These include herrings, sardines, anchovies, tarpons, bonefishes, and deep-sea slickheads. The poison does not impart any unusual appearance, odor, or flavor to the fish.

Signs and Symptoms
1. Onset abrupt, within 30 to 60 minutes of ingestion
2. Initially, marked metallic taste, xerostomia, nausea, vomiting, diarrhea, and abdominal pain
3. Next symptoms: chills, headache, diaphoresis, severe paresthesias, muscle cramps, vertigo, malaise, tachycardia, peripheral cyanosis, and hypotension
4. Death can occur within 15 minutes of onset of symptoms

Treatment
1. Therapy is supportive and based on symptoms.
2. Because of the severe nature of the intoxication, early gastric emptying is desirable. However, the affliction is so unusual that the victim may die before the diagnosis is suspected.

▶ SCOMBROID FISH POISONING

Scombroid fish (dark fleshed; predominantly tuna) and some nonscombroid fish (e.g., Hawaiian dolphin or "mahi mahi") are affected with this toxin. L-Histidine within muscle tissue is decarboxylated to form histamine and similar compounds. Thus the poisoning is also known as "pseudoallergic" fish poisoning. Affected fish typically have a sharply metallic or peppery taste. However, they may be normal in appearance, color, and flavor. Not all persons who eat a contaminated fish become ill, possibly because of an uneven distribution of histamine within the fish. The toxin is not destroyed by cooking.

Signs and Symptoms
1. Onset within 15 to 90 minutes of ingestion
2. Flushing (sharply demarcated, exacerbated by ultraviolet exposure, particularly of the face, neck, and upper trunk); sensation of warmth without elevated core temperature; conjunctival hyperemia; pruritus; urticaria; angioneurotic edema; bronchospasm; nausea; vomiting; diarrhea; epigastric pain; abdominal cramps; dysphagia; headache; thirst; pharyngitis; burning of the gingivae; palpitations; tachycardia; dizziness; hypotension; localized numbness of the oropharynx; and rare arrhythmias
3. If untreated, resolution of symptoms generally within 8 to 12 hours
4. Reaction much more severe in a person who is concurrently ingesting isoniazid

Treatment
1. Administer an antihistamine (diphenhydramine, 25 to 50 mg PO or IV; cimetidine, 300 mg, or ranitidine, 50 mg IV). Alternatives are nizatidine, 150 mg PO, or famotidine, 20 mg PO. Combination therapy with both a histamine-1 receptor antagonist and a histamine-2 receptor antagonist may be more effective than either alone.
2. If the victim is severely ill with facial swelling indicative of an airway obstruction, hypotension, or significant bronchospasm, treat as for an allergic reaction with epinephrine and inhaled bronchodilators in addition

to antihistamines. Corticosteroids are of no proven benefit.
3. Control nausea and vomiting that do not remit after anti-histamine administration with an antiemetic (prochlorper-azine, 2.5 mg IV; promethazine, 25 mg IM; or ondansetron 4 mg IV or PO dissolving tablet).
4. Treat persistent headache with acetaminophen or an anti-histamine (such as cimetidine).

Prevention
1. Make sure that all captured fish are gutted, cooled, and refrigerated or placed on ice or frozen immediately.
2. Do not consume fish that has been handled improperly or carries the odor of ammonia. Fresh fish generally has a sheen or oily rainbow appearance; avoid "dull" fish or those that do not smell fresh.

▶ **TETRODOTOXIN FISH POISONING**

Tetrodotoxin is a potent nonprotein poison that interferes with central and peripheral neuromuscular transmission. It is found in pufferfish (blowfish, globefish, swellfish, toad-fish, balloonfish), and porcupine fish. "Puffers" are prepared as delicacies (fugu) and when ingested may cause paresthe-sias, a sensation of "floating," flushing of the skin, general-ized warmth, and mild weakness with euphoria. The toxin is concentrated in the liver, viscera, gonads, and skin of the fish.

Signs and Symptoms
1. Onset possibly as rapid as 10 minutes or delayed for up to 4 hours; usually occurs within 30 minutes of ingestion; death may occur within 20 minutes
2. Initial symptoms: oral (lips and tongue) paresthesias, light-headedness, and then general paresthesias
3. Rapidly developing symptoms: hypersalivation, diaphoresis, lethargy, headache, nausea, vomiting, diarrhea, abdominal pain, weakness, ataxia, incoordination, tremor, paralysis, cyanosis, aphonia, dysphagia, seizures, bradycardia, dysp-nea, bronchorrhea, bronchospasm, respiratory failure, coma, hypotension, and coagulopathy
4. Gastrointestinal symptoms may be severe and include nau-sea, vomiting, diarrhea, and abdominal pain
5. Miosis progressing to mydriasis with poor papillary light reflex
6. When mechanical ventilation maintained and no anoxic brain injury present, full mentation maintained with total flaccid paralysis

Treatment
1. Be aware that the toxin is stable in gastric acid and partially inactivated in alkaline solutions.
2. Secure the airway and administer oxygen.
3. Perform gastric lavage with 2 L of 2% sodium bicarbonate in 200-mL aliquots, followed by placement of 50 to 100 g of activated charcoal in 70% sorbitol solution (or 30 g of "highly activated" charcoal in sorbitol).
4. Further therapy is supportive and based on symptoms.

▶ PARALYTIC SHELLFISH POISONING

Paralytic shellfish poisoning (PSP) is induced by ingesting toxic filter-feeding (on certain dinoflagellates) organisms such as clams, oysters, scallops, mussels, chitons, limpets, murex, starfish, and sand crabs. The toxins that cause PSP are water soluble and stable in heat and gastric acid. They inhibit neuromuscular transmission. One phytoplankton that is implicated as the origin of PSP toxin is *Protogonyaulax*.

Signs and Symptoms
1. Within minutes (usually 30 to 60) to a few hours after ingestion of contaminated shellfish, onset of intraoral and perioral paresthesias, notably of the lips, tongue, and gums, which progress rapidly to involve the neck and distal extremities; early onset of vertigo
2. Tingling or burning sensation that becomes numbness
3. Gastroenteritis in only 25% of victims
4. Lightheadedness, sensation of "floating," disequilibrium, incoordination, weakness, hyperreflexia, incoherence, dysarthria, sialorrhea, dysphagia, dysphonia, thirst, diarrhea, abdominal pain, nausea, vomiting, nystagmus, dysmetria, headache, diaphoresis, loss of vision, sensation of loose teeth, chest pain, and tachycardia
5. Flaccid paralysis and respiratory insufficiency 2 to 12 hours after ingestion
6. Unless there is a period of anoxia, victim often awake and alert, although paralyzed

Treatment
1. Secure the airway and administer oxygen.
2. Do not induce emesis. If the airway is secure, perform gastric lavage with 2 L of 2% sodium bicarbonate in 200-mL aliquots, followed by placement of 50 to 100 g of activated charcoal in 70% sorbitol solution (or 30 g of "highly activated" charcoal in sorbitol).
3. Further therapy is supportive and based on symptoms.

▶ *Vibrio* FISH POISONING

Vibrio organisms can cause gastroenteric disease and soft tissue infections, particularly in immunocompromised hosts. The most common vector is raw oysters, shrimp, or fish. Although some variation in clinical presentation exists depending on the particular *Vibrio* species (e.g., *vulnificus*, *parahaemolyticus*, *mimicus*), a general description of the signs and symptoms and an approach to therapy will suffice for the initiation of field therapy. Persons particularly prone to septicemia and rapid demise are those with elevated serum iron levels, achlorhydria, chronic liver disease, diabetes, human immunodeficiency virus (HIV) infection, alcoholism, cancer, and various forms of immunosuppression.

Signs and Symptoms
1. Gastroenteric manifestations
   a. Ingestion of raw or partially cooked seafood products followed in 6 to 76 hours by explosive diarrhea, nausea, vomiting, headache, abdominal pain, fever, chills, and prostration in the case of *V. parahaemolyticus.* This is not likely to be the case with *V. vulnificus.*
   b. Blood in stools
   c. Hypotension initially secondary to dehydration and then, in immunocompromised individuals, to sepsis
2. Soft tissue infection
   a. Ingestion of raw or partially cooked seafood products or direct skin (wound) contact with ocean water followed in 12 to 48 hours by skin erythema, vesiculation, and hemorrhagic or contused-appearing bullae, progressing rapidly to necrotizing fasciitis and tissue necrosis *(V. vulnificus)*
   b. Hypotension secondary to sepsis

Treatment
1. Treat dehydration and hypotension with intravenous crystalloid fluid replacement.
2. Administer an appropriate antibiotic as soon as a *Vibrio* infection is suspected.
   a. Appropriate antibiotics for sepsis include doxycycline (100 mg IV q12h), certazidime (2 g IV q8h), or ciprofloxacin (400 mg IV q12h). Other antibiotics that have been suggested include trimethoprim-sulfamethoxazole, ciprofloxacin, tetracycline, carbenicillin, chloramphenicol, tobramycin, gentamicin, imipenem-cilastatin, meropenem, and many third-generation cephalosporins. A course of oral ciprofloxacin, trimethoprim/sulfamethoxazole,

or doxycycline may shorten the course of severe gastro-enteritis.
  b. For information about antibiotic prophylaxis for marine-acquired wounds, see Chapter 51.

▶ ANISAKIASIS

Anisakiasis is caused by penetration of the *Anisakis* nematode larva through the gastric mucosa. The nematode originates from the muscle tissue of raw fish.

Signs and Symptoms
1. Within 1 hour of ingestion of raw fish: severe epigastric pain, nausea, and vomiting, mimicking an acute abdomen
   a. If the worm does not implant, it may be coughed up, vomited, or defecated, usually within 48 hours of the meal
   b. If the worm is felt in the oropharynx or esophagus, "tingling throat" sensation
2. Intestinal anisakiasis more often delayed in onset (up to 7 days after ingestion) and marked by abdominal pain, nausea, vomiting, diarrhea, and fever

Treatment
Unfortunately, no effective field treatment exists. Until the worm is rejected or endoscopically removed, give symptomatic therapy (e.g., an antacid). Albendazole, 200 mg PO bid for 3 days, has been recommended, but is of questionable efficacy.

▶ DOMOIC ACID INTOXICATION (AMNESTIC SHELLFISH POISONING)

Shellfish, particularly certain species of mussels and razor clams, that have concentrated domoic acid (glutamate agonist) generate in humans a syndrome of amnestic shellfish poisoning.

Signs and Symptoms
1. Initial symptoms of nausea, vomiting, abdominal cramps, and diarrhea 1 to 24 hours after ingestion
2. In 15 minutes to 38 hours (median 5 hours) after ingestion of contaminated shellfish, rapid onset of arousal, confusion, disorientation, and memory loss
3. Severe headache, hiccoughs, arrhythmias, hypotension, seizures, ophthalmoplegia, hemiparesis, mutism, grimacing, agitation, emotional lability, coma, copious bronchial secretions, and pulmonary edema

Treatment
1. Therapy is supportive and based on symptoms.
2. For seizures, administer a potent rapid-acting anticonvulsant such as diazepam.

▶ GEMPYLOTOXICATION

Gempylotoxic fishes are the pelagic mackerels, which produce an oil with a pronounced purgative effect. The "toxin" is contained in both musculature and bones.

Signs and Symptoms
1. Within 30 to 60 minutes of ingestion, abdominal cramping, bloating, mild nausea, and diarrhea
2. Fever, bloody or foul-smelling stools, or protracted vomiting suggests infectious gastroenteritis

Treatment
1. Therapy is supportive and based on symptoms.
2. Antimotility agents are not recommended unless the diarrhea is debilitating because inhibition of peristalsis may increase the duration of the disorder.

▶ BOTULISM

Botulism is a paralytic disease caused by the potent natural toxins of *Clostridium botulinum*. Seafood-related botulism can be caused by raw, parboiled, salt-cured, or fermented meats from marine mammals or fish products. Toxin types A, B, and E predominate.

Signs and Symptoms
1. Within 12 to 36 hours of ingestion: nausea, vomiting, abdominal pain, and diarrhea, followed by dry mouth, dysphonia (hoarseness), difficulty swallowing, facial weakness, ptosis, nonreactive or sluggishly reactive pupils, mydriasis, blurred or double vision, descending symmetric muscular weakness leading to paralysis, and bulbar and respiratory paralysis

Treatment
1. Provide ventilatory support.
2. Consider a cathartic if airway is maintained.
3. Administer equine trivalent antitoxin A, B, and E as soon as possible. Initial dose is 10 mL (one vial) every 2 to 4 hours for 3 to 5 doses or longer if symptoms persist. Anticipate an anaphylactic reaction to antitoxin.

▶ *Pfiesteria* (POSSIBLE ESTUARY-ASSOCIATED) SYNDROME

Pfiesteria piscicida is a toxic dinoflagellate that inhabits estuarine and coastal waters of the eastern United States and has been associated with fish kills and possibly with human illness. The route of exposure is unknown, although it is thought to be either by prolonged direct skin contact with toxin-laden water or via aerosols after breathing air over areas where fish are dying.

Signs and Symptoms
Headache, erythematous and edematous skin papules on the trunk or extremities, muscle cramps, eye irritation, upper respiratory irritation, and neuropsychologic symptoms (forgetfulness, difficulties with learning)

Treatment
1. Therapy is symptomatic and supportive.
2. Empirical-based recommendations state that cholestyramine may be effective in patients with persistent syndromes.

Aquatic Skin Disorders

54

Among the disorders acquired in water that affect the skin are various dermatoses, cutaneous larva migrans, infections, sensitivity to diving equipment, pseudomonal folliculitis, and otitis externa.

DISORDERS

▶ SEA CUCUMBER DERMATITIS

Signs and Symptoms
1. Skin erythema, pain, and pruritus

Treatment
1. Prompt washing with soap and water to remove toxins.
2. Treat a mild to moderate reaction with a topical low or medium potency corticosteroid preparation (Table 54-1).
3. Treat a severe reaction with an oral corticosteroid, specifically prednisone, 60 to 100 mg for adults and 1 mg/kg for children, with a 2-week taper.

▶ SEA MOSS DERMATITIS (DOGGER BANK ITCH)

Sea moss dermatitis is caused by a plant *(Fragilaria striatula)* or sea chervils (genus *Alcyondium*), which appear in seaweed-like animal colonies (mosses or "mats"), usually drawn up within fishing nets.

Signs and Symptoms
1. Irritation, first appearing on the hands and forearms (see Plate 33)
2. Recurrent exposures are more severe, characterized by vesiculated and edematous eruption of the hands, arms, legs, and face

Treatment
1. Treat as for mild poison oak dermatitis (see Chapter 39).
   a. Depending on the severity of the reaction, apply calamine lotion or a topical medium or high-potency corticosteroid preparation.
   b. Give an oral antihistamine to help control itching.
2. Treat a severe reaction with an oral corticosteroid, specifically prednisone, 60 to 100 mg for adults and 1 mg/kg for children, with a 2-week taper.

TABLE 54-1. Potency Ranking of Topical Steroids

POTENCY	BRAND	GENERIC	SIZES
Super high	Temovate Cream, Ointment 0.05%;	Clobetasol propionate	15, 30, 45, 60 gm
	Psorcon Ointment	Diflorasone diacetate	15, 30, 60 gm
Medium	Westcort Cream 0.2%	Hydrocortisone valerate	15, 45, 60 gm
	Locoid Cream 0.1%	Hydrocortisone butyrate	15, 45 gm
Low	Aclovate Cream, Ointment 0.05%;	Alclometasone dipropionate	15, 45, 60 gm
	DesOwen Cream, Lotion 0.05%	Desonide	15, 60, 118 mL

These topical steroids must be applied twice daily. However, the actual application rate can vary upward a maximum of 3 to 4 times per day according to the prescriber's discretion.

▶ **SEAWEED DERMATITIS**

Seaweed dermatitis is almost always secondary to irritation from contact with algae. For instance, the stinging seaweed *Microcoleus lyngbyaceus* is green or olive colored, drab, and finely filamentous. The typical victim does not remove a wet bathing suit for a time after leaving the water.

Signs and Symptoms
1. In minutes to hours after exposure, a pruritic, burning, moist, and erythematous rash developing in bathing suit distribution, followed by bullous escharotic desquamation in the genital, perineal, and perianal regions (see Plate 34)
2. Lymphadenopathy, pustular folliculitis, and local infections
3. Oral and ocular mucous membrane irritation, facial rash, conjunctivitis

Treatment
1. Wash the skin vigorously with soap and water.
2. Apply a brief soak of isopropyl alcohol 40%.
3. Apply a topical corticosteroid preparation. This may need to be medium to high potency.

4. Treat a severe reaction with an oral corticosteroid, specifically, prednisone, 60 to 100 mg for adults and 1 mg/kg for children, with a 2-week taper.

▶ PROTOTHECOSIS

The genus *Prototheca* consists of nonpigmented algae from the family Chlorellaceae. *Prototheca wickerhamii* and *Prototheca sopfii* are the most commonly isolated pathogens in human protothecosis.

Signs and Symptoms
1. Superficial cutaneous lesions present as papulonodules or verrucous plaques with or without ulcerations. Bullous lesions or, rarely, eczematous and cellulitis-like lesions may occur (see Plate 35).
2. Olecranon bursitis, with or without spontaneous drainage. A history of preceding trauma should suggest protothecosis.
3. Systemic infection, particularly in immunosuppressed persons.
4. A case of esophageal protothecosis has been reported.

   In cases associated with a traumatic episode, the initial lesion is a nodule or tender red papule, which enlarges, becomes pustular, and ulcerates. There may be a purulent, malodorous, and blood-tinged discharge. Satellite lesions surround the primary lesion and may become confluent. Regional lymph nodes may develop metastatic granulomas.

Treatment
1. Localized lesions can be excised.
2. Topical medications are unsatisfactory.
3. Algaecidal agents including ketoconazole, itraconazole, fluconazole, and miconazole may inhibit or kill the organisms.

▶ AQUAGENIC URTICARIA

Signs and Symptoms
1. Urticaria on exposure to water of any temperature
2. Eruption usually confined to the neck, upper trunk, and arms, whereas the face, hands, legs, and feed are spared (see Plate 36)

Treatment
1. Prevent or inhibit the reaction by applying petroleum ointment to the skin before water exposure.
2. Consider prophylaxis with an antihistamine 1 hour before exposure.

3. In persons with recurrent aquagenic urticaria, consider stanazol 10 mg/day for symptom control.

▶ AQUAGENIC PRURITUS

Signs and Symptoms
1. Intense disabling itching without visible cutaneous changes on exposure to water of any temperature
2. Reaction within minutes of exposure and lasting between 10 minutes and 2 hours
3. Lack of concurrent skin disease or drug exposure
4. Symptoms may occur only in areas exposed to water. Typically, the head, palms, soles, and mucosa are spared.

Treatment
1. Alkalinization of water and application of petroleum ointment to skin have had limited success.
2. Antihistamines may have limited success.

▶ SCHISTOSOMIASIS (CERCARIAL DERMATITIS, "SWIMMER'S ITCH")

Swimmer's itch is caused by penetration of the epidermis by the cercariae of avian, rodent, or ungulate schistosomes. The cercariae are immature larval forms, usually microscopic, of the parasitic flatworms. Although penetration of cercariae may occur in the water, it usually occurs as the film of water evaporates on the skin. The eruption occurs primarily on exposed areas of the body.

Signs and Symptoms
1. Initial symptom: prickling sensation (sometimes burning and itching sensations)
2. Itching 4 to 60 minutes after the cercariae penetrate the skin, accompanied by erythema and mild edema
3. Subsidence of the initial urticarial reaction over 60 minutes, leaving red macules that become papular and more pruritic over the next 10 to 15 hours; discrete and highly pruritic papules 3 to 5 mm in diameter are surrounded by a zone of erythema (see Plate 37)
4. Vesicles, which may become pustules, frequently forming within 48 hours and possibly persisting for 7 to 14 days
5. Peak inflammatory response within 3 days and subsidence slowly over 1 to 2 weeks

Treatment
1. In a mild case, apply isopropyl alcohol 40% or equal parts of isopropyl alcohol and calamine lotion to control the itching.
2. Oral antihistamines may be helpful.

3. For a severe case, give an oral corticosteroid, specifically prednisone, 60 to 100 mg for adults and 1 mg/kg for children, with a 2-week taper.
4. Manage secondary bacterial infection, which is frequently caused by *Staphylococcus aureus* or *Streptococcus* species, with a topical antiseptic ointment (mupirocin, bacitracin) or a systemic antibiotic (e.g., erythromycin, dicloxacillin).

Prevention
Obtain some prevention by brisk rubbing with a rough, dry towel immediately on leaving the water to remove moisture that harbors the cercariae. Washing the skin with rubbing alcohol or soap and water is not effective.

▶ SEA BATHER'S ERUPTION

See Chapter 52.

▶ LEECHES

Leeches attach to the skin of the victim with jaws that allow the introduction of an anticoagulant, which causes moderate painless bleeding at the site of removal. Leeches feed until they are engorged, then fall off.

Signs and Symptoms
1. In unsensitized individual, freely bleeding wound that heals slowly
2. In sensitized victim, urticarial, bullous, or necrotic reaction to the bite
3. With rapid onset of bullae, necrosis, and sepsis, suspect *Aeromonas hydrophila* infection (see later)

Treatment
1. To remove a leech, apply a few drops of brine, alcohol, or strong vinegar, or hold a flame near the site of attachment. Do not rip the leech off the skin because its jaws may remain and induce intense inflammation.
2. After removal of the leech, inspect the wound site closely for retained mouth parts.
3. Hasten hemostasis by the application of a styptic pencil, topical thrombin solution, or oxidized regenerated cellulose absorbable hemostat.
4. Clean wounds several times daily with an antiseptic. Treat any secondary infection that develops with an antibiotic.

▶ SEA "LOUSE" DERMATITIS

Sea "lice" are small, biting marine crustaceans often buried in the sandy bottom that attach to fish, feet, or hands.

Signs and Symptoms
1. Immediate sharp pain, with noticeable punctate hemorrhage
2. Injury resolving over 5 to 7 days

Treatment
1. Clean the acute wound with a brisk soap and water scrub or brief hydrogen peroxide application; then cover lightly with antiseptic ointment.
2. Inspect daily for secondary infection.

▶ CUTANEOUS LARVA MIGRANS

Cutaneous larva migrans ("creeping eruption") is caused by the larvae of various nematode parasites for which humans are an abnormal final host. The larvae penetrate the epidermis but are unable to penetrate the dermis. The feet and buttocks are most often involved with the superficial serpiginous tunnels.

Signs and Symptoms
1. Thin, wandering, linear or serpiginous, raised, and tunnel-like lesion 2 to 3 mm in width (see Plate 38)
2. Severe itching
3. Creeping eruption as the larvae move a few millimeters to a few centimeters each day
4. Older lesions that are dry and crusted

Treatment
1. Use cryotherapy with ethyl chloride for a mild infestation, topical thiabendazole in a more refractory case, and oral thiabendazole (25 to 50 mg/kg) for 2 to 4 days in a more severe case. Alternative drugs are albendazole (400 mg/day PO for 7 days) or ivermectin (12-mg single dose).
2. Secondary infection may occur and require incision and drainage of pustules or furuncles and the use of topical and systemic antibiotics.

▶ SOAPFISH DERMATITIS

The soapfish *Rypticus saponaceus* (Fig. 54-1) releases a soapy mucus when handled or disturbed.

Signs and Symptoms
Skin irritation with redness, itching, and mild swelling

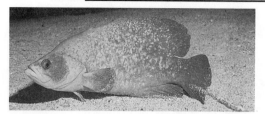

Figure 54-1. Soapfish *(Rypticus saponaceus)*. Skin contact with soapy mucus causes dermatitis. (Courtesy of Carl Roessler.)

Treatment
1. Apply cold compresses of Burow's solution to alleviate the burning and itching.
2. For a severe case, apply a topical steroid preparation.

▶ *Mycobacterium marinum* INFECTION

Infection occurs after exposure to fresh or salt water. *Mycobacterium marinum* invades skin through a preexisting skin lesion. Most lesions heal spontaneously within 2 to 3 years.

Signs and Symptoms
1. Development of localized area of cellulitis 7 to 10 days after sustaining puncture wound or laceration, particularly of the cooler distal extremity; may progress to localized arthritis, bony erosion, formation of subcutaneous nodules, and superficial desquamation
2. Development of red papule within 3 to 4 weeks after inoculation that transforms into hard purple nodule, with scaling, ulceration, and verrucous appearance; may enlarge to 6 cm in diameter, although 1 to 2 cm more common
3. New lesions developing in pattern that resembles sporotrichosis, with dermal granulomas in linear distribution (see Plate 39) along the superficial lymphatics

Treatment
1. Administer trimethoprim/sulfamethoxazole or ethambutol plus rifampin as first-line therapy.
2. Subsequent treatment is determined by culture and drug sensitivity testing. Effective antibiotics have included minocycline, tetracycline, levofloxacin, azithromycin, amikacin, amoxicillin/clavulanate, and tuberculostatic drugs.
3. Therapy is continued from months to years.

▶ *Erysipelothrix rhusiopathiae* INFECTION

Erysipelothrix rhusiopathiae, the causative agent of erysipeloid, enters the skin through a puncture wound or abrasion, usually on the finger or hand.

Signs and Symptoms
1. Appearance of violaceous, raised area within 2 to 7 days after inoculation
2. Enlarged area, accompanied by pain and itching
3. Low-grade fever, malaise
4. Hallmark lesion: purplish skin irritation or paronychia, with edema and small amount of purulent discharge
   a. Surrounded by area of relative central fading, in turn surrounded by centripetally advancing, raised, well-demarcated, and marginated erythematous or violaceous ring (see Plate 28)
   b. Lesion warm and tender, with progression up the dorsal edge of the finger into the web space and descent along the adjoining finger
5. Infection seldom affecting the palm; absence of pitting or suppuration
6. Regional inflamed lymph nodes
7. Malaise, fever
8. Arthritis

Treatment
1. For skin involvement, administer penicillin VK (250 to 500 mg PO qid), cephalexin (250 mg PO qid), or ciprofloxacin (500 mg PO bid) for 10 days. Erythromycin is not recommended.
2. If arthritis is present, give IV aqueous penicillin G (2 to 4 million units q4h for 4 to 6 weeks).

▶ SEAL FINGER

This is usually an infection of a digit after exposure to the skin or mucous membranes of a seal or sea lion, thought to be secondary to infection with strains of *Mycoplasma.*

Signs and Symptoms
1. Swollen and painful digit, preceded by an inflammatory papule that develops into a nodule with swelling, purulence, and pain (see Plate 40)
2. Stiff digit with occasional fever

Treatment
1. Tetracycline 1.5 g initial oral dose, followed by 500 mg PO qid for 4 to 6 weeks

▶ *Aeromonas hydrophila* INFECTION

Aeromonas hydrophila poses a threat to freshwater aquarists in the same manner that *Vibrio* species do to marine aquarists.

Signs and Symptoms
1. Within 24 hours, wound (particularly of puncture variety) that becomes cellulitic, with erythema, edema, and purulent discharge (see Plate 41)
   a. Most frequently affects the lower extremity
   b. Appearance indistinguishable from streptococcal cellulitis
2. Localized pain, lymphangitis, fever, chills
3. Rapidly advancing, gas-forming, soft tissue reaction, with bullae formation and necrotizing myositis

Treatment
1. Administer an antibiotic such as chloramphenicol, gentamicin, tobramycin, tetracycline, trimethoprim/sulfamethoxazole (co-trimoxazole), ciprofloxacin, cefotaxime, ceftazidime, moxalactam, imipenem-cilastatin, or meropenem.
2. For severe infection, administer IV antibiotics as soon as possible. Aggressive wound débridement may be necessary.

▶ *Vibrio* SP. INFECTION

For information on antibiotic prophylaxis against *Vibrio* sp. infection, see Chapter 51. For information on antibiotic therapy for established *Vibrio* sp. infection, see Chapters 51 and 53.

▶ REACTIONS TO DIVING EQUIPMENT

Some chemical components in the plastic and rubber used to create masks and mouthpieces can cause irritant or allergic dermatitis.

Signs and Symptoms
1. "Mask burn," which may appear as reddish imprint of the mask on the face or a severe, vesicular, and weeping eruption
2. Glossitis
3. Redness and lichenification over exposed surfaces of the feet (contact with swim fins)

Treatment
1. Treat acute facial dermatitis with cool compresses of Burow's solution.
2. For a severe skin reaction, treat with an oral corticosteroid, specifically, prednisone, 60 to 100 mg for adults and 1 mg/kg for children, with a 2-week taper.

3. For a serious intraoral reaction, use a twice-daily mouthwash of equal parts of antihistamine (diphenhydramine) elixir and magnesium salts (milk of magnesia). Coat individual sores twice daily and at bedtime with triamcinolone acetonide (0.1%) dental paste (Kenalog in Orabase) for 5 to 7 days.

▶ PSEUDOMONAL FOLLICULITIS

Pseudomonas aeruginosa is the most common microbe causing skin disorders in occupational saturation divers and can occur after recreational use of diving suits. It is also a cause of folliculitis in occupants of heated recreational water sources.

Signs and Symptoms
1. Follicular rash appearing within 48 hours of exposure, most pronounced in areas covered by a wet suit or bathing garment (see Plate 42)
2. External otitis, conjunctivitis, tender breasts, enlarged and tender lymph nodes, fever, malaise

Treatment
1. Apply drying lotions such as calamine, with or without oral antihistamines.
2. Treat local infection with antimicrobial ointment such as polymyxin B or gentamicin, until resolved.
3. Treat systemic infection with ciprofloxacin or an aminoglycoside.

▶ OTITIS EXTERNA (SWIMMER'S EAR)

Otitis externa is inflammation and infection (often polymicrobial) of the external ear canal caused by constant moisture, warm body temperature, and introduction of microorganisms.

Signs and Symptoms
1. Initial symptoms: itching, mild pain; rarely, decreased hearing
2. Possibly sensation of "fullness" in the affected ear
3. Pain that worsens as the inflammation progresses until it is uncomfortable to push on the tragus or pull on the earlobe
4. Severe infection: possible cellulitis, with purulent discharge (see Plate 43), occlusion of the ear canal, cervical lymphadenopathy, headache, nausea, fever, and toxemia

Treatment
1. The most important topical therapy is re-acidification and desiccation of the ear canal, which can be accomplished with a 50:50 mixture of isopropyl alcohol 40% and acetic acid 5% (vinegar) or with Burow's solution (Domeboro: aluminum sulfate and calcium acetate).

2. Avoid oily solutions.
3. Administer appropriate pain medications.
4. For a mild infection (slight pain and discharge), use ear drops such as nonaqueous acetic acid (VoSol Otic). Colistin sulfate has been recommended to combat *Pseudomonas*. Using acetic acid or acetic acid with hydrocortisone 1% (VoSol Otic HC) avoids sensitization that may occur with neomycin-containing products.
5. If suppuration occurs, antibiotic ear drops such as hydrocortisone 1%, polymyxin B, and neomycin (Cortisporin otic) or ofloxacin otic are indicated.
6. If the ear canal is so swollen that drops will not penetrate the debris, place a gauze or foam wick and keep it soaked with the topical solution for 24 to 72 hours.
7. If adenopathy, profuse purulent discharge, or fever is present, give oral co-trimoxazole, ciprofloxacin, or amoxicillin-clavulanate.

Prevention
1. The most important preventive measure is to diminish moisture retention in the external ear canal.
2. Do not use cotton-tipped applicators to extract moisture because they can damage the ear canal lining or press cerumen deeply into the canal.
3. Acidifying and desiccating agents are effective prophylaxis.
4. Achieve prevention by briefly rinsing with common rubbing alcohol, vinegar, or a mixture of these after each entry into the water. Avoid petroleum jelly or other substances intended to form a watertight seal because they may act as a moist trap for debris.

Search and Rescue

55

Wilderness settings are usually relatively inaccessible or not serviced by maintained roads, and they encompass a wide range of terrain and environmental conditions. Rescuers find themselves working in hot, dry, desert conditions or snowy, thin-air, or alpine environments, and anything in between. It is a fortunate rescuer who is able to work in a controlled environment, with clean cliffs rather than steep and unstable rock, ice, thin gullies, and loose scree.

This chapter addresses broad concepts of wilderness search and rescue; responders should evaluate their particular circumstances and seek specific training for the types of incidents that they may encounter.

Not all rescuers need to be trained to the most advanced levels of wilderness operations, and individuals should always operate within the limits of their experience and training. Before attempting to respond to any rescue incident, responsible persons should ensure that every field team has a breadth and depth of experience to enable personnel to operate safely and make sound decisions. The safety of the rescuer(s) and rescue team should always be the first priority.

▶ OVERVIEW

During any search and rescue (SAR) the following rudiments are essential for a safe and efficient operation:
1. Provide for the safety of rescuers and victims. This must include injury prevention from environmental and rescuer causes; provision of water, shelter, and possibly food; and providing a mechanism for personal hygiene.
2. Communicate needs and changes during all phases of the operation. Call for backup at the earliest possible time. Ensure that rescuers are apprised of the activities and needs of others when there is a need to know. Keep command, base camp, medical control, and incoming rescuers informed. Communication seems to be the most frequently missed or most poorly managed item.
3. Locate and reach the victim with medical-rescue personnel and equipment. Implement organized and methodical procedures for finding the victim as soon as the safety of rescuers and victims has been ascertained.
4. Treat and monitor the victim during evacuation. Support basic personal hygiene and physiologic functions. Psychologic support is also essential. This may be as basic as hand-holding

with verbal encouragement by a familiar and constant voice. Help the victim to feel involved with the rescue by communicating as often as the situation permits.

▶ PREPLANNING

1. Before engaging in any type of technical or advanced rescue, responsible individuals should perform a risk assessment to identify necessary skills and capabilities.
2. The preplan should consider the types of terrain in the response area, people exposed to that terrain, types of accidents likely to occur, and available resources.
3. Exposed personnel must be specifically trained for terrain and environmental considerations commonly encountered in the areas in which they may work. For example, a rescuer responding to a fallen ice climber incident in the wilderness must be trained in both high-angle ice rescue and in wilderness SAR.
4. Having wilderness skills also enables rescuers to work independently of external support and resources in nonwilderness incidents. For example, self-sufficiency and an ability to function with minimal external resources are beneficial when working in the aftermath of an earthquake, or in responding to a transmission tower incident far from a road.

Research the Location
1. Review all geographic and medical concerns specific to the rescue location, identifying in advance any hazards that pose a threat.
2. Determine the topography and potential evacuation routes (and nearest phones) before beginning any travel.
3. Make certain that the location of cached equipment and supplies and the phone numbers of available rescue resources and local hospitals are communicated to each member of the party.

Rescue Resources
1. The outdoor recreation and rescue communities emphasize personal responsibility. If the group has the skills and technical abilities to accomplish self-rescue, the participants must know their limitations. If necessary, members must be capable and willing to mobilize organized rescue resources. Organized rescue is often more expeditious and may reduce the number of participants who are injured or killed.
2. Rescuers not familiar with a particular environment or type of response should operate only under the direct

supervision and care of appropriately trained personnel. Placing an untrained person in a high-angle rope rescue situation to perform patient care, for example, endangers that person, the victim, and others involved in the operation.

3. Within the United States, law enforcement agencies are generally responsible for the command structure and direction of an operation. Mutual aid contracts or interagency agreements may give certain agencies responsibility for specific incidents. When adventuring outside the United States, always discuss rescue issues (e.g., forms of payment, available resources, notification systems) with the foreign U.S. embassy. In the United States, follow these guidelines:

   a. County sheriffs have jurisdiction in unincorporated county areas and in most Bureau of Land Management (BLM) and U.S. Forest Service (USFS) lands, by congressional mandate.

   b. The city police have jurisdiction on city lands and, in some cases, adjacent watersheds.

   c. Fire districts and city fire departments may have jurisdiction over hazardous materials or urban SAR operations.

   d. Emergency medical services (EMS) usually have jurisdiction over medical care of sick or injured persons.

   e. The National Park Service has jurisdiction over its lands except where otherwise mandated.

Support Services

Any single responsible agency may not have the most efficient means of conducting a rescue operation. It may delegate or request help from other groups that are more capable of performing the actual rescue such as the following:

1. Volunteer SAR and sheriff's SAR groups usually have both responsibility and authority to conduct an operation.

2. Technically specialized volunteer teams, in addition to the regular SAR teams, may be available and may be certified by national organizations. Examples include local ski patrols and the National Ski Patrol System, National Cave Rescue Commission, Mountain Rescue Association, and National Association for Search and Rescue (NASAR).

3. Do not overlook commercial enterprises or professional individuals or teams, even if they are not specifically certified. Such groups include mountain, river, and bicycle guides, commercial mine rescue teams, and military units.

Personal Preparation

Rescue operations are inherently dangerous. No amount of preparation can completely remove all dangers. To effect a rescue in the backcountry, rescue party members must possess personal skills specific to the terrain where they will operate.

Fitness
1. Participate in a regular physical fitness program.
2. Psychologic fitness includes the following:
   a. The victims are responsible for their own predicament.
   b. Rescuers must ensure their own safety during both training and rescue operations.
- Have backups available whenever possible.
- Use appropriate safety equipment for the environment. Make sure that anchors are secure. Tie in anyone near an edge or precipice. Make sure that helmets are worn by persons exposed to falls or falling objects. Wear personal flotation devices when performing rescues near or in the water.
- Double-check everything.
- Practice using all systems before they are needed in an actual rescue operation.
   c. Rescuers must be aware of their exposure to such risks as rockfalls, avalanches, dangerous plants and animals, faulty equipment, violent victims, untrained personnel, unrealistic personnel or victims, weather, exposure to falls, and water hazards.
   d. Rescuers must be realistic about life and death situations in the backcountry. Victims may die if they are seriously injured and definitive care is far away. The death or significant injury of a friend, trip member, or child may cause profound psychologic impact such as post-traumatic stress syndrome. A Critical Stress Debriefing Team may be requested through the local EMS agency or sheriff's office.

Training (Box 55-1)
1. As a rescuer, participate in wilderness medical and rescue conferences and practice regularly under realistic conditions.
2. Basic survival, navigation, and first-aid skills are essential for all team members. Although complete information on these areas is beyond the scope of this field guide, two basic items essential for survival bear mention: procurement of drinking water and maintenance of body temperature.
   a. Dehydration is a major problem for both rescuer and victim. Take the following steps to prevent problems:
- Drink before you are thirsty, and monitor rescuer and victim hydration status by observing urine output and color

---

Box 55-1.   Rescue Personnel and Training in the United States

1. Most technical rescue personnel in the United States are climbers or skiers who have added rescue techniques and medical training to their skills.
2. Approximately 600,000 EMTs work in the United States.
3. A growing number of wilderness EMTs have been trained in the skills of extended victim care in the backcountry environment.
4. Key skill elements of medical training for wilderness medical and rescue training include the following:
   a. Thorough victim assessment skills and monitoring
   b. Technical skills and the authority to perform the following:
   * Airway management, to include endotracheal intubation
   * Shock management to include intravenous therapy
   * Use of the military antishock trousers (MAST) garment or other pelvic stabilization device
   * Oxygen administration
   * Use of appropriate medications:
     Epinephrine for anaphylactic reactions
     Antibiotics for open fractures
     Acetazolamide, nifedipine, and other drugs used for acute high-altitude problems
   * Pain medications for musculoskeletal trauma
   * Field rewarming techniques
   * Field reduction of fracture-dislocations
   * Victim packaging and transportation skills
5. Key skill elements of technical training for rescue personnel in the United States include the following:
   a. Appropriate climbing skills for terrain (rock, ice, snow, glacier)
   b. Radio communications skills and protocols
   c. Helicopter and fixed-wing protocols
   d. Training and expertise in using the Incident Command System in field protocols

---

(minimum urine output should consist of a third of a liter every 6 hours, and urine should remain light or "straw" colored).

* Disinfect drinking water (see Chapter 44). In winter, insulate water bottles with commercial foam wrap or cover them with old socks or Ensolite and duct tape. Use petrolatum (Vaseline) on bottle threads to keep the cap from freezing closed. Melt snow for water (average water-to-snow yield is 1:7). On mild days, spread snow on a dark plastic sheet to melt. Use a straw or piece of intravenous tubing to access trickles of water under the snow's surface.

- Derive electrolytes from food and maintain energy stores by eating before you become hungry.
    b. Evaporation exacerbated by wind can cause significant heat loss. Use garbage bags to create a hasty personal shelter and vapor barrier (carry two for yourself and two for the victim). For an improvised bivouac, place one bag over the legs from the bottom and the other bag over the top, covering the head except for a small area cut out for the face. Use duct tape to join the bags for a complete seal. "Space blankets" (reflective lightweight Mylar tarps) flap in the wind and are not as useful as "space bags" into which the victim can be placed.

Personal Equipment

1. Your pack should be lightweight but rugged. An external frame snags trees and is generally less stable than an internal frame. Remember that the person with the largest pack usually carries the most.
2. Footwear may be anything from sneakers to double mountain boots, depending on the environment and situation.
3. Shell material should protect from wind, evaporative heat loss, and external moisture. Because of the moisture and temperature difference (vapor pressure) between the inside and outside, breathable waterproof products work best in cold weather under conditions of little physical exertion. As temperature and physical activity increase, the practical differences between these products and simple coated nylon decrease. Sweating and condensation are uncomfortable but, if minimized, are not dangerous. They can be controlled by venting and modifying work load and pace. Excessive body moisture can cause increased evaporative heat loss, increased conductive heat loss (through wet clothes), and noticeable symptoms of dehydration and hypothermia.
4. Insulation guidelines are as follows:
    a. Layer clothing for easy changing as weather and exertion change.
    b. Avoid materials such as down or cotton that lose their insulating qualities when wet. "Water-compatible" materials (e.g., pile, wool, Polypro) absorb less water and lose less loft.
5. Great amounts of heat can be lost from the uncovered head and neck. Put on or take off your hat, "neck gaiter," or balaclava to compensate for underheating or overheating. Wear a helmet (UIAA approved). Carry a wide-brimmed hat for sun protection. A baseball cap does not cover the ears or back of the neck.

6. For hand protection, use water-compatible material with a windproof, water-resistant shell as needed.

7. For eye protection, 100% ultraviolet (UV) filtering is suggested for exposure to snow or altitude. Side shields are essential in the snow at high altitude. Make sure that each person is carrying a spare pair of sunglasses.

8. Miscellaneous gear can include the following:

   a. Bivouac ("bivi") and survival gear (garbage bags/bivi sack, duct tape, whistle, candles and fire source, flares, smoke signal, signal mirror, etc.) (Box 55-2)

   b. Personal care items (hygiene, personal first-aid kit that includes sun block, blister care, etc.)

   c. Self-evacuation and rescue equipment. Comprehensive information on these areas is beyond the scope of this field guide. Familiarity and competency with the use of the following items are recommended:

- Tubular webbing (2.5 cm [1 inch] in diameter) for an improvised chest and seat harness
- Kernmantle (5 to 7 mm [$\frac{1}{5}$ to $\frac{1}{3}$ inch] in diameter) rope for lowering or raising if the terrain has a potential for ledges that are too steep or high for a simple climb up or down
- Carabiners to improvise lowering (rappelling) or climbing devices on the ropes
- Tubular webbing (2.5 cm) or 4-mm rope for making improvised breaking devices (e.g., Prusik knot) for use with ropes and carabiners

---

Box 55-2. Bivouac Kit

Two large garbage bags (emergency shelter or raingear), 10 × 10 ft sheet of plastic, and 100 ft of parachute cord (shelter)
Emergency space blanket (shelter, ground cloth)
Stocking cap (warmth)
Spare socks (warmth and can act as spare mittens)
Metal cup (to warm liquids)
Gelatin (to make a drink)
Two plumber's candles (to warm water or start fire)
Waterproof matches or lighter
Knife
Compass
Whistle
All of these items fit neatly into a small stuff sack that is 6 × 6 inches and weighs less than 1 lb when filled.

▶ RESCUE OPERATIONS

Sequence of Events in Backcountry Rescue
(Box 55-3)
Occurrence of the Critical Event
The critical event occurs when an individual participating in an activity away from immediate help is suddenly stricken by injury or illness.

Making the Decision to Get Help
Before anyone leaves to seek assistance, the victim's companions should do the following:
1. Perform a physical examination.
2. Record vital signs.
3. Determine the level of consciousness.
4. Provide appropriate emergency care, which may entail moving the victim into a protective shelter.
5. Summarize victim information in a note that accompanies the individual(s) going for help.
6. Prepare a map depicting the victim's exact location and a list of the other party members, noting their level of preparedness to endure the environmental conditions.
7. Assemble appropriate provisions.

Box 55-3. Sequence of Events in Backcountry Rescue

1. The critical event occurs: an injury or illness that requires assistance and evacuation.
2. A decision is made to "get help," and someone goes for help.
3. The emergency medical system is notified of the emergency.
4. The emergency medical system is activated, or "dispatched."
5. Eventually, the "extended rescue team" is notified and mobilized.
6. The rescue team assembles and organizes, then leaves the trailhead (may be preceded by a "hasty team").
7. The team locates the victim.
8. The team provides appropriate "extended emergency care."
9. The team organizes and evacuates the victim to the appropriate facility.
10. The team returns to base, is debriefed, and prepares for the next rescue.

Notifying and Mobilizing the Rescue Team
The first step is to notify team members.
1. Notification of an emergency usually occurs via pagers worn by individual members.
2. An alert tone is followed by an oral message describing the emergency, its location, and the type of response required.

Organizing the Rescue Team
Rescue team members assemble at a common location (rescue station) to organize the rescue effort. The first task is to define the type of rescue to establish equipment needs. Estimating the time it will take to effect the rescue and assessing the need for other agency involvement and assistance are also primary tasks. The first person on scene should ask these kinds of questions to determine necessary resources. The questions to be answered and the variables to be considered may include the following:
1. Assessment of time required and time of day. Will this be a night rescue? How long will the evacuation take? Will there be darkness and lighting considerations? How physically demanding will the operation be, and how often will rescuers need to be rotated for rest? The answers will influence resource requirements and may indicate that additional resources must be called in from farther away.
2. What are the current weather conditions at the rescue location, and what is the forecast?
3. When did the accident occur? Do we know the exact location, or is this a SAR?
4. Number of known and potential victims. How many victims are there? What are the supposed injuries? How many people are in the party? How well prepared are they? Does anyone in the party have medical expertise? When the potential of additional victims becomes a reality, the number of rescuers needed increases, and other stresses emerge. A new sense of urgency arises, and there is a need for triage, more equipment, more time, and more resources for evacuation. Additional potential victims must be anticipated.
5. Scope and magnitude of wilderness influence. Is the incident 100 yards from a vehicle access point or several miles into the backcountry? If high angle, is the best evacuation route at the top or bottom of the slope or cliff?
6. Scope and magnitude of technical rescue considerations. Is it high angle? How technical? What are the anchor points, rock types, etc.? The scope and magnitude of the

incident will affect the type and number of resources requested.

7. Assessment of manpower needs. Given the time and work to be done, will changing shifts be a consideration? Is it necessary to keep responders available for a second incident in the area? Are there sufficient resources within the organization, or will external resources be required? If multiple agencies are involved, are radio frequencies coordinated?

8. Dedicating all resources in a given area to one incident requires consideration in advance. Prearranged agreements with nearby agencies can be useful in staffing a large incident or for backup in case of another call.

9. Specific environmental factors involved. Are available personnel suitably trained and equipped for the terrain that will be encountered? Is there a river or lake in the area that will require additional personnel? What is the time of year? Is snow or ice a consideration? The steepness of terrain, as well as groundcover, must be considered when estimating whether personnel are adequately prepared to function.

10. Integrity and stability of the environment. Is a storm coming? Will night fall before the operation is done? Planning to accommodate for changes in weather, ground instability, and other environmental factors must be done several hours in advance.

11. Is a "hasty team" needed? Has it left for the scene yet?

12. Is each of the team members prepared? Does each have personal equipment, a bivouac kit, headlamp, food, and water? Is each member trained and skilled in this particular type of rescue?

13. Who is on the medical team? Who is on the evacuation team?

14. Is the team equipment organized and divided up?

15. How urgent is the situation? Is a helicopter required? Is one available? Are the weather conditions appropriate for an air rescue?

16. Will multiple agencies be involved? If so, are radio frequencies coordinated?

Beginning the Search

1. Once the team is assembled and all pertinent issues have been addressed satisfactorily, the team is transported to the trailhead (launch point) to begin the search.

2. Commonly, a hasty team starts out ahead of the main team. Once the hasty team has enough information to locate the victim, team members travel as lightly as possible,

with only enough gear to ensure their own safety and to equip them to manage the victim's primary injuries. The goal is to reach the victim as quickly as is reasonably possible and deliver primary care, and then apprise the rest of the team of the victim's condition, equipment needs, and environmental concerns.

Locating the Victim

How long it takes to locate the victim varies tremendously, depending on:
1. Distance
2. Terrain
3. Weather conditions
4. Mode of transportation
5. Whether the victim's exact location is known

A general rule of thumb for a team responding on foot is that it will take 1 hour for each mile through the backcountry. If a search is involved, all bets are off.

Scene Safety

Identify any factors that could immediately threaten the safety of the team or victim (e.g., avalanche, rockfall, swift water).

Victim Access

1. Be certain that all rescuers are aware of the fall line. This virtual line represents the path of travel for rocks, avalanches, or drifting boats and is the direction a rescuer may fall if footing is lost. Always avoid approaching the victim from directly above the fall line when working on loose ground or snow.
2. Accessing the victim usually requires one to possess the skills essential for navigation, travel, and survival in the rescue environment.
3. The first person to the victim must have the medical skills required to stabilize the victim's condition.

Victim Evaluation and Treatment at Scene
(Box 55-4)

1. In most cases, it takes at least 2 hours for an outside rescue or transport team to arrive. Use the time well. Carefully assess the situation and arrange efficient packaging. It is difficult to redo systems once an evacuation has begun. If time and circumstances allow, test the system on an uninjured party member before using it on the victim.
2. Reduce the danger and minimize the risks to rescuers first, victims second. Make sure that safety officers (to watch for and halt high-risk activity) and equipment backups (e.g., belay or fixed safety lines) are in place when possible.

Box 55-4. Victim Assessment

PRIMARY SURVEY: LOCATING AND TREATING LIFE-THREATENING PROBLEMS

A—AIRWAY MANAGEMENT
Is the airway open?
Is the airway going to stay open?

B—BREATHING
Is air moving in and out?
Is the airway quiet or silent?
Is breathing effortless?
Is the respiratory system intact?
Is breathing adequate to support life?

C—CIRCULATION
Is there a pulse?
Is bleeding well controlled?
Is capillary refill normal (<2 seconds)?
Is circulation adequate to support life?

D—DISABILITY
Conscious versus unconscious
Level of consciousness—awake/verbal/painful/unconscious (AVPU) or Glasgow Coma Scale
Cervical spine stabilization

E—ENVIRONMENT
Internal versus external
Is the victim warm and dry?
Protected from the cold ground
Protected from the elements

SECONDARY SURVEY: WHAT IS WRONG AND HOW SERIOUS IS IT?

VITAL SIGNS: INDICATE THE CONDITION OF THE VICTIM
RR—respiratory rate and effort
PR—pulse rate and character
BP—blood pressure (systolic/diastolic)
LOC—level of consciousness (AVPU or Glasgow Coma Scale)
TP—tissue perfusion: skin color, temperature, and moisture
Capillary refill (<2 seconds)

VICTIM EXAMINATION: HEAD-TO-TOE EXAMINATION TO LOCATE INJURIES

AMPLE HISTORY:
Allergies
Medicines
Past medical history
Last food/drink
Events leading up

Continued

Box 55-4. Victim Assessment—*cont'd*

SOAP NOTE: To Record and Organize Victim Data
Subjective: age, gender, mechanism of injury, chief complaint
Objective: vital signs, victim examination, AMPLE history
Assessment: problem list
Plan: plan for each problem

---

3. Perform the initial assessment and treatment essential to salvage or stabilize the victim's condition. This includes the primary survey:
   A: Airway
   B: Breathing
   C: Circulation
   D: Disability determined (mental status checked and spine stabilized if any potential for injury)
   E: All areas of the victim requiring further evaluation exposed (with consideration for environmental factors)
4. Perform a detailed head-to-toe assessment (secondary survey) of the victim before litter packaging. Continue to reevaluate the victim throughout the evacuation. Note the following:
   a. Mechanism of injury or illness. Debilitating preexisting medical conditions, trauma, environmental stress, or any combination of the three raises your index of suspicion for a serious injury (e.g., a fall from three times the victim's height would mean great potential for head, spine, and internal injuries; chest pain in a 45-year-old man before a snowmobile accident [vs. a tree accident] occurring 12 hours earlier would suggest the possibility of spine, head, and internal injuries; hypothermia; frostbite; and myocardial infarction).
   b. Victim medical history (SAMPLE):
      S: Signs, symptoms, and chief complaint
      A: Allergies
      M: Medications taken currently
      P: Past medical history
      L: Last oral intake to suggest fuel or fluid deficiency
      E: Events leading up to the illness, i.e., history of present injury or illness
   c. Initial vital signs, with subsequent monitoring at regular intervals. Vital sign changes occurring over time, coupled with the victim's mechanism of injury, help to direct treatment.
5. Take time to determine short-term and long-term plans, as well as contingencies for victim management and evacuation. Situations usually change, requiring a dynamic approach to problem solving.

Victim Evacuation Considerations
While providing emergency care, part of the team is designated the evacuation team.

1. To properly evaluate the situation, the first information needed by this team is provided by the medical team leader.
2. If the victim's condition is stable, time is less important; if the victim's condition is critical, time is critical.

The evacuation team must explore different options:

1. If speed is a consideration, weather conditions are reviewed and the availability of a helicopter-assisted rescue is determined.
2. If a helicopter is not an option, the fastest route out is established.
3. If time or speed is not critical, the safest means of evacuation that is easiest on the victim and rescuers is defined.
4. A general rule for the duration of an evacuation is that it will take 1 to 2 hours for every mile to be covered, requiring six well-rested litter bearers for every mile. Thus a 4-mile carryout will require a 24-member litter team and can take 4 to 8 hours to complete.
5. Eventually, the team reaches a trailhead and the victim is transferred to an ambulance for transport to a hospital emergency facility.

Termination Criteria
1. Termination criteria should be identified and in place before the start of a rescue. Criteria should center on the probability of success weighed against the risk to rescuers.

Additional Victim Evacuation Considerations
On the basis of scene and victim assessments, evacuation may be divided into the following four methods:

1. No evacuation. Definitive care either is not necessary or is available at the scene.
2. Assisted evacuation. Definitive therapy is necessary, but the victim is ambulatory and needs moderate support. Consider walking assists, with either one or two persons.
3. Simple carries. The victim can sit, or the injuries allow positioning other than horizontal. Examples would include a victim with exhaustion and dehydration and an uncomplicated limb fracture.
4. Litter carries (see Chapter 56). The victim is unable to sit or injuries require a horizontal position. Examples would be a femoral fracture and spine immobilization. This type of transport usually requires a minimum of six rescuers. The longer the transport, the more necessary are additional party members. Depending on the terrain, this type of

carry may also present significant risk to victim and rescuers. Two general types of litters are found on rescues: commercial and improvised.

a. The most common commercial litter is the Stokes litter (wire or plastic), which may be found with or without leg dividers; the latter is preferable because of flexible packaging configuration based on injuries.

b. Another commercial litter is the SKED, which is popular among SAR teams and the military because it is easily carried rolled up in its own backpack, slides easily, and has flotation capability. It is narrower than the Stokes litter and somewhat flexible. A short spine immobilization device is necessary if spinal injury is possible.

c. Other specialized litters such as cave-evacuation litters may be found in particular environments. You can construct improvised litters from the external frames of packs, saplings, or ropes.

d. Litter packaging should provide for victim comfort and protection from trauma and environmental impact. Secure the victim in the litter by attaching harnesses to side rails, using pretied foot loops hitched to rails or torso immobilizing devices (e.g., KED, OSS), which may then be attached to the litter.

e. Monitor the victim. Protect the face from falling objects and passing branches. You can cover the head and face with a plexiglass (Lexan) shield or a helmet and goggles or fashion a piece of closed-cell foam (Ensolite) for this if necessary. Package and adequately pad the victim to prevent pressure sores during prolonged transport. Protect the victim from insects with netting, repellent, or a secure outer wrap. Environmental concerns relate primarily to temperature regulation. The goal is warmth without overheating. Immobility reduces heat production. Extra insulation and an external heat source may be necessary. In a cold environment, a double-vapor barrier system may be necessary, with less insulation in a hot environment. A mixed system may be necessary in the high desert to allow venting of the package during the day and sealing at night. You can set up a double-vapor barrier system as follows:

• Place the outside vapor barrier on the ground first (e.g., the victim's tent fly or ground cloth).

• Place the insulation layer(s) such as a sleeping bag or a number of blankets on top.

• Strip the victim down to a Polypro layer (or just skin), dry off, and place any instrumentation (e.g., blood pressure cuff, stethoscope, Foley catheter) properly.

- Cover the victim and seal him or her in an inner vapor barrier (two garbage bags).
- Place the victim in the insulation layer.
- Wrap the victim like a burrito with the outer vapor barrier.
  f. Because the litter carry is strenuous and requires great focus, designate a route finder to find the most efficient trail. Choose a medical leader to direct victim monitoring and communication. Litter carries are best performed by at least six persons. Make sure the victim is level (head or feet up as indicated by injuries) and is transported feet first. On level terrain with few obstructions, position any extra rescuers behind the litter. Rotate the carriers through the three litter-carrying positions on one side until they have finished their forward-most carry, and then have them rotate to the rear of the line on the opposite side. This allows for a change in sides to limit rescuer fatigue.
- On terrain with short drops or obstructions, have extra rescuers place themselves in the direction of travel. This allows for a litter pass with rescuers in a stable, nonmoving position. When a rescuer has finished a pass, have the person move to the front of the line, in the direction of travel, on the opposite side.
- On steeper terrain, set up a simple belay using a tree wrap as the lowering device or an anchored lowering device such as a Muenter hitch attached to a rock. Leave an extra length of rope, or "tag" line, at the head of the litter to tie off the litter and rescuers during belay transfers. Remind rescuers to lean downhill so that their legs are perpendicular to the hillside. Trying to stand upright usually results in feet slipping out from under the rescuer and dropping the litter.

Victim Evaluation and Treatment During Transport
Victim Communication and Monitoring
1. Minimize the number of rescuers who are directly over the victim's head. Limit the number of rescuers who communicate directly with the victim. This reduces perceived chaos and helps keep the victim become oriented and calm.
2. Monitor pulses at the temporal or carotid artery with a packaged victim. Unless the pulse's character changes significantly, blood pressure probably does not have to be measured.
3. Monitor blood pressure by placing a cuff over a flat-diaphragm stethoscope that is taped to the victim's upper arm. Run the cuff bulb, gauge, and stethoscope ear pieces

through a hole in the vapor barriers to the outside for easy access. Reseal access holes with duct tape after placement.

4. Monitor respirations using a small pocket mirror or noting condensation on the facemask or in the endotracheal tube.

5. Obtain rectal temperature using an indoor/outdoor remote thermometer. Insert the "outdoor" probe into the rectum after covering with a lubricated finger cot, latex glove finger, or condom. The "indoor" reading reflects the victim's local environment. During the preplanning phase, test the thermometer's accuracy against glass thermometers in water of varying temperatures. Thermometry is an essential component of a double-vapor barrier system because of the potential for raising the victim's core temperature.

6. Skin color, temperature, and moisture are difficult to monitor in a litter-packaged victim. Other vital signs, especially pulse rate, are used more frequently.

7. Mental status is extremely sensitive to perfusion changes. If the rescuers continue to interact with a conscious victim, they will perceive subtle changes.

Respiratory Guidelines

1. Protect the airway.

2. The definitive airway is an endotracheal (ET) tube. Neither oropharyngeal nor nasopharyngeal airways protect the trachea from upper airway bleeding or vomitus.

3. Improvise suction devices using a turkey baster or a 60-mL irrigating syringe with 1.5-cm ({5/8}-inch) surgical tubing or an inverted nasal airway. A commercial device (V-VAC hand-powered suction unit) is compact and works well. Remember that gravity is readily available. A well-packaged victim can be quickly rolled to the side or downward without compromise of spinal alignment.

4. LSP makes a bag refill-valve that is a demand valve for the bag-valve-mask, delivers 100% oxygen, and shuts off flow once the bag is filled. This prolongs a 30-minute E cylinder for up to 1{1/2} hours at high flow.

5. Remote ventilation systems, mouth-to-mask ventilation, or even a bag-valve-mask may be difficult to manipulate when a victim is packaged in a litter, being carried over steep or rough terrain, or transported in a confined space. For a victim needing ventilation, consider the following system:

a. Mask or ET tube (preferable). A mask can be taped to the face (with quick-release capability), or an anesthesia mask and rubber spider strapping may be used (airway must be constantly monitored).

b. One-way valve. This is placed in-line near the facemask to limit dead space. In cold weather, this may freeze from condensation, so always carry a spare valve inside your coat or pack.

c. Oxygen

d. Ventilator tube

e. Bag-valve-mask

f. One-way valves purchased through MDI, Respironics, Life Support Products (LSP), or their distributors may be taped to the ventilator tubing, which can be purchased from most hospital respiratory therapy departments. Dan White (Independence, MO) manufactures the White Pulmonary Resuscitator (WPR), which is a commercial version of the improvised system.

Circulatory Considerations

1. Because of weight and space restrictions, intravenous (IV) fluid therapy in the field is usually reserved for SAR teams or large expeditions.
2. Intravenous fluids are typically infused by bolus during stops or when needed.
3. Do not leave any IV lines hanging during transport. They get in the way and are pulled out too easily.
4. Blood pressure cuff and body weight methods of pressure infusion are usually inadequate for high-volume fluid replacement.
5. Prewarm IV bags by carrying them inside your coat, and then protect lines from freezing by placing the fluids inside the litter package or your coat. To set up a non–gravity-feed field IV system, proceed through the following steps:
   a. Invert the bag and squeeze out the air.
   b. Start the IV line using a saline lock and a large-bore catheter.
   c. Run in the amount of fluid desired using a pressure IV sleeve, with the quantity measured with the bag.
   d. Disconnect the IV tubing from the saline lock and cap the needle.
   e. Package the remaining fluids with the victim.

Nervous System Considerations

1. Vomiting is a classic sign of head injury. Monitor and protect the airway.
2. Compartment syndrome may be a problem with inadequate padding. Pad the system wherever possible (without compromising spine immobilization).

Musculoskeletal System Considerations

1. Skin and soft tissues may develop pressure sores. Use adequate padding.
2. Compartment syndrome from tissue edema is often overlooked because of the intensity of the evacuation. Perform ongoing assessment of injured extremities.

3. When packaging for a long evacuation, place the victim's knees and elbows in slight flexion to achieve maximum comfort.

Gastrointestinal and Genitourinary Considerations

1. Although the fasting status of victims who may require surgery is a consideration, hydration of the victim during the extended evacuation is important. Persuade victims whose injuries or illness do not preclude fluids by mouth to take small sips of water. Encourage them to eat and drink regularly.

2. With proper double-vapor barrier packaging and long transport delays unlikely, allow the victim to defecate or urinate freely inside the litter packaging. An improvised diaper helps to reduce discomfort.

3. For the unconscious victim, insert a Foley catheter and use a leg bag to allow for the assessment of urine output. In a conscious male, you may use a "condom catheter."

4. For the conscious victim, the litter can be inverted or stood on end for urination if the packaging arrangement allows. A bedpan or urinal can also be used.

5. Female victims may benefit from an improvised funnel made from an inverted pocket mask held against the perineum. Attach this to 1.5-cm (⅝-inch) surgical tubing and drain it outside the litter. The Whiz Freedom or Lady J are manufactured devices that may also be used.

6. For defecation, you can cut a foam pad into a toilet seat (donut-shaped) and place the pad over a hole dug into the ground or snow (this method assumes the victim can be moved out of the litter). Constipation and fecal impaction may become problematic in the immobile and dehydrated victim. Adequate hydration is the best prevention.

▶ ADDITIONAL RESCUE CONSIDERATIONS

Communication

1. Fire is probably the most effective signaling method during darkness. The international distress signal is three fires in a triangle or in a straight line with about 25 m (80 feet) between fires. It is better to be able to maintain one signal fire if it is too difficult to keep three going. Using a small campfire for a signal conserves fuel and energy. Keep a good supply of rapid-burning materials to throw on the fire quickly if needed.

2. Make sure that smoke signals contrast to the surrounding area. Dark-colored smoke can be made with oil-soaked rags, rubber, plastic, or electrical insulation. Light-colored

smoke can be made with green leaves, moss, ferns, or water sprinkled on the fire.

3. You can make a signal mirror from shiny metal or glass; this is probably the most effective method for signaling on a bright, sunny day. Extend your arm while sighting the reflection between your thumb and forefinger on the outstretched arm. Slowly move your arm direction until an aircraft or vehicle comes into sight between your thumb and forefinger, and then move the reflection to signal the vehicle.

4. Emergency radio communications usually occur on the following bands:

a. Common public safety bands
   - Very high frequency (VHF), 32 to 50 MHz: good for two-way communication and paging; follows the terrain; susceptible to manmade and natural interference; uses more power and a longer (45-cm [18-inch]) antenna
   - VHF high band, 140 to 170 MHz: less distance; more line of sight; short (15-cm [6-inch]) antenna
   - Ultra high frequency (UHF), 460 to 470 MHz or higher: least distance, more penetration of buildings, almost always needs repeaters, shortest (5-cm [2-inch]) antenna

b. Civilian radio bands
   - Ham (amateur): many bands used; high power and good distance; phone patch and relay possible (IMARS); emergency nets already in place (RACES); worldwide
   - CB (citizens band): crowded high-frequency (HF) band with poor distance; heavy interference; common and inexpensive

c. The basic parts for all mobile, hand-held, and fixed (base) radios are as follows:
   - PTT (push-to-talk). Push the key, and then talk.
   - Volume/on-off. Adjust the volume so that the speaker does not distort an incoming broadcast.
   - Squelch (signal sensitivity). Turn the squelch until the noise just stops for optimum, nonirritating sensitivity. You may need to turn sensitivity up to be able to hear a poor transmission.

d. The protocol for use is as follows:
   - Turn off transmitter locator beacons because they may interfere with the radio broadcast.
   - Use normal, "clear" speech. Code signal meanings vary from location to location.
   - Identify the receiver (Rx) first and the transmitter (Tx) second.
   - Battery life is limited. Keep batteries warm and as dry as possible. Keep transmissions limited to short periods on a regular basis rather than transmitting

continuously. Energy consumption while transmitting is much greater than when receiving.
  • Speak from written notes.
5. With cellular phones, it is important to know your location. The actual cell picking up your call may be many miles from your location, particularly if your location is at high altitude. Keep this in mind when placing a 911 call.

Helicopter Operations (see Chapter 57)

General Safety Rules
1. Approach the helicopter from the front, where the pilot can see and direct you, not from the rear.
2. If on a slope, approach from the downhill side; if the rear is the downhill side, approach from the right or left in view of the pilot.
3. The main and tail rotors are invisible when in operation. Stay clear of the tail rotor area. The main rotor on some helicopters is not fixed and can rise or dip. Keep your head low.

Personnel Safety
1. Remove unsecured hats or helmets, and secure any loose or lightweight equipment. Unless directing the actual landing or takeoff, stay at least 30 m (100 feet) from the landing zone (LZ).
2. Wear eye protection.
3. In cold weather, cover any exposed skin during takeoff and landing. Do the same for the victim.

Setting Up the Landing Zone
1. Most helicopters require a square area for touchdown of 30 m (100 feet) per side. Make sure that this area is free of hazards such as trees, wires, and poles and of loose objects that can blow into the rotor system.
2. Position the guide (rescuer) for the landing helicopter far enough from the touchdown point for the pilot to stay in eye contact. Have this individual wear eye protection and keep his or her back to the wind because helicopters take off and land into the wind.
3. Night landings should have the corners of the LZ illuminated with one light indicating wind direction. Red lighting is best because it does not have the blinding effect of white lights on the pilot. If automobile lights are used, use one vehicle to indicate wind direction, aiming low beams at the center of the LZ and tail-lights in the direction from which the wind is coming. Use any other vehicles to illuminate hazards such as trees.
4. If you have a radio and know your frequency, let the helicopter pilot know this at the time of dispatch. You can

more easily direct them into the LZ (see back azimuth in Land Navigation, next) and warn of potential hazards. Wires are almost impossible to see during the daytime and virtually invisible at night.

Land Navigation

Map
1. Basic information
   a. Obtain topographic maps from the U.S. Geological Survey (USGS), U.S. Forest Service, college bookstores, outfitters, sporting goods stores, or engineers.
   b. Topographic maps are available from 1:250,000 (1 degree latitude or 60 minutes) to 1:24,000 (7.5 minutes). For navigation, the 7.5-minute or 15-minute (1:62,500) quads are most convenient. Military topographic maps are 1:25,000.
2. Margin information: declination, year, grid
   a. Declination is the magnetic deviation from true north caused by geographic magnetic loading. An example in the continental United States is Hudson Bay, which has a large magnetic load and therefore reduces your reading of true north if you are east of the bay (and increases your reading if west of the bay). Therefore you must add for true north (west declination) if you are east of Hudson Bay and subtract for true north (east declination) if you are west of Hudson Bay. For instance, Denver is 15 degrees east declination; true map north is 15 degrees less magnetic compass north.
   b. Grid is measured on an x (longitude) versus y (latitude) axis, using longitude and latitude lines. Extrapolation to find your location on a map is essential to give a helicopter or rescue party your exact location. A helicopter can input longitude and latitude and fly directly to the location.

Compass
1. Simple travel by map and compass
   a. Orient the map to the terrain, with the magnetic north arrow of the map pointing in the same direction as the magnetic needle of the compass.
   b. Place the straight edge of the base plate along a line between the starting and destination points on the map (the direction-of-travel arrow pointing to the point of destination).
   c. Holding the base plate firmly, rotate the housing so the orienting needle arrow is in line with north on the compass needle.
   d. Look at the terrain and see where the direction-of-travel arrow is pointing. Use a landmark in direct line with the direction of travel.

e. Hike in that direction. Leapfrog with a companion if necessary. Repeat.

2. Terminology

a. Azimuth: compass bearing (direction from north) to a target

b. Back azimuth: 180 degrees plus or minus azimuth (opposite direction). Bringing in a helicopter using back azimuth: Line your north sign or your declination tick mark up with the direction-of-travel arrow. Turn the compass around until the direction-of-travel arrow is pointing at you. Point the rear of the compass toward the sighted or heard helicopter. The number noted at the direction-of-travel arrow is the back azimuth to the aircraft, but it is the pilot's azimuth to you. Tell the pilot, "we are at X degrees from your location." Updates will bring him directly to your location quickly.

c. Pacing: number of steps per distance per individual

d. Timing: time per distance; this changes with terrain and elevation (group on a trail travels about 2 mph plus 1 hour per 300 m [l000 ft] gain, 1 half-hour per 1000 feet loss; multiply by 2 to 4 for "bushwhacking")

e. Triangulation: plotting compass bearings to multiple landmarks on the map to pinpoint an exact map location. (Location can also be determined by intersecting a plot with a known line, such as a road or stream.)

Altimeter

1. Knowledge of weather patterns and cloud types is helpful. A falling barometric pressure may mean an incoming storm, not just a rise in altitude, because a 150- to 300-m (500- to 1000-feet) change occurs with a large storm.

2. An altimeter can be extremely useful for navigation. To use an altimeter for pinpointing or narrowing down a map location, use known geographic features, and then determine where they intersect with a contour line of measured altitude.

Global Positioning System

1. The global positioning system (GPS) may give you the exact longitude and latitude of your position.

2. It is battery dependent and can be dropped and broken, so you should also have other means of navigation.

Ropes (also see Chapter 59)

1. Laid rope is easily abraded, has great stretch, and spins when loaded.

2. Braided and plaited rope is used for lighter loads, is pliable, and is easily abraded.

3. Kernmantle rope has a braided mantle that covers and protects the core (kern) strands. Kernmantle ropes have variable stretch:
   a. Static: low stretch (1% to 5% for 75-kg [165-pound] load, <20% at failure); used for rescue, top roping
   b. Dynamic: high stretch (5% to 15% for 75-kg load, 20% to 60% at failure); used for lead climbing
4. Working strength is about 15% of static (tested) strength (relates to working load).
5. Fall factor is a measure of fall severity and is found by dividing the distance fallen by the length of rope used to control the fall.
6. Impact force is the amount of force transmitted to the load when the rope stops the fall.

Webbing
1. The two types of webbing are tubular and flat.
2. Webbing is easily abraded and is slippery for knot tying.

Rope and Web Fibers
1. Nylon is strong and heavy and has low stretch.
2. Spectra is a hybrid nylon with extreme strength; it is slippery for knotting.
3. Polypro fiber is lightweight and floats; it has low strength and high stretch, is easily abraded, and has a low melting temperature.
4. Kevlar has extreme strength in line and is stiff; some debate surrounds its large strength loss when knotted or bent.

Maintenance
1. Rope running on hardware and rope running across a stationary rope can produce melt and weld abrasion. Avoid rapid descents or lowers with sudden stops. However, two ropes running across each other do not generate damaging heat at any single spot along either rope.
2. Store rope in a cool, dry place with no exposure to chemicals or sun.
3. Clean with cold water without detergent, followed by air drying.
4. Inspect ropes before and after use, checking for lumpiness, 50% or more of the sheath fibers broken, stiff spots, a gap under tension, or visible strains.
5. Consider rope retirement when appropriate. The decision to retire the rope is usually subjective, based on hours of service, number of falls versus fall rating, written rope logs, and manual inspection.

Improvised Litters and Carries

56

▶ SIZE-UP

To select the best method for bringing a victim to definitive care, the rescuer must make a realistic assessment of several factors:

1. Scene safety is the initial priority.
2. The necessary evaluation, called the size-up (Box 56-1), involves a (usually hasty) determination of whether the victim, rescuer, or both are immediately threatened by either the environment or the situation.
3. Proper immobilization and victim packaging are always preferable, but sometimes the risk of aggravating existing injuries is outweighed by the immediate danger presented by the physical environment. In such a situation, the rescuer may choose to immediately move the victim to a place of safety before definitive care is provided or packaging is completed.
4. Evacuation options are limited by three variables:
   a. Number of rescuers
   b. Fitness of rescuers
   c. Technical ability of rescuers
5. Carrying a victim, even over level ground, is an arduous task. At an altitude where walking requires great effort, carrying a victim may be impossible.
6. Complex rescue scenarios requiring specially trained personnel and special equipment are called *technical rescues* and often involve dangerous environments such as severe terrain, crevasses, avalanche chutes, caves, or swift water. To avoid becoming victims themselves, rescuers must realistically evaluate their abilities to perform these types of rescues.

▶ DRAGS AND CARRIES

A drag or carry may be the best option when a person cannot move under his or her own power, injuries will not be aggravated by the transport, resources and time are limited, the need for immediate transport outweighs the desire to apply standard care criteria, travel distance is short, or the terrain makes use of multiple rescuers or bulky equipment impractical. Spine injuries generally prohibit the use of drags or carries because the victim cannot be properly immobilized. Drags are particularly useful for victims who are unconscious or incapacitated and unable to assist their rescuer (or rescuers) but may be uncomfortable for conscious victims. When a drag is used, padding should be placed beneath the victim, especially

709

when long distances are involved. The high fatigue rate of rescuers makes carries a less attractive option when long distances are involved.

Blanket Drag (Fig. 56-1A)
1. This can be performed on relatively smooth terrain by one or more rescuers rolling the victim onto a blanket, tarp, or large coat and pulling it along the ground.
2. This simple technique is especially effective for rapidly moving a person with a spinal injury to safety because the victim is pulled along the long axis of the body.

Fireman's Drag
1. In an extreme circumstance, the "fireman's drag" (see Fig. 56-1B) can be used.
2. In this method, the rescuer places the bound wrists of the victim around his or her neck, shoulders, or both and crawls to safety.

Fireman's Carry (Fig. 56-2)
Two-Hand Seat
1. Two carriers stand side by side. Each carrier grasps the other carrier's wrists with opposite hands (e.g., right to left).
2. The victim sits on the rescuers' joined forearms.
3. The carriers each maintain one free hand to place behind the back of the victim for support (support hands can be joined).
4. This system places great stress on the carriers' forearms and wrists.

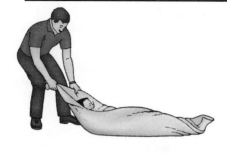

A

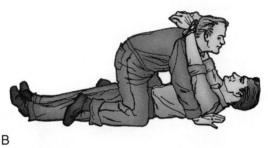

B

Figure 56-1. A, Blanket drag. **B,** Fireman's drag. Both techniques are intended to be used when expeditious transport over a short distance is required. (From Auerbach PS: Medicine for the Outdoors: The Essential Guide to Emergency Medical Procedures and First Aid, 3rd ed. New York, Lyons Press, 1999.)

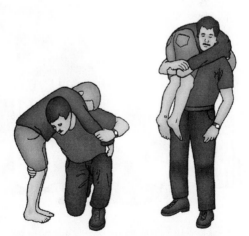

Figure 56-2. Classic fireman's carry: a single rescuer technique for short-distance transport only. The rescuer must use his or her legs for lifting. (From Auerbach PS: Medicine for the Outdoors: The Essential Guide to Emergency Medical Procedures and First Aid, 3rd ed. New York, Lyons Press, 1999.)

Four-Hand Seat (Fig. 56-3)

1. Two carriers stand side by side. Each carrier grasps his or her own right forearm with the left hand, palms facing down.
2. Each carrier then grasps the forearm of the other with his or her free hand to form a square "forearm" seat.
3. With the forearm seat, the victim must support himself or herself with a hand around the rescuers' backs.

Ski Pole or Ice Ax Carry (Fig. 56-4)

1. Two carriers with backpacks stand side by side with four ski poles or joined ice ax shafts, resting between them and the base of the pack straps. The ski poles or ice ax shafts can be joined with cable ties, adhesive tape, duct tape, wire, or cord.
2. Because the rescuers must walk side by side, this technique requires wide-open, gentle terrain.
3. The victim sits on the padded poles or shaft with his or her arms over the carriers' shoulders.

Split-Coil Seat ("Tragsitz") (Fig. 56-5)

1. The split-coil seat transport uses a coiled climbing rope to join the rescuer and victim together in a piggyback fashion (Fig. 56-6).

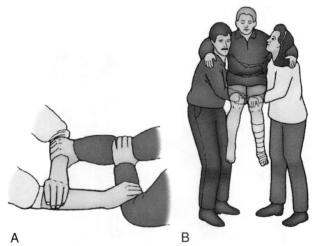

A　　　　**B**

Figure 56-3. **A,** Four-handed seat used to carry a person. In this technique the upper body is not supported. **B,** Alternative four-handed seat that helps support the victim's back. (From Auerbach PS: Medicine for the Outdoors: The Essential Guide to Emergency Medical Procedures and First Aid, 3rd ed. New York, Lyons Press, 1999.)

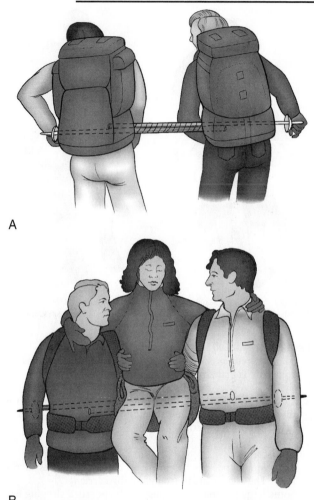

Figure 56-4. Ski pole seat. **A,** Ski poles are anchored by the packs. **B,** The victim is supported by the rescuers.

2. The victim must be able to support himself to avoid falling back or must be tied in.

Commercial Tragsitz Harness (Fig. 56-7)
A few commercial harnesses allow a lone rescuer and single victim to be raised or lowered together by a technical rescue system.

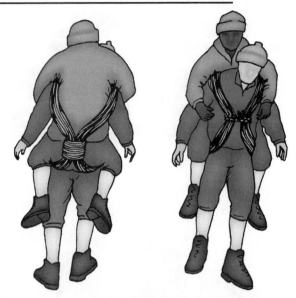

Figure 56-5. Single-rescuer split coil carry. Note that the coil can be tied in front of the rescuer and the wrists of the victim can be bound and wrapped around the rescuer's neck for more stability.

Two-Rescuer Split-Coil Seat (Fig. 56-8)

1. The two-rescuer split-coil seat is essentially the same as the split-coil Tragsitz transport, except that two rescuers split the coil over their shoulders.
2. The victim sits on the low point of the rope between the rescuers (Fig. 56-9). Each rescuer maintains a free hand to help support the victim.

Backpack Carry

1. A large backpack is modified by cutting leg holes at the base. The victim sits in it like a baby carrier.
2. Some large internal frame packs incorporate a sleeping bag compartment in the lower portion of the pack that includes a compression panel. With this style of pack, the victim can sit on the suspended panel and place his or her legs through the unzipped lower section without damaging the pack, or the victim can simply sit on the internal sleeping bag compression panel without the need to cut holes.

Nylon Webbing Carry (Fig. 56-10)

1. Nylon webbing can be used to attach the victim to the rescuer like a backpack.

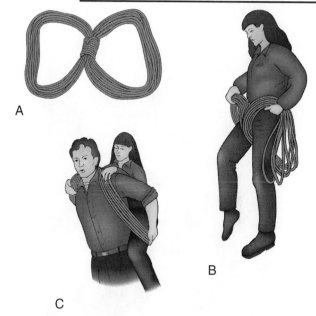

Figure 56-6. Split-coil seat. **A,** Rope coil is split. **B,** Victim climbs through rope. **C,** Rescuer hoists the sitting victim.

2. At least 4.6 to 6.1 m (15 to 20 feet) of nylon webbing are needed to construct this transport.
3. The center of the webbing is placed behind the victim and brought forward under the armpits. The webbing is then crossed and brought over the rescuer's shoulders, then down around the victim's thighs.
4. The webbing is finally brought forward and tied around the rescuer's waist. Additional padding is necessary for this system, especially around the posterior thighs of the victim.

Three-Person Wheelbarrow Carry
1. This system is extremely efficient and can be used for prolonged periods on relatively rough terrain.
2. The victim places his or her arms over two rescuers' shoulders (the rescuers stand side by side). The victim's legs are then placed over a third rescuer's shoulders.
3. This system equalizes the weight of the victim very efficiently.

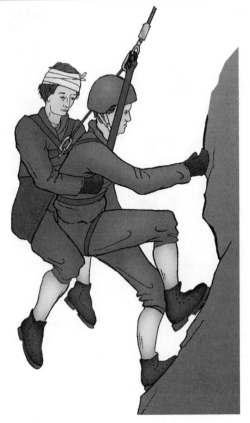

Figure 56-7. Tragsitz harness in use.

Papoose-Style Sling
1. For carrying infants and small children, a papoose-style sling works well and can easily be constructed by the rescuer tying a rectangular piece of material around his or her waist and neck to form a pouch.
2. The infant or child is then placed inside the pouch, which can be worn on the front or back of the rescuer's body.

▶ LITTER IMPROVISATION

Litters (Nonrigid)
Nonrigid litter systems are best suited for transporting non–critically injured victims over moderate terrain. They should never be used for trauma victims with potential spine injuries.

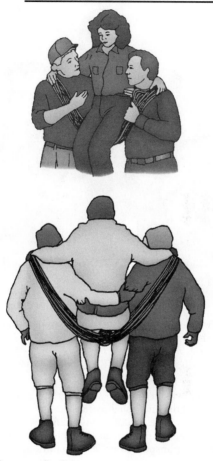

Figure 56-8. Two-rescuer split-coil seat.

1. When victims are transported in improvised litters, especially over rough terrain, they should be kept in a comfortable position, with injured limbs elevated to limit pressure and movement.
2. For a victim with a head injury, the head should be elevated slightly.
3. For persons with dyspnea, pulmonary edema, or myocardial infarction, the upper body should be elevated. Conversely,

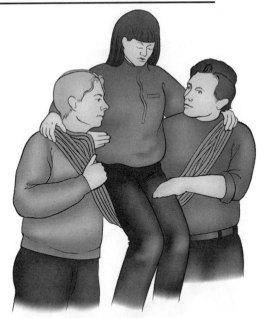

Figure 56-9. Two-rescuer split-coil seat. Balance could be improved by using a longer coil to carry the victim lower.

when the victim is in shock, the legs should be elevated and the knees slightly flexed.
4. Whenever possible, unconscious victims with unprotected airways should be positioned so that they are lying on their sides during transport to prevent aspiration.

Blanket Litter (Fig. 56-11)
1. A simple, nonrigid litter can be fabricated from two rigid poles, branches, or skis and a large blanket or tarp.
2. The blanket or tarp is wrapped around the skis or poles as many times as possible, and the poles are carried.
3. The blanket or tarp should not be simply draped over the poles. For easier carrying, the poles can be rigged to the base of backpacks.
4. Large external frame packs work best, but internal frame packs can be rigged to do the job.
5. Alternatively, a padded harness to support the litter can be made from a single piece of webbing, in a design similar to a nylon webbing carry.

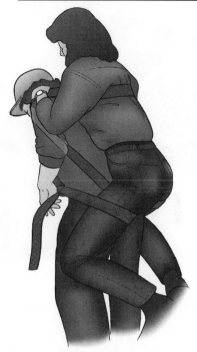

Figure 56-10. Webbing carry. Webbing crisscrosses in front of the victim's chest before passing over the shoulders of the rescuer.

6. Another improvised blanket litter can be made from a heavy plastic tarpaulin, tent material, or large polyethylene bag (Fig. 56-12).
7. By wrapping the material around a rock, wadded sock, or glove and securing it with rope or twine, the rescuer can fashion handles in the corners and sides to facilitate carrying.
8. The beauty of this device is its simplicity, but it can be fragile, so care must be taken not to exceed the capabilities of the materials.
9. This type of nonrigid, "soft" litter can be dragged over snow, mud, or flat terrain but should be generously padded, with extra clothing or blankets placed beneath the victim.

Tree Pole Litter
1. The tree pole litter is similar to the blanket litter.
2. In the tree pole litter, instead of a blanket or a tarp, the side poles are laced together with webbing or rope and then padded.

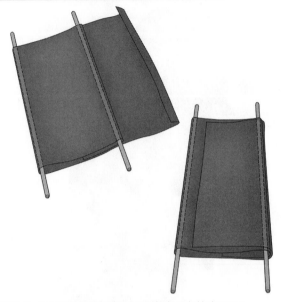

Figure 56-11. Improvising a stretcher from two rigid poles and a blanket or tarp.

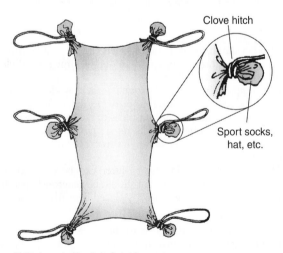

Figure 56-12. Improvised handled soft stretcher.

3. The poles may be fitted through pack frames to aid carrying.
4. To give this litter more stability and to add tension to the lacing, the rescuer should fabricate a rectangle with rigid cross-bars at both ends before lacing.

Parka Litter
1. Two or more parkas can be used to form a litter (Fig. 56-13).
2. Skis or branches are slipped through the sleeves of heavy parkas, and the parkas are zipped shut with the sleeves inside.
3. Ski edges should be taped first to prevent them from tearing through the parkas.

Internal Frame Pack Litter
1. The internal frame pack litter is constructed from two to three full-size internal frame backpacks, which must have lateral compression straps (day packs are suboptimal).
2. Slide poles or skis through the compression straps. The packs then act as a support surface for the victim.

Life Jacket Litter
Life jackets can be placed over paddles or oars to create a makeshift nonrigid litter.

Rope Litter (Fig. 56-14)
1. On mountaineering trips the classic rope litter can be used, but this system offers little back support and should never be used for victims with suspected spine injuries.
2. The rope is uncoiled and staked onto the ground with sixteen 180-degree bends (eight on each side of the rope center).
3. The rope bends should approximate the size of the finished litter.
4. The free rope ends are then used to clove hitch off each bend (leaving 2 inches of bend to the outside of each clove hitch).

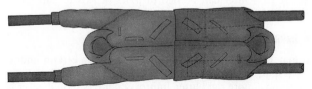

Figure 56-13. Parka litter. On the right the sleeves are zipped inside to reinforce the litter.

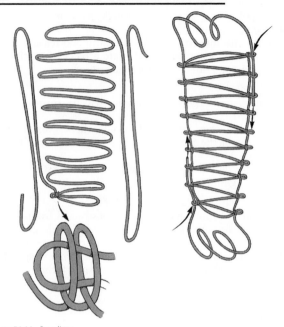

Figure 56-14. Rope litter.

5. The leftover rope is threaded through the loops at the outside of each clove hitch.
6. This gives the rescuers a continuous handhold and protects the bends from slipping through the clove hitches.
7. The rope ends are then tied off.
8. The litter is padded with packs, Therm-a-Rest pads, or foam pads.
9. This improvised litter is somewhat ungainly and requires six or more rescuers for an evacuation of any distance.
10. A rope litter can be tied to poles or skis to add lateral stability if needed.

▶ IMPROVISED RIGID LITTERS

It may be necessary to transport victims with certain injuries (i.e., spine injuries, unstable pelvis, or knee or hip dislocations) on a more rigid litter. Improvised litters should never be used for victims with suspected spine injuries unless no alternative for professional rescue exists.

Continuous Loop System (Daisy Chain Litter, Cocoon Wrap, Mummy Litter) (Fig. 56-15)

For the continuous loop system, the following items are necessary:

1. Long climbing or rescue rope
2. Large tarp
3. Sleeping pads (Ensolite or Therm-a-Rest)
4. Stiffeners (e.g., skis, poles, snowshoes, canoe paddles, tree branches)

To construct the continuous loops system:

1. Lay the rope out with even U-shaped loops as shown in Figure 56-15A.
2. The midsection should be slightly wider to conform to the victim's width.
3. Tie a small loop at the foot end of the rope and place a tarp on the laid rope.
4. On top of the tarp, lay foam pads the full length of the system (the pads can be overlapped to add length).
5. Lay stiffeners on top of the pads in the same axis as the victim (see Fig. 56-15B).
6. Add multiple foam pads on top of the stiffeners, followed optionally with a sleeping bag (see Fig. 56-15C).
7. Place the victim on the pads.
8. To form the daisy chain, bring a single loop through the pretied loop, pulling loops toward the center and feeding through the loops brought up from the opposite side. It is important to take up rope slack continuously.
9. When the victim's armpits are reached, bring a loop over each shoulder and tie it off (or clip it off with a carabiner) (see Fig. 56-15D).
10. One excellent modification involves adding an inverted internal frame backpack. This can be incorporated with the padding and secured with the head end of the rope. The pack adds rigidity and padding, and the padded hip belt serves as an efficient head and neck immobilizer (Figs. 56-16 and 56-17).
11. Although this type of litter offers improved support, strength, and thermal protection, careful thought must be given to the physical and psychologic effects that such a restrictive enclosure may have on the victim (see Fig. 56-15).

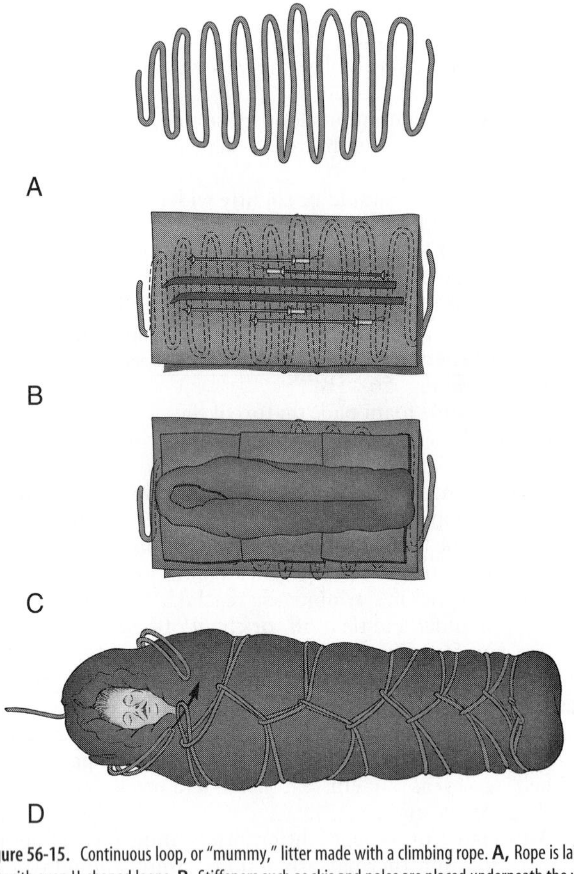

Figure 56-15. Continuous loop, or "mummy," litter made with a climbing rope. **A,** Rope is laid out with even U-shaped loops. **B,** Stiffeners such as skis and poles are placed underneath the victim to add structural rigidity. It is important to pad between the stiffeners and the victim. **C,** A sleeping bag may be used in addition to the foam pads. **D,** Loop of rope is brought over each shoulder and tied off (see text).

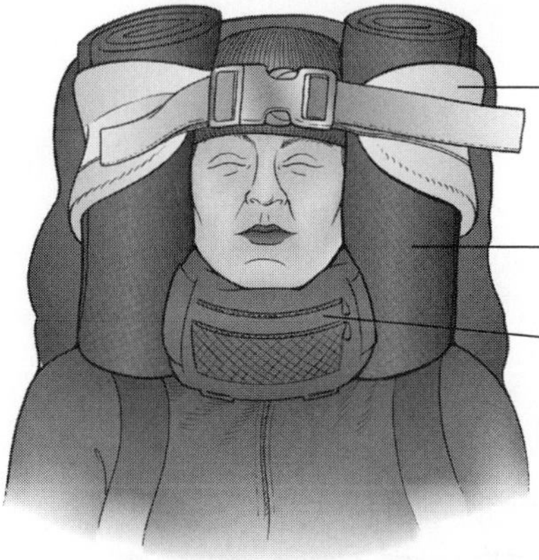

Hip belt
of inverted
backpack

Cervical
stabilizer

Fanny pack as
cervical collar

Figure 56-16. Inverted pack used as spine board.

Backpack Frame Litters (Fig. 56-18)

1. Functional litters can be constructed from external frame backpacks.
2. Traditionally, two frames are used, but three or four frames (Fig. 56-19) make for a larger, more stable litter.
3. Cable ties or fiberglass strapping tape simplifies this fabrication.
4. These litters can be reinforced with ice axes or ski poles.

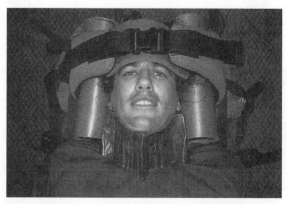

Figure 56-17. Short board using an inverted pack system. The backpack waistbelt can be seen encircling the head.

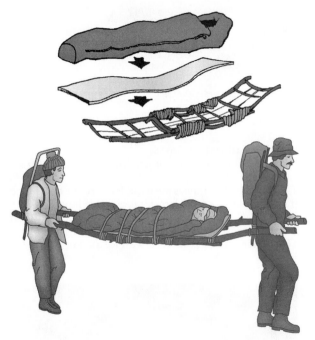

Figure 56-18. Packframe litter. Note that the sapling poles on the litter can be attached to the rescuer's pack frames to help support the victim's weight.

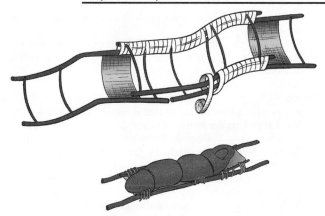

Figure 56-19. Backpack frame litter.

Sledge (Fig. 56-20)

1. If long distances must be traveled or if pack animals are available, a litter may be constructed so that it can be dragged or slid along the ground like a sled. One such device is known as a *sledge* (see Fig. 56-20).
2. This litter is fashioned out of two forked tree limbs, with one side of each fork broken off.
3. The limbs form a pair of sled-like runners that are lashed together with cross members to form a victim platform.
4. The sledge offers a solid platform for victim support and stabilization. If sufficient effort is put into fashioning a smooth and curved leading edge to the runners, a sledge

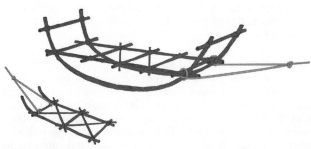

Figure 56-20. A "sledge."

can be dragged easily over smooth ground, mud, ice, or snow.

5. Ropes also can be attached to the front of the platform for hauling and to the rear for use as a brake when traveling downhill.

Travois

1. A travois is a similar device that is less like a sled and more like a travel trailer (without wheels).
2. A travois is a V-shaped platform constructed of sturdy limbs or poles that are lashed together with cross members or connected with rope or netting.
3. The open end of the V is dragged along the ground, with the apex lashed to a pack animal or pulled by rescuers.
4. Although the travois can be dragged over rough terrain, the less smooth the ground, the more padding and support necessary for comfort and stabilization.
5. A long pole can be passed through the middle of the platform and used for lifting and stabilization by rescuers when rough terrain is encountered.

Kayak System

1. Properly modified, the kayak makes an ideal rigid, longboard improvised litter.
2. First, remove the seat along with sections of the upper deck if necessary.
3. A serrated river knife (or camp saw) makes this improvisation much easier.
4. Open deck canoes can be used almost as they are, once the flotation material has been removed.

Canoe System

1. Many rivers have railroad tracks that run parallel to the river canyon.
2. The tracks can be used to slide a canoe by placing the boat perpendicular to the tracks and pulling on both bow and stern lines.

Improvised Rescue Sled or Toboggan

A sled or toboggan can be constructed from one or more pairs of skis and poles that are lashed, wired, or screwed together. Many designs are possible. Improvised rescue sleds may be clumsy and often bog down hopelessly in deep snow. Nonetheless, they can be useful for transporting victims over short distances (to a more sheltered camp or to a more appropriate landing zone). They do not perform as well as commercial rescue sleds for more extensive transports.

1. To build an improvised rescue sled/toboggan, the rescuer needs a pair of skis (preferably the victim's) and two pairs of ski poles; three 2-foot-long sticks (or ski pole sections); 24.4 m (80 feet) of nylon cord; and extra lengths of rope for sled hauling.
2. The skis are placed 0.6 m (2 feet) apart.
3. The first stick is used as the front cross-bar and is lashed to the ski tips.
4. Alternately, holes can be drilled into the stick and ski tips with an awl and bolts can be used to fasten them together.
5. The middle stick is lashed to the bindings.
6. One pair of ski poles is placed over the cross-bars (baskets over the ski tips) and lashed down.
7. The second set of poles is lashed to the middle stick with baskets facing back toward the tails.
8. A third rear stick is placed on the tails of the skis and lashed to the poles. The lashings are not wrapped around the skis; the cross-bar simply sits on the tails of the skis under the weight of the victim.
9. Nylon cord is then woven back and forth across the horizontal ski poles.
10. The hauling ropes are passed through the baskets on the front of the sled.
11. The ropes are then brought around the middle cross-bar and back to the front cross-bar. This rigging system reverses the direction of pull on the front cross-bar, making it less likely to slip off the ski tips.
12. Another sled design incorporates a predrilled snow shovel incorporated into the front of the sled. A rigid backpack frame can also be used to reinforce the sled. This requires drilling holes into the ski tips and carrying a predrilled shovel. This system holds the skis in a wedge position and may offer slightly greater durability.

▶ VICTIM PACKAGING

Victims on stretchers must be secured, or "packaged," before transport.

Packaging consists of the following:
1. Stabilization
2. Immobilization
3. Preparation of a victim for transport

Physically strapping a person into a litter is relatively easy, but making it comfortable and effective in terms of splinting can be a challenge.

The rescuer's goals are as follows:
1. Package the person to avoid causing additional injury.
2. Ensure the victim's comfort and warmth.
3. Immobilize the victim's entire body in such a way as to allow continued assessment during transport.
4. Package the victim neatly so that the litter can be moved easily and safely.
5. Ensure that the victim is safe during transport by securing him or her within the litter and belaying the litter as needed.

Generally, proper victim packaging must provide for physical protection and psychologic comfort.
1. Once packaged in a carrying device, a person feels helpless, so transport preparation must focus on alleviating anxiety and providing rock-solid security.
2. Rescuers must provide for the victim's ongoing safety, protection, comfort, medical stabilization, and psychologic support.

Splinting and spinal immobilization are usually achieved by using a full or short backboard.
1. The victim is secured to the board, and then the victim (on the board) is placed into the litter.
2. When the immobilized victim is placed into the litter, adequate padding (e.g., blankets, towels, bulky clothing, sleeping bags) placed under and around him or her contributes to comfort and stability.

Improvised Short Board Immobilization

Internal Frame Pack and Snow Shovel System
1. Some internal frame backpacks can be easily modified by inserting a snow shovel through the centerline attachment points (the shovel handgrip may need to be removed first).
2. The victim's head is taped to the lightly padded shovel (Fig. 56-21); in this context the shovel blade serves as a head bed.
3. This system incorporates the remainder of the pack suspension as designed (i.e., shoulder and sternum straps with hip belt) and works well with other long-board designs such as the continuous loop system (see earlier).

Inverted Pack System
1. An efficient short board can be made using an inverted internal or external frame backpack.
2. The padded hip belt provides a head bed, and the frame is used as a short board in conjunction with a rigid or semirigid cervical collar (see Fig. 56-17).

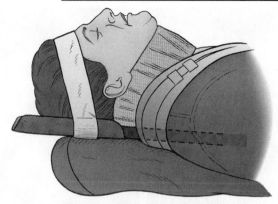

Figure 56-21. Head immobilized on a padded shovel.

3. Turn the pack upside down, and lash the victim's shoulders and torso to the pack. Fasten the waist belt around the victim's head, as in the top section of a Kendrick extrication device.
4. The hip belt is typically too large, but you can eliminate excess circumference with bilateral Ensolite rolls.
5. Unlike the snow shovel system, this system requires that the victim be lashed to the splint.

Snowshoe System
1. A snowshoe can be made into a fairly reliable short spine board (Fig. 56-22). Pad the snowshoe and rig it for attachment to the victim as shown.

During Transport
1. During transport, victims like to have something in their hands to grasp, to have pressure applied to the bottom of their feet by a footplate or webbing, and to be able to see what is happening around them.
2. Because persons are vulnerable to falling debris when packaged in a litter, especially in a horizontal high-angle configuration, a cover of some type should always be used to protect the victim. A blanket or tarpaulin works well as a cover to protect most of the body, but a helmet and face shield (or goggles) are also recommended to protect the head and face.
3. Alternatively, a commercially available litter shield can be used and allows easy access to the airway, head, and neck (Fig. 56-23).

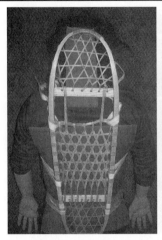
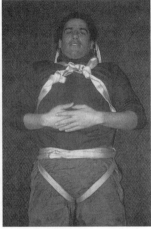

Figure 56-22. Improvised snowshoe short board. A well-padded snowshoe is prerigged with webbing and attached to the victim as shown. This system can also be used in conjunction with long-board systems such as the continuous loop system.

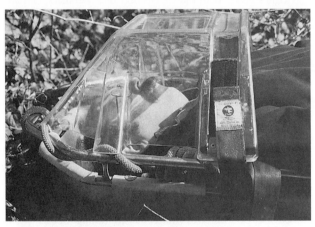

Figure 56-23. The CMC Litter Shield protects the victim from falling debris, while allowing access to the head and face. Litter shields can also be improvised.

4. Remember also that the conscious victim desires an unobstructed view of his or her surroundings.

Securing a Person within the Litter

Carrying a person in the wilderness often requires that the litter be tilted, angled, placed on end, or even inverted. In all of these situations the victim must remain effectively immobilized and securely attached to the litter, the immobilizing device within the litter, and any supporting rope. Poor attachment can cause victim shifting, exacerbation of injuries, or complete failure of the rescue system. Manufacturers have taken several approaches to securing a person within the litter.

1. Most integrate a retention or harness system directly into the litter.
2. A few require external straps to secure the victim to the device.
3. Many users suggest that an independent harness be attached directly to the victim to provide a secondary attachment point in case there is failure of any link in the attachment chain.
4. When a harness is not available, tubular webbing, strips of sturdy material, or rope can be used to secure the victim.
5. One approach uses tubular webbing slings in a figure-of-eight at the pelvis and shoulders to prevent the victim from sliding lengthwise in the litter. A 10-m (30-foot) piece of 5-cm (2-inch) webbing or rescue rope can be used to achieve the same goal (Fig. 56-24).
6. The rope or web is laced back and forth between the rails of the litter in a diamond pattern until the victim is entirely covered and secure.
7. Such a technique also easily incorporates a protective cover and support of the victim's feet.
8. For any high-angle evacuation, be certain the victim is also secured via a harness (commercial or improvised) to the litter.
9. Regardless of the techniques and equipment used, frequently check vital signs (i.e., distal pulse and capillary refill) during transport to help ensure that strapping does not obstruct circulation.

Carrying a Loaded Litter

High Angle or Vertical

1. An evacuation is defined as high angle or vertical when the weight of the stretcher and tenders (stretcher attendants) is

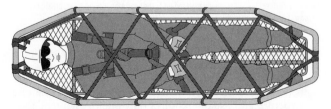

Figure 56-24. One 10-m (30-foot) web or rope can be used to secure a person into a litter.

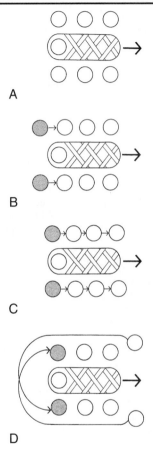

Figure 56-25. Litter-carrying sequence. **A,** Six rescuers are usually required to carry a litter but may need relief over long distances (farther than ¼ mile). **B,** Relief rescuers can rotate into position while the litter is in motion by approaching from the rear. As relief rescuers move forward **C,** the forwardmost rescuers can release the litter (peel out) and move to the rear **D.** Rescuers in the rear can rotate sides so that they can alternate carrying arms. Carrying straps (webbing) can also be used to distribute the load over the rescuers' shoulders. In most cases the litter is carried feet first with a medical attendant at the head monitoring airway, breathing, level of consciousness, and so forth.

primarily supported by a rope and the angle of the rope is 60 degrees or greater.
2. This type of situation is often encountered when a rescue is performed on a cliff or overhang or over the side of a structure and usually requires only one or two tenders.

3. In high-angle rescue, most often the stretcher is used in the horizontal position to allow only one tender and to keep the victim supine and comfortable.

4. When the packaged victim and stretcher must be moved through a narrow passage or when falling rock is a danger, the stretcher may be positioned vertically.

Low-Angle

1. In a scree or low-angle evacuation, the slope is not as steep (<60 degrees), the tenders support more of the weight of the stretcher, and a rope system is still necessary to help move the load. In this type of rescue, more tenders (usually four to six) are required and the rope is attached to the head of the stretcher.

2. The head of the litter is kept uphill during a low-angle rescue.

Nontechnical Evacuation

1. In a nontechnical evacuation, tenders completely support the weight of the stretcher during a carry out.

2. Generally, the terrain dictates the type of evacuation. If the stretcher can be carried without the support of a rope, it is a nontechnical evacuation.

3. If rope is necessary to support the load or to move the stretcher, it is either a low- or high-angle evacuation, depending on the angle of the slope.

▶ **CARRYING A LITTER IN THE WILDERNESS**

1. It takes at least six rescuers to carry a person in a litter a short distance (0.4 km, or ¼ mile, or less) over relatively flat terrain.

2. With six rescuers, four can carry the litter while the other two clear the area in the direction of travel and assist in any difficult spots.

3. However, depending on the terrain and the weight of the victim, all six rescuers may be necessary to safely carry the litter any distance.

4. If the travel distance is longer, many more rescuers are required (Fig. 56-25).

Aeromedical Transport 57

Because aeromedical transport involves medical care delivered in a hostile environment, the patient and crew are at risk of injury or death in the event of a mishap. Flight crew training must emphasize safety. A helicopter mountain rescue operation is a high-risk endeavor for the pilot and crew, as well as for the patient. Dangerous mistakes are easy to make around working helicopters. Therefore aeromedical transport is not always the proper choice for rescue. Risk versus benefit must always be evaluated.

▶ COMMON AEROMEDICAL TRANSPORT PROBLEMS

Pretransport Preparation

1. Once the decision is made to transport a victim by air and the appropriate aeromedical service is contacted, preparations must be made to ensure safety and comfort and to aid the flight crew in patient care.
2. To minimize delays, pretransport preparations should be made for victims of acute trauma (Box 57-1).

Patient Comfort

Motion, vibration, noise, temperature variations, dry air, changes in atmospheric pressure, confinement to a limited position or backboard, and fear of flying may cause patient discomfort.

Patient Movement

1. Victim handling and movement can contribute to morbidity and mortality in unstable persons.
2. All transported victims should be adequately secured to the stretcher with safety straps to prevent sudden shifting of position or movement of a secured fracture.
3. During transport from the ground to the aircraft cabin, attempts should be made to limit sudden pitching of the stretcher.
4. U.S. Department of Transportation guidelines recommend design of cabin access such that no more than 30 degrees of roll and 45 degrees of pitch may occur to the victim-occupied stretcher during loading.
5. The stretcher, in turn, should be adequately attached to the floor.
6. Motion sickness in the victim may be treated with an antiemetic such as promethazine (25 mg PO, IV, or IM) or prochlorperazine (5 to 10 mg PO, IV, or IM).

Box 57-1. Pretransport Preparations

Scene Response
Airway secured
Stabilization on a rigid spine board with cervical immobilization device, neck rolls, and tape
Two large-bore intravenous lines
Antishock garment applied but not inflated unless indicated
Landing zone selected and secured

Interhospital Transport
Airway secured
Stabilization on a rigid spine board with cervical immobilization device, neck rolls, and tape
Two large-bore intravenous lines
Tube thoracostomy for pneumothorax/hemothorax
Bladder catheterization (if not contraindicated)
Nasogastric catheterization (if not contraindicated)
Lactated Ringer's solution hanging
Typed and cross-matched blood if available
Extremity fractures splinted (traction splinting for femur fractures)
Copies of all available field and emergency department records and laboratory results including a description of the mechanism of injury

---

7. Transdermal scopolamine patches are useful for prolonged flights and do not require parenteral or oral administration. Scopolamine's antiemetic effects are not always uniform and may not occur until 4 to 6 hours after application of a patch. Patches may best be used to decrease motion sickness in the flight crew because they are nonsedating.

Noise
1. Noise can be avoided with hearing protectors, which are devices similar to headphones but without internal speakers.
2. Inexpensive hearing protectors are available as moldable foam earplugs. In some cases, headphones may be used in the awake patient if the crew wants the patient to be able to communicate on the intercom system.

Cold
1. For winter and cold weather operations, remember that rotor wash can produce wind speeds of 80 mph under the rotor.
2. Always adequately dress or protect the victim from freezing rotor wash when loading under power ("hot loading")

or for winch or short haul operations (patient outside the aircraft).
3. Use goggles to protect from blowing snow, along with full head and hand protection.

Eye Protection
1. Serious eye injuries can result from debris blown into the air.
2. When a victim is loaded onto or off a helicopter with the rotors turning, the victim's eyes must be protected.
3. The eyes must be protected even if the victim is unconscious.
4. Lightweight skydiver goggles ("boogie goggles") or ski goggles are effective and inexpensive.
5. Taping temporary patches over the eyes is also effective.

Respiratory Distress
1. Persons with respiratory disease or distress should have immediately treatable conditions addressed before takeoff.
2. Endotracheal (ET) intubation is essential if airway patency is threatened or if adequate oxygenation cannot be maintained with supplemental oxygen.
3. It is better to err on the side of caution when making a decision about a victim's airway.
4. During flight it is easier to treat restlessness in an intubated person than airway obstruction or apnea in a non-intubated person.
5. Nearly all victims should receive supplemental oxygen.
6. FIO_2 should be increased with increasing cabin altitude to maintain a stable PO_2.
7. When oxygen saturation monitoring is unavailable and pretransport arterial oxygen content unknown, 100% oxygen may be administered throughout the flight to ensure adequate oxygenation.
8. Persons with chronic lung disease who are prone to hypercapnia may undergo deterioration in condition if the hypoxic drive is eliminated. In these victims the least oxygen necessary to maintain saturation above 90% is advisable.
9. Close in-flight monitoring is essential.
10. Altitude changes may affect ET cuff volume, so cuff pressure must be checked frequently.

Transport of Dive-Related Injuries (e.g., Decompression Sickness, Arterial Gas Embolism)
1. Aircraft selection is crucial because the stricken diver should not be exposed to a significantly lower atmospheric pressure in the aircraft.

2. Ideally, transport only by pressurized aircraft.
3. For nonpressurized aircraft (i.e., helicopter), the flight altitude must be maintained as low as possible, not to exceed 1000 feet (305 m) above sea level, if possible.

Cardiopulmonary Resuscitation and Cardiac Defibrillation

1. CPR in an aircraft is difficult. The rescuers must perform several tasks simultaneously while ventilating the lungs or compressing the chest, all in a physically confining space.
2. There should be no concern with airborne defibrillation if all electronic navigational equipment on the aircraft has a common ground, as mandated by Federal Aviation Agency standards.
3. Despite cramped quarters and sensitive electrical equipment, defibrillation can be safely performed in all types of aircraft currently used for emergency transport utilizing standard precautions routinely used during defibrillation on the ground.
4. In the interest of safety, it is best to notify the pilot before performing defibrillation.

Patient Combativeness

1. Patients may be combative to the point that they pose a threat to the safety of the flight and crew.
2. An uncontrollable person may cause sudden shifts in aircraft balance or may strike a crew member or important flight instruments or equipment.
3. Any combative person should be properly restrained in advance.
4. If sedation is necessary, document a thorough neurologic examination before administering medication.
5. Useful sedative-hypnotic agents include diazepam (5 to 20 mg IV) or a shorter-acting agent such as midazolam (2 to 5 mg IV or IM).
6. Paralyzing agents such as pancuronium, vecuronium, and succinylcholine have the advantage of not altering the sensorium, but they require airway control with ET intubation. In addition, it is humane to sedate a victim who is paralyzed to facilitate intubation and transport.

Endotracheal Intubation

1. ET intubation may be difficult to perform while airborne, especially in a confining cabin, and should be done before departure if possible. This is especially true in trauma victims with head injuries and in burn victims who have carbonaceous sputum or hoarseness.

2. Special techniques are available to supplement standard methods of intubation, including a lighted stylet, ET tubes with controllable tips, and digital intubation.

3. Sedation and/or pharmacologic paralysis may be necessary.

4. Induction of paralysis before intubation in the aeromedical setting is controversial. Besides the need for a surgical airway if intubation is unsuccessful, concerns exist about cervical spine manipulation during intubation in the paralyzed patient, unrecognized esophageal intubation in a nonbreathing patient, and the relative contraindications to the use of paralyzing agents in certain patients. Determination of paralysis before ET intubation is made by the crew and medical control physicians taking into account all relevant factors including safety of the patient and crew in flight.

5. Shorter-acting nondepolarizing paralytic agents (e.g., mivacurium) may have advantages, but they have not yet been thoroughly validated in the aeromedical setting.

6. In some flight programs, nonphysician crew members are taught to perform emergency cricothyrotomy. Although occasionally lifesaving, this procedure is often difficult to perform and should be undertaken only as a final method to secure an emergency airway.

Thrombolysis

Air transport of victims with acute myocardial infarction may involve thrombolytic therapy. Bleeding is a major adverse effect of thrombolysis. However, helicopter transport of persons with acute myocardial infarction after initiation of thrombolysis is comparatively safe and without a clinically significant increase in bleeding complications.

▶ FLIGHT SAFETY

The pilot is ultimately responsible for the safety of the aircraft's occupants and is trained not only to operate the aircraft skillfully and safely but also to provide necessary safety instructions and guidance to crewmembers and passengers. Safety practices vary depending on the type of aircraft but include common guidelines. All medical personnel involved in loading and off-loading patients from helicopters should be aware of the following safety concepts.

Approaching the Aircraft

Helicopters (Fig. 57-1 and Box 57-2)

1. Approach helicopters with turning rotor blades only from the front and sides and only while under pilot observation.

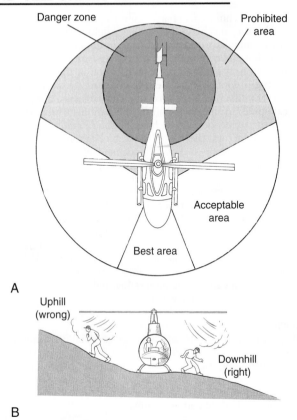

Figure 57-1. Helicopter safety. **A,** Safe approach zones. **B,** Proper way to approach or depart a helicopter.

2. Give the tail rotor a wide berth, especially on helicopters with rear doors.
3. Station a crewmember in a safe position to direct approaching individuals away from the tail rotor.
4. Shut down the helicopter's engines completely, when the situation allows, before patient loading and unloading.
5. Approach the helicopter in a crouched position to minimize the risk of contact with the rotor blades should a sudden gust of wind or movement of the aircraft cause them to dip.
6. Loose clothing and debris should be secured.

Box 57-2. Helicopter Safety

Do:
Approach and depart downhill
Use crouched position
Approach after visual contact and approval from pilot
Await direction of flight crew
Approach from the front or the sides
Secure area first of people and then of loose debris

Don't:
Approach or depart uphill
Use tall intravenous poles or other objects
Use loose sheets or clothing
Smoke tobacco within 50 feet
Run near the aircraft
Drive a vehicle within 30 feet
Shine headlights or flashlights toward the aircraft

Fixed-Wing Aircraft
1. Fixed-wing aircraft should be approached with similar precautions regarding propellers.
2. This is especially important in aircraft with access doors in front of the wing and engine nacelles.
3. Engine shutdown on the side of entry enhances safety of loading and unloading.

Safety Belt Use
1. Use of safety belts (preferably with shoulder harnesses, especially in helicopters) is an important safety measure. Certain patient care activities (e.g., ET intubation, CPR), however, may be impossible to perform with safety belts secured.
2. Design and selection of aircraft and interior configurations should allow maximal access to the victim with the crew members properly restrained.
3. Throughout the flight the crew members and patient should remain restrained as much as possible in smooth air and at all times in rough air.
4. Movement inside the cabin affects aircraft balance. An aircraft loaded near its aft center-of-gravity (CG) limit may exceed its limits if a crewmember moves to a new position within the cabin.
5. Changes in position should be preceded by consultation with the pilot.
6. Light aircraft are sensitive to turbulent air, and appropriate precautions must be taken to avoid being injured from sudden motion.

Proper Use of Aircraft Equipment

1. Crew members must be familiar with all aircraft equipment they may be required to operate in flight or in an emergency. This includes aircraft doors, fire extinguisher, communications equipment, emergency locator transmitters (ELT), oxygen equipment, and electrical outlets.
2. The crew must be familiar with emergency shutdown procedures.
3. Before takeoff, door security must be confirmed by a crew member familiar with the operation of the door.

In-Flight Obstacle Reporting

1. An extra pair of eyes can be invaluable to a pilot in a busy airspace or on a scene approach complicated by trees and electrical or phone wires.
2. Primarily important in visual flight (VFR) conditions, assistance with obstacle identification can enhance the safety of the mission; however, flight should not occur under conditions in which obstacle reporting by a crew member is essential to safety because the person must then divide attention between patient care and obstacle reporting.

Ground Coordination and Control

1. Enthusiastic rescue personnel or curious onlookers may approach the aircraft in a hazardous manner.
2. Flight crew members must be able to communicate with ground units during the landing phase to ensure adequate scene preparation; they may be required to perform crowd control while on the ground. This requires directing individuals away from the rotor blades, propellers, or other hazardous equipment.
3. If loading or unloading the victim while the rotors or propellers are still turning ("hot loading" or "hot offloading") is necessary, special precautions must be undertaken for ground crews, the flight crew, and the patient.

Emergency Procedures

All crew members should memorize and routinely practice emergency procedures that address in-flight fires, electrical failures, loss of pressurization, engine failure, emergency landing with and without power, precautionary landing away from an airport, and other in-flight emergencies.

Survival

1. An emergency or precautionary landing away from an airport necessitates survival before rescue.

2. Under adverse environmental conditions and with injured victims, survival may depend on specific actions by the crew.

3. The crew should be proficient in emergency egress from the aircraft, including escape after crashes and water landings, especially in helicopters.

4. After water landings, helicopters usually roll inverted and sink rapidly. Helicopter "dunker" training is required for all military helicopter crews and should be practiced by any crew involved in over-water operations.

5. All crew members should be trained in the use of emergency signaling devices such as ELTs, flares, signal fires, and ground emergency signals.

6. Survival skills taught to all crew members include advanced first aid, building emergency shelters, fire starting, and obtaining water and food from the environment.

Ground-to-Air Signaling

1. It is best to have radio communication between the ground party and the helicopter crew. If this is not possible, hand signals may be necessary.

2. Standard hand signals are used by military rescue personnel for communication between a deployed rescue swimmer and the helicopter (Table 57-1). These same signals can be used while on land. To acknowledge the signals, the hoist operator gives a thumbs up or the pilot flashes the rotating beacon.

TABLE 57-1. Swimmer to Helicopter and Ground-to-Air Signals

INTENTION	ACTION
Deploy medical kit	Arms above head, wrists crossed
Situation okay	Thumbs up
Lower rescue cable with rescue device attached	Arm extended over head, fist clenched
Lower rescue cable without rescue	Climbing-rope motion with hands device attached
Helicopter move in/out	Wave in/out with both hands
Cease operations	Slashing motion across throat
Deploy litter	Hands cupped, then arms outstretched
Personnel secured, raise cable	Vigorously shake hoist cable or thumb up; vigorous up motion with arm
Team recall	Circle arm over head with fingers skyward

Landing Zone Operations

1. The ideal helicopter landing zone is a wide, flat, clear area with no obstacles in the approach or departure end.
2. Vertical landings and takeoffs can be accomplished, but it is safer for the helicopter to make a gradual descent while flying forward.
3. Higher altitudes and higher temperatures require larger landing zones.
4. The center of the landing zone can be marked with a V, with the apex pointing into the prevailing wind.
5. Any obstacles can be marked with brightly colored, properly secured clothing.
6. The size of the landing zone depends on the weather conditions, type of helicopter involved, altitude, temperature, and types of obstacles in the area. Small helicopters, such as the Jet Ranger, can usually land safely in a 60 × 60-foot landing zone. Larger helicopters such as the Bell 412 require a 120 × 120-foot zone. Large military helicopters may require even more space.
7. The condition of the ground (e.g., loose snow, dust, gravel) should be communicated to the pilot before the final approach.
8. Before the helicopter lands, all loose clothing and equipment should be secured.
9. During approach, no personnel or vehicles should move on or near the landing zone.
10. Once the helicopter is on the ground, it must be approached only from the front and side, and then only while under direct observation of the pilot.
11. The aft portion of the aircraft and areas around the tail rotor must be avoided at all times. Some helicopters (e.g., BK-117) have rear doors for loading and unloading patients, and ground personnel should wait for directions from the crew before approaching the rear area. A safety person should be assigned to prevent anyone from inadvertently walking toward the tail rotor.
12. If the ground is uneven or sloped, all personnel should approach and depart from the helicopter on the down slope side.
13. It is safest to load the victim into the helicopter with the engines off and the rotors stopped ("cold load").
14. If the victim must be loaded with the engines on and blades turning ("hot load"), eye and ear protection should be worn by all personnel approaching the helicopter including the victim.

15. Once the victim is loaded, all persons should leave the landing zone, take cover, and stay in place until the helicopter has departed.
16. It is best to be off to the side, not directly in the takeoff path.

Hoist Operations

If a helicopter is not able to land and has a rescue hoist installed, hoist operations may be the only means to evacuate the victim. In most circumstances, a helicopter crew member rides the hoist down to the site to rig the survivor into the rescue device and to oversee the hoist operation, using the following guidelines:

1. Do not touch the hoist, rescue device, or cable until after it has touched the ground (or water). A helicopter can build up a powerful static electricity charge that will be grounded through whatever the hoist first touches. This has been known to knock rescuers and survivors off their feet.
2. Once the rescue device and cable have touched the ground, put the victim into the rescue device, taking care to keep the hoist cable clear of all persons.
3. Do not allow the hoist cable to loop around any person or around the rescue device because serious injury is possible when the cable slack is taken up.
4. Make sure that the victim is properly secured in the rescue device, with all safety straps tightened.
5. When the victim is secured, move away from the rescue device and signal "up cable."
6. If the rescue device is a basket (Stokes) litter, use a tag line with a properly installed weak link to prevent the litter from spinning during the hoist.

Night Operations

1. Night helicopter rescue operations are considerably more dangerous than daylight operations. It is preferable to delay helicopter insertion or extraction operations until daylight.
2. The landing zone should be clearly marked, and the pilot allowed to make the approach. All personnel should stay clear of the landing zone until the pilot has made a safe landing.
3. Persons approaching the landing zone should have a small light or reflective material attached to outer clothing so that it can be clearly seen.
4. A minimum number of people should approach the helicopter, and a safety observer is mandatory to keep the

ground team together and clear of the tail rotor and rotor blades.
5. The landing zone should be as large as possible, preferably at least 50% larger than a daylight landing zone.
6. Any obstacles should be clearly marked with light-colored streamers, small lights, or even light-colored clothing.
7. The landing zone can be illuminated with flashlights at the corners, with another flashlight at the center point. These flashlights should be pointed at the ground, not into the air; flashlights pointed at the helicopter during landing and takeoff may distract or momentarily blind the crew. If flashlights are not available, small fires can be used to illuminate the edges of the landing zone, although the helicopter can scatter burning embers for many meters.
8. If crewmembers are using night vision equipment, lights must never be flashed at the helicopter. Even the amount of white light from a small flashlight may be sufficient to overload the night vision equipment, functionally blinding the crew.

Dispatch and Communications
1. The dispatch center is the focal point for communications during aeromedical transport operations.
2. Dispatchers receive incoming requests for service; obtain necessary information relative to the launch decision: coordinate the interaction between essential parties; "scramble" the flight crew; assemble and maintain necessary information regarding destination, weather, local telephone numbers and frequencies; follow the progress of the flight; input data into the system database; and communicate with ground emergency medical services (EMS) units and hospitals.
3. Communication may occur through a combination of methods: land telephone lines into a dispatch switchboard, hospital-EMS net transceiver, discrete frequency transceiver (communications with aircraft), or walkie-talkie radios.
4. Familiarity with the EMS system and EMS communications is essential for successful dispatch.
5. Flight following is an important part of aeromedical safety and involves tracking the position of the aircraft during a mission by plotting the location according to reports from the pilot at 10- to 15-minute intervals. If an accident or in-flight emergency occurs, the dispatcher is soon aware and can initiate search and rescue to a precise location, which enhances the chances of survival.

▶ APPROPRIATE USE OF AEROMEDICAL SERVICES

1. Aeromedical transport combines skilled treatment and stabilization capability with rapid access to definitive care, but not without risk and at a cost approximately four times that of ground transport.
2. The comparative risk of aeromedical transport must be placed in perspective against the risk of patient death from less timely ground transport with limited medical capability en route.
3. In isolated rural or wilderness locations, a helicopter may be the only means of expedient access.
4. Prolonged victim extrication allows time for a helicopter to arrive at the scene, decreasing total transport time and thereby increasing the advantage of helicopter transport.
5. Victim comfort must be considered, especially on long transports over rough roads. Although a helicopter moves in three dimensions, fore and aft acceleration is usually steady, without the starting and stopping motions present during ground transport. However, helicopters typically travel within 914 m (3000 feet) of the ground's surface and are more subject to turbulence than are high-flying fixed-wing aircraft.
6. The decision to transport a patient by air requires judgment and a realistic appraisal of the risks. A victim should be transported by air only if he or she is so ill that transport is necessary; if ground transport is unavailable, delayed, or unable to reach the patient; or if aeromedical transport would reduce the risk of death by permitting more rapid access to definitive care, providing greater medical skill en route, or both.

Survival

58

The term survival means "to continue to live or exist" and implies the presence of adverse conditions that make this more difficult. Survival scenarios frequently accompany wilderness medical events.

▶ COLD WEATHER SURVIVAL

Shelter

Anyone who spends time in the wilderness should practice the construction of emergency survival shelters. The function of a shelter is to provide protection from environmental elements. In a cold environment a shelter becomes an extension of the microclimate of still, warm air created from body heat and trapped by insulated clothing. All shelters need adequate ventilation, especially important to consider when building a snow shelter.

Choosing the type of survival shelter to build depends on why the shelter is necessary and the availability of resources. Considerations include the following:

1. How quickly is the shelter needed? (Or, how much time do you have to build the shelter?)
2. Is there a sick or injured person that needs shelter?
3. How many people will be in the shelter at one time? (How big does the shelter need to be?)
4. What is the length of time you anticipate using the shelter? (One should always overestimate.)
5. Against what elements of nature are you protecting?

A properly designed shelter should permit easy and rapid construction with simple tools and give good protection from adverse elements, whether they be wind, rain, snowfall, or sun. The type and size of shelter also depend on the presence or absence of snow and its depth, on natural features of the landscape, and on whether firewood or a stove and fuel are available. If external heat cannot be provided, a shelter must be small, waterproof, and windproof to preserve body heat.

When choosing a location for a shelter, ask what needs to be accomplished and estimate the exposure risks. General guidelines and considerations for choosing a location include the following:

1. Is the shelter needed solely for warmth or also for protection from wind and snow?
2. Where should the shelter be built?
3. What are the avalanche or rock-fall risks in the area?

4. Avoid exposed windy ridges.
5. Avoid any areas at risk for flooding (drainages, dry river-beds).
6. Avoid low-lying areas such as basins that tend to collect the colder night air.
7. A timbered area provides protection from foul weather but can also block the sun.
8. Select a shelter site where there is access to water.
9. In windy conditions, a shelter should be built with the entrance at 90 degrees to the prevailing winds.
10. Shelters can be built in small caves or indentations in a rock outcropping, in a tree well, or under downed trees.
11. Environmental resources that can be used for building and insulating a shelter include small trees, branches, thick grass, or leaf piles.
12. Snow is a good insulator because it traps the warmed air generated by body heat; however, direct contact with snow must be avoided.
13. An insulation barrier between the snow and an individual can be created by using equipment such as a closed cell foam pad or backpack, or it can be created by piling up small tree branches and boughs.
14. The insulation layer if using tree boughs should be 10 to 12 inches thick to allow for compression when sitting or lying on this layer.

▶ TYPES OF SHELTERS

Natural Shelters
1. Caves and alcoves under overhangs are good shelters and can be improved by building barrier walls with rocks, snow blocks, or brush to protect from wind.
2. In deep snow, large fallen logs and bent-over evergreens frequently have hollows underneath them that can be used as small snow caves.
4. Cone-shaped depressions around the trunks of evergreens ("tree wells") can be improved by digging them out and roofing them over with evergreen branches or a tarp (Fig. 58-1).

Constructed Shelters
Shelters can be built of small trees, branches, brush, boughs, or snow. They can be constructed with two easy-to-carry survival tools:
- A 3- to 4-mil large, heavy duty plastic bag (cut open to form a tarp)
- 50 feet of cordage

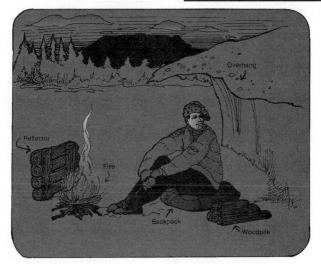

Figure 58-1. Natural shelter.

1. A tarp can be rigged into either a lean-to or an A-frame shelter. In cold weather, an A-frame provides the best method for retaining heated air.
2. Tie cordage between two trees situated approximately 10 feet apart. The tree at the entrance end should be a large tree if a fire is going to be made (see later). If there is a slight slope to the terrain, the head end of the shelter should be uphill.
3. Tie the foot end of the cord 18 to 24 inches above the ground.
4. Tie the head end of the cord 3.5 to 4 feet above the ground.
5. Fold the tarp in half over the cord, and secure both ends to the cord.
6. Ideally, place the foot end next to a large tree, which offers a natural closure for that end of the shelter.
7. Secure the edges of the sides of the tarp to the ground by tying them to rocks or other trees.
8. To prevent heat from escaping along the edges of the A-frame, the sides should have an overlapping flap on the ground that can be secured with dirt, snow, or rocks.
9. Close the foot end to prevent heat escape.
10. Leave the front end, or entrance, open if a fire is going to be built.

11. If there will be no fire, the entrance can be at least partially closed off by stacking a backpack or tree branches in the opening.
12. Insulate the sides of the constructed shelter by thatching brush, branches, or broad leaves (e.g., the first layer is placed at ground level, with each successive layer overlapping the one below it).

Tents and Bivouacs
1. Tents are generally comfortable and dry, but in very cold weather they are not as warm as snow shelters.
2. Tents are preferable to snow shelters at mild temperatures, during damp snow conditions at temperatures above freezing, or when the snow cover is minimal.
3. Bivouac sacs are carried by climbers on long alpine-style climbs or for emergencies. They are usually made of Gore-Tex or waterproof fabric and hold one or two persons. They pack small, are lightweight, and can easily be carried for an emergency shelter on any trip into the backcountry.
4. Many modern packs have extensions, so when used with a cagoule or mountain parka, they form acceptable bivouac sacs. The cagoule is donned, and the backpack is pulled on the feet and legs, extending the top of the pack as high up the body as it can be placed.

▶ **SNOW SHELTERS** (Fig. 58-2)

Snow Trenches
1. A snow trench is the easiest and quickest survival snow shelter and the one least likely to make the diggers wet.
2. If a shovel; large tarp; structural support items (skis, poles, trees); and a small fire, candle, or stove are available, a trench can be created that is as comfortable as a snow cave.
3. It is easiest to dig a trench in a flat area. However, if the snow is deep enough, it can be dug out on an incline, keeping the trench itself level.
4. If possible, dig all the way to the ground. If the snow is too deep to dig to the ground, dig to a depth of 3 feet. If the snow is not deep enough, pile snow up around all four sides of the trench to make walls until the total depth of the trench is 3 feet.
5. The trench width should be just slightly wider and 2 to 3 feet longer than the person(s) that will be lying in the shelter. The additional length allows for a fire pit at one end of the shelter.

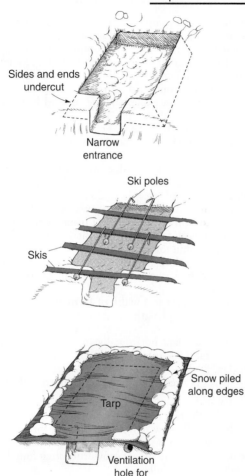

Sides and ends undercut

Narrow entrance

Ski poles

Skis

Snow piled along edges

Tarp

Ventilation hole for cookstove

Figure 58-2. Three-person snow trench.

6. Ski poles, skis, or long tree branches are placed perpendicular to the length of the trench.
7. The trench is then covered with a tarp, leaving one end open for the entrance.
8. Secure the tarp on all sides by packing the edges into the snow.
9. Gently toss snow on top of the reinforced tarp to provide insulation to the shelter.

10. The snow pack on top should be 8 or more inches.
11. The object is to keep the maximal amount of snow around and over the trench for optimal insulation.
12. If the trench is going to be wide enough to accommodate more than one person, the entrance should still be only wide enough for one person to pass through at a time. A narrow entrance is easier to close off and helps contain heat within the shelter.
13. A barrier can be created at the entrance by stacking backpacks or snow blocks or hanging a tarp across the opening.
14. When the entrance is closed, a small votive size candle or stove and the occupants' body heat will raise the interior temperature to $-4°$ to $-1°$ C (25 to 30° F).
15. Higher temperatures should be avoided so that clothing and bedding will not become wet from melting snow.
16. Ventilation is necessary to prevent build-up of carbon monoxide within the shelter.
17. Anywhere that deep snow has been wind-packed, as happens above timberline, the trench can be roofed with snow blocks.
18. The blocks are cut to a width of 18 to 20 inches, a depth of 4 inches, and a length equal to the length of the snow saw.
19. They are then laid horizontally for a narrow trench or vertically for a wider trench, set as an A-frame, or laid on skis (Fig. 58-3).
20. Any spaces between the blocks are chinked with snow.

Snow Caves

1. A shovel is the best item to use when digging a snow cave, although small snow caves large enough for one person can be dug with a ski or cooking pot.
2. The optimum site is a large snowdrift, often found on the lee side of a small hill.
3. Areas in avalanche zones must be avoided.
4. Ski poles, skis, or tree branches are poked in the snowdrift to a depth of 18 inches around the area that will be the outside walls of the cave.
5. The entrance is dug just large enough to crawl through and is angled upward toward the sleeping chamber (Fig. 58-4).
6. After the entrance is dug with the shovel, the digger crawls inside, lies supine, and uses the shovel to excavate the chamber, which should be large enough for a stove and the number of occupants requiring shelter.
7. The snow is removed from the walls inside the shelter until the ends of the ski poles, skis, or tree branches are met.

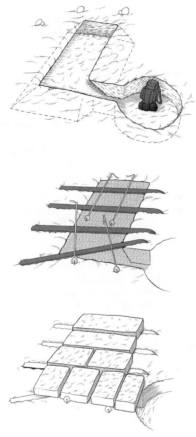

Figure 58-3. Above timberline snow trench.

This assures that the snow cave walls maintain a depth of 18 inches, necessary to prevent collapse of the walls.

8. Because diggers tend to become wet, water-resistant or waterproof jackets and pants should be worn.

9. Pine branches or other natural materials can be used to cover the floor if a sleeping pad is not available.

10. The entrance to the snow cave can be blocked off using backpacks or blocks of snow.

11. If the group is large and there are several people available to dig out the cave, a larger entrance can be created, providing room for multiple diggers to excavate the interior.

12. The disadvantage is the larger opening that needs to be closed to maintain warmth inside the snow cave.
13. The cooking area for the snow cave can be in the entrance area outside the cave itself.
14. If cooking is going to be done inside the cave, a ventilation hole as large as a ski pole basket must be cut in the roof over the cooking area to provide adequate ventilation.
15. A snow cave large enough for two persons takes several hours to dig and therefore is not the primary choice of shelter in an emergency.
16. It can be built after a faster improvised shelter is provided for the safety and well-being of the group (see Fig. 58-4).

Quinzhee (Snow Dome)
A quinzhee is an artificially created pile of snow that is dug out to create a snow cave. It is an alternative method available when a snow cave is desired and a natural snowdrift cannot be located, as occurs when the ground is flat or the snow cover is shallow.
1. The snow is piled into a large dome 6 to 7 feet in height and width and left to harden for a few hours. The waiting time allows the snow crystals to adequately consolidate so that the dome will not collapse when it is excavated.
2. After the settling time, the dome is dug out in the same method as described earlier for the snow cave.
3. This size of dome will accommodate two or three persons.

Igloos
Igloos are the most comfortable arctic shelters but require time, experience, and engineering skill. They are not recommended for the novice but may be worth the effort if the party will be stranded for any length of time.
1. An igloo requires one, or ideally two, snow saws and snow that is well packed and easy to cut into multiple uniform blocks.
2. This type of packed snow is found in wind-blown, treeless areas
3. Packed, consolidated snow can be created by stamping a large area of snow and letting it settle and harden for several hours
4. To mark the diameter of the igloo, a ski pole is held by the handle and the body turned so that the pole basket makes a large circle. This will outline the base of an igloo suitable for three people. The first snow blocks are cut from inside the circle. This will lower the floor so that fewer blocks are required for the dome.

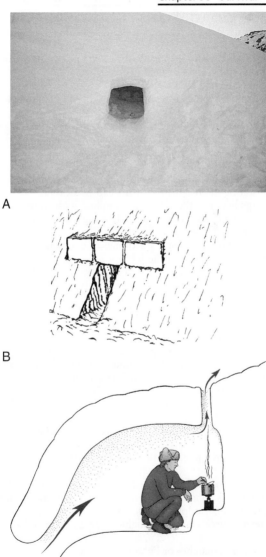

Figure 58-4. A, Snow cave entrance. **B,** Snow cave partly closed with snow blocks. **C,** Interior of snow cave.

5. At least two persons are needed for this project; one to cut and carry the blocks and the other inside the igloo to lay the blocks.

6. The blocks should be about 18 inches wide, 30 inches long, and 8 inches thick.

7. They are laid in a circle leaning in 20 to 30 degrees toward the center of the igloo, with the sides trimmed for a snug fit.

8. The tops of the first few blocks in the first circle are beveled so that a continuous line of blocks is placed down, with the first few blocks of each succeeding circle cocked upward (Fig 58-5A).

9. A common error is to not lean the blocks inward enough, resulting in an open tower instead of a dome.

10. Gaps between the blocks are caulked with snow.

11. The dome should be 5 to 6 feet high inside and can be closed with a single capstone of snow.

12. The entrance is dug as a tunnel underneath rather than through the edge of the igloo, preventing warm air from escaping (see Fig. 58-5B and C).

▶ FIRE

Fire Building

The ability to build a fire under adverse conditions is an essential skill that should be practiced by persons who engage in outdoor activities. One needs about 10 armloads of wood logs to keep a fire burning all night. The area in which to build a fire should be carefully chosen so that the fire can provide warmth to the shelter and not create danger of spreading to the surrounding area.

Mandatory equipment for starting a fire includes the following:

1. A heat source (e.g., spark from a striker)
2. Tinder

Two other helpful items for fire preparation are as follows:

1. Solid shank, nonfolding knife with a 4- to 6-inch blade
2. Waterproof/windproof matches

A **heat source** can be thought of as a spark to start the fire.

1. Obviously, matches or lighters are the easiest way to create the spark.

2. However, in adverse conditions in wilderness environments, matches and lighters do not always work and are not reliable 100% of the time.

3. The heat source that is always reliable is a metal match. Like a regular match, it needs to strike against something.

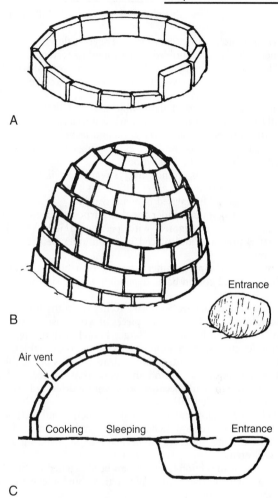

Figure 58-5. **A** to **C,** Stages of igloo construction.

A knife blade, when scraped briskly against a metal match, produces a spark that readily lights a piece of tinder.
4. Other strikers similar in appearance to a 2-inch piece of hacksaw blade are often packaged with a metal match.
5. A metal match and striker are the perfect fire starting tools for a survival scenario, as they will work in any weather

condition, at any altitude, and last for 10,000 or more strikes.

6. Metal matches are a composite of several different types of metals heated and molded into a round or rectangular bar.
7. This molded metal is usually joined to a piece of wood or a magnesium bar, which then acts as a handle for the match.

Tinder is any type of flammable material that ignites instantly when spread out and a spark is applied.

1. Natural tinder includes dry grass and leaves, dry pine needles, inner bark of birch trees, shavings from dry sticks, and pitch wood (or "fat wood").
2. Natural materials are not always readily available when a fire is necessary.
3. Tinder should be carried in a survival kit.
4. The most practical tinder for this purpose is a cotton ball generously impregnated with petroleum jelly (Vaseline) that is prepared and placed in a container before leaving home.
5. Small screw top containers the size of a film canister can hold 8 to 12 cotton balls, depending on the size of the cotton ball.

Kindling and fuel are necessary to maintain the fire.

1. Kindling is small to medium pieces of wood, usually sections of small dead branches or larger branches that have been split lengthwise with a knife or ax (if one is available).
2. In a wet environment, standing dead wood is preferable to wood lying on the ground and wood that has lost its bark to wood with bark because both will be drier and less rotten than the alternatives.

Fuel is the largest material, usually branches and sections of dead tree trunks several inches or more in diameter.

1. Several times more fuel than the predicted need should be collected.
2. Long, dead sections of trees can be shortened by first laying them across a fire. When they burn through, two shorter sections result.
3. Fires generally should be kept small to conserve wood, to allow them to be approached more closely, and to be able to easily extinguish the flames should the wind pick up and threaten the safety of having a fire.
4. Firewood for the kindling and fuel must be gathered and prepared before lighting the fire.
5. It is helpful stack the wood by the designated fire site, arranging it into piles according to size, beginning with pine needle kindling, progressing to pencil size, then thumb size, and then up to wrist and arm size.

6. Wood that is too big will not burn as efficiently unless the fire is very hot.
7. Some logs can be split with the knife or ax.
8. If a knife is used, the knife blade is placed on the end of a piece of wood. Another log or rock is used to hammer the knife until a piece of the log splits off.
9. The fuel supply should be protected from rain and snow.
10. The fire needs a platform and a brace to protect it from the natural earth contact surface (snow or grasses).
11. The platform can be as simple as several logs of similar diameter laid side by side.
12. The brace is laid perpendicular to the platform logs.
13. Wind direction also needs to be considered when placing the brace.
14. The brace should be placed parallel to the direction of the wind.
15. The fire can also be built behind a rock or log.
16. In a snow environment, if possible, dig to the ground to build the fire.
17. If the snow is too deep and it is not possible to dig to the ground, build the fire on the platform on the snow.

Fire Starting
Once the fire site is chosen; the platform is prepared; and the wood for fuel is gathered, split, and arranged, it is time to light the fire. An impregnated cotton ball spread out to enable air to reach the fibers is placed on the platform. The metal match is positioned next to the cotton ball, which allows the spark from the striker to fall onto the cotton ball. Once the cotton ball is ignited, the pine needle–size kindling is then placed on the burning cotton ball as it catches on fire. Large pieces of kindling are then added. Fuel is added after the kindling is burning well. Too much smoke from a fire indicates the fire is not getting enough air and the fuel should be spread out, allowing for better airflow.

1. A fire should be built in such a way that heat reflects onto the occupant, regardless of the type of shelter. If the shelter is a natural cave or underneath a rock overhang, the fire should be 5 to 6 feet from the back of the shelter. A reflector wall of logs or stones on the opposite side of the fire should be constructed. The occupant should sit between the fire and the back of the shelter (see Fig. 58-1).
2. For an A-frame type shelter, the fire is built in the 3- to 4-foot space between the entrance and the large tree. If reflective material is available, it is secured to the tree. This fire is a small fire and needs to be monitored at all times.

3. Fires can be built in tree well but should not be positioned under snow-laden branches. Fires can be built on a platform at the entrance of a trench. The entrance area needs to be large enough to allow ingress and egress from the trench without risk of coming in contact with the fire.
4. All fires should be observed and carefully controlled. It is imperative that water, sand, dirt, or snow be readily available should the fire need to be immediately extinguished.

Food

Although most persons in a survival situation worry more about food than anything else, food is usually less important than are shelter and water because a person can survive for weeks without food, even in cold weather. Bare ridges, high mountains above timberline, and dense evergreen forests are difficult places to find wild food, even in summer. Success is more likely on river and stream banks, on lakeshores, in margins of forests, and in natural clearings. The specifics of finding edible wild plants are not within the scope of this book. In most cases the amount of wild food found by an untrained individual will not provide enough calories to replenish the energy expended in searching for it. Therefore it is important to carry extra food for emergencies.

Water

1. You can survive 3 to 5 days without water. Because about 800 mL of water per day are contained in food and 300 mL produced by metabolism, a minimum daily intake of 1200 mL is necessary in a temperate climate at sea level to avoid dehydration.
2. In a hot, dry climate, at high altitude, or with exertion, insensible losses and sweating increase considerably, so fluid intake should be increased proportionally.
3. Electrolyte drinks and salt tablets are generally unnecessary in cold weather because the electrolytes lost in sweat are easily replaced by a normal diet.
4. Whenever open water is encountered, individuals should drink their fill of disinfected water and then top off all water bottles.
5. Almost all surface water should be considered contaminated by animal or human wastes, with the possible exception of small streams descending from untracked snowfields; springs erupting from underground; or high, uninhabited areas.
6. If survival forces you to drink from a stagnant or muddy pool, remember that it is always better to drink dirty water than to die of dehydration.

7. Let water filled with particulates settle and then strain it through a cloth.
8. Water can be disinfected by heat, filtration, or addition of chemicals (see Chapter 44). At altitudes below 5488 m (18,000 feet), simply bringing water to a boil will kill *Giardia* cysts and most harmful bacteria and viruses.
9. Rainwater can be collected by spreading out a survival tarp and channeling it into a container.
10. On a sunny day in a snow environment, snow can be spread on a dark plastic sheet to melt and then be channeled into a container.
11. On cloudy days, in subfreezing temperatures, and in locations above the snow line where liquid water is difficult to find, snow or ice must be melted to obtain water. This requires a metal pot (which should be included in every survival kit), fire-starting equipment, and wood for fuel.
12. If it is possible to melt the snow and heat the water, enough snow should be melted to provide water for rehydration and to fill a water bottle. The water bottle is placed in the bottom of the sleeping bag to keep it from freezing and is ready for drinking during the night or the next day.
13. Melting ice or hard snow is more efficient than melting light, powdery snow.
14. Melting enough snow to maintain hydration in harsh winter environments requires a significant amount of vigilance.
15. Enough snow should be melted to provide everyone with at least 1 or 2 water bottles for the day. Adding fruit flavors and making hot drinks improve the palatability of water.

Several general guidelines apply when water supplies are limited:
1. Overexertion is avoided, and energy expenditure is kept to a minimum.
2. Do not drink seawater, alcohol, or urine.
3. Thirst is not an adequate indicator of dehydration. Monitoring urine output determines whether intake is adequate; 1 to 1.5 L of light-colored urine should be excreted per day.
4. Food intake should be kept to a minimum (i.e., do not overeat).
5. You may eat snow or ice, but only if hypothermia is not a risk. There is significant heat loss when melting snow in one's mouth.

Emergency Snow Travel

Travel in deep snow is almost impossible without skis or snowshoes.

1. Emergency snowshoes (Fig. 58-6A) can be made from poles that are 6 feet long, ¾ to 1 inch thick at the base, and ¼ inch thick at the tip, and sticks ¾ inch thick and 10 inches long.

2. Snowshoes require 12 long poles and 12 short sticks. For each snowshoe, six long poles are placed side by side on the ground, and the middle point of the poles is marked.

3. One short stick is lashed crosswise to the tail (base) of the poles, and three short sticks are lashed side by side just forward of the midpoint of the poles where the toe of the boot will rest.

4. Two sticks are lashed where the heel of the boot will strike the snowshoe. The tips of the six poles are tied together.

5. Each binding (see Fig. 58-6B) is made of a continuous length (about 6 feet) of nylon cord, preferably braided, because it will eventually fray.

6. The midpoint of the cord is positioned at the back of the boot above the bulge of the heel.

7. Each end of the cord is run under the three side-by-side short sticks at the side of the boot, then up and across the

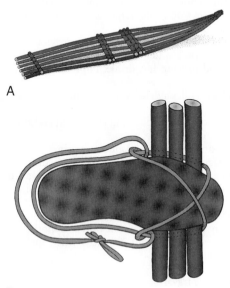

Figure 58-6. A, Emergency snowshoe. **B,** Detail of snowshoe binding.

boot toe so that it crosses the other end on top of the toe, forming an X.

8. Then, each end is looped around the cord running along the opposite side of the boot, and the ends are brought around the back of the boot heel.

9. The cord is pulled tight around the boot, and the ends are tied together at the lateral side of the heel.

10. When walking, the tip of the snowshoe should rise, the boot heel should rise, and the boot sole should remain on the snowshoe.

11. Snow travelers should avoid stepping close to trees (because of funnel-shaped "tree wells" around tree trunks), large rocks (because of weak snow or moats around them), and overhanging stream banks.

12. The person who falls into a stream or lake should roll repeatedly in powdery snow to wick the water from clothing, brushing the snow off each time. A fire completes the drying process.

Stalled or Wrecked Vehicle

Persons stranded in an automobile or downed airplane can often survive using the equipment in the vehicle. Usually, the survivors should stay with the vehicle rather than go for help because a vehicle is much more visible to rescuers than is a person. Floor mats and upholstery can be used for insulation, but it is much better to have a vehicle survival kit containing extra clothing, blankets, and gear listed in Appendix N.

Automobile

1. Survival equipment should be removed from the trunk as soon as possible if it cannot be accessed via the back seat of the automobile.

2. The marooned driver should tie brightly colored flagging tape to the antenna and at night should leave the inside dome light on to be seen by snowplow drivers and rescuers (headlights use too much battery current).

3. If there are people only in the front seat of the car, a space blanket is duct-taped to the back of the front seat, cutting in half the amount of space in the car that needs to be heated via body heat or the candle.

4. One 36-hour candle is placed on the dashboard and lit. Although variation occurs depending on the air tightness of the vehicle and the outside air temperature, a candle can raise the interior temperature above freezing.

5. A window should be cracked 1 to 2 inches to prevent build-up of carbon monoxide.

6. Reusable carbon monoxide detectors are available and can be carried in the survival kit.
7. Running the motor and heater for a couple of minutes each hour has its disadvantages. Someone will need to regularly get out of the automobile to check if the exhaust pipe is free of snow. In doing so, too much heat from the interior of the car is lost, negating the benefit of running the engine and heater.

Airplane
1. In most circumstances, it is advised to remain with the aircraft.
2. Sizeable parts from the aircraft can be used for the shell of a shelter.
3. Because aircraft often do not provide sufficient insulation, a fire is optimal for providing warmth in a cold environment.
4. Cloth and stuffing from the seats and life vests can be used for insulation.
5. Seat belts can be cut away from the aircraft, clipped together, and used for rope.
6. Any accessible baggage should be investigated for useful supplies.
7. Creating a signal in clear weather is important.
   a. The area of the crash site should be made visible from the air.
   b. Anything of color and contrast that will help to identify the site should be tied to trees around the area or laid out in a large X on the ground.
   c. Words can be stomped in snow and then lined with tree branches.
   d. Rocks can be arranged to form SOS or HELP.
   e. A smoke signal can be made by white or black smoke from a fire. Black smoke can be created by burning a chunk of tire, gasoline, or oil.
   f. Dried wood creates white smoke.
   g. The color of smoke desired depends on the environment.
   h. Black smoke is preferred in contrast with snow.
   i. Oil and gasoline are more safely ignited when poured over a container full of dirt or sand.

▶ HOT WEATHER/DESERT SURVIVAL

The body adapts better to heat and altitude than to cold. It acclimatizes to heat by increasing the blood volume, dilating skin blood vessels, and improving cardiac efficiency in order to carry more heat from the body core to the shell. The process of acclimatization takes about 10 days, during which the subject begins to perspire at a lower temperature, the volume of perspiration increases, and the perspiration contains fewer electrolytes (see Chapter 5). The following discussion emphasizes survival in a desert environment.

Practical Methods for Adjusting to Hot Weather

1. Heat loss by conduction, convection, and radiation can be increased by exposing the maximum amount of skin to the circulating air. This should be done only when in the shade; when in the sun, skin should be completely protected by clothing.
2. Wearing clothing when exposed to hot sun also reduces water loss by reducing sweating.
3. Because heat loss and sweating may be impaired by sunscreens, a good compromise is to cover the face and hands with sunscreen and to wear a long-sleeved shirt and long trousers of tightly woven, loose-fitting, and light-colored (preferably white) cotton.
4. Consider special clothing with an SPF of 30 or greater (e.g., Solumbra). T-shirts have an SPF of only 5 to 9.
5. If desired, ventilation holes can be cut at the axillae and groin.
6. Hydration is maintained by drinking adequate fluids, some of which can contain electrolyte supplements. Optimal hydration maintains blood volume and shell circulation and supports the sweating mechanism.
7. Enough water must be carried or be available in the field. Water bottles may be wrapped with clothing to insulate them and be buried in the backpack.
8. The layer principle of clothing is recommended in the desert, as well as in cold weather. Layers can be taken off during the heat of the day and added at night when the dry desert air cools rapidly.
9. Because high winds and sandstorms occur frequently in desert areas, a wind-resistant parka and pants are desirable; because rains occasionally occur as well, the garments should also be water repellent.
10. Because of its high thermal conductivity, poor insulating ability, and good wicking ability, cotton—which is avoided in cold weather—is the fabric of choice for hot weather clothing.
11. Clothing should be loose to promote air circulation.
12. Before exposure to prolonged or strenuous hot weather exertion, individuals should allow time for acclimatization.
13. Heat gain from the environment can be minimized by using clothing to protect the head and body from the direct rays of the sun.

14. A hat with a wide brim or a Foreign Legion–style cap with a neck protector and ventilation holes in the crown is recommended.
15. A neck protector can be improvised from a large bandanna by placing it on the head with the point just above the forehead, bringing the two tails around in front of the ears, tying them under the chin, and then replacing the hat.
16. Travelers should seek shelter during the hottest part of the day.
17. Caves and overhangs can be used.
18. Be aware that gullies and other dry watercourses can flash flood.
19. A sun shelter can be made by suspending a tarp from brush or cacti or by laying the tarp on a framework of poles.
20. Travelers who become stranded in a vehicle should lie under it, not in it.
21. Because desert air is much cooler a foot above or a few inches below the ground surface, the desert traveler should lie on a platform or in a scooped-out depression rather than directly on the ground.
22. Direct contact with the hot ground and other hot objects, particularly hot metal, should be avoided.
23. Sturdy hiking or climbing boots should be worn to protect the feet, not only from the hot ground but also from sharp rocks, the spines of cacti, and snakes.
24. Gaiters should be worn or improvised from strips of cloth to keep sand and insects out of boots and socks.
25. Rest periods should be taken in the shade rather than in the direct sun.
26. High-quality sunglasses should be used to protect the eyes; if necessary, sunglasses can be improvised from a piece of cardboard or wood with a narrow slit cut for each eye.
27. Body heat production can be minimized by avoiding muscular exertion during periods of high heat and humidity. Persons should travel only early in the morning, late in the evening, or at night.

Desert Water Procurement

Table 58-1 shows the expected days of survival in the desert in relation to the amount of water available.

1. There is no substitute for water in the desert, although a person can prolong life in a survival situation by decreasing water loss.
2. Waterholes and oases are rare in deserts. They occasionally may be located by watching the behavior of animals and birds, which travel toward water at dawn and dusk.
3. Animal trails tend to lead to water and may be joined by other trails and become wider as they approach it.

TABLE 58-1. Expected Days of Survival at Various Environmental Temperatures and with Varying Amounts of Available Water

MAXIMUM DAILY TEMPERATURE IN SHADE (° F)	AVAILABLE WATER PER PERSON (U.S. QUARTS)					
	0	1	2	4	10	
No walking						
120	2	2	2	2.5	3	
110	3	3	3.5	4	5	
100	5	5.5	6	7	9.5	
90	7	8	9	10.5	15	
80	9	10	11	13	19	
70	10	11	12	14	20.5	
60	10	11	12	14	21	
50	10	11	12	14.5	21	
Walking at night and resting thereafter						
120	1	2	2	2.5	3	
110	2	2	2.5	3	3.5	
100	3	3.5	3.5	4.5	5.5	
90	5	5.5	5.5	6.5	8	
80	7	7.5	8	9.5	11.5	
70	7.5	8	9	10.5	13.5	
60	8	8.5	9	11	14	
50	8	8.5	9	11	14	

From Adolph et al: Physiology of Man. New York, Interscience, 1947.

4. Birds may circle before landing at a waterhole, especially in the morning. A pool of water with no animal tracks or droppings may be poisonous.
5. Muddy and dirty water should be filtered through cloth, and all water should be treated chemically or by filtration or boiling before drinking (see Chapter 44).
6. Persons should not drink urine or water from a vehicle radiator.
7. A device often mentioned for producing potable water is a solar still (Fig. 58-7). Be advised that water output may be negligible if materials are desiccated.
   a. The materials needed include a 6 × 6 foot piece of sturdy, clear plastic sheeting (preferably reinforced with duct tape in the center), a shovel, a 6- to 8-foot piece of surgical tubing, a 1-quart plastic bowl, duct tape, and a knife.
   b. A cone-shaped hole about 3½ feet in diameter and 18 to 20 inches deep should be dug in a low area where water would stand the longest after a rain.
   c. With the surgical tubing taped securely to its bottom, the bowl is placed in the center of the hole.
   d. The plastic sheet is positioned loosely on top of the hole and weighted with a fist-sized rock in the center so that it sags into a cone whose apex is just above the bowl.
   e. Crushed desert vegetation, preferably barrel and saguaro cactus parts, is placed inside the hole to provide additional moisture.

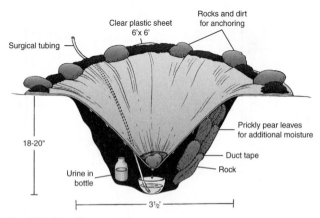

Figure 58-7. Solar still.

   f. Unknown or possibly poisonous plants are avoided.

   g. Dirt and rocks are piled around the rim on top of the plastic sheet to seal the edges of the hole (see Fig. 58-7).

   h. Urine can be placed inside the hole in an open container.

   i. Contaminated surface water can also be purified inside a solar still, but water from a vehicle radiator should not be used because the glycols will distill along with the water.

   j. The still is not opened once it starts operating.

   k. Optimally it will produce 1 pint to 1 quart of water per 24 hours without added urine or vegetation and up to 4 quarts with it.

   l. The surgical tubing is used to suck water from the bowl periodically as it collects.

8. If vegetation is plentiful, another type of solar still can be made from a large, clear plastic bag:

   a. On a slope, a hole several feet in diameter is dug with a crater-like rim surrounded by a moat that drains downhill into a small hole.

   b. The bag is centered on the large hole with its edges over the moat and its mouth downhill at the small hole.

   c. An upright stick is placed inside the bag in the middle and clean rocks along the crater rim inside the bag to keep the bag anchored and ballooned out.

   d. Duct tape reinforces the bag where the stick tents it. After the bag is filled with vegetation, its mouth is tied shut.

   e. The vegetation should not touch the sides of the bag or spill into the part of the bag that is over the moat.

   f. The warmth of the sun causes water to evaporate from the vegetation and condense on the inside of the bag, run down into the part of the bag that is over the moat, run downhill toward the mouth of the bag, and collect in the part of the bag's neck that is in the small hole.

   g. Survivors open the mouth of the bag and pour out the water as needed.

▶ NAVIGATION

Anyone venturing into the wilderness should be proficient in basic navigation skills. It is outside the scope of this book to endeavor to teach map and compass or global positioning system (GPS) navigation. The following are a few simple suggestions on safety and what should be carried into the wilderness.

Compass

1. Even if in a familiar area, backcountry travelers should always carry a compass, map, and altimeter.
2. The best type of compass for the layperson is an orienteering compass that adjusts for magnetic declination.
3. It is important to note that not all compasses work all over the world. Many compasses purchased in the northern hemisphere will not work south of the equator. A compass that works anyplace in the world is called a "global compass."
4. The compass is always followed even if at odds with "gut feelings" about direction.
5. Some navigation experts recommend carrying two compasses. The second compass can be part of a GPS unit, a watch, or another regular compass. That way, if there is concern about a compass not working, it can be checked against the other compass.

Topographic Maps

1. Topographic maps in a 1:24,000 to 1:50,000 scale are the best maps to use for land navigation.
2. The 1:24,000 scale provides more terrain detail than a 1:50,000 scale.
3. Topographic maps are available at most outdoor stores in both the 7.5- and 15-minute series.

Global Positioning System (GPS)

1. GPS units are small electronic devices that can mark a traveler's position by receiving signals from satellites.
2. Although very useful and a worthy adjunct to navigation, it is important to note that they should never be relied on as the only source for navigation.
3. Drawbacks include the fact that they are battery dependent, they require at least three satellites to mark a position, and the satellite system is provided by our government.
4. The government is at liberty to "take away" our access to GPS information at any time and without warning.
5. GPS also requires some prior practice in order to accurately translate output into a position on a map.
6. The backcountry traveler should be expert with map and compass and not rely solely on a GPS unit for navigation safety.

▶ WEATHER

1. Blue sky, a few cirrus or cumulus clouds, cold temperatures, low to medium winds, and a steady or dropping altimeter are predictors of good weather.

2. A lowering cloud pattern (cirrus followed by cirrostratus, altostratus, and nimbostratus), rising temperatures, wind freshening and shifting to blow from the southeast or south, and an altimeter rise of 152 to 244 m (500 to 800 feet) indicate a possibly severe winter storm.

3. Building cumulus congestus clouds changing to cumulonimbus clouds indicate probable thunderstorms and possible hail. A thunderstorm is often immediately preceded by a rush of cold air (gust front).

4. Signs that a severe winter storm is abating include clouds thinning, cloud bases rising, temperature falling, altimeter dropping (i.e., pressure rising), and winds shifting to originate from the north or northwest.

▶ GENERAL ASPECTS OF SURVIVAL

Injured Team Member

1. A person with a minor injury or illness should be encouraged to self-evacuate, accompanied by at least one healthy party member.

2. When a person with a severe injury or illness needs to be evacuated, the party must decide whether to use the resources at hand or send for help.

3. The decision will depend on the weather; party size; training; available equipment; distance; type of terrain involved; type of injury or illness; victim's condition; and availability of local search and rescue groups, helicopters, and other assistance.

4. Unless the weather is excellent, the party strong and well equipped, the route short and easy, and the victim comfortable and stable, the best course of action generally is to make a comfortable camp and send the strongest party members for help.

5. A written note should include each victim's name, gender, age, type of injury or illness, current condition, and emergency care; the party's resources and location (preferably map coordinates); and names, addresses, and telephone numbers of relatives.

6. The victim who must be left alone should have an adequate supply of food, fuel, and water.

As soon as you realize that you are lost, do the following:

1. Stop, sit down in a sheltered place, calmly go over the situation, and make an inventory of your survival equipment and other resources.

2. If it is cold or becoming dark, start a fire and eat if you have food.

3. Take out your map or draw a sketch of your route and location on the basis of natural features.

4. Unless you know your location and can reach safety before dark, prepare a camp and wait until morning.
5. Do not allow yourself to be influenced by a desire to keep others from worrying or the need to be at work or keep an appointment.
6. Your life is more important than anyone else's peace of mind.
7. If you are alone and unquestionably lost, and especially if injured, you must decide whether to wait for rescue or attempt to walk out under your own power.
8. Almost always, it is better to use the time to prepare a snug shelter and conserve strength if rescue is possible.
9. If you decide to leave, mark the site with a cairn or bright-colored material such as surveyor's tape; leave a note at the site with information about your condition, equipment, and direction of travel; and then mark your trail.
10. These actions will aid rescuers and enable you to return to the site if necessary. Travel should never be attempted in severe weather, desert daytime heat, or deep snow without snowshoes or skis.
11. If no chance of rescue exists, prepare as best possible, wait for good weather, and then travel in the most logical direction.

▶ SIGNALING

1. Besides radios, cell phones, and other electronic equipment, signaling devices are either auditory or visual.
2. Three of anything is a universal distress signal: three whistle blasts, three shots, three fires, or three columns of smoke.
3. The most effective auditory device is a whistle. Blowing a whistle is less tiring than shouting, and the distinctive sound carries farther than a human voice.
4. A very effective visual ground-to-air signal device is a glass signal mirror, which can be seen up to 10 miles away but requires sunlight.
5. Smoke is easily seen by day, and a fire or flashlight is visible at night. On a cloudy day, black smoke is more visible than white; the reverse is true on a sunny day.
6. Black smoke can be produced by burning parts of a vehicle such as rubber or oil and white smoke by adding green leaves or a small amount of water to the fire (see airplane section earlier).

7. Ground signals (e.g., SOS, HELP) should be as large as possible—at least 3 feet wide and 18 feet long—and should contain straight lines and square corners, which are not found in nature.

8. They can be tramped out in dirt or on grass or can be made from brush or logs. In snow, the depressions can be filled with vegetation to increase contrast.

9. Many pilots do not know the traditional 18 international ground-to-air emergency signals, so remember the following two:
   a. (**X**) I require medical assistance
   b. (↑)Am proceeding in this direction

10. When using cell phones, radios, and other electronic devices, persons should move out of valleys and gullies to higher elevations if possible.

11. Operational pay phones in campgrounds closed for the season or other facilities can be used to call for help.

12. Most will allow 911 or another emergency number to be dialed without payment, but carrying the right change and memorizing your telephone credit card number are recommended.

Knots

59

PRACTICE BEFORE YOU REALLY NEED TO USE THEM

▶ TERMINOLOGY

1. Stopper knot—a knot tied at the end of a rope to keep something from slipping off the rope (e.g., figure-eight knot)
2. End-of-line knot—a knot used to form a loop or other construction in the end of a rope to anchor, tie in, or attach the rope to something (e.g., double bowline knot)
3. Midline knot—a knot used to form a loop in the middle of the rope, for clipping into, grasping, or bypassing a piece of damaged rope (e.g., butterfly knot)
4. Knots to join two ropes—a knot used to connect two ropes, of equal or unequal diameter (e.g., double fisherman's bend)
5. Safety knot—a final knot tied into the tail of the rope after the original knot is tied to keep the original knot from deforming or unraveling (e.g., barrel knot)
6. Hitch—a knot that is tied around something, which conforms to the shape of the object around which it is tied and that does not keep its shape when the object around which it is tied is removed (e.g., Prusik hitch)
7. Tied loop—a knot that forms a fixed eye or loop in the end of a rope (e.g., bowline knot)

▶ ANATOMY OF A KNOT

1. The working end of the rope is the section used to tie or rig the knot.
2. The standing part of the rope is the section not actively used to form the knot or rigging.
3. The running end of the rope is the free end.
4. A line is a rope in use.
5. A bight of rope is formed when the rope takes a U-turn on itself so that the running end and standing end run parallel to each other. The U portion, where the rope bends, is referred to as the *bight*.
6. A loop of rope is made by crossing a portion of the standing end over or under the running end. Note that a loop closes, as compared with a bight. Many knots that form a loop from a bight in the standing part of the rope are named *something on a bight*, such as *figure eight on a bight*.
7. The tail of a rope is the (usually) short, unused length of rope that is left over once the knot is tied.

Examples of knots are presented in Figures 59-1 through 59-26.

Stopper Knots (Figs. 59-1 and 59-2)
A stopper knot is typically tied into the end of a rope to prevent the rope from exiting the system (e.g., tying a stopper on the end of a rappel line to prevent the rappeler from rappeling off the end).

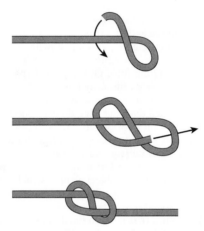

Figure 59-1. Figure-eight stopper knot.

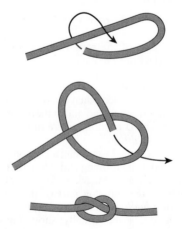

Figure 59-2. Overhand stopper knot.

End-of-Line-Knots (Figs. 59-3 to 59-6)
These knots form a loop or bight in the end of the rope. The bight can then be used to attach the rope to something (e.g., an anchor).

The **double bowline** (see Fig. 59-3) is preferred for rescue over the less secure single bowline above (see Fig. 59-4).

A **figure eight** on a bight (see Fig. 59-5) creates a preformed loop, so it will only function if you can clip into the loop (e.g., with a carabiner).

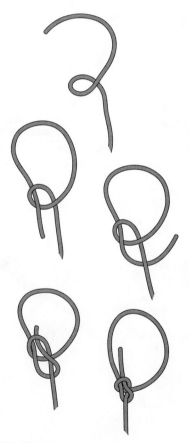

Figure 59-3. Double bowline.

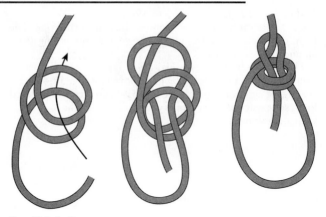

Figure 59-4. Bowline.

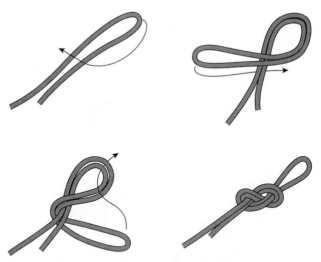

Figure 59-5. Figure eight on a bight.

The **figure eight on a bight** is probably the single knot every potential rescue worker should know. Climbers and rescue personnel across the world use it. It is strong and easy to undo when loaded. It can be tied directly into a bight (see Fig. 59-5), or it may be tied as a retrace (or follow-through) (see Fig. 59-6). It is easy to tell when it has been tied correctly by quick visual inspection.

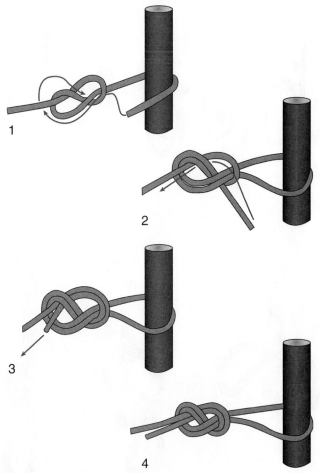

Figure 59-6. Retrace figure eight on a bight.

Midline Knots

These knots are used to form loops in the middle of a rope. They are used for clipping into, grasping, or bypassing a piece of damaged rope. A **figure eight on a bight** may be used (see Fig. 59-4). In addition, the following knots can be used:

Butterfly knot (Fig. 59-7)
Overhand on a bight (Fig. 59-8)
Bowline on a bight (Fig. 59-9)

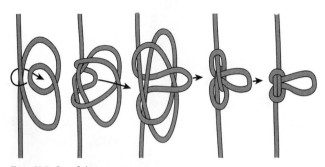

Figure 59-7. Butterfly knot.

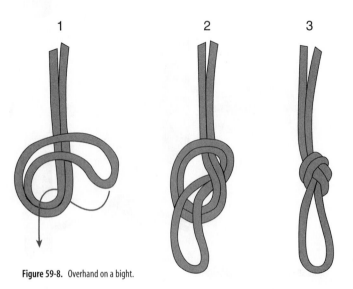

Figure 59-8. Overhand on a bight.

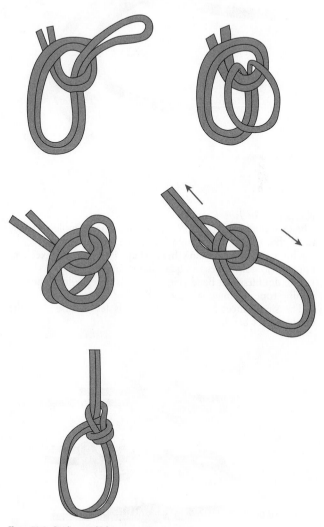

Figure 59-9. Bowline on a bight.

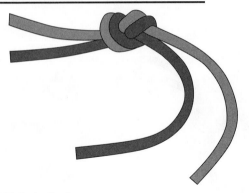

Figure 59-10. Overhand bend.

Knots to Join Two Ropes
The overhand bend (Fig. 59-10) is functional, simple and easy to tie, but not secure enough for rescue.

This **double fisherman's bend** (Fig. 59-11) is an excellent knot for joining ropes of equal diameter.

The **double-sheet bend** (Fig. 59-12) is an excellent knot for joining ropes of unequal diameter.

The **single-sheet bend** (Fig. 59-13) is less secure than the double-sheet bend.

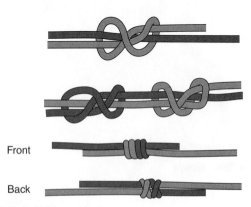

Front

Back

Figure 59-11. Double fisherman's bend.

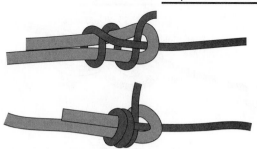

Figure 59-12. Double-sheet bend.

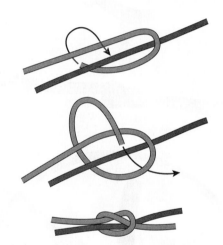

Figure 59-13. Single-sheet bend.

The **figure-eight bend** (Fig. 59-14) is a reasonable choice if tied with the rope ends exiting from opposite ends of the bend. Do not tie it as in Figure 59-15.

The **ring bend** (Fig. 59-16) is the ideal knot for joining flat or tubular webbing. It is also used to tie loops of webbing (runners).

Hitches (Figs. 59-17 to 59-20)

Additional Knots and Hitches (Figs. 59-21 to 59-24)

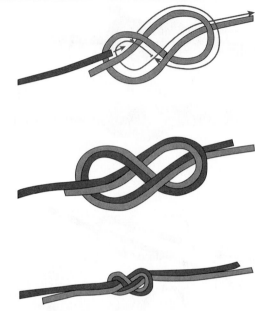

Figure 59-14. Figure-eight bend.

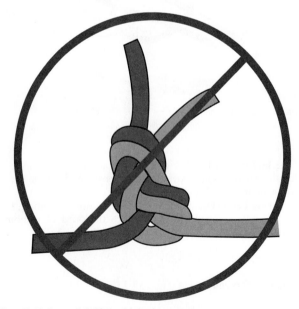

Figure 59-15. Incorrectly tied figure-eight bend.

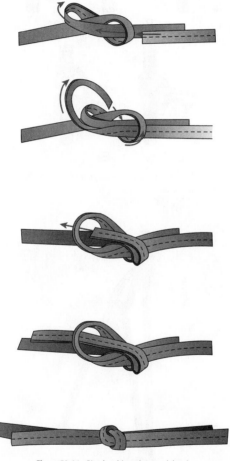

Figure 59-16. Ring bend (tape knot, web knot).

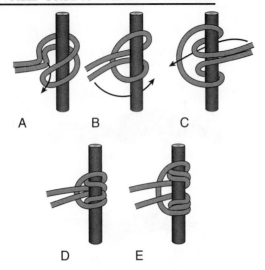

Figure 59-17. Prusik hitch. **A** to **C,** Tying sequence for the Prusik knot. **D,** Two-wrap Prusik knot. **E,** Three-wrap Prusik knot.

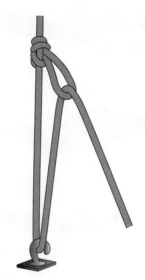

Figure 59-18. Trucker's hitch.

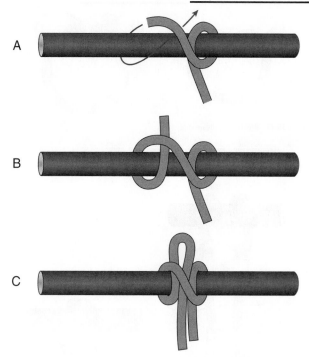

Figure 59-19. A and **B,** Clove hitch. **C,** Clove hitch with draw loop for temporary attachment.

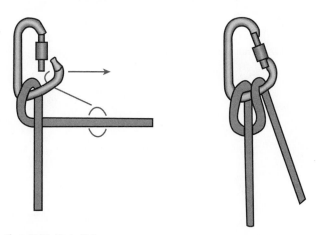

Figure 59-20. Munter hitch.

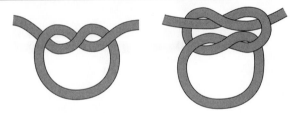

Figure 59-21. Reef knot, or square knot.

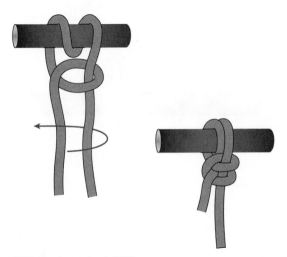

Figure 59-22. Round turn and two half-hitches.

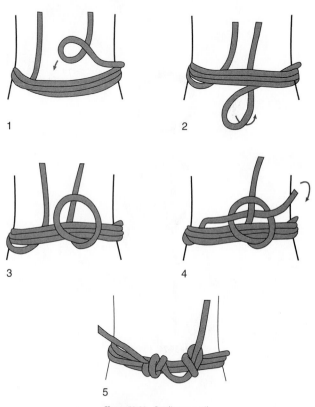

1

2

3

4

5

Figure 59-23. Bowline on a coil.

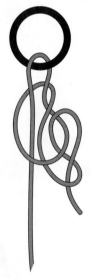

Figure 59-24. Halter hitch.

Wilderness Medical Kits

60

Organizing the medical equipment for an expedition requires an enormous amount of planning and forethought. No matter how much equipment is hauled in, one cannot possibly prepare for every conceivable illness or accident. The variables on any expedition or wilderness excursion are complex, making generic advice on "what to take" difficult without an operational context. Major considerations should include the following:

1. Environmental extremes of the trip
   a. Arctic, high altitude, tropical, desert, etc.
2. Time of year (e.g., climatic conditions) and disease conditions
3. Specific endemic diseases
4. Medical expertise of the intended user
5. Medical expertise of other trip members
   a. Neophyte tourists, a group of guides, other doctors, etc.
6. Total number of expedition members including ancillary staff
   a. Porters, local guides, expedition staff, etc.
7. Duration of trip
8. Age and sex of participants
9. Known preexisting medical problems of the group
10. Distance from definitive medical care
11. Availability of communications
    a. Cell phones, radios, satellite phones, telemedicine capability, etc.
12. Availability and time frame of rescue
    a. Organized rescue groups, proximity of airfields, availability and capability of helicopters, and fixed-wing aircraft
13. Medical kit weight and volume limitations
    a. Will the kit be carried on your back, on others' backs, on pack animals, sleds, rafts, boats?
14. Responsibility for local health care
    a. On the trek in and out

▶ **GENERAL GUIDELINES FOR EXPEDITION DRUGS**

1. When possible, choose medications with low side effect profiles.
2. Choose medications with limited contraindications (e.g., amoxicillin-clavulanate is contraindicated in penicillin-allergic patients).

3. When possible, choose medications that have multiple indications (e.g., drugs like diphenhydramine and prednisone have multiple uses on expeditions).
4. Choose medications that have favorable dosing schedules (e.g., azithromycin over erythromycin). Compliance will markedly improve, and the weight and volume of the medical kit will be greatly reduced.
5. Carry enough medications to treat multiple persons over the course of the expedition.

▶ Kit

1. The wilderness medical kit should be well organized in a protective and convenient carrying case or pouch. For backpacking, trekking, or hiking, a nylon or Cordura organizer bag is optimal.
2. Newer-generation bags with clear, vinyl compartments have proved superior to mesh-covered pockets for protecting the components from the environment.
3. Clear vinyl protects the components from dirt, moisture, and insects and keeps the items from falling out when the kit is turned on its side or upside down.
4. For aquatic environments, store the kit in a waterproof dry bag or watertight container such as a Pelican or Otter box. Inside, seal items in resealable plastic bags with "zippers" (e.g., Ziploc) because moisture will invariably make its way into any container.
5. Some medicines may need to be stored outside of the main kit to ensure protection from extreme temperatures. Capsules and suppositories melt when exposed to temperatures above 37° C (99° F), and many liquid medicines (e.g., insulin) become useless after freezing.
6. Commercially produced kits are available, either prestocked or unfilled.
7. Fragile items and injectable medications can be carried in small, portable plastic containers (e.g., Tupperware).

Organization

Dividing the kit into a group kit and personal kits is helpful.

Each trip member should be responsible for and carry a personal kit. This avoids constant disruption of the group kit, which can play havoc over time. Personal kits are variable but should include commonly used items. A personal kit might contain the following:

1. Non-narcotic analgesics and/or nonsteroidal antiinflammatory drugs (NSAIDs)
2. Throat lozenges or hard candy
3. Sunscreen and lip protection
4. Water disinfection equipment or chemicals

5. Blister care
6. Duct tape
7. Minor wound care (e.g., bandages [Band-Aids])
8. Insect repellent
9. Malaria prophylaxis (if risk exists)
10. Vitamins
11. Personal medications (for preexisting problems)

Contents

The possible variations in kit design and organization are infinite; choose a logical system that is efficient for you, your group, and your environmental needs and constraints.

The following is a sample medical kit for a multiweek trek or climb into a remote location.

Antibiotics

Even in a hospital setting two doctors seldom agree on the optimum antibiotic for treating a given disease. Prepare for the common infectious disease problems listed here, and choose antibiotics accordingly. Examples follow:

1. **Upper and lower respiratory infections:** newer-generation macrolide (e.g., azithromycin [Zithromax, Z-Pak, etc.])
2. **Skin and soft tissue infections:** Consider a first-generation oral cephalosporin: cephalexin (e.g., Keflex) or dicloxacillin (e.g., Dycill). Cefadroxil (e.g., Duricef) has the advantage of an q12–24h dosing schedule, which means less bulk. On longer trips also carry trimethoprim-sulfamethoxazole or another methicillin-resistant *Staphylococcus aureus* (MRSA) appropriate antibiotic. Unfortunately MRSA has become ubiquitous and has already appeared in community-acquired backcountry settings.
3. **Gastrointestinal tract (bacterial diarrhea):** A fluoroquinolone antibiotic (e.g., ciprofloxacin [Cipro] or levofloxacin [Levaquin]) should be included.
4. **Urinary tract infections (UTIs):** Use a fluoroquinolone or trimethoprim-sulfamethoxazole (see earlier).
5. **Additional considerations** on longer or more remote trips:
   a. Protozoal infections (e.g., *Giardia:* tinidazole or metronidazole)
   b. Rickettsial illness, tropical fever of unknown origin, sexually transmitted diseases: tetracycline or doxycycline
   c. Helminthic infections (hookworm, roundworm, and tapeworm): mebendazole or other antihelminthic
   d. Malaria (prophylaxis or presumptive treatment): check the Centers for Disease Control for specific guidelines on area of travel (see Chapter 46)
   e. Injectable antibiotics such as ciprofloxacin, ceftriaxone, cefazolin, etc.

Analgesics (see Chapter 24)
1. Acetaminophen (Tylenol), 500-mg tablets
2. Aspirin, 325-mg tablets
3. NSAIDs such as ibuprofen 800 mg or naproxen 500 mg. On longer expeditions, long-acting (qd) preparations (e.g., oxaprozin (Daypro]) might be considered for persons requiring chronic antiinflammatory therapy.
4. Acetaminophen with hydrocodone (Vicodin), oxycodone and acetaminophen (Percocet), or other potent oral narcotic
5. For stronger analgesia consider the following:
   a. Fentanyl (Fentanyl Oralet). This works well but requires a long time to administer (e.g., lick) and tends to cause nausea.
   b. A promising recent development is fentanyl buccal tablets (Fentora) intended for buccal mucosal administration. The tablets are placed and retained within the buccal cavity for a period sufficient to allow disintegration of the tablet and absorption of fentanyl across the oral mucosa.
   c. Butorphanol tartrate (Stadol) nasal spray (may cause dysphoria and profound sedation)

Respiratory/Allergy
1. Beta-agonist metered-dose inhaler (MDI) and spacer (for asthma and other allergic reactions): albuterol MDI (Ventolin, Proventil). Advair contains a beta-agonist and steroid in combination.
   a. Commonly overlooked medical item; essential for cold or exercise-induced bronchoconstriction, a common malady on mountaineering expeditions at higher altitudes
   b. Serves as an important adjunct in the treatment of lower and upper respiratory tract infections accompanied by reactive airway component
   c. Now also indicated for high-altitude pulmonary edema
2. Prednisone is a "must have" for the treatment of asthma exacerbations, or any number of inflammatory conditions (e.g., severe poison oak, severe marine cutaneous exanthems, insect envenomation).
3. Diphenhydramine (Benadryl) 25-mg tablets are useful for mild allergic reactions, as well as for mild sedation in higher doses.

Ear, Nose, and Throat
1. Nasal tampon (Rhino Rocket) and tonsil sponge (Wecksorb). A light-weight, simple method for anterior nasal packing
2. Oxymetazoline (Afrin) or other topical nasal decongestant
   a. Essential for epistaxis

    b. Helpful for eustachian tube dysfunction during altitude or pressure changes

    c. Helpful for nasal congestion

3. Ofloxacin 0.3% solution (Floxin Otic), 2% acetic acid otic solution with hydrocortisone (VoSoL HC), Cortisporin otic or other topical anti-infective. Necessary for external otitis, common on aquatic trips

4. Loratadine (Claritin) or other nonsedating antihistamine for treatment of mild allergic symptoms

5. Throat lozenges or hard candy (e.g., Ricola) for the omnipresent "altitude throat" or "Khumbu cough"

6. Pseudoephedrine (Sudafed) or other oral decongestant

Eye

1. Generic topical ophthalmic antibiotic (e.g., erythromycin ophthalmic solution [Ilotycin])

2. Topical ophthalmic fluoroquinolone (e.g., moxifloxacin [Vigamox] or gatifloxacin [Zymar])

    a. Essential for treatment of corneal ulcers and should be carried if immediate definitive care is not an option

3. Cyclopentolate HCl (Cyclogyl) or other intermediate-acting cycloplegic for relieving the ciliary spasm of photokeratitis or uveitis

4. Topical ophthalmic anesthetic (e.g., tetracaine)

    a. Essential for corneal examination

    b. May be useful in extreme conditions for allowing a climber with disabling photokeratitis to get off the mountain (suboptimal treatment!)

    c. Should not be overused because chronic application can cause corneal sloughing

5. Ketorolac ophthalmic solution (Acular) for painful UV photokeratitis or minor irritation

6. Fluorescein strips for staining corneal defects

7. Eye patches for corneal abrasions improvised from cloths or gauze bandages

8. Irrigation solution: use clean drinking water (e.g., filtered and preferably disinfected)

8. Penlight with cobalt blue filter or small cobalt blue LED

Central Nervous System

1. Lorazepam (Ativan), diazepam (Valium), or alprazolam (Xanax) for mild to moderate sedation

2. Haloperidol (Haldol) for major sedation. NOTE: Transient psychosis is not uncommon under the extremes of expedition life and wilderness rescue

3. Sumatriptan (Imitrex) for migraine headache

4. Caffeine citrate (e.g., NoDoz, useful for a little extra "get-up-and-go" or to relieve caffeine withdrawal headaches, or modafinil [Provigil])

5. Modafinil for alertness on all night rescues, survival scenarios, etc.
6. Motion sickness medications and solutions (antihistamines, wristbands, scopolamine, ginger, etc.). Consider for any trip involving ocean travel, small aircraft or long mountainous bus rides

Cardiovascular
1. Aspirin, essential for chest pain or myocardial infarction (MI)
2. Nitrostat/transdermal nitroglycerin, for chest pain or MI
3. Beta-blocker such as metoprolol (Lopressor) or atenolol (Tenormin), for chest pain or MI
4. Nifedipine, useful for high-altitude pulmonary edema (HAPE), angina, and hypertension, and possibly effective for Raynaud's phenomenon

Gynecologic
1. Urine pregnancy test: an important addition to the medical kit, essential for ruling out ectopic pregnancy in a reproductive age female with lower quadrant/pelvic pain and/or vaginal bleeding
2. Oral contraceptive pills (e.g., Ovral) for hormonal cycling of dysfunctional uterine bleeding
3. Fluconazole (Diflucan) tablets, 200 mg single-dose treatment for candidal vaginitis

Gastrointestinal/Proctology
1. Bismuth subsalicylate (Pepto-Bismol) tablets, for symptomatic treatment of nondysenteric mild diarrhea
2. Loperamide (Imodium) 2-mg tablets—irreplaceable for long bus rides or summit bids
3. Metamucil for adding bulk to fiber-poor expedition diets
4. Bisacodyl 10-mg suppositories (Dulcolax); one suppository daily for relief of constipation and irregularity
5. Antiemetics
   a. Ondansetron (Zofran) 4 mg orally disintegrating tablets and solution for injection
   b. Prochlorperazine 25-mg suppositories (Compazine) for severe nausea and vomiting; one suppository q8h
   c. Promethazine 25-mg suppositories (Phenergan) for severe nausea and vomiting; one suppository q8h
   d. A suppository may melt at high temperatures. Though less ergonomic, it can still be used after cooling
6. Antacids (reflux is common at altitude)
   a. Histamine-2–adrenergic blocking medication (e.g., famotidine [Pepcid])
   b. Calcium carbonate and magnesium hydroxide (Mylanta)

7. Oral rehydration solution (dehydrated packets) such as oral rehydration salts, Infalyte, or sports drink mixes. Homemade oral rehydration salts can also be prepared. Any of these is often better tolerated and absorbed when diluted to half strength.

8. Hydrocortisone acetate with cortisone (Anusol-HC) 25-mg suppositories. For inflamed hemorrhoids, one suppository is placed in the rectum morning and night for 2 weeks.

9. Tucks pads (containing 50% witch hazel) or baby wipes. Rectal inflammation from protracted diarrhea is extremely common on expeditions.

Topicals

1. Ketoconazole (Nizoral), tolnaftate (Tinactin) or nystatin cream or ointment (or other antifungal agent)

2. Triamcinolone acetonide (Kenalog 0.1% cream or other intermediate-potency steroid)

3. Insect repellent with DEET; consider picaridin, lemon eucalyptus, and other repellents

4. Silvadene cream for burns

5. Bacitracin, mupirocin, and/or bacitracin and polymyxin (Polysporin) for topical antibiotic

6. Aloe vera gel, excellent for minor burns and inflammation

7. Vaseline or other ointment such as Aquaphor or Blistex for treatment of chapped lips and fever blisters (some choose to include zidovudine [Zovirax] or other antiviral ointment for suspected herpes labialis)

8. Lip balm (Labiosan or other occlusive sun protection for lips)

9. Povidone-iodine (Betadine) solution

10. Small packets of K-Y Jelly (optional) for rectal or vaginal examinations

11. Foot powder

12. 5% acetic acid (vinegar) if risk of marine envenomation

Blisters

1. Moleskin, a thin, padded adhesive material for protecting skin from developing blisters

2. Adhesive foam, for fashioning donuts and padding for boots

3. Compeed, an excellent product that is durable and indispensable for painful, ulcerated bases of deroofed blisters or other severe blisters

4. Blistoban, an effective product for reducing friction and preventing blisters

5. Spenco 2nd Skin, good for burns and abrasions

6. Adhesive tape

7. Duct tape—suitable for blister prophylaxis

Wound Care Supplies
1. Povidone-iodine solution 10% (Betadine)
   a. Sterilize wound edges
   b. When diluted tenfold, can be used for wound irrigation
   c. Emergency disinfection of backcountry water
2. Wound closure strips (Steristrips), assorted sizes
3. Tincture of benzoin
4. First-aid cleansing pads with lidocaine; textured surface ideal for scrubbing dirt and embedded objects out of abrasions
5. Antiseptic towelettes with benzalkonium chloride
6. Sutures, multiple sizes, both nylon and absorbable
7. Cyanoacrylate glue ("super glue") for treatment of painful skin fissures
8. 2-octyl cyanoacrylate (Dermabond) tissue adhesive or over-the-counter alternative
9. Miscellaneous gauze, bandages (Band-Aids), etc.:
   a. 8 × 10 inch or 5 × 9 inch sterile trauma pads
   b. 4 × 4 inch sterile dressings
   c. Nonadherent sterile dressings such as Aquaphor, Xeroform, Adaptic, or Telfa; Spenco 2nd Skin is an excellent alternative and provides an ideal covering for burns, blisters, abrasions, and cuts. This polyethylene oxide gel laminate is composed of 96% water that cools and soothes on contact and can be left in place for up to 48 hours.
   d. Gauze rolled bandages or Kling bandages
   e. Elastic rolled bandage (Ace wrap)
   f. Assortment of strip and knuckle adhesive bandages
   g. Woven net-style bandage for holding dressings in place over joints

Instruments and Equipment
1. 14-gauge IV catheter for emergency tube thoracostomy
2. Chest tubes (28 to 36 French) include a Heimlich valve (or condom/rubber glove finger, for improvising a one-way "Heimlich" valve)
3. Urinary (Foley or Opticon) catheter: 16 French with 30-cc balloon—can be used as urinary catheter, suboptimal improvised chest tube, posterior nasal pack
4. "Uncle Bill's" tweezers or "sliver pickers" for foreign body removal
5. Disposable skin stapler (15 Shot Precise, 3M), especially useful for scalp lacerations; staple remover
6. No. 11 scalpels for incision and drainage
7. Bandage scissors, which are designed with a blunt tip to protect the victim while cutting through clothes, boots, or bandages

8. Tissue scissors
9. Needle driver for suturing
10. Forceps
11. 20- or 30-cc syringes with 18-gauge IV catheters for wound irrigation
12. Tuberculin (TB) syringes for administration of lidocaine
13. Stethoscope
14. Oto-ophthalmoscope
15. Blood pressure cuff
16. Regular thermometer
17. Hypothermia thermometer, which ideally should be able to read temperatures down to 29.4° C (85° F)

Orthopedics
1. SAM splints, full-length and optional extra-wide
2. Kendrick Traction Device (KTD) for femoral traction
3. Adhesive tape
4. Ensolite pads or Thermarest pads, not for the medical kit, but mentioned because they make excellent improvised universal knee immobilizers, ankle splints, cervical collars, etc.
5. Ace wraps for providing compression; also useful for holding pressure over taped extremities (Coban also works well)
6. Stiff neck extrication collar
7. Lightweight stirrup splints (Air Casts) for sprained ankles that allow near-normal ambulation and can be used inside of boot

Altitude (see Chapter 1)
1. Acetazolamide (Diamox) 125-mg tablets
2. Dexamethasone (Decadron) 4-mg tablets
3. Prochlorperazine (Compazine) 10-mg tablets
4. NSAIDs
5. High-altitude pulmonary edema (HAPE) treatment:
   a. Albuterol or salmeterol metered dose inhaler
   b. Sildenafil (Viagra) or Tadalafil (Cialis)
   c. Nifedipine 10 mg and 30 mg long acting
6. Ginkgo biloba
7. Portable hyperbaric bag (Gamow Bag)
8. Medical oxygen

Injectable Medications
1. Epinephrine 1:1000 solution: (Ana-Kit, Epi-Pen auto injector, Twinject auto injector, or epinephrine with TB syringe)
2. Morphine sulfate
3. Lorazepam (Ativan) or diazepam (Valium)

4. Dexamethasone (Decadron)
5. Antinausea
   a. Ondansetron (Zofran): oral disintegrating tablet or IV 4-mg dose
   b. Prochlorperazine (Compazine): 2.5 to 10 mg (0.5 to 2 mL) by slow IV injection or infusion at a rate not to exceed 5 mg per minute; must be into a clearly patent vessel or IV
   c. Promethazine (Phenergan) 12.5 to 25 mg by slow IV or IM injection
   d. Diphenhydramine (Benadryl)
      i. Allergic reactions or motion sickness: 25 to 50 mg IM q6h
      ii. Treatment of dystonic reactions secondary to prochlorperazine or haloperidol
      iii. Substitute for lidocaine (Xylocaine) for local anesthesia: a 50-mg (1-mL) vial diluted in syringe with 4 mL of normal saline to produce 1% solution; local infiltration carried out as usual
      iv. Mild sedation in higher doses
6. Depo-Medrol (or other injectable steroid): trigger point injections or treatment of severe tendinitis
7. Lidocaine 1% to 2% for wound infiltration
8. Ketorolac (Toradol) 30 or 60 mg, injected IV or IM q6h
9. Injectable antibiotics, for treatment of serious infections including meningitis, severe lower respiratory tract infection (pneumonia), pyelonephritis, and severe skin and soft tissue infections
7. Injectable antibiotics covering anaerobic infections:
   a. Anaerobes should be considered for all intra-abdominal infections. Examples include ruptured appendix, bowel perforation, and intra-abdominal abscess. These drugs can often temporize patients until evacuation is complete (in the absence of surgical resources).
   b. Examples include cefotetan (Cefotan), cefoxitin (Mefoxin), metronidazole (Flagyl), clindamycin (Cleocin), and imipenem-cilastatin sodium (Primaxin).

Intravenous Equipment
1. Multiple sizes of catheters
2. Intraosseous needle (for IO infusions); when intravenous access is difficult to establish, consider user-friendly device (e.g., the "BIG" bone injection gun [www.waismed .com])
3. Microdrip administration sets
4. Heparin locks
5. Bacteriostatic normal saline and/or heparin flushes

6. IV fluids, crystalloid for volume resuscitation (e.g., normal saline or lactated Ringer's solution); dextrose 5% in water (D5W) for administration of medication
7. Alcohol swabs

Airway
1. CPR Microshield or pocket mask. These are compact, easy-to-use, clear, flexible barriers or masks with a one-way air valve for performing mouth-to-mouth rescue breathing; prevents physical contact with a victim's secretions.
2. Oral airways
3. Laryngeal mask airway (LMA Fastrach), designed to facilitate tracheal intubation with an endotracheal tube
4. Endotracheal tubes, assorted sizes, to use with LMA or blind nasotracheal intubations. (NOTE: some expeditions carry laryngoscopes, but they are heavy and bulky; lightweight plastic units are a good alternative.)
5. V-VAC or other portable suction device—bulky but effective
6. Medical oxygen tanks with regulators, nasal cannulas, and 100% nonrebreathing masks

Dental Kit
1. Minimal kit includes:
   a. Cavit (temporary filling)
   b. Eugenol (topical analgesic) with zinc oxide for temporary fillings and repair
   c. Dental floss: multiple uses including reinforcing splint for avulsed teeth
2. More extensive kit to include the following:
   a. Benzocaine (Orabase-B); topical anesthetic, antiinflammatory
   b. Intermediate restoration material (IRM) powder for recementing crowns and repair
   c. Dental syringe with bupivacaine (Marcaine) ampules
   d. Mouth mirror and explorer
   e. Filling instrument
   f. Probe
   g. Universal extractor
   h. Elevator
   i. Cotton rolls

Miscellaneous Medical
1. Duct tape
2. Paper and pencil or commercial accident report form, essential for medical communication if patient is transported, as well as for medical record keeping
3. Headlamp, essential for any nighttime operations or surgical procedures requiring extra lighting

4. Tongue blades
5. Sterile applicators
6. Sterile gloves
7. Nonsterile examination gloves
8. Cotton-tipped applicators, which may be used to remove insects or other foreign material from the eye; also useful to evert an eyelid and for many other applications
9. Safety pins, many uses
10. Urine test strips (Chemstrips)
11. Water disinfection system
12. Fluorescent surveyors tape for marking helicopter landing zone, finding your way back to a victim, alerting rescuers, etc.
13. Spare sunglasses (protective eyewear can also be improvised if necessary)

Children in the Wilderness 61

▶ **WHAT MAKES CHILDREN DIFFERENT**

1. Medications and fluids must be calculated on the basis of the weight of the child (Table 61-1). One should also be aware of normal ranges of vital signs according to age (Table 61-2).
2. Children experience greater toxicity from envenomation because of the increased dose of venom per kilogram of weight.
3. Children experience greater exposure to environmental factors such as cold, heat, and solar radiation because they have a larger body surface area–to–mass ratio than do adults.
4. Thermoregulation is less efficient in children, making them more susceptible to heat illness and hypothermia.
5. Children experience a greater number of infections than do adults.
6. Children are at greater risk of dehydration than are adults.
7. Small children tend to explore their environment with hands and mouths.

▶ **AGE-SPECIFIC EXPECTATIONS FOR WILDERNESS TRAVEL**

See Table 61-3.

▶ **ENVIRONMENTAL ILLNESSES**

Dehydration

Signs and Symptoms
1. Mild-moderate dehydration (5% to 10% weight loss)
   a. Irritability
   b. Sunken eyes
   c. Dry mucous membranes
   d. Thirst
   e. Dark urine
   f. Tachycardia
2. Severe dehydration (>10% weight loss)
   a. Lethargy
   b. Extremely sunken eyes
   c. Extremely dry mucous membranes
   d. Cool, mottled extremities
   e. Rapid thready pulse
   f. Tachypnea
   g. Absent tears
   h. No urine output

TABLE 61-1. Average Weight for Age

AGE (yr)	WEIGHT	
	kg	lb
1	10	22
3	15	33
6	20	44
8	25	55
9.5	30	66
11	35	77
13	45	100

From U.S. Centers for Disease Control and Prevention, National Center for Health Statistics (www.cdc.gov/nchs/).

TABLE 61-2. Age-Specific Resting Heart Rate and Respiratory Rate*

AGE	HEART RATE (Beats/Min)	RESPIRATORY RATE (Breaths/Min)
0-5 mo	140 ± 40	40 ± 12
6-11 mo	135 ± 30	30 ± 10
1-2 yr	120 ± 30	25 ± 8
3-4 yr	110 ± 30	20 ± 6
5-7 yr	100 ± 20	16 ± 5
8-11 yr	90 ± 30	16 ± 4
12-15 yr	80 ± 20	16 ± 3

*Mean rate, ± 2 standard deviation.

Treatment
1. Replace fluids and electrolytes.
   a. Oral rehydration with water and oral rehydration salts (ORS) is the most important treatment for dehydration in the backcountry. Simply drinking plain water is inadequate replacement.
   b. Gatorade can be used but should be diluted to half-strength with water.
   c. Add commercial ORS (Jianas Brothers, Kansas City, MO; http://rehydrate.org/resources/jianas.htm, 816-421-2880) containing sodium chloride, 3.5 g; potassium chloride, 1.5 g; glucose, 20 g; and sodium bicarbonate, 2.5 g to 1 L (quart) of drinking water.
   d. Improvise an oral rehydration solution by adding one teaspoon (5 mL) of table salt and eight teaspoons (40 mL) of table sugar to 1 L (quart) of drinking (disinfected)

TABLE 61-3. Age-Specific Expectations for Wilderness Travel

AGE	EXPECTATION	SAFETY ISSUES
0-2 yr	Distance traveled depends on adults Use child carriers	Provide "safe play area" (e.g., tent floor, extra tarp laid out), bells on shoes, ipecac syrup
2-4 yr	Difficult age; stop every 15 min, hike 1-2 miles on own	Dress in bright colors, teach how to use whistle; ipecac syrup
5-7 yr	Hike 1-3 hr/day, cover 3-4 miles over easy terrain, rest every 30-45 min	Carry whistle (three blows for "I'm lost"), carry own pack with mini first-aid kit and water
8-9 yr	Hike a full day with easy pace, cover 6-7 miles over variable terrain; if over 4 feet tall (1.2 m), can use framed pack	As for 5-7 yr, plus teach map use and route finding, precondition by increasing maximal distances by <10%/wk, watch for overuse injuries, keep weight of pack <20% of bodyweight
10-12 yr	Hike a full day at moderate pace, cover 8-10 miles over variable terrain	As for 8-9 yr
Teens	Hike 8-12 miles at adult pace; may see a decrease in pace or distance with growth spurt	As for 8-9 yr

water. A rice cereal–based rehydration solution is made by adding one teaspoon (5 mL) of table salt and 1 cup (50 g) of rice cereal to 1 L (quart) of drinking (disinfected) water.

e. For rapid treatment of mild to moderate dehydration, 50 to 100 mL/kg (1 to 1.5 oz/lb) of ORS should be administered over the first 4-hour period, followed by maintenance fluid volumes (75 to 150 mL/kg/day or 1 to 2 oz/lb/day). An additional 10 mL/kg, or 4 oz, can be given for each diarrhea stool and 5 mL/kg, or 2 oz, for each episode of emesis. If vomiting develops, most children will still tolerate ORS if given small volumes (5 to 10 mL) every 5 minutes. Severe dehydration requires prompt medical attention and administration of IV fluids for rehydration.

Hypothermia (see Chapter 3)

Children cool more rapidly than adults because of their proportionally large body surface area and because they lack the knowledge and judgment to initiate responses that will maintain warmth in a cold environment.

Signs and Symptoms (Table 61-4)
1. Ataxia
2. Altered mental status
3. Inappropriate remarks
4. Shivering is not a reliable marker of hypothermia in children

Treatment
1. Remove any wet clothing and replace with dry, insulating garments. Cover child's head and neck.
2. Place child in a sleeping bag with a normothermic person.
3. Place hot water bottles insulated to prevent burns at the axillae, neck, and groin.
4. If the child is alert, administer oral hydration with warm fluids containing glucose.

Hyperthermia (see Chapter 5)

Children generate more heat per kilogram and are less able to dissipate heat from the core to the periphery.

Signs and Symptoms
1. Early signs and symptoms include flushing, tachycardia, weakness, headache, and nausea.
2. Late signs are confusion, ataxia, or any altered mental state.
3. Sweating is either present or absent.
4. Temperature is elevated.

Treatment
1. Remove child from sources of heat and remove clothing.
2. Spray the victim with warm water and fan vigorously.
3. Place ice packs or cold compresses at the neck, axillae, scalp, and groin.
4. If the child is alert and not vomiting, administer oral fluids (see earlier).

High-Altitude Illness (see Chapter 1)

Prevention
1. Avoid abrupt ascent to a sleeping altitude higher than 3000 m (9843 feet).
2. Spend two or three nights at 2500 to 3000 m (8202 to 9843 ft) before going higher.

3. Avoid abrupt increases of greater than 500 m (1640 feet) in sleeping altitude per night.
4. Acetazolamide prophylaxis (5 mg/kg/day, in two divided doses, up to a maximum daily dose of 250 mg started 24 hours before ascent and continued while at altitude) in children with a history of recurrent acute mountain sickness despite graded ascent.

Signs and Symptoms
1. Bitemporal, throbbing headache
2. Anorexia
3. Nausea and vomiting
4. Dizziness, dyspnea on exertion, and fragmented sleep
5. Infants may display irritability, poor feeding, and sleep disturbance.
6. Ataxia, altered mental state

Treatment
1. Descend at least 500 to 1000 m (1640 to 3281 feet).
2. Administer acetaminophen for headache.
3. Promethazine (Phenergan) may be administered to relieve nausea and vomiting. The dose is 0.2 to 0.5 mg/kg every 6 hours, preferably per rectum.
4. Administer oxygen if available.
5. Administer acetazolamide (Diamox), 5 mg/kg/day divided bid up to 250 mg/day if symptoms persist despite descent.
6. Administer dexamethasone, 0.6 mg IM/IV/PO q6h, for children with deterioration of consciousness, truncal ataxia, or severe vomiting.

Travelers' Diarrhea
Young children are at greater risk for travelers' diarrhea and its complications because of relatively poor hygiene, immature immune systems, lower gastric pH, more rapid gastric emptying, and difficulties with adequate hydration.

Signs and Symptoms
1. Greater than three unformed stools a day
2. Fever
3. Abdominal cramps
4. Vomiting
5. Blood or mucus in the stool

Treatment
1. Provide oral rehydration to correct dehydration and electrolyte losses (see earlier).
2. Give rice, bananas, and potatoes as supplements to oral rehydration solutions. Fats, dairy products, caffeine, and alcohol should be avoided.

3. If the victim is older than 2 years of age and does not have bloody diarrhea or fever, administer loperamide (Imodium). Weight-adjusted dose is 13 to 20 kg (1 mg tid); 20 to 30 kg (2 mg bid); greater than 30 kg (2 mg tid).
4. In a severe case (fever, bloody stool, or abdominal distention), consider giving an antibiotic (azithromycin, 10 mg/kg on day 1, then 5 mg/kg once daily for 2 days).
5. Consider using a probiotic agent such as *Lactobacillus acidophilus* for prevention and treatment. This is available over the counter with dosing of one tablet or capsule a day for children younger than 2 years old and two capsules a day for children older than 2 years. Capsules can be opened and placed into food or drink for children unable or unwilling to take pills.

Medications (Table 61-4)

Most children can chew tablets once their first molars are present (15 months of age). Before that time, chewable medications or tablets can be crushed between two spoons and mixed with food. Liquid medications add excess weight and the potential for leaks; they should be carried in powder form only for children younger than 6 months of age. Medication can be camouflaged in a food such as instant pudding.

TABLE 61-4. Signs and Symptoms of Hypothermia*

RECTAL TEMPERATURE	SIGNS AND SYMPTOMS
Mild (33-35° C)	Sensation of cold, shivering (91-95° F), increased heart rate, progressive inco-ordination in hand movements, developing poor judgment
Moderate (28-32° C) (82-90° F)	Loss of shivering, difficulty walking or following commands, paradoxical undressing, increasing confusion, decreased arrhythmia threshold
Severe (<28° C) (<82° F)	Rigid muscles, progressive loss of reflexes and voluntary motion, hypotension, bradycardia, hypoventilation, dilated pupils, increasing risk of fatal arrhythmias, appearance of death

*Data from adult subjects.

Wild animals may stalk support animals. Wild (and occasionally domestic) animals are most likely to respond adversely if:
1. Approached too closely
2. Handled improperly
3. They are fearful for their lives
4. Their young are approached too closely
5. They are cornered or otherwise threatened
6. They are protecting their territory
7. They are breeding
8. They are wounded or ill (diseased)
9. They are being fed by hand

▶ PRETRIP ANIMAL HEALTH CONSIDERATIONS

Carry proper health certificates of travel. Perform a proper pretrip examination. Condition and train animals for the expected environment and terrain. Do not travel with immature animals. Dogs should be at least 1 year old. Llamas and horses should be older than 3 years. Well-conditioned and trained horses, mules, burros, and dogs can carry approximately 30% of their body weight. Llamas usually carry only 25% of their body weight.

The normal vital statistics of trek animals are itemized in Table 62-1.

▶ HORSES, MULES, AND DONKEYS

A tetanus booster should have been given within the past year. Vaccinate against rabies if appropriate. Encephalomyelitis vaccine should be used in endemic areas. Determine internal parasite levels by fecal flotation and use medication if needed to reduce the parasite burden. Feet should be trimmed and shod properly at least 2 weeks and not more than 4 weeks before a trek begins. Use sole pads if sharp, rocky terrain is expected.

▶ LLAMAS

Tetanus immunization should be current within the past 6 months. Other basic immunizations should include *Clostridium perfringens* toxoid, types C and D, within the past 6 months, and vaccinations against leptospirosis and rabies if entering an endemic area. Toenails should have been trimmed within the past 2 months. Ova levels should be checked, but usually treatment

TABLE 62-1. Vital Statistics of Trek Animals

ANIMAL	BODY WEIGHT		HEART RATE	RESPIRATORY RATE	BODY TEMPERATURE		WEIGHT CARRIED BY WELL-CONDITIONED ANIMAL	
	lb	kg	(beats/min)	(breaths/min)	°C	°F	kg	lb
Horse	800-1200	360-540	28-40	10-14	37.2-38	99-100.5	110-136	240-300
Mule	600-1200	275-540	28-40	10-14	37.2-38	99-100.5	82-136	180-300
Donkey	300-600	136-275	28-40	10-14	37.2-38	99-100.5	40-82	90-180
Llama	300-450	136-200	60-90	10-30	37.2-38.7	99-101.8	34-50	75-110
Dog	20-100	9-45	65-90	15-30	37.5-38.6	99.5-101.5	3-14	6-30
Camel	880-1200	400-550	40-50	5-12	36.4-42	97.5-107.6	225	500
Elephant	5000-8000	2300-3700	25-35	4-6	36-37	97.5-99	900	2000
Yak	2200	1000	55-80	10-30	37.8-39.2	100-102.5	235	550

*Sustained trekking for 24-40 km (15-25 miles) per day on moderately difficult trails. The weight includes tack. Animals in training should be expected to carry only one half to two thirds of this weight.

with an antihelmintic (ivermectin, 0.2 mg/kg, subcutaneously, or fenbendazole (10 mg/kg orally) is desirable within the previous 2 months.

▶ DOGS

Immunize dogs against canine distemper, canine adenovirus, leptospirosis, and rabies. Check for internal parasites and fleas. Bathe with a pyrethrin insecticide-containing shampoo and carry a dusting powder.

▶ EMERGENCY RESTRAINT

Know how to create a halter tie (Fig. 62-1) and a temporary rope halter (Fig. 62-2).

For horses, mules, and burros, if the animal is down and entangled in rope, wire, or bushes, approach it from its back and keep the head held down until it can be extricated. Stay out of reach of the fore and hind limbs. If the animal is standing, stand close to the left shoulder. If examining the feet and legs of a standing animal, keep your head above the lower body line to avoid having the animal reach forward and strike with a rear limb. You can "ear" the animal by grasping one or both ears. Stand at the left shoulder and grasp the halter or lead rope with the left hand. Place the right hand palm down with the fingers together and the thumb extended, on top of the neck. Slide the hand up the neck until the thumb and fingers surround the base of the ear. Squeeze tightly, but do not twist the ear. Be prepared to move with the horse while maintaining a firm grip.

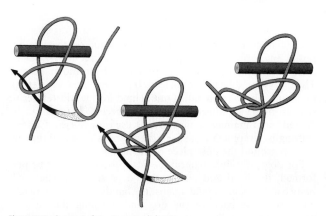

Figure 62-1. Sequence of steps to create a halter tie.

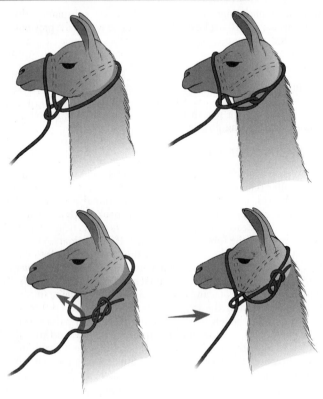

Figure 62-2. Temporary rope halters.

For llamas, one or two people should stand on the side opposite any limb to be lifted, or the animal should be placed next to a tree or large rock to prevent it from moving away. The limb should be firmly grasped. If a llama refuses to get up, the rear limbs may be pulled out behind it. If it still refuses to rise, an injury or illness should be suspected. Llamas can be "eared" in a manner similar to that used for horses. Control spitting by draping a cloth over the animal's nose and tucking the top around the nose piece of the halter.

For dogs, if a mild painful medical procedure must be performed, the head and mouth should be secured. The dog's body can be securely held against the handler's body by reaching across the back of the dog and grasping the base of the neck while pulling the opposite shoulder with the elbow toward the handler. The other hand should tuck the dog's head under the handler's arm. Alternatively, a muzzle can be constructed from a nylon cord or even a shoelace. A loop should be formed with an overhand knot on one side. The loop is placed over the muzzle of the dog, with the knot on top, and tightened. The ends of the loop should be wrapped around the muzzle, crossed beneath the jaw, and tied behind the ears.

▶ CONDITIONS COMMON TO ALL SPECIES

Trauma

Hair or wool should be trimmed from the margins of wounds before treatment or suturing to prevent matting with exudate. The skin may be sutured with any suture material suitable for humans. Antibiotics are not necessary unless vital structures such as synovial or serosal membranes are exposed. Therapy for rope burns is similar to that for human burns.

Foot, Hoof, and Nail Problems

Foot and limb trauma is accompanied by varying degrees of lameness (limping). It may be difficult to establish which leg is painful, but the principles are similar to evaluation of such pain in humans, with the obvious differences of two extra limbs to evaluate and the animal's inability to communicate.

Cellulitis may develop on the limbs or body. The signs include heat, swelling, and redness and are the same in all species, as is therapy.

Therapy for foot injuries includes providing drainage of infected lesions, disinfection, and protection of exposed sensitive structures. Antibiotics are not indicated for most wounds unless a joint surface is exposed. It may be necessary to bandage the foot to provide protection while in camp and to fashion special shoes or boots to keep an animal functioning on the trail. Special booties are available commercially for dogs, but a temporary moccasin may be constructed from soft leather (such as the leather used by crafts people to make moccasins).

Hyperthermia (Heat Stress, Heat Exhaustion)

Clinical Signs
Signs may vary according to species and the stage of hyperthermia, but all affected animals have an increased heart and respiratory rates, usually accompanied by open-mouth breathing. Rectal temperatures may vary from 106° F to 110° F (41.1° C to 43.3° C). Horses, mules, burros, and llamas sweat in the early stages of hyperthermia, but sweating may cease if the animal becomes severely dehydrated. Sweating is evident in horses

but imperceptible in llamas because most sweating occurs on the ventral abdomen in what is known as the *thermal window,* where the fibers are less dense and the fiber length is short.

Dogs cool themselves by evaporation of respiratory fluids while panting. The mouth is held open, and the tongue lolls from the mouth. The respiratory rate increases from a normal of 30 breaths/minute up to 200 to 400 breaths/minute. Moisture may be observed dripping from the tongue. As dehydration intensifies, salivation and dripping may slow or cease.

Hypotension causes hypoxemia of the brain, resulting in dullness, restlessness, and incoordination. Hypoxemia may lead to convulsions and collapse. The shift of blood from the gastrointestinal tract may cause decreased motility and the potential for ileus and tympany. Signs of colic in horses and llamas (kicking at the belly, looking back at the side, treading, attempting to lie down and roll) may be noted.

Treatment
Cessation of excessive muscular activity may be all that is necessary if hyperthermia is mild. If streams or lakes are nearby, the animal can be walked into the water and water splashed on its underbelly. Contingencies for hyperthermia are part of all plans for capture operations for wildlife translocation and reintroduction projects. Water is carried for cooling and intravenous fluids to deal with heat stress. Cold water enemas are the most effective and rapid way to cool the body of a large animal.

Tick Paralysis

Clinical Signs
Signs may not appear for 5 to 7 days following the tick bite. Initially, there is paresis of the legs; progressing to unsteady gait; knuckling; ataxia; and, ultimately, flaccid paralysis of the hind limbs. Loss of motor function ascends cranially, causing paralysis of the forelimbs. Pain perception remains. Even with paralysis of the limbs the animal is bright and alert and able to eat and drink if feed is placed within reach. Ultimately, paralysis involves the neck, throat, and face, causing difficulties in chewing, swallowing, and breathing. Respiratory failure is the cause of death.

Diagnosis
The sequence of clinical signs is the only sure method of diagnosis, unless the tick or ticks are found. That may be quite difficult on an animal the size of a horse. Differential diagnoses should include encephalitides, head or spinal trauma, and hyperthermia.

Management
No antidote is available for the toxin. The offending tick or ticks must be removed, which may produce a dramatic response. Look in the lightly haired areas of the axillary space, perineum, and behind the ears if tick paralysis is suspected.

Skunk Odor Removal

In addition to the obvious odor, skunk musk is nauseating to some people and may also cause retching in dogs. If a person or pet is sprayed in the face, the musk is an irritant that causes conjunctivitis, keratitis, lacrimation, temporary impairment of vision, glossitis, slobbering, and foaming at the mouth.

Management of Odor Removal
Quick flushing of the face and eyes with copious quantities of cold water will restore vision and minimize persistent irritation. If conjunctivitis persists, instill contact lens solution or a drop of olive oil into the conjunctival sac.

The objective of odor removal is to wash away the offending oily liquid and neutralize the compound. Simple bathing will not completely eliminate the odor, which is pungent in a remarkably dilute concentration.

One of the most effective oxidizing agents is a dilute solution of household bleach (Clorox); however, this may bleach clothing and hair and is harsh on the skin of people and animals. Skunk musk is alkaline, so mild acidic solutions may be at least partially effective and will reduce the pungency of the odor. Tomato juice, white vinegar, and ammonia in water are all touted but may not completely eliminate the odor.

A formula that is mentioned most frequently is a combination of hydrogen peroxide (347 mL, 3%), water (1 cup, 237 mL), baking soda (sodium bicarbonate, ¼ cup or 60 mL), and a dog detergent (1 tablespoon or 15 mL). Mix the peroxide with the water, and then add the baking soda and shampoo. Mix and pour into a squirt bottle/sprayer. This solution may be sprayed onto a dog or horse but should not be sprayed directly into the eyes or nose. The solution should be allowed to remain on the coat for 10 minutes, while being worked into the coat with a gloved hand.

Washable clothing should be washed with a strong soap or heavy-duty detergent. In a permanent camp, items that cannot be washed (shoes, leather goods) may be buried in sandy soil for a few days. The soil will adsorb the odorous chemicals.

A number of commercial products are available that have been formulated to completely eliminate the skunk odor:
1. Neutroleum alpha is nontoxic and may be used on clothing and pets. It may be obtained from USDA, Damage Control,

P.O. Box 81886, Lincoln, NE, 68501, phone (402) 434-2340.

2. Skunk Off is nontoxic and nonirritating, even to mucous membranes, and safe to use on pets and clothing.

3. Odor-Mute is available in granular form and easy to transport. It is nontoxic and may be applied to pets and clothing after being dissolved in water.

All of the products mentioned are for use on pets or fabric and not recommended for use directly on people. The trek physician is the only one qualified to make such a recommendation. However, washing with soap and copious amounts of cold water will wash away considerable musk.

Plant Poisoning

Certain highly toxic plants that grow in wilderness areas of the United States should be recognized (Table 62-2).

Lightning Strike

During an electrical storm, animals on the trek should be positioned in the safest environment possible, away from tall trees and exposed hills. Llamas may be encouraged to lie down in a small ravine or a depression or against a rock face, with the head tied close to the ground. A picket line stake may be used for the tie-down. Avoid tying an animal to a tree; however, using a small bush for a tie-down may be safe. Horses are more difficult to deal with because it is impossible to get them to lie down unless they are specially trained to do so. Get them into a ravine, a depressed area, or near a rock face.

If the strike is witnessed and the heart has stopped beating, chest compression (cardiac massage) may be performed if it is determined that it is safe for a human to be in the open. With the animal in lateral recumbency, pull the forelimb as far cranially as possible and press on the chest wall just caudal to the triceps muscle. Cardiac massage may be required for a number of minutes.

Snakebite

Llamas and, to a lesser extent, young horses are curious animals and may stick their noses out to investigate strange animals in their area. Thus it is not uncommon for an animal to be struck on the nose. Leg bites may occur in any animal.

Clinical Signs

Venom injection results in pronounced swelling in the area of the bite, beginning 1 to 3 hours after the bite. The most serious consequence of being bitten on the nose is swelling that

TABLE 62-2. Poisonous Plants That May Affect Horses or Llamas on Trek

COMMON NAME	SCIENTIFIC NAME	POISONOUS PRINCIPLE	SIGNS OF POISONING	HABITAT	SPECIES	THERAPY*
False hellebore, corn lily	*Veratrum californicum*	Alkaloids	Vomiting, salivation, convulsions, fast irregular pulse	High mountains, meadows	Llama	Symptomatic
Death camas, sandcorn	*Zigadenus* species	Alkaloids	Foaming at mouth, convulsions, ataxia, vomiting, fast weak pulse	Hillsides, fields, meadows, in spring of year	Horse, llama	Symptomatic
Water hemlock	*Cicuta douglasii*	Resin	Frothing at mouth, muscle twitching, convulsions, death in 15-30 min	Standing or running water, obligate aquatic	Horse, llama	Symptomatic
Nightshade	*Solanum* species	Alkaloidal glycoside, solanine	Vomiting, weakness, groaning	Ubiquitous	Horse, llama	Symptomatic
Jimson weed	*Datura stramonium*	Alkaloid, atropine	Dry mucous membranes, dilated pupils, mania	Waste places	Horse, llama	Parasympathomimetics
Tobacco, tree tobacco	*Nicotiana* species	Alkaloid, nicotine	Stimulation of CNS, then depression; sweating; muscle twitching, convulsions	Waste places	Horse, llama	Symptomatic
Lupine, blue bonnet	*Lupinus* species	Alkaloid	CNS depression, dyspnea, muscle twitching, ataxia, frothing, convulsions	Ubiquitous	Horse, llama	Symptomatic

Continued

TABLE 62-2. Poisonous Plants That May Affect Horses or Llamas on Trek—cont'd

COMMON NAME	SCIENTIFIC NAME	POISONOUS PRINCIPLE	SIGNS OF POISONING	HABITAT	SPECIES	THERAPY*
Dogbane, Indian hemp	*Apocynum cannabinum*	Cardioactive glycoside (similar to digitoxin)	Dyspnea, cardiac arrhythmias, agonal convulsions, vomiting, diarrhea	Ubiquitous	Horse, llama	Symptomatic
Oleander	*Nerium oleander*	Same as for dogbane	Same as for dogbane	Ornamental	Horse, llama	Symptomatic, gastrotomy
Castor bean	*Ricinus communis*	Ricin, water solution	Anaphylactic shock, diarrhea	Ornamental	Horse, llama	Treat for shock; fluids
Rhododendron	*Rhododendron* species	Andromedotoxin glycoside	Vomiting, colic, severe depression	Shrubs in meadows and moist places	Llama	Activated charcoal, time

*In most cases of poisoning from ingestion of poisonous plants, no specific antidote exists. Victims are treated symptomatically. The critical factor is to empty the digestive tract of the plant material with cathartics, parasympathomimetic stimulation, and enemas. Activated charcoal, given orally, may be of value.

occludes the nostrils, making it virtually impossible for horses and llamas to breathe. Dogs are not obligate nasal breathers, but the effects of a bite may be more severe in them than in the larger animals. A rattlesnake bite on the nose is an emergency.

Management
A 10-cm segment of a 1-cm diameter flexible plastic tube should be in the first aid kit of the trek. This should be inserted into a nostril before any swelling occurs. The swelling will be in the area of the nostril, and the tube will prevent occlusion of the nostril, providing a passageway for air. It is not possible to insert a tube after the swelling has developed. If swelling has already developed, the only life-saving procedure is a tracheotomy.

DO NOT attempt to cut the skin and suck out the venom with your mouth. This procedure is not effective.

The only specific treatment for pit viper envenomation is the administration of antivenom. The same product used for humans is used in animals. One to three vials should be administered intravenously once signs of envenomation have appeared.

Choke

"Choke" in animals usually refers to lodging of food or other objects in the esophagus. The signs of choke may be alarming, but an animal will rarely die unless feed is regurgitated and inhaled into the lungs. Choke is most often caused by overly rapid ingestion of pellets and/or grain. Importantly, animals must be accustomed to any supplemental feed to be used on the trek. Ingestion may be slowed by placing rock pebbles in the container used to feed the animal, causing it to separate the rocks from the feed. Metallic or wooden objects will rarely be swallowed. Llamas and horses are too fastidious in their eating habits to consume such objects.

Retching is the principle sign of choke, as the animal attempts to dislodge the mass. Choked animals are able to breathe, but they are obviously in distress. Saliva may flow from the mouth, and the victim may cough up particles of the material (grain or pellets). It may be possible to feel a mass on the left side of the neck if the obstruction occurs in the cervical area. Peristaltic waves may be observed moving up and down the left side of the neck. The mass may lodge anywhere along the course of the esophagus, but generally it lies within the chest and is not visible externally.

Management
Water may be offered, but feed should be withheld until the problem has corrected itself. Palpate along the lower neck to determine if a bulge is present. If so, gently massage it to

determine if it can be moved. Sometimes, moderate exercise may cause the object to move toward the stomach. In some cases, passage of a stomach tube and application of gentle pressure may push the mass into the stomach. Medication (acepromazine 0.05 mg/kg IV or xylazine 0.05 to 0.25 mg/kg IV for a llama and 1.1 mg/kg IV for a horse) may be necessary to relax esophageal spasm.

Wound Dressing and Bandaging
The principles of wound dressing are basically the same as for humans, to provide uniform pressure over a variably shaped surface.

The foot requires special consideration. When dressing a foot wound, make certain that the spaces between the digits of dogs or llamas are padded with cotton. The easiest bandage to apply is a Vetrap elastic bandage that conforms to the odd shape. If a severe foot wound occurs while trekking in the back country, additional protection may be necessary to allow the animal to continue on the journey. The author carries a sheet of pliable leather of the type used to construct moccasins. The dressed foot is placed in the center of the sheet, and then the leather is gathered up around the pastern and held in place by duct tape or another bandage, to form a roughly shaped boot.

Cardiopulmonary Resuscitation

Rescue Breathing
The procedure is different than that employed in humans because mouth-to-mouth breathing cannot be performed on an adult llama or horse. Mouth-to-mouth breathing could be performed in a dog by clamping the mouth and lips shut and breathing through the nostrils. A llama or horse should be placed in lateral recumbency, preferably on the right side. Stand at the animal's withers (top of the shoulder) and reach across the body to grasp and lift the arch of the rib cage. This maneuver will flatten the diaphragm and expand the chest, producing inspiration. Do not press in this same area to force expiration because this will put pressure on the stomach and possibly cause regurgitation. Instead, press over the heart area just above the elbow and caudal to the muscles of the upper limb. The rate for the horse or llama is 10 to 15 breaths per minute. Rescue breathing in the dog is performed by compressing the chest at the widest segment of the thorax at a rate of 20 to 30 breaths per minute.

Cardiac massage may be performed by placing the llama or horse on its right side, if not already there. Have an assistant pull the upper foreleg forward and press the chest in the area vacated by pulling the leg forward. Kneel next to the bottom of the chest. Position the heels of both hands against the chest approximately 6 inches (15 cm) above the sternum, with the fingers directed toward the spine. Press firmly with the arms held straight and release quickly. Repeat the movement every second. After 15 compressions, check for a pulse in the saphenous artery on the medial aspect of the stifle in a llama, or listen for the heart beat with a stethoscope. After 15 heart compressions, administer five cycles of rescue breathing, as described previously. It is futile to continue cardiac massage if no oxygen is available to the heart or the general circulation. Massage must be continued until heartbeat returns and the victim begins to breathe, or when signs indicate that the victim is dead (pupils dilated, no response to touching the cornea).

For a dog, cardiac massage is performed in lateral recumbency in the type of dogs that are likely to be on a trek (small dogs or those that are round-chested are placed on their back and compression exerted over the sternum).

West Nile Viral Encephalitis

Transmission is via mosquito bites (*Culex, Aedes, Anopheles* species) and possibly other blood-sucking insects.

Signs in Horses, Llamas, and Humans
The incubation period is 6 to 10 days. Although most infections are subclinical in horses and humans, 10% of affected individuals develop fever and the encephalitic signs of depression, ataxia, and paresis, particularly of the hind limbs. More advanced signs include head shaking, incessant chewing, paralysis of the lower lip or tongue, severe ataxia, ascending paralysis, and terminal recumbency.

Management
Two vaccines are approved for use in horses in the United States but have also been used in camelids (West Nile-Innovator killed, Fort Dodge Animal Health, Overland Park, KS, and Recombitek live, Merial, Athens, GA). If a trek is planned for an area where WNV is endemic and when mosquitoes are prevalent, trek horses and llamas should be vaccinated, consisting or one injection followed by another one month later. If trek managers are contracting for animals, they should insure that the animals they hire have been properly immunized.

▶ UNIQUE DISORDERS OF HORSES, MULES, AND DONKEYS

Laminitis (Founder)

Clinical Signs
Laminitis usually develops on both fore feet, but rear feet may also be affected in severe cases. The horse shifts its center of gravity to the hind limbs to minimize pressure on the fore feet, standing with the hind limbs forward under the body and the fore limbs extended in front of the body (camped forward in front), as seen in Figure 62-3. The feet are warm or hot to palpation, and there is a pounding digital artery pulse. The horse is reluctant to move.

Management
Prevention or minimizing the effects of the inciting causes of laminitis is vitally important. Once clinical signs occur, the objectives of treatment are to eliminate the predisposing factors, decrease inflammation, and maintain or reestablish blood flow to the laminae.

If laminitis is the result of a digestive upset, it is imperative to administer a cathartic (magnesium sulfate [Epsom salts], 1 kg in 4 L of water via nasogastric tube). Phenylbutazone (Butazolidin 6 mg/kg IV daily) should always be administered

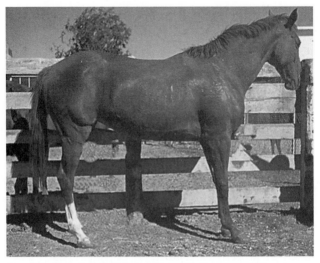

Figure 62-3. Stance of a horse with laminitis. Front and hind legs are extended forward.

to relieve pain so that the horse will move. Acepromazine maleate 0.04 mg/kg IM every 6 hours is used as a vasodilator to enhance blood flow to the laminae. If available, heparin (60 units/kg subcutaneously) helps to prevent platelet aggregation and thrombus formation.

In acute laminitis, the feet are warm or hot, so the inclination would be to soak the feet in cold water. This is actually contraindicated because it is desired to increase circulation to the foot and not inhibit circulation.

Experts now believe that mild exercise is an important aid in preventing damage to the laminae. The horse should be exercised slowly on soft ground for 10 to 15 minutes every hour for 12 to 24 hours, and then exercise should be stopped. Even slow walking may be quite painful. A low volar nerve block relieves pain and inhibits vascular constriction within the foot. This is accomplished by palpating the pulsating artery on the posterior lateral aspect of the fetlock (Fig. 62-4). The nerve lies posterior to the artery.

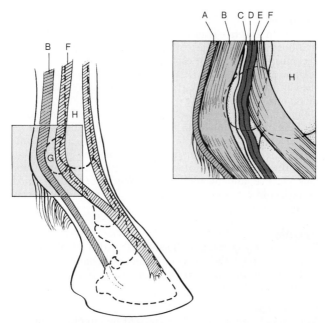

Figure 62-4. Diagram of the anatomy of the equine fetlock. **A,** Skin. **B,** Flexor tendons. **C,** Volar nerve. **D,** Palmar digital artery. **W,** Digital vein. **F,** Suspensory ligament. **G,** Sesamoid bone. **H,** Metacarpal bone (cannon).

With a 20- to 22-gauge needle, 3 mL of 2% lidocaine is injected over each nerve. It may be necessary to repeat nerve blocks two or three times daily for several days. Corticosteroids are contraindicated.

Saddle, Cinch, and Rigging Sores

If the lesion is rested and treated as inflamed tissue, complete healing may occur. However, if the saddle is reapplied, it overlies a lump that is subject to abrasion. The injury can extend through the dermis, resulting in severe ulceration. Cinch and rigging sores are usually caused by friction, leading to blister formation.

Clinical Signs

Hot and tender swellings are the primary signs of acute saddle sores. The hair or epidermis may be rubbed off. General sensitivity over the back is usually caused by muscle soreness.

Evidence of previous sores includes white hairs in spots over the withers or saddle bed, scars that may or may not be haired over, thickening of the dermis, and alopecia with or without swelling.

Treatment

Prevention is better than treatment. Toughening the backs of trail horses is a major job of the trainer. Proper pads or blankets must be selected for each horse.

Upon arrival at a rest area, the girth should be slowly loosened at intervals of 10 to 15 minutes to prevent rapid flow of blood into ischemic areas.

Once a sore has developed, the horse must be rested or the tack changed to eliminate pressure or friction on the lesion. Holes are often cut in pads to accommodate a saddle sore, but spot pressure at the ring edge may be as detrimental as the original cause of the saddle sore. Riders must keep tack cleaned and in good repair. When the saddle is removed, cold water poured over the back for 15 minutes may minimize swelling.

Myopathy

Exertional myopathies of horses vary from simple muscle soreness, through the "tying up" syndrome (similar to "Charlie horses" in humans), to paralytic myoglobinuria (rhabdomyolysis, azoturia).

Clinical Signs

Mild muscle soreness is characterized by alterations in gait that indicate muscle weakness. As severity increases, the gait becomes progressively altered until the horse is in obvious

pain and reluctant to move. The horse has an anxious expression and may sweat excessively. Affected muscles are
painful to palpation and may be swollen. Skin temperature
over the muscle may be elevated. Muscle spasms may occur,
but not consistently. Myoglobinuria is observed grossly in
moderate to severe cases and should be considered prima
facie evidence for stopping and resting or treating the
horse.

Treatment
Rest is paramount in all cases. A rider may have difficulty
differentiating the pain associated with myopathy from that
seen with colic until the horse is allowed to lie down, look
at its side, or kick at its belly). It is disastrous to force the
severely myopathic horse to walk, as is done with a suspected case of colic. If there is doubt, the horse should not
be exercised.

Horses in inaccessible locations should not be walked out
until all possible recovery has taken place. Horses with mild
muscle soreness may improve if walked slowly, but rest from
ride exertion is the primary recommended therapy.

Dehydration
The horse must have an adequate amount (10 to 15 gallons)
of water each day during a trek.

Clinical Signs
Signs of mild dehydration (3% body weight loss) are low
urine output, dry mouth, and mild loss of skin elasticity.

Moderate dehydration (5% body weight loss) is characterized by marked loss of skin elasticity. The eyes become
sunken. Blood pressure may fall as a result of decreased
plasma volume. Weakness, fever, and weak pulse may be
observed. Sweating is not possible, even with elevated body
temperature.

Marked dehydration (10% body weight loss) may involve
circulatory failure from decreased plasma volume.

Treatment
During 3 hours of hard work, a 450-kg horse may lose as
much as 45 L of fluid. If this degree of dehydration is not corrected quickly, death may result. The horse should be allowed
to drink along the trail if water is available. Small amounts of
cool, but not cold, water should be offered. If the horse refuses
to drink, gastric intubation may be indicated. Fluid is also
absorbed from the colon; thus enemas (10 to 20 L of water)
are effective in rehydration. Electrolyte replacement is encouraged, but for the usual case of dehydration, it is not critical.

Packaged electrolytes are available in veterinary supplies shops.

Heat stress usually accompanies dehydration, so cooling (such as shade or a water bath) is important. Administration of intravenous fluids, if available, is routine therapy.

Camels are uniquely adapted to desert conditions. They are able to survive a week without water. Optimally, a camel should be watered daily, just as are horses and llamas. Camels do not store water but conserve it by enduring a diurnal fluctuation of body temperature, from a normal 37.0° C (98.6° F) up to 42° C (107.6° F). The body acts as a heat-sink during the heat of the day, thus conserving vital water that would otherwise be lost through evaporative cooling. During the cool desert night, the heat is dissipated by conduction. Camels are able to concentrate urine to a syrup consistency to avoid water loss through urine. Fecal pellets are passed that are dry enough to be used for fuel immediately following defecation.

The camel is able to tolerate a 40% reduction in body weight from dehydration, and after such severe dehydration is able to drink sufficient water at one session to rehydrate. The shape of the camel erythrocyte is elliptical, allowing circulation in the face of significant hemoconcentration. This elliptical shape allows expansion of the cell to 250% of normal volume without hemolysis when rehydration occurs.

Exhausted Horse Syndrome

The term *exhausted horse syndrome* (EHS) was coined to describe a complex metabolic disease occurring when horses are pushed beyond endurance limits.

Clinical Signs

Although a composite picture exists, the individual horse may show only a few signs. The severely affected horse is depressed and exhibits lethargic movements, holding its head low. The ears are expressionless. Facial grimacing creates an anxious expression that may progress to a painful expression if colic or muscle spasms accompany the syndrome. The horse takes no interest in its surroundings. Anorexia is typical, and frequently the horse has no inclination to drink, even though dehydrated. The corneas appear glazed.

Body temperature is usually elevated and may reach 41° C (106° F). The horse does not cool properly. Usually, body temperature continues to rise. Temperature measured rectally may be inaccurate in the exhausted horse because the anal sphincter loses tone and allows air to enter the rectum.

Cardiovascular and respiratory systems are markedly affected by endurance riding. Heart and respiratory rates are elevated. The rates depend on the prior condition of the horse, pace, length of action, and amount of work performed in climbing or walking on soft footing. Heart rates of 150 beats/minute are not uncommon after a grueling climb. With 10 to 15 minutes of rest, the heart rate of a conditioned horse should drop below 60 beats/minute, whereas in the exhausted horse, tachycardia and tachypnea may persist. The exhausted horse may have a respiratory rate faster than the heart rate. Respiration under these circumstances is shallow and inefficient. Additional cardiopulmonary signs may include synchronous diaphragmatic flutter, arrhythmias, murmurs, and visible jugular pulses. Auscultation of the thorax may reveal moist rales and, in extreme cases, frank pulmonary edema.

Severe dehydration is the most consistent sign of EHS. Loss of skin elasticity, sunken eyeballs, and dry mouth and mucous membranes reflect a 7% to 10% loss of body weight, after loss of 30 to 40 L of fluid. Serious electrolyte and acid-base imbalances are associated with dehydration. Alkalosis is common.

Muscular manifestations of EHS include fatigue; trembling; spasm; stiffness; muscles painful to palpation; and, rarely, exertional rhabdomyolysis (stiff gait, excessive sweating, high respiratory rate, firm, and painful muscles of the back and rump).

Horses suffering from EHS are prone to colic, which also may occur independently. When colic accompanies EHS, it is of the spasmodic type, with diminished or absent borborygmus.

Treatment

Rest, rehydration, and electrolyte supplementation are the keys to recovery. If the horse is drinking and will take electrolytes in the water, the effect is nearly as beneficial as the administration of intravenous fluids. Packaged electrolyte powders can be carried.

If the horse is hyperthermic, shows evidence of shock, and refuses to drink, more drastic steps must be taken. The horse may require 40 to 50 L of fluid. Besides intravenous fluid (80 mL/kg/hour) administration, gastric intubation may be employed to give fluids orally. Enemas are also effective because fluid is absorbed from the colon (it is essentially impossible to instill water into the rectum too rapidly or in too great a volume as long as the fluid is allowed to be pushed out by peristaltic activity.

Synchronous Diaphragmatic Flutter

Synchronous diaphragmatic flutter (SDF) is a clinical sign observed in endurance horses while on long-distance rides and may be seen on an expedition. SDF is defined as a spasmodic contraction of the diaphragm synchronous with the heartbeat. It is not life threatening in itself but indicates mild to serious metabolic conditions that may be or become life threatening. Overexertion with excessive sweating produces metabolic alterations. The development of SDF at any point on a trek should be ample reason to prevent the horse from going farther until the metabolic alteration is resolved.

Contrary to what is seen in acute exertional stress characterized by acidemia, SDF is associated with alkalemia. Electrolyte imbalances may also be involved.

Clinical Signs
SDF may develop after 20 to 30 miles of riding. No sex, age, or breed predilection exists. The primary sign is spasmodic contraction in the flank area. The "thump" is easily felt by light palpation in the flank area. A person who auscultates the heart while holding a hand over the dorsocaudal rib area can tell that diaphragmatic contraction is synchronous with the heartbeat. SDF may be the only clinical sign noted, or it may be seen as part of EHS.

The degree of thumping may vary from a barely perceptible quiver to a contraction that seems to rock the horse's body and is observable from a distance. The flutter may be continuous or intermittent, especially in degree.

Treatment
Rest and rehydration are required.

Colic

Colic is the clinical manifestation of abdominal pain, usually the result of a gastrointestinal disorder. The most likely inciting causes on a trek are overeating of nonregular forages, ingestion of poisonous plants, or exhaustion.

Clinical Signs
Horses express colic by looking back at one side, stamping the feet, getting up and down, rolling, and pressing the head against trees or rocks. The pulse rate may exceed 100 beats/minute with severe pain. The conjunctival membranes are congested and cyanotic.

Treatment

Only superficial emergency measures are discussed. Treatment is variable, depending on the anatomic location of the obstruction or spasm. Mild obstructions may be relieved by hydration and administration of a cathartic. Cold water enemas may stimulate sluggish intestinal peristalsis and relieve impaction of the small (terminal) colon.

Pain and spasms may be relieved by administration of flunixin meglumine (Banamine), 1.1 mg/kg intramuscularly twice a day. Walking the horse may prevent it from lying down and rolling, which may result in a torsion of the intestine.

▶ UNIQUE MEDICAL PROBLEMS OF PACK LLAMAS

Nose bites from rattlesnakes are especially hazardous to llamas because local swelling may occlude the nostrils. Llamas are primarily obligate nasal breathers, so dyspnea and suffocation may ensue. Rattlesnake bites of the limbs cause edema and in severe cases local tissue necrosis and ulceration. Many cases are diagnosed as trauma unless the bite is observed. The signs of snakebite in llamas are essentially the same as for horses.

Therapy for a nose bite may require tracheotomy (in the upper third of the neck, the surgical approach is similar in all species) and insertion of an improvised tube to allow breathing. Edema may persist for 2 to 3 days. If the bite is observed and progressive swelling noted, a small tube (1-cm diameter) can be inserted 15 cm into the ventral meatus of the nasal passage and sutured to the nares. An alternative improvisation is to insert a woman's hollow plastic hair curler into the nostril. Swelling occurs around the tube or curler, but patency of the nasal passage is maintained.

▶ UNIQUE PROBLEMS OF DOGS

Porcupine Quills

When dogs are brought into porcupine country, the risk of an encounter is great. Some dogs fail to learn from experience and are repeatedly quilled. The dog must have physical contact with the porcupine for the tail to introduce the quills. The muzzle and face are the usual sites of penetration, and a dog can be blinded by perforation of the eyeball.

The quills must be removed physically. A pair of pliers should be included in supplies and equipment. The process is painful, and sedation with diazepam is indicated. The quill should not be broken because the retrograde barbs on the quill foster migration and abscess formation.

Grass Awns

Numerous species of grass awns ("foxtails") may become attached to the dog's hair coat or lodged in the external ear canal, nasal passage, conjunctival sac, or interdigital space.

Signs depend on the location of the foreign body. When it is within the ear canal, the dog paws at its ear and shakes its head. The head may be held tilted. Exudate may flow from the ear. Awns in the nostril cause sneezing and nasal exudate. Awns in the conjunctival sac cause lacrimation, photophobia, and corneal edema and ulceration. The dog paws at the eye. Awn penetration between the digits and at other locations through the skin is more difficult to diagnose because the awn may be at some distance from the fistula.

Awns must be removed physically. Sedation, topical anesthesia, or both may be necessary. Although topical ophthalmic anesthetics are desirable in the eye, lidocaine may be used in an emergency. A pair of small alligator forceps is most suitable for reaching into otherwise inaccessible places. An otoscope may be necessary to visualize awns in the nostril or ear canal. Instillation of an antiseptic or antibiotic ointment is desirable after removal of the awn.

Stinging Nettle Poisoning

Stinging nettle (*Urtica* species) is common along streams and lakes in wilderness areas. Humans vary in sensitivity when the plants accidentally contact exposed skin. Leaves and stems are covered by harsh hairs, some of which have a tiny ball tip that breaks off just before penetration. The specialized hairs are hollow. A base gland produces histamines and acetylcholine, which are injected into the victim.

Short-haired dogs that move through patches of stinging nettle are at risk of poisoning from the cumulative effect of thousands of minute injections of acetylcholine. Weakness, dyspnea, and muscle tremors are characteristic of the action of acetylcholine on peripheral nerves. Parasympathomimetic effects include salivation, diarrhea, tachycardia, and pupillary dilation. Atropine sulfate (0.04 mg/kg) subcutaneously is a specific treatment.

Medication Procedures

A list of medications and indications for their use is provided in Table 62-3. In the horse, intramuscular injections are given in the neck or rump. Subcutaneous injections are given by lifting a fold of skin just cranial to the scapula. Intravenous injections are given in the jugular vein, which is easily distended along the jugular groove on the ventral aspect of the neck.

In the llama, intramuscular injections are given in the relatively hairless area at the back of the upper rear leg, by standing against the body in front of the rear limb while facing the rear and reaching around the back of the animal to give the injection. Subcutaneous injections are given in the relatively hairless area of the caudal abdomen, just in front of the rear limb or by lifting a fold of skin just cranial to the scapula.

In the dog, intramuscular injections may be administered in the triceps muscles caudal to the shoulder or in the muscle masses on the upper rear limb. Subcutaneous injections are made by lifting a fold of loose skin on the neck near the withers. Intravenous administration is via the jugular vein or the cephalic vein. For the latter, an assistant grasps the limb at the elbow to occlude the vein, which courses on the dorsal aspect of the forearm. The vein is more visible if the hair is wetted down with water.

▶ EUTHANASIA

Indications for euthanasia include compound and comminuted fractures of long bones; falling or sliding into inaccessible places from which the animal is unable to extricate itself or trek participants are unable to aid the animal; lacerations exposing abdominal or thoracic organs (e.g., wild animal attacks or ramming tree branches into the body); head injuries resulting in persistent convulsions or coma; and protracted colicky pain unrelieved by analgesics or mild catharsis, usually associated with a pulse rate greater than 100 beats/minute, rolling, and congested conjunctival membranes.

The expedition may carry a bottle of euthanasia solution, which must be given intravenously or intraperitoneally. If firearms are carried, a properly placed bullet to the head produces a fast and humane death. For placement, the shooter stands in front of the animal's head and draws an imaginary line from the medial canthus of each eye to the base of the opposite ear. The shot should be aimed where those lines cross and approximately perpendicular to the contour of the forehead (Fig. 62-5). The tip of the barrel should be no more than 6 inches from the head. A heavy blow to the head at the same location is equally effective.

TABLE 62-3. Medications for Trek Animals

GENERIC NAME	TRADE NAME (COMPANY)	CONCEN-TRATION IN VIAL	ROUTE OF ADMINIS-TRATION
Acepromazine maleate	Prom Ace (Fort Dodge)	10 mg/mL	IM or IV
Ampicillin sodium	Generic	—	IM
Atropine sulfate	Generic	2 mg/mL	IM, SC
Benzathine penicillin G	Benza Pen (Pfizer)	150,000 U/mL	IM
Charcoal (activated)	Generic	—	PO
Dexamethasone	Azium (Schering-Plough)	2 mg/mL	IM
Diazepam	Generic	5 mg/mL	IV, IM
Epinephrine	Generic (Bayer)	1:1000, 1 mg/mL	IV, IM
Fenbendazole	Panacur (Hoechst Roussel)	—	PO
Flunixin meglumine	Banamine (Schering-Plough)	—	IM
Ivermectin	Ivomec (Merck AGVET)	—	PO, SC
Ketamine	Vetelar (Pfizer)	100 mg/mL	IV, IM
Lidocaine	Generic	2%	SC
Magnesium oxide	Carmilax (Pfizer)	361 g/lb	PO
Magnesium sulfate	Generic	—	PO
Phenylbutazone	Butazolidin (Schering-Plough)	200 mg/mL 1-g tab	IV, PO
Trimethoprim/ sulfamethoxa-zole	Tribrissen (Schering- Plough)	24%	IV, SC
Xylazine	Rompun (Bayer)	100 mg/mL	IV, IM
Euthanasia solution	T-61 (Taylor)	—	IV

IM, intramuscular; IV, intravenous; PO, oral; SC, subcutaneous; q, every; bid, twice daily; tid, 3 times daily; qid, 4 times daily.

DOSAGE AND INTERVAL

HORSE	LLAMA	DOG	INDICATION
0.04-0.1 mg/kg	Not indicated	0.05-0.22 mL/kg	Tranquilizer
10-50 mg/kg qid	10-25 mg/kg tid	25 mg/kg q6hr	Infection
0.04 mg/kg	0.04 mg/kg	0.04 mg/kg	Stinging nettle
Not recommended	5000-15,000U/kg q 2 days	40,000U/kg q 5 days	Infection
60-250 g	100 g	3-5 g	Toxins
2-4 mg/kg	1-2 mg/kg	4 mg/kg q8hr	Shock
0.05-0.1 mg/kg	0.2-0.4 mg/kg	2-5 mg/kg	Sedation
0.1-0.4 mg/kg	0.1-0.5 mg/kg	0.1-0.5 mg/kg	Anaphylaxis
5-20 mg/kg	10-15 mg/kg single dose	50 mg/kg	Parasites
1 mg/kg daily	1 mg/kg daily	0.3 mg/kg daily	Colic pain, inflammation
0.2 mg/kg single dose	0.2 mg/kg single dose	Not indicated	Parasites
2 mg/kg	2-5 mg/kg	Not indicated	Anesthesia
As needed	As needed	As needed	Local anesthesia
—	10-20 g total dose	—	Cathartic
20-100 g	Not indicated	8-25 g	Cathartic
1-2 g/450 kg, 2-4 g/450 kg daily	2-4 mg/kg daily	15 mg/kg q8hr	Pain, inflammation
2 mg/kg bid	2 mg/kg bid q12hr	2.2 mg/kg	Infection
0.5-1 mg/kg	0.25-0.5 mg/kg	1.1 mg/kg	Sedation
40 mL total dose	25 mL total dose	0.3 mL/kg	Euthanasia

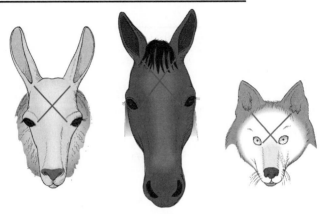

Figure 62-5. Location for euthanasia blow or shot.

The blow may be administered with the blunt edge of a single-bladed ax or hatchet. A large rock held in the hand may also be used. A less desirable but sometimes expedient method is to sever the jugular vein to allow exsanguination. This would probably be used on an animal that is already unconscious.

Avalanche Resources

▶ **GENERAL AVALANCHE INFORMATION**

www.avalanche-center.org
The CyberSpace Avalanche Center: The avalanche center is a source of worldwide avalanche information including news, conditions, forecasts, accidents, education, and forums.

www.americanavalancheassociation.org
American Avalanche Association (AAA): The national professional association for avalanche workers in the United States maintains a website with information about the study, forecasting, control, and mitigation of snow avalanches.

www.avalanche.org
Avalanche Org: Avalanche.org provides global, high-level avalanche information to public and professional avalanche workers. It is also a link to current avalanche conditions throughout the United States.

www.fsavalanche.org
The U.S. Forest Service National Avalanche Center: fsavalanche.org provides technology transfer and education for the U.S. avalanche community.

www.avalanche.ca
Canadian Avalanche Center: The Canadian Avalanche Center provides Canadian-based reports, information, and conditions.

▶ **REGIONAL AVALANCHE INFORMATION**

Twenty-four-hour regional avalanche information is available, generally from November through April, from the following Internet Web sites or recorded telephone messages.

California
Internet: www.sierraavalanchecenter.org
Truckee: 530-587-2158
Internet: www.esavalanche.org
Mammoth Lakes: 760-924-5500
Internet: www.shastaavalanche.org
Mount Shasta: 530-926-9613

Colorado
Internet: http://avalanche.state.co.us
Denver/Boulder: 303-275-5360
Fort Collins: 970-482-0457
Colorado Springs: 719-520-0020
Summit County: 970-668-0600

Crested Butte: 970-349-4022
Aspen: 970-920-1664
Durango: 970-247-8187

Idaho
Internet: www.avalanche.org/~svavctr/
Sun Valley: 208-622-8027

Montana
Internet: www.mtavalanche.com/
Bozeman: 406-587-6981
Missoula: 406-549-4488

New Hampshire
Internet: www.mountwashington.org/avalanche

Utah
Internet: www.avalanche.org/~uac
Salt Lake City: 801-364-1581
Provo: 801-378-4333
Ogden: 801-626-8600
Park City: 435-658-5512
Logan: 801-797-4146
Alta: 801-742-0830
Moab: 801-259-7669

Washington and Oregon
Internet: www.nwac.us
Seattle: 206-526-6677
Portland: 503-808-2400

Wyoming
Internet: www.jhavalanche.org/
Jackson: 307-733-2664

Canada
Internet: www.avalanche.ca

Glasgow Coma Scale

This scale evaluates the degree of coma by determining the best motor, verbal, and eye-opening response to standardized stimuli.

Eye Opening	
Spontaneous	4
To voice	3
To pain	2
None	1
Verbal Response	
Oriented	5
Confused	4
Inappropriate words	3
Incomprehensible words	2
None	1
Motor Response	
Obeys command	6
Localizes pain	5
Withdraw (pain)	4
Flexion (pain)	3
Extension (pain)	2
None	1
TOTAL:	

C

Contingency Supplies for Wilderness Travel

ITEM	DESCRIPTION, QUANTITY (NO.; WEIGHT)*	COMMENT
1. Whistle	Nonmetal, shrill (1 oz)	Emergency signal (bursts of 3)
2. Knives	A sturdy folding or straight knife plus a multitool knife	e.g., Swiss Army knife
3. Maps	Trail and topographic (1 oz) (as needed per group)	Plastic coated or with cover
4. Compass, fluid-filled	≤2° gradations (1-2 oz)	Know area declination
5. Headlamp	LED most efficient; lithium or alkaline spare batteries attachment (one; 3-6 oz)	Headlamp if using flashlight
6. Sunglasses	With side and nose blocks; polycarbonate or glass lens (1-3 oz)	>99% UVB filtering; >85% light absorption
7. Rescue and survival guide	Condensed (3-6 oz) (one per group)	Learn basic air-to-ground signals
8. Pencil and paper	Waterproof paper preferred (2 oz)	
9. Quarters	Two (1 oz)	Phone calls; wrap in plastic and tape inside kit
10. Accident report forms	Waterproof preferred, (1 oz) (two per group)	
11. Spare sunglasses	(1-3 oz) (two per group)	May improvise—make slits in cardboard, cloth
12. Toilet paper, small roll	One (1 oz)	Store in plastic bag
13. Matches, waterproof	"Strike-anywhere" type, 12	Store in plastic bag
14. Spare bulb, batteries	(1-3 oz)	Store in plastic bag

ITEM	DESCRIPTION, QUANTITY (NO.; WEIGHT)*	COMMENT
15. Closed-cell foam pads	1 × 1 ft sections; 1-3 (3 oz)	e.g., Ensolite; to insulate stove, seats, use as cervical collar or splint pads
16. Avalanche cord	Red; metal arrows (2 oz)	Attach to body
17. "Space" blanket	56 × 84 inches, two to three (1 oz)	Emergency insulation (replace every 3 yr)
18. Surveyor's trail tape	Bright color, 50 ft (1 oz) (per group)	Trail, avalanche site markers
19. Utility cord	Nylon 25-50 ft (2 oz)	Shelter; utility
20. Heat source	Candle; fuel tabs, one or two (2 oz)	
21. Emergency toboggan kit	Variable (per 2-3 persons)	Convert skis and poles; e.g., NSP
22. Goggles	Rose or amber (4 oz)	Double lens, polarized preferred
23. Radio beacon	(8 oz); e.g., Pieps, Skadi, Ortovox	Use in avalanche terrain
24. Scraper	Metal edged (1 oz)	Ice and wax removal
25. Shovel	Lexan or aluminum (16-32 oz) (per 1-3 persons)	e.g., REI
26. Facemask	Leather, silk, or synthetic (1 oz)	
27. Aerial flares; ground smoke bombs	Red smoke, two to four (1 oz) (per group)	Rescue signal
28. "Bungie" elastic cords with hooks	6-12 inch (1-2; 1 oz)	Pack compression; lash equipment to pack
29. Swami belt	1-inch webbing 10-20 ft (4-8 oz)	Waist, seat harness
30. Carabiner, locking type	Aluminum, (2-3; 3 oz)	Climbing or rappel harness; rope brake; Prusik handle
31. Rescue pulley	Small, (1-2; 2 oz)	Cliff, crevasse rescue

Continued

ITEM	DESCRIPTION, QUANTITY (NO.; WEIGHT)*	COMMENT
32. Rope, Perlon or Goldline	5.5-9 mm, 50-75 ft (8-16 oz) (per group)	Rescue, evacuation
33. Magnifying lens	8-15 × (1 oz) (per group)	Snow crystal examination; map reading; splinter removal; fire starter
34. Altimeter	≤20-ft accuracy (2 oz) (per group)	Altitude orienteering; barometric changes
35. Saw	Wire or blade (2-15 oz) (per 1-4 persons)	Fuel or shelter (cuts wood, snow, ice)
36. Extra food and candy	1-day supply (8-16 oz)	Prevent hypothermia
37. Extra clothing	Wool preferred	Sock doubles as mitten
38. Signal mirror	Unbreakable preferred (1 oz)	
39. Road flare	5-minute, (1-3; 3 oz)	Rescue signal; emergency fire starter
40. Extra ski wax	Klister or two-wax system (3 oz)	
41. Emergency shelter	"Tube" tent, tarp, or bivvy sack (3-16 oz)	May improvise with large plastic bags
42. Extra water	1 pint, metal container preferred (18 oz)	Metal canteen can be heated directly
43. Thermometer, outdoor	In protective case (0.5 oz) (per group)	Snow, water, air temperature
44. Lens antifogger	Liquid or stick (1 oz)	For glasses, goggles
45. Climbing skins, adhesive	"Skinny" type (11-16 oz)	Urgent snow climbing, or slowing descent

*Quantity is per person per trip, unless otherwise specified; weight given is per individual item, in ounces (35 oz = 1 kg = 2.2 lb).

Repair Supplies for Wilderness Travel

1. Duct tape (lots)
2. Parachute cord
3. Cable ties (large and small)
4. Extra plastic hardware (e.g., cord locks, Fastex buckles, d-rings)
5. Safety pins
6. Heavy-duty needle or sewing awl and thimble
7. Nylon thread
8. Multitool or screwdrivers (flat and Phillips No. 2)
9. Wire (e.g., braided steel, i.e., picture hanging wire or paper clips)
10. Awl (on multifunction knife)
11. Glue (e.g., two-component epoxy, meltable nylon glue stick)
12. Seam sealer
13. Adhesive ripstop nylon (and alcohol swabs)
14. Tent pole splint
15. Knife sharpener

▶ BACKCOUNTRY SKIING OR CLIMBING

1. Spare bale and screws (for repair of ski binding)
2. "P-tex" ski base repair
3. Spare ski tip (if lightweight or fragile skis)
4. Spare crampon wrench
5. Crampon file

Priority First-Aid Equipment

Airways
Antiseptic towelettes
SAM splint
Dressings, bandages, Kling, tape, cravats, Ace wrap
Flashlight
Germicidal soap
Notebook and pencil, tags
Pain medications
Plastic bags (for snow, sprain and contusion treatment)
Pocket mask
Safety pins
Bandage scissors or trauma shears
Syringe (20 mL) for irrigating with 18-gauge catheter tip
Thermometers (low reading for cold weather and high altitude; regular for hot weather)
Xeroform or Vaseline gauze
Nitrile examination gloves
Wound closure strips
Tincture of benzoin
Dermabond tissue glue
Scalpel with No. 11 blade
Tourniquet
Cotton-tipped applicators
Moleskin and Molefoam
Duct tape
Adhesive cloth tape
CPR mouth barrier
Cavit
Paraffin (dental wax) stick
Dental floss
Disposable skin stapler and remover
4 × 4 inch sterile dressing pads
3-inch sterile gauze bandage
Elastic bandage with Velcro closures

▶ FOR EXPEDITIONS AND THE MEDICALLY TRAINED

Bag-mask
Chest tube set (Heimlich valve, McSwain dart)
Cricothyrotomy set
Foley catheter, gloves, lubricant, clamp, and plug
For allergic reactions and anaphylaxis: bee sting kit, EpiPen or Twinject, diphenhydramine (Benadryl)

For high altitude: acetazolamide (Diamox), dexamethasone (Decadron), furosemide (Lasix)

For pneumonia and other infections: antibiotics

IV solutions, sets, needles

Oxygen

Suction device (mechanical)

Instant glucose

Stethoscope

Urine pregnancy test

Urine test strips (e.g., Clinitek)

Gamow Bag for travel to high altitude

Pulse oximeter for travel to high altitude

Amoxicillin: adult dose, 250 to 500 mg q8h; pediatric dose, 8 to 15 mg/kg (2.2 lb) q8h (tid).

Amoxicillin/clavulanate (Augmentin): adult dose, 500 to 875 mg bid; pediatric dose, 25 to 45 mg/kg in two divided doses per day. For otitis media in children, use the higher dose.

Ampicillin: same dose as phenoxymethyl penicillin (see later).

Azithromycin (Zithromax): adult dose, 500 mg day 1, then 250 mg/day for 4 additional days; pediatric dose, 10 mg/kg day 1, then 5 mg/kg for 4 additional days.

Cefadroxil (Duricef): adult dose, 500 mg to 1 g bid. For pharyngitis, to eradicate group A *Streptococcus,* an acceptable dose is 1 g/day for 10 days. Pediatric dose: for skin infections, 30 mg/kg/day in two divided doses; for pharyngitis, administer in a single dose or two divided doses for 10 days.

Cefdinir (Omnicef): adult dose, 300 mg bid for 10 days; pediatric dose, 14 mg/dg/day bid for 5 to 10 days.

Cefixime: adult dose, 400 mg/day; pediatric dose, 8 mg/kg/day; no refrigeration needed; discard 14 days after the dry powder is reconstituted with water.

Cefuroxime axetil: adult dose, 500 mg bid; pediatric dose, 30 mg/kg in two divided doses per day.

Cefpodoxime (Vantin): adult dose, 200 to 400 mg bid for pneumonia.

Cephalexin (Keflex): adult dose, 250 mg q4-6h or 500 mg q12h; pediatric dose, the same as for phenoxymethyl penicillin. *Avoid use in a person with penicillin allergy* because 5% to 10% of persons allergic to penicillin are allergic to cephalosporins.

Chloroquine (Aralen): adult dose, 500 mg q wk for prevention; 1500 mg on day 1, then 500 mg daily × 2 days for treatment.

Ciprofloxacin (Cipro): adult dose, 500 mg bid for 3 days to treat infectious diarrhea. *This drug should not be given to pregnant women or children younger than age 18.*

Clarithromycin (Biaxin): adult dose, 500 mg bid; pediatric dose, 15 mg/kg in two divided doses per day.

Clindamycin (Cleocin): adult dose, 150 to 450 mg PO qid; pediatric dose, 8 to 25 mg/kg/day suspension divided tid/qid.

Dicloxacillin: same dose as phenoxymethyl penicillin (see later).

Doxycycline (Vibramycin): adult dose, 100 mg bid for treatment or once a day for prevention of infectious diarrhea. *Do not give to pregnant women or children up to age*

7 *years* because this drug may cause permanent dark discoloration of the teeth.

Erythromycin: same dose as phenoxymethyl penicillin (see later). A common side effect is stomach upset and diarrhea. This drug is the first alternative for penicillin in penicillin-allergic individuals.

Erythromycin/sulfisoxazole (Gantrisin): pediatric dose, 50 mg/kg based on the erythromycin component in four divided doses a day.

Fleroxacin: adult dose, 400 mg/day for 3 days for the treatment of infectious diarrhea.

Fluconazole (Diflucan): adult dose, 150 mg daily.

Levofloxacin (Levaquin): adult dose, 250 to 500 mg PO/IV qd.

Metronidazole (Flagyl): adult dose, 250 mg tid. *Do not drink alcohol when taking this medication and for 3 days afterward. The interaction would cause severe abdominal pain, nausea, and vomiting.*

Nitazoxanide (Alinia): adult dose 500 mg bid for 3 days; pediatric dose, 100 mg bid for 3 days.

Noroxin: adult dose, 400 mg q12h.

Ofloxacin: adult dose, 300-400 mg q12h.

Phenoxymethyl penicillin (Penicillin Vee K): adult dose, 250 to 500 mg q4-6h; pediatric dose: 2 to 6 years, 125 mg q6-8h, 6 to 10 years, 250 mg q6-8h. For pharyngitis, to eradicate the group A *Streptococcus,* an acceptable adult dose is 1 g bid for 10 days.

Quinine: adult dose 650 mg tid × 7 days for malaria in chloroquine-resistant areas.

Tetracycline: adult dose, 500 mg 4 qid. *Do not give to pregnant women or children up to age 7 years* because this drug may cause permanent dark discoloration of the teeth.

Trimethoprim with sulfamethoxazole (Bactrim or Septra double strength): adult dose, 1 pill (80 mg TMP with 400 mg SMX) bid for infectious diarrhea or bladder infection; 1 pill once a day for prevention of traveler's diarrhea. The pediatric dose for an ear infection or severe infectious diarrhea (caused by *Shigella* bacteria) is 1 tsp of the pediatric suspension per 10 kg body weight q12h (bid), not to exceed 4 tsp (the adult dose) per dose. More precisely, the pediatric dose is 4 mg/kg/dose TMP with 20 mg/kg/dose SMX.

Wilderness Eye Kit

▶ OPHTHALMIC ANTIBIOTIC SOLUTIONS

Fluoroquinolones
Fluoroquinolones provide excellent coverage for serious corneal infections. These drugs should be considered for remote expeditions with potential for prolonged evacuation times. They are very expensive and not mandatory for less severe infections (e.g., bacterial conjunctivitis). Examples include the following:

Gatifloxacin ophthalmic solution (Zymar)
Moxifloxacin (Vigamox) ophthalmic solution

Other Topical Antibiotic Solutions
Gentamicin (Garamycin) 3 mg/mL ophthalmic solution
Tobramycin (Tobrex) 0.3% ophthalmic solution

Topical Antiseptic/Antibiotic Ointments
Bacitracin (AK-Tracin) 500 U/g ophthalmic ointment
Erythromycin (Ilotycin) 5 mg/g ophthalmic ointment
Gentamicin (Garamycin) 3 mg/g ophthalmic ointment
Tobramycin (Tobrex) 0.3% ophthalmic ointment

Antiviral Agent
Trifluridine (Viroptic) 1% ophthalmic solution

Systemic Antibiotics
Although not specific to ocular infection, fluoroquinolones are ideal because of their high intraocular tissue penetration (e.g., levofloxacin [Levaquin] 500 mg or ciprofloxacin [Cipro] 500 mg or 750 mg tablets).

Systemic Steroid
Prednisone 20 mg tablets

▶ TOPICAL ANESTHETIC AGENT

Proparacaine hydrochloride (Ophthaine) 0.5% ophthalmic solution
The ocular examination is better tolerated after administration of a topical anesthetic agent. Do not use a topical anesthetic agent repeatedly because it can delay corneal re-epithelialization. A few drops of a topical anesthetic can help differentiate a superficial (corneal or conjunctival) process from a deeper intraocular cause of pain. Do not use a topical anesthetic with a suspected open globe injury.

▶ MYDRIATIC-CYCLOPLEGIC

Cyclopentolate hydrochloride (Cyclogyl) 1% ophthalmic
  solution, intermediate duration, or homatropine (Isopto
  homatropine) 5% ophthalmic solution, longer duration
  (@ 1 to 2 days)
Homatropine has greater efficacy than cyclopentolate, but
there are times when the longer duration of homatropine
may be excessive (e.g., when the victim needs to negotiate
difficult terrain the next morning). Ciliary muscle spasm is
thought to play a role in the pain of many ocular conditions.
A mydriatic paralyzes the pupillary constrictor muscle
(sphincter), causing pupillary dilation. A cycloplegic relaxes
the ciliary muscles.

▶ TOPICAL STEROID

Prednisolone acetate (Pred Forte) 1% ophthalmic solution
  Note: Use of ocular steroids may cause exacerbation of infectious keratitis (herpes simplex); increase intraocular pressure; and cause cataract formation with prolonged use. A
topical steroid will probably not cause significant side effects
if given to a victim with a fluorescein-negative eye disorder for
no more than 2 to 3 days.

▶ TOPICAL NONSTEROIDAL ANTIINFLAMMATORY DRUGS (NSAIDS)

Diclofenac (Voltaren) ophthalmic solution
Ketorolac (Acular) ophthalmic solution)

▶ TOPICAL VASOCONSTRICTOR AND DECONGESTANT

Pheniramine maleate 0.3% plus 0.025% naphazoline ophthalmic solution (Naphcon-A)
  This combination helps control the inflammatory symptoms
of conjunctivitis. It is most useful for the treatment of allergic
symptoms.

▶ ADDITIONAL SUPPLIES

Fluorescein Strips

Strips are lighter in weight than drops and avoid the potential
for contamination. When examining an eye with a possible
infectious process, always use a separate fluorescein strip for
each eye to avoid cross-contamination.

Artificial Tears

Polyvinyl alcohol 1% (Hypo Tears) ophthalmic solution

Hypertonic Ophthalmic Saline Solution (Muro 128 Solution)

This is used for corneal erosion (relatively rare but difficult to treat; see later).

Headlamp

Penlight with cobalt blue filter or small blue LED

Small magnifying lens; small, lightweight, Fresnel-type hand lenses can be purchased at many office supply stores

▶ OPTIONAL AGENTS FOR TREATMENT OF ANGLE-CLOSURE GLAUCOMA

(This is an unlikely presentation.)

Timolol 0.5% (Timoptic) ophthalmic solution

Pilocarpine hydrochloride (Pilocar) 2% ophthalmic solution

Acetazolamide (Diamox) 250-mg tablets

Recommended Oral Antibiotics for Prophylaxis of Domestic Animal and Human Bite Wounds

▶ **FOR ESTABLISHED INFECTIONS WHEN THE ORGANISMS ARE KNOWN**

Treat according to specific antibiotic sensitivities of cultured organism(s).

▶ **WHEN ORGANISMS ARE UNKNOWN (DOG AND MOST OTHER BITES)*†**

DRUG	CHILD	ADULT
Standard:		
Amoxicillin-clavulanate‡	30-40 mg/kg/day in 3 divided doses	250 mg PO tid or 500 mg PO bid
or		
Second-generation ceph-alosporin with anaerobic activity		
or		
Penicillin and first-generation cephalosporin		
or		
Clindamycin *plus*		300 mg PO qid
Ciprofloxacin		500 mg PO bid
or		
Azithromycin	10 mg/kg PO day 1, then 5 mg/kg days 2-5	500 mg PO day 1, then 250 mg days 2-5
or		
Trovafloxacin (restrict use to seriously ill, hospitalized patients)		
or		
BMS-284756 (garenoxacin)		

Continued

DRUG	CHILD	ADULT
or Experimental ketolide antibiotics: HMR 3004 (RU64004) or HMR 3647 (RU 66647)		

*This regimen is effective for most potential pathogens. No single antibiotic covers everything.

†Penicillin is excellent for *Pasteurella* but is not optimal for many other significant pathogens. Most patients can take an oral cephalosporin such as cephalexin without adverse effect. Erythromycin is not effective against *Staphylococcus* or *Pasteurella*, so close clinical observation is necessary if this antibiotic is chosen.

‡In the case of pig bite, ciprofloxacin, when not contraindicated, should be added to amoxicillin-clavulanate.

Therapy for Parasitic Infections

ETIOLOGIC AGENT	DRUG AND DURATION
Giardia lamblia	Quinacrine,* 100 mg tid for 7 days for adults, 7 mg/kg/day in 3 divided doses for 7 days for children; albendazole 400 mg qd for 7 days; tinidazole (Tiniba), 2 g PO single dose; nitazoxanide, 500 mg bid for 3 days (100 mg bid for 3 days for children 1-4 yr; 200 mg bid for 3 days for children 4-11 yr); or metronidazole, 250 mg tid for 7 days for adults, 15 mg/kg/day in three divided doses for children Infants: furazolidone, 1.5 mg/kg qid for 7 days
Entamoeba histolytica	Carrier/no symptoms: iodoquinol, 650 mg tid for 20 days for adults and 40 mg/kg/day in 3 divided doses for 20 days for children; or paromomycin, 500 mg tid for 7 days Intestinal disease: metronidazole, 750 mg tid for 5-10 days for adults, or metronidazole, 50 mg/kg/day in 3 divided doses for 10 days for children; or tinidazole 1000 mg bid for 3 days, followed by iodoquinol 650 mg tid for 20 days; or paromomycin 500 mg tid for 7 days
Dientamoeba fragilis or *Balantidium coli*	Tetracycline, 500 mg qid for 10 days, or iodoquinol, 650 mg tid for 20 days for adults
Entamoeba polecki	Metronidazole, 250 mg tid for 10 for adults
Blastocystis hominis	Iodoquinol, 650 mg tid for 20 days, or metronidazole, 750 mg tid for 10 days for adults
Cryptosporidium parvum	Nitazoxanide 500 mg bid for 3 days or paromomycin, 500 mg tid for 7 days, plus azithromycin, 500 mg/day for 5 days; for adults in severe cases or patients with AIDS, consider nitazoxanide 500 mg bid for 2 wk, paromomycin 500-750 mg tid or qid for 2 wk, or azithromycin 1200 mg qd for 4 wk

Continued

ETIOLOGIC AGENT	DRUG AND DURATION
Isospora belli	Trimethoprim/sulfamethoxazole (TMP/SMX), 160 mg/800 mg qid for 10 days, followed by same dose bid for 3 wk; or pyrimethamine 75 mg qd with folinic acid 10 mg qd for 2 wk
Cyclospora or *Sarcocystis*	TMP/SMX, 160 mg/800 mg bid for 7 days for adults, and TMP, 5 mg/kg, SMX, 25 mg/kg bid for 7 days for children; for patients with AIDS, follow with same dose in adults and children 3 times per wk until cured
Angiostrongylus cantonensis	Mebendazole, 100 mg bid for 5 days for adults and 100 mg bid for 5 days for children
Ascaris lumbricoides	Mebendazole, 100 mg bid for 3 days or 500 mg once for adults and 100 mg bid for 3 days for children
Babesia spp.	Clindamycin, 600 mg tid for 7 days, plus quinine, 650 mg tid for 7 days for adults
Schistosoma (bilharziasis)	Praziquantel, 40-60 mg/kg/day in 2 doses for 1 day in adults and 40-60 mg/kg/day in 2 doses for 1 day for children
Microsporidiosis	Albendazole 400 mg bid for 2-4 wk, followed by chronic suppression in patients with AIDS
Tapeworms: *Diphyllobothrium latum* (fish), *Taenia saginata* (beef), *Taenia solium* (pork), *Dipylidium canium* (dog)	Praziquantel, 5-10 mg/kg once for adults and for children
Strongyloides stercoralis	Ivermectin, 200 μg/kg/day for 1-2 days for adults and for children
Trichomonas vaginalis	Metronidazole, 2 g once; or 250 mg tid for 7 days for adults and 15 mg/kg/day in 3 doses for 7 days for children
Trichuris trichiura (whipworm)	Mebendazole, 100 mg bid for 3 days for adults and for children
Trypanosoma cruzi	Nifurtimox, 8-10 mg/kg/day in 3-4 doses for 90-120 days for adults

*If available; otherwise, use metronidazole or tinidazole.

Sample Basic Wilderness Survival Kit

Everyone traveling away from paved roads should develop the habit of carrying, at the very least, a minimalist survival kit consisting of basic equipment for shelter, fire craft, and signaling. This kit is a piece of equipment that is easily transported on a bike ride, an afternoon hike, or a trail run. It is one of those "Don't leave home without it" pieces of equipment. Each person in the group should have their own basic survival kit.

This kit is contained in its own small pack and consists of the following:

Shelter-building equipment:

> 3- or 4-ml plastic bag, nylon tarp, or blue polyethylene tarp (not a "space blanket")
>
> Parachute cord, 50 to 100 feet

Fire-building equipment:

> Metal match and striker
>
> Petroleum-impregnated cotton balls in a screw-top container
>
> Waterproof and windproof matches

Sharp, solid shank hunting knife with a 4- to 6-inch blade (NOTE: Other types of tinder include steel wool, dryer lint, magnesium shavings, and a variety of commercial products. The items listed here (metal match and striker, petroleum-impregnated cotton balls, and the method of waterproof and windproof matches) are the most reliable and easiest to carry. They burn the longest (steel wool and magnesium burn quickly) and are therefore recommended for a survival scenario.)

Signaling equipment:

> Whistle
>
> Signal mirror, preferably glass with sighting device
>
> Flagging tape

Other:

> Headlamp (small LED) with spare batteries and bulb (also for signaling)
>
> Multitool
>
> Small roll of duct tape
>
> Goat skin leather gloves for working with wood
>
> Two days of personal prescription medications

For multiday trips into the wilderness, the following can be added to the basic kit:

> Pencil and small waterproof paper notebook
>
> Spare eyeglasses
>
> Sunglasses
>
> Sunblock

Lip balm with high SPF number
Compass
Map of area of travel
Toilet paper
Spare clothing (wool hat, mittens, fleece or down jacket, cagoule)
Emergency food
First-aid kit
Water container
Water disinfection equipment: chemicals or filter
Insect repellent (in season)
Folding saw

Emergency repair tool kits should be carried and adapted to type of travel (e.g., ski, snowshoe, kayak):
Small screwdriver with multiple tips
Picture wire
Fiberglass tape
Steel wool for shimming
Assorted nuts, bolts, and screws
Ski tips
More duct tape

Additional considerations:
Emergency personal locator beacon (PLB)
GPS
Altimeter
Thermometer (plastic alcohol type clipped to loop on outside of pack)
Fishhooks and line
No. 28 piano wire for snares
Cellular or satellite telephone
.22-caliber rifle and ammunition
Cigarette lighter

Sample Winter Survival Kit

In addition to basic survival items from Appendix J, take the following:
1. Winter sports repair kit
2. Spare wool or fleece clothing for severe weather (at least four layers total):
   a. A hat, neck gaiter, and neoprene face cover or balaclava
   b. Spare mittens
3. Snow shovel: small grain-scoop type with detachable handle
4. Piece of Ensolite or Therm-a-Rest mattress
5. In avalanche terrain:
   a. Avalanche beacon
   b. Probe poles
6. Optional items:
   a. Sleeping bag
   b. Gore-Tex bivouac sac
   c. Stove and fuel
   d. Light ax
   e. Snow saw

Sample Desert Survival Kit

In addition to basic survival items from Appendix J, take the following:

Fold-up steel shovel with short handle

Items for construction of four solar stills:

1. Four sheets of clear plastic, 6 × 6 feet, reinforced in center by cross of duct tape
2. Four pieces of surgical tubing, 6 to 8 feet long
3. Four 1-quart plastic bowls
4. 5-gallon water jug, full (when space and weight conditions permit)

1-L wide-mouth bottle for use as urinal

Large sun hat and/or cotton cravat, bandana, or large handkerchief for fashioning a head covering

Spare sunglasses

Heavy leather gloves

Citizens band radio

Light rifle or target pistol with ammunition

Sample Camp and Survival Gear for Jungle Travel

1. Trail shoes (1 pair)
2. Camp boots (1 pair)
3. Special cleats (e.g., Covell Ice Walker Quick Clip Cleats)
4. Socks, lightweight cotton or thin nylon (3 pairs)
5. Hat (1)
6. Pullover garment, polyester (1)
7. Shirts, cotton
   a. Long sleeved (2)
   b. Short sleeved (2)
8. Pants, lightweight cotton or Supplex or Taslan (2 pairs)
9. Undergarments
   a. Underpants, lightweight polyester mesh (3)
   b. Sports bra, cotton or cotton-Lycra blend mesh (2)
10. Poncho, nylon (1)
11. Flannel sheet
12. Hammock or Therm-a-Rest
13. Mosquito net
14. Backpack for porter
15. Personal backpack
16. Antifogging solution for eyeglasses
17. Batteries
18. Binoculars
19. Camera equipment and film
20. Campsuds
21. Candles, dripless
22. Cup (Lexan polycarbonate)/plate (melamine)
23. Duct tape, 1 small roll
24. Ear plugs
25. Fishing supplies
26. Garbage bags
    a. 30-gallon size (4)
    b. 13-gallon size (4)
27. Headlamp
28. Inflatable cushion
29. Insect repellent
30. Laminated maps
31. Machete (Collins style)
32. Waterproof matches or butane piezo ignition lighter
33. Pen
34. Toilet paper
35. Leatherman pocket survival tool
36. Polycarbonate wide-mouth bottles (2)
37. Razor/battery-operated shaver
38. Spoon
39. Sport sponge
40. Sunglasses
41. Umbrella
42. Whistle, plastic
43. Zipper-lock bags
    a. Gallon size (5)
    b. Quart size (5)
    c. Pint size (5)

N

Vehicle Cold Weather Survival Kit

In addition to basic survival items from Appendix J, take the following:

Sleeping bag or two blankets for each occupant

Extra winter clothing including snow boots, wool or fleece hat, and mittens for each occupant

Emergency food

Two 36-hour candles in a can

Space blanket

First-aid kit

Spare doses of personal medications—enough for 3 or more days

Two plastic water jugs, full

Large, heavy-duty, zipper-lock plastic bags

Extra toilet paper

Citizens band radio or cell phone

Flashlight with extra batteries and bulb (if LED spare bulb not applicable)

Battery booster cables

Tire chains

Snow shovel

Tow chain or strap, at least 20 feet long

Small sack of sand

Tool kit

Gas line deicer

Signal flares

Long rope

Carbon monoxide detector

Ax

Folding saw

Full tank of gas

1. Experts generally recommend that individuals in a vehicle caught in a snowstorm stay inside the vehicle. It is the best source of shelter available. Minimizing exposure is important. In a severe storm, going outside the car to find firewood, and then maintaining the fire, would be nearly impossible.

2. If in deep and accumulating snow, it is important NOT to run the car engine and heater for warmth. The exhaust pipe(s) can become blocked by blowing/drifting snow, causing carbon monoxide to enter the car. The candles will provide adequate heat in combination with the sleeping bags and extra clothing for 72 hours.

3. Some authorities recommend running the engine for a few minutes in order to operate the vehicle's heater, then having a quiet period until the temperature drops. If this technique is used, it is necessary to check the exhaust pipe(s) before running the motor, for the reason stated earlier.
4. After the storm abates and it becomes safe to exit the vehicle, flares and smoke from a fire (e.g., burning oil in a hubcap) can be used for signaling as needed.

O

Pediatric Wilderness Medical Kit: Basic Supplies

Assorted adhesive bandages
Butterfly bandages or Steri-Strips
Gauze pads
Cotton-tipped applicators
Gauze roll
Nonadherent dressings
Tape
Moleskin or Spenco 2nd Skin
Eye patches
Triangular bandage or sling
Elastic bandage
Povidone-iodine solution 10% (use to cleanse wounds and disinfect water)
Antiseptic wipes (benzalkonium chloride)
Antibacterial soap
Tincture of benzoin
Alcohol wipes
Lightweight malleable splint (SAM splint)
Needles
Safety pins
Syringe, 20 to 35 mL (for wound irrigation)
Plastic catheter or irrigation tip, 18-gauge (for wound irrigation)
Bulb syringe
Digital thermometer
Scissors
Tweezers
Sunscreen waterproof cream, SPF of at least 15
Insect repellent (no more than 35% DEET)
First-aid book
Whistle
Identification card with basic health information (past medical history, medications, allergies, blood type, weight, immunizations)
Surgical stapler, suture material, and suturing supplies
Dermabond (2-octyl cyanoacrylate) tissue glue

Medicines Specific to Women's Health

INDICATION	MEDICATION*	DOSE
Dysmenorrhea	Ibuprofen	200 mg 1-4 tabs q4-6h
Headache, pain, fever	Acetaminophen	325-500 mg
Nausea and vomiting	Promethazine (Phenergan) (tablet or suppository)	25 mg q4-6h
	Ondansetron (Zofran) oral dissolving tablet	4 mg q4-6h
Urinary tract infection	Nitrofurantoin	100 mg bid × 7 days
	Ciprofloxacin	250-500 mg bid × 3 days
	Trimethoprim-sulfamethoxazole	160 mg/800 mg bid × 3 days
Urinary analgesic	Pyridium	200 mg tid PRN
Pyelonephritis	Ciprofloxacin	500 mg bid × 14 days
Yeast vaginitis	Miconazole cream or suppository	One applicator HS × 3-7 days
	Fluconazole	150 mg single dose
Bacterial vaginosis	Metronidazole tablets	250-500 mg bid to tid
	Metronidazole vaginal gel; clindamycin vaginal cream	One applicator HS × 3-7 days
Menstrual regulation or breakthrough bleeding	Oral contraceptive pills	As directed
	Conjugated estrogen	2.5 mg qd
	Medroxyprogesterone acetate	5-10 mg qd
Nutritional supplements	Ferrous sulfate	300 mg qd-tid
	Calcium carbonate multivitamin	1250 mg qd

*Suggested medications or equivalent depending on tolerance, allergy history, and patient preferences.

qd, daily; bid, twice daily; tid, three times daily; qid, four times daily; HS, at bedtime; PRN, as needed.

Q   Drug Storage and Stability

Sarah R. Williams, David A. Nix, and Ketan H. Patel

▶ BACKGROUND

Stability data on drug products are generally derived from studies done under controlled and artificial environmental conditions. However, drug stability in the setting of "real-world" variable climate conditions is more difficult to study. Only limited research in this area has been published.

This appendix reviews the data currently available on drugs likely to be carried in field and expedition medical kits. The list is extensive, and for smaller expeditions only a fraction of the more critical medications will be required. However, it is also useful for medical professionals who are setting up field hospitals and clinics in suboptimal climate conditions.

Most medications, as indicated in the following sections, have strict temperature ranges at which they should be maintained to assure their potency. Other factors including light, humidity, and packaging also influence the shelf life and sterility of a drug. Strong packaging is critical; if a parenteral drug (packaged in a syringe for ready use) is frozen, the drug may be fully potent, but its sterility may have been lost due to hairline cracks in the plastic caused by freezing. Polyvinyl (plastic) containers often used to package drugs may affect product stability. Glass containers, although considered the most inert of storage vessels, may leach alkali and associated decomposition products into the product, thereby initiating chemical reactions that alter drug potency. The inclusion of preservatives in the drug formulation and the actual processes used by the manufacturer may also make products more or less resilient in the face of prolonged storage. Thus for most of the drug products listed, stability and sterility cannot be guaranteed if products are stored under conditions deviating from those recommended by the manufacturer. The following guide should be supplemented with drug packaging information provided by the manufacturer.

▶ EXPIRATION DATES

Drug manufacturers usually set shelf life by calculations of drug potency under ideal conditions. Shelf life is the time during which the potency is expected to be greater than or equal to 90% of the drug's initial potency at manufacture. Shelf life assumes that the drug is maintained at optimal storage conditions.

866

Extremes of temperature, high humidity, loss of integrity of original packaging, and exposure to light can all potentially shorten this period. In addition, some drugs may actually have decreased bioavailability after exposure to nontemperate climate conditions. This is because the rate of dissolution is often the rate-limiting step in the absorption of many medications taken by mouth and further complicates a drug's pharmacodynamics. High heat and humidity conditions can affect the rate of product dissolution.

▶ STORAGE OPTIONS

Unfortunately, the wilderness setting leaves few options for the storage of drugs under ideal environmental conditions. Vehicular storage, although a convenient option in many cases, can expose drugs to temperature variations much greater than ambient conditions unless efforts are actively undertaken to control the temperature swings.

Vehicle-powered cooling devices are a viable option in this setting, assuming the vehicle battery is kept charged. Styrofoam or plastic cooler boxes with cooling packs are an adequate storage modality as well but can be somewhat cumbersome on a trekking expedition. Many small coolers are available, however, so medications that require cooling or darkness can be separated out and stored in a manageable small unit.

Portable refrigeration units may be required for long-term storage of products that require strict constant refrigeration, especially if ice is not going to be readily available. Many of these units require electricity and are equipped with enough insulation to prevent their contents from becoming too warm in the event of a power failure for up to several hours if unopened. A few products can also run on natural gas or kerosene, thereby ameliorating the problem of unreliable electricity supply. Systems with passive cooling such as ice packs tend to be lighter, whereas those with active cooling systems can be much heavier (over 50 kg [110 lb]).

An important consideration in choosing these devices and other, simpler ice coolers is the thickness of their foam insulation and the durability of the surrounding encasement, often constructed of metal or plastic. The amount of snow or ice used for cooling varies depending on the ideal temperature storage range for each drug. A thermometer should be kept inside the box near the medications and monitored regularly.

Portable generators can weigh as little as 12 kg (26.5 lb), but careful consideration of the power needs for the expedition should be made before purchase because the weight to be carried can increase quickly with increased power requirements. Additional weight is also incurred for the generator's power source. Power types include batteries, liquid fuel, and solar panels. Solar has the added advantage of being lightweight and renewable. Several solar products are ideal for portable heating and cooling equipment and for recharging car batteries.

Many medications suggest storage at "room temperature" of 15° C to 30° C (59° F to 86° F). For these, standard refrigeration is not appropriate. Electric medication storage boxes are available and for long expeditions are a reasonable solution. A more inexpensive, lightweight solution for short-term medication storage problems is to use chemical heat packs or instant cold packs (both widely commercially available) to heat or cool the ambient temperature inside a cooler. Confirm appropriate temperature range with a thermometer. Chemical heat packs can produce up to 150° F (70° C) of heat and last for several hours, so do not place them directly on the medication. Otherwise, the medication may "cook"; also avoid direct ice application to avoid inadvertent freezing. Routinely recheck the medication thermometer.

Whatever storage container is chosen should be waterproof and, if possible, airtight. Consider adding a desiccant to decrease damage from humidity. Many medications need to be protected from light, so if the box is transparent, place it in a dark bag. Place loose tablets in a bottle or blister pack to avoid breakage. If product packaging is discarded to save space, retain the product information leaflet and dosing information in a plastic bag.

No formal consensus on the long-term effect of humidity and other climate changes on many medications is available. Anticipate that any gel-encased medication such as a suppository may melt in high humidity and/or warmth, making it challenging to use even if it is still medically active.

After longer trips, consider replacing medications with a fresh stock.

▶ DRUG STABILITY INFORMATION

The following drugs and other medical products are nearly always based on studies done in controlled environmental conditions. It is often difficult to ascertain whether a drug product can be safely used after storage under conditions other than those specified by the manufacturer.

The question of stability of drug products pertains not only to the drug itself but also to the container in which it is packaged. If, for example, a parenteral drug packaged in a syringe for ready use is frozen, the drug itself may be fully potent, but the sterility of the product may be lost due to hairline cracks from freezing of the syringe.

Thus for most of the drug products listed, stability and sterility cannot be guaranteed if stored under conditions other than those recommended by the manufacturers.

Slight variations in packaging and formulation between brands may influence the drug's stability. The following guide should be supplemented with drug packaging information provided by the manufacturer.

Any deviation from the manufacturer's recommendations is the choice of the treating medical professional and is neither condoned nor approved by the authors of this chapter.

Medications are listed by their generic names. Where trade names are given, no endorsement of a particular product is implied unless explicitly stated.

By pharmaceutic convention, "room temperature" is defined as between 15° C and 30° C (59° F and 86° F) and "controlled room temperature" is defined as between 20° C and 25° C (68° C and 77° F).

Availability in the United States is subject to Food and Drug Administration (FDA) and Drug Enforcement Agency (DEA) regulations and annotated as OTC (over-the-counter), Rx (prescription required), DEA Schedule (Schedule [S] II to S IV), or NA (not available in the United States).

▶ **ACETAMINOPHEN TABLETS, ELIXIR, AND SUPPOSITORIES (OTC)**

Store at room temperature and definitely below 40° C (104° F). Avoid freezing because stability after freezing is unknown. This medication is not known to be light sensitive. Keep suppositories refrigerated below 27° C (81° C).

▶ **ACETAMINOPHEN WITH CODEINE TABLETS AND ELIXIR (S III)**

Store at room temperature and definitely below 40° C (104° F). Do not refrigerate or freeze. Protect from light and moisture.

▶ **ACETAMINOPHEN WITH HYDROCODONE TABLETS (S III)**

Store at room temperature and definitely below 40° C (104° F). Do not refrigerate or freeze. Protect from light and moisture.

► ACETAZOLAMIDE TABLETS, SUSTAINED-RELEASE CAPSULES, INJECTION, AND ORAL FORMULATION (Rx)

Store tablets at room temperature; store capsules at controlled room temperature.

Oral formulation: a studied extemporaneous oral formulation of acetazolamide 25 mg/mL in a 1:1 mixture of Ora-Sweet, Ora-Plus, and in cherry syrup (diluted 1:4 with simple syrup) was stable at 94% of initial concentration for up to 60 days. Temperatures tested were 5° C and 25° C (41° F and 77° F), and the solutions were protected from light.

Store powder for injection at room temperature. Manufacturer labeling states that the reconstituted drug is stable for 12 hours at room temperature and for 3 days if refrigerated (36° F to 46° F). Other research, however, has demonstrated 90% potency for 1 week at room-temperature conditions, 4 weeks when refrigerated, and 8 weeks when frozen (admixed with 50 mL D5W, 100 mL sodium chloride injection, 50 mL lactated Ringer's injection, or 45 mL lactated Ringer's injection with 5 mL sodium bicarbonate 5%). Do not freeze if combined with lactated Ringer's with sodium bicarbonate because the solution becomes turbid. Do not administer if discoloration, cloudiness, or particulate matter is observed.

► ACETIC ACID SOLUTION (OTC)

Store in airtight containers at controlled room temperature. Protect from light.

► ALBUTEROL TABLETS, SYRUP, AND INHALED FORMULATIONS (RX)

Tablets and syrup: store between 2° C and 25° C (36° F and 77° F). Protect tablets from excessive moisture. Refrigeration of syrup can improve taste.

Aerosol inhalers: store at room temperature. Do not expose to excessive temperatures (49° C, 120° F) for more than 1 to 2 days because of the explosive danger of chlorofluorocarbons. Do not puncture or incinerate aerosol containers.

Inhalation solution and capsules for inhalation: store between 2° C and 30° C (36° F and 86° F). Inhalation solution is light yellow to clear; discard if discolored.

► ALOE GEL, OINTMENT, LAXATIVES (OTC)

Topical: *Aloe vera* has been used for burns, wounds, and as an antipruritic. Pharmacologically it is composed of substances capable of producing topical anesthesia, bactericidal activity, and increased local microcirculation, but actual therapeutic capability is not clear. Lotions are for external use only. Product stability in extremes of temperature is not well studied.

Laxatives: Aloe acts as a stimulant laxative if taken internally because of anthraquinone glycosides. Aloe laxatives (e.g., Nature's Remedy) should be stored at room temperature in airtight containers. Avoid humidity and temperatures higher than 38° C (100° F).

▶ ALUMINUM ACETATE OTIC AND TOPICAL PREPARATIONS (OTC)

Otic solution: a clear colorless liquid comprised of acetic acid 2% in aqueous aluminum acetate solution. Store below 30° C (86° F) but protect from freezing.

Topical solution: stable virtually indefinitely, but partially used irrigation solutions have high potential contamination rates. Label extemporaneously prepared solutions with a 7-day expiration date, which is consistent with the shelf life recommended by the manufacturer.

▶ AMIODARONE TABLETS AND VIALS (Rx)

Store tablets and vials for intravenous (IV) administration at room temperature. Protect both from light during storage. The IV form does not need to be protected from light during infusion itself. Note that dosing studies were performed using polyvinyl chloride (PVC) tubing. The use of other plastic tubing may affect dosing because as amiodarone IV has been found to leach out plasticizers. This effect is exacerbated by higher drug concentrations and lower flow rates than recommended by the manufacturer.

▶ ANTACIDS (OTC)

Avoid freezing aluminum hydroxide or milk of magnesia products. If frozen, many antacids separate into water and gel layers on thawing. Freezing is not known to affect the therapeutic value of the product, but anecdotally it affects taste and prevents reformation of the emulsion, even with shaking.

▶ ASPIRIN TABLETS, ORAL SOLUTION, AND SUPPOSITORIES (OTC)

Tablets: Aspirin is stable in dry air but gradually hydrolyzes to salicylate and acetate and gives off a vinegar odor. Most manufacturers recommend storage at room temperature.

Oral solution: An extemporaneous oral solution can be made from a commercial buffered effervescent tablet (Alka Seltzer) with 90 mL of water.

Suppositories: Store between 2° C and 15° C (36° F and 59° F).

▶ ATENOLOL TABLETS (Rx)

Store at controlled room temperature, 20° C to 25° C (68° F to 77° F). Dispense in well-closed, light-resistant containers.

▶ ATROPINE INJECTION (Rx)

Store at room temperature and protect from light. Atropine sulfate 1 mg/mL solutions packaged in Tubex (0.5 mL and 1 mL) have been shown to be stable for 3 months. Atropine methylnitrate 10 mg/mL solutions are stable for 6 months when stored in dark bottles at room temperature. Inspect solution before administration for the presence of particulate matter, cloudiness, or discoloration and discard if present.

▶ AZITHROMYCIN TABLETS, CAPSULES, SUSPENSION, AND INJECTION (Rx)

Tablets and capsules: Store below 30° C (86° F).

Suspension: Single-dose packets should be refrigerated if possible (5° C to 30° C, 41° F to 86° F) and, if reconstituted with 60 mL of water, used immediately. Discard multiple dose suspension after 10 days.

Injection: Store under 30° C (86° F). After preparation, it is stable for 24 hours at room temperature and for 7 days if refrigerated.

▶ BACITRACIN TOPICAL (OTC) AND INJECTION (Rx)

Topical: Store at room temperature. If in ointment form, it is stable but rapidly inactivated in water. Calamine, benzocaine, and zinc oxide have been combined with bacitracin without affecting its stability. If in aqueous solution, it must be refrigerated. Bacitracin is stable for only 1 week due to oxidation.

Injection: Store sterile powder for injection between 2° C and 15° C (36° F and 59° F), and protect from light. Solution is stable for 1 week after reconstitution if refrigerated.

▶ BISMUTH SUBSALICYLATE TABLETS AND SUSPENSION (OTC)

Store at room temperature and avoid heat greater than 40° C (104° F). Suspension should not be frozen.

▶ BRETYLIUM TOSYLATE (Rx)

Store at room temperature. Protect from freezing.

▶ BUPIVACAINE INJECTION (Rx)

Bupivacaine is a relatively stable drug, but excessive heat or cold decreases its shelf life. Store between 15° C and 40° C (59° F and 104° F). If frozen, bupivacaine may be used after thawing provided the container is completely intact and the solution remains clear. Bupivacaine with epinephrine exposed to light and/or temperatures higher than 40° C (104° F) for a long period should not be used due to loss of epinephrine effect.

▶ BUTORPHANOL TARTRATE INJECTION AND NASAL SOLUTION (S IV)

Store below 30° C (86° F). Protect from light, and do not freeze. Inspect parenteral drug for particulate matter or discoloration before use and discard if present.

▶ CALCIUM CHLORIDE INJECTION (Rx)

10% solution: Drug pH is altered significantly if frozen or exposed to temperatures higher than 40° C (104° F). The product should be considered unusable if either occurs.

▶ CEFTRIAXONE INJECTION (Rx)

Store powder for injection at or below 25° C (77° F). Protect from light. The color of solution ranges from light yellow to amber, depending on concentration, length of storage, and diluent. Once mixed, intramuscular (IM) and IV solutions remain greater than 90% potent for up to 10 days if refrigerated at 4° C (39° F). Potency is affected by diluent, concentration, and temperature. IM and IV preparations may maintain greater than 90% stability for as little as 1 or 3 days, respectively, at room temperature. If reconstituted with 5% dextrose or 0.9% sodium chloride solution and then frozen at −20° C (−4° F), preparations have been stable for 26 weeks in PVC or polyolefin containers. Thaw at room temperature before using. Unused thawed solutions should be discarded. Do not refreeze. Ceftriaxone may be incompatible with other antimicrobials; do not mix.

▶ CEPHALEXIN CAPSULES, TABLETS, AND ORAL SUSPENSION (Rx)

Capsules and tablets: Store at room temperature.
Suspension: Stable after reconstitution for up to 14 days if refrigerated, ideally between 2° C and 8° C (36° F and 46° F). Keep tightly closed. Shake well before using.

▶ CHARCOAL, ACTIVATED (OTC)

Sealed aqueous suspensions may be stored for at least 1 year in tightly sealed containers. For longest shelf life, keep in well-sealed metal or glass containers.

▶ CIPROFLOXACIN CAPSULES, TABLETS, SUSPENSION, AND INJECTION (Rx)

Oral: Store tablets at room temperature, and store capsules and suspension diluent below 25° C (77° F), but do not freeze. Discard unused suspension after 14 days. Protect from light.

Injection: Store flexible containers between 5° C and 25° C (41° F and 77° F) and IV infusion vials between 5° C and 30° C (41° F and 86° F). Avoid temperatures higher than 40° C (104° F) and protect from light. When injection is diluted for injection, it is stable for 2 weeks at either room temperature below 30° C (86° F) or when refrigerated between 2° C and 8° C (36° F and 46° F). Do not freeze.

▶ CYCLOPENTOLATE HYDROCHLORIDE OPHTHALMIC SOLUTION (Rx)

Store between 5° C and 25° C (41° F and 77° F). Keep in tightly capped airtight container.

▶ DEET-CONTAINING (*N,N*-DIETHYL-META-TOLUAMIDE, DIETHYLTOLUAMIDE) INSECT REPELLENTS (OTC)

Store at room temperature and in airtight containers. Avoid exposures of propellant cans to temperatures of 49° C to 54° C (120° F to 130° F) because of explosion danger. Do not store or use near fire or open flame. Avoid contact with plastic or rayon. DEET may be toxic internally, so store away from other consumables.

▶ DERMABOND (2-OCTYL CYANOACRYLATE) TOPICAL SKIN ADHESIVE (Rx)

Store below 30° C (86° F). Protect from moisture, direct heat, and incidental crushing. The product should be used immediately after crushing the glass ampule because it will not flow freely after a few minutes.

▶ DEXAMETHASONE INJECTION (Rx)

Injection: a clear, colorless to light yellow solution that is sensitive to light and extremes of temperature. Do not store at high temperature for long periods. It maintains full potency for 6 months at 40° C (104° F) and up to 3 months at 50° C (122° F). Do not use after freezing and protect from light except while injecting.

▶ DEXTROAMPHETAMINE TABLETS, ELIXIR, AND CAPSULES (S II)

Tablets: Store in well-sealed containers at room temperature.
Elixir and extended-release capsules: Store in tight, light-resistant containers, below 40° C (104° F), preferably at room temperature. Do not freeze elixir.

▶ DEXTROSE ORAL (OTC) AND INJECTION (Rx)

Oral: Store in well-airtight containers.
Injection: Store 50% parenteral dextrose below 25° C (77° F). Do not freeze or expose to extreme heat. Do not use if cloudy. Discard unused portions.

▶ DIAZEPAM TABLETS, ORAL SOLUTION, SUPPOSITORIES, AND INJECTION (S IV)

Tablets and elixir: Store at controlled room temperature. Protect from moisture and avoid freezing.
Oral solution: Store at controlled room temperature. Protect from moisture and avoid freezing. The solution is available as both a regular dose and concentrated solution requiring calibrated dropper for accurate dosing. Do not prepare and store doses for future use.
Suppository: Store at controlled room temperature and protect from moisture.
Injection: Store at controlled room temperature. If frozen, diazepam tends to flocculate and precipitate. Rewarm with warm water and, if no precipitate is visible, the product may be used. Do not inject if solution is cloudy, contains particulate matter, or is darker than slightly yellow.

▶ DIGOXIN INJECTION (Rx)

Digoxin has been shown to be stable at room temperature for 3 months in Tubex cartridges. Protect from light and store between 15° C and 25° C (59° F and 77° F). Use diluted injection immediately. This product is compatible with most IV infusion fluids.

▶ **DILTIAZEM CAPSULES, ORAL SOLUTION, AND INJECTION (Rx)**

Capsules: Store at room temperature. Protect from excess humidity.

Oral solution: 12 mg/mL solution prepared in Ora-Sweet, Ora-Sweet SF, Ora-Plus, or in a 1:4 mixture of cherry syrup and simple syrup was more than 92% potent for up to 60 days at either 5° C or 25° C (41° F or 77° F). In another study, 1 mg/mL solution prepared from dextrose, fructose, mannitol, and sorbitol (but NOT lactose) remained potent for a minimum of 50 days at 25° C (77° F).

IV solution: Preferably, store at between 2° C and 8° C (36° F and 46° F), without freezing, but may store at room temperature for up to 1 month, then discard.

▶ **DIPHENHYDRAMINE TABLETS, ELIXIR (OTC), AND INJECTION (Rx)**

Store at room temperature if possible in airtight containers. Tablet, elixir, and injection (10 mg/mL) forms are stable after freezing, but injection containers should be checked for cracks or leakage. Protect injection form from light.

▶ **DOMEBORO ASTRINGENT AND OTIC SOLUTIONS (OTC)**

Astringent solution: Do not cover compress or wet dressing with plastic; allow to breathe.

Otic solution: A clear colorless liquid. Store below 30°C (86°F). Avoid freezing.

▶ **DOPAMINE HYDROCHLORIDE INJECTION (Rx)**

Store at room temperature and protect from light. Brief exposure to temperatures of 40° C (104° F) is tolerated, but excessive heat should be avoided. Do not freeze. Do not use if there is yellow, pink, purple, or brown discoloration of the solution because this indicates decomposition. The diluted form is stable for injection for at least 24 hours after dilution.

▶ **DOXYCYCLINE CAPSULES, TABLETS, SYRUP, SUSPENSION, AND INJECTION (Rx)**

Oral formulations: Store capsules, tablets, syrup, and suspension below 30° C (86° F), preferably at room temperature. Store delayed-release capsules between 15° C and 25° C

(59° F and 77° F). Suspension is stable for 2 weeks after reconstitution if stored at room temperature.

Injection: Frozen, reconstituted 10 mg/mL solution for injection in sterile water is stable for 8 weeks when stored at −20° C (−4° F). After thawing, excess heating is not recommended. Do not refreeze. Protect from light. The infusion should be completed within 6 to 48 hours (brand and diluent dependent) if not refrigerated.

▶ EPINEPHRINE INJECTION (SALTS AND SOLUTIONS) (Rx)

Store at controlled room temperature and protect from light and air. Avoid freezing.

Heat above 40° C (104° F) and exposure to light may inactivate the product. Oxidation causes a color change to pink, then brown. Do not use if epinephrine is discolored or cloudy or contains precipitate.

▶ ERYTHROMYCIN TABLETS, SUSPENSIONS, TOPICAL, AND INJECTION (Rx)

Oral formulations: Erythromycin estolate and erythromycin ethylsuccinate (EES 200 and 400) liquid suspensions maintain their potency for 14 days at room temperature. Refrigeration maintains optimal taste. Tablets should not be crushed.

Topical: Stable for 2 years when stored at room temperature. Gel and pledgets should be stored at room temperature while ointment should be stored below 27° C (81° F). An extemporaneous topical solution made from tablets with hydroalcoholic vehicle as a 2% solution was stable for 60 days at 25° C (77° F). A 2.7% preparation in E-Solve was stable for 4 months when refrigerated between 4° C and 8° C (39° F and 46° F).

Injection: Stable at room temperature in dry form. Reconstituted IV solution should be used within 8 hours after preparation or within 24 hours if refrigerated. Drug stability may be maintained up to 2 weeks if refrigerated but carries significant risk of contamination. Solution may be frozen for 30 days and is stable if used within 8 hours of thawing under refrigeration conditions. Do not refreeze thawed solution.

▶ ESTAZOLAM TABLETS (S IV)

Store below 30° C (86° F). Stable for 3 years after date of manufacture.

▶ FLUOCINOLONE ACETONIDE OINTMENT AND SHAMPOO (Rx)

Ointment: Store in a tight container below 40° C (104° F), preferably at room temperature. Avoid freezing.
Shampoo: Stable for 3 months after extemporaneous formulation.

▶ FURAZOLIDONE TABLETS AND LIQUID (NA)

Store in light-resistant container. Exposure to strong light may cause darkening. Do not expose to excessive heat. May crush tablets and administer in spoonful of corn syrup.

▶ FUROSEMIDE ORAL FORMULATIONS AND INJECTION (Rx)

Oral, tablets and solutions: Store in tightly closed, light-resistant container at room temperature. Discard oral solution bottles 60 days after opening. Do not use if discolored.
Injection: Protect containers from light. When packaged in Tubex cartridges (2 mL of 10 mg/mL), potency was retained for 3 months at room temperature. If exposed to refrigeration, solution may be used barring evidence of cracking, leaking, or other damage to glass containers. All intact ampules or syringes, when returned to room temperature, should be vigorously shaken to redissolve any constituents that may have crystallized out of solution; stability should not be affected. Do not use if discolored.

▶ GLUCAGON INJECTION (Rx)

In powder form, glucagon should be refrigerated but is stable at room temperature for several weeks. When diluent is added to powder, the resulting solution may be refrigerated for up to 3 months. Thawing will not affect activity. Cloudy or thick diluent should not be used. Do not use if stored at temperatures greater than 35° C (95° F) for an extended period.

▶ HYDROCORTISONE TABLETS, SUSPENSION, TOPICAL CREAM, AND INJECTION (Rx)

Oral preparations: Store below 40° C (104° F), at room temperature. Protect suspension from light and freezing.
Topical: Do not refrigerate.
Injection: Do not freeze. Only use reconstituted solutions if clear and discard after 3 days.

▶ **HYDROMORPHONE TABLETS, ELIXIR, SUPPOSITORIES, AND INJECTION (S II)**

Tablets and elixir: Store at room temperature and protect from light.

Suppositories: Keep refrigerated.

Injection: Store at room temperature. Avoid refrigeration/freezing as precipitation or crystallization can occur, but product may be redissolved at room temperature without affecting stability. A slight yellowish discoloration does not affect potency. Polypropylene infusion syringes containing hydromorphone hydrochloride in normal saline were stable for 30 days when stored at 30° C (86° F).

▶ **IBUPROFEN TABLETS (OTC)**

Store at room temperature and protect from light.

▶ **INTRAVENOUS SOLUTIONS (D5W, D5NS, etc.)**

The effects of freezing these solutions are unknown. Incomplete resolubility, especially with electrolyte-containing solutions, seems a real danger.

▶ **ISOPROTERENOL HYDROCHLORIDE (Rx)**

Store at room temperature 15° C to 30° C (59° F to 86° F). Protect from light. Do not use if solution is pinkish to brownish in color.

▶ **KETOCONAZOLE SHAMPOO AND TABLETS (Rx)**

Shampoo: Store at or below 25° C (77° F). Protect from light.

Oral tablets: Store at room temperature. Protect from moisture.

▶ **LACRISERTS (HYDROXYPROPYL METHYLCELLULOSE) TOPICAL OCULAR SOLUTION (Rx)**

Store drops at room temperature in airtight containers. Protect from freezing.

▶ **LEVOFLOXACIN TABLETS AND INJECTION (Rx)**

Tablets: Store at room temperature and protect from light.

Injection: Store concentrate at room temperature and protect from light. Reconstituted form can be stored up to 3 days if kept below 25° C (77° F), 14 days if refrigerated between 2° C and 8° C (36° F and 46° F), and up to 6 months if frozen. Thaw at room temperature or under refrigeration conditions, but do not thaw by immersion in water or by microwave. A mild yellow/greenish color is normal and not indicative of contamination or breakdown. However, do not use if particulate matter or other discoloration is noted.

▶ LIDOCAINE INJECTION (Rx)

Lidocaine is a relatively stable drug, but excessive heat or cold decreases its shelf life. Store between 15° C and 40° C (59° F and 104° F). If frozen, it may be used after thawing provided the container is completely intact and the solution remains clear. Lidocaine with epinephrine exposed to light and/or temperatures higher than 40° C (104° F) for a long period should not be used because of loss of epinephrine effect.

▶ LIDOCAINE/EPINEPHRINE/TETRACAINE (LET) TOPICAL (Rx)

Anesthetic solution stored in amber glass (light-shielding) containers is stable for 4 weeks at approximately 18° C (65° F) and for 26 weeks if refrigerated (4° C, 39° F).

▶ LINDANE (GAMMA-HEXACHLOROCYCLOHEXANE) LOTIONS AND SHAMPOO (Rx)

The lotion and shampoo become thick when frozen but do not lose effect. The effect of high temperatures is unknown. Protect from light. Spray should not be exposed to temperatures below −2° C (28° F) or above 54° C (129° F).

▶ LOPERAMIDE HYDROCHLORIDE CAPSULES (OTC)

Store at room temperature. Do not mix oral solution with other solvents.

▶ LORAZEPAM TABLETS, ORAL SOLUTION, AND INJECTION (S IV)

Tablets: Store at room temperature and protect from moisture.
Oral solution: Refrigerate between 2° C and 8° C (36° F and 46° F). Protect from light.
Injection: Refrigerate between 2° C and 8° C (36° F and 46° F). Protect from light. Do not use if cloudy, discolored, or if particulate matter is present.

▶ MANNITOL INJECTION (Rx)

Injection form (5% to 25% solution): Store at controlled room temperature. Solutions of 15% or higher may crystallize at temperatures below 25° C (77° F) but will resolubilize when warmed to 70° C to 80° C (158° F to 176° F) in a water bath. A reheated solution must be allowed to cool to body temperature before administration. Microwaves had been used to reheat mannitol, but extreme caution is indicated because explosions of ampules have been reported. Sterility cannot be guaranteed if frozen.

▶ **MEPERIDINE HYDROCHLORIDE ORAL SOLUTION AND INJECTION (S II)**

Oral solution: Store at room temperature. Protect from moisture, light, and freezing.

Injection: Store at room temperature. Protect from moisture, light, and freezing. If frozen, injection form may be used after thawing if the solution shows no signs of precipitation or cloudiness and if the ampules or vials show no signs of cracking or leaking.

▶ **METOPROLOL ORAL PREPARATIONS AND INJECTION (Rx)**

Store at 25° C (77° F). Excursions permitted to 15° C to 30° C (59° F to 86° F). Do not freeze. Protect from moisture. Store in a tight, light-resistant container.

▶ **MIDAZOLAM ORAL SOLUTION AND INJECTION (S IV)**

Oral solution: An oral solution of 2.5 mg/mL, made from injectable midazolam and a flavored, dye-free syrup, maintained at greater than 90% of the original concentration throughout a 56-day trial period at temperatures of 7° C, 20° C, and 40° C (45° F, 68° F, and 104° F).

Injection: Store in syringes or glass at room temperature and protect from light. Parenteral midazolam of 2 mg/mL (hydrochloride salt) in 0.9% sodium chloride injection was stable in polypropylene infusion-pump syringes at both 5° C and 30° C (41° F and 86° F) for 10 days. A 3 mg/mL concentration is maintained with at least 90% stability for 1 week when stored in disposable polypropylene syringes in 20° C, 32° C, and 60° C (68° F, 90° F, and 140° F). Midazolam 40 mg/L in 0.9% sodium chloride was stable when protected from light at 21° C (70° F) over 24 hours, with no loss in glass or laminate containers and less than 2% loss in PVC bags.

▶ **MODAFINIL TABLETS (S IV)**

Store at controlled room temperature. Not known to be light sensitive.

▶ **MORPHINE SULFATE INJECTION (S II)**

Store at room temperature in airtight containers. Protect from light. When exposed to air, morphine sulfate loses its water and concentration may change, producing higher than expected dosing. Avoid freezing. If freezing occurs, it does not affect potency but may form precipitate. Solution should be colorless to pale yellow. Do not inject if cloudy, discolored, or contains precipitate. May use if precipitate resolubilizes with shaking. Most studies of morphine stability have been limited to 30 days, but one study noted stability after 14 weeks of frozen storage. However, intentional freezing cannot be recommended.

▶ **MOXIFLOXACIN TABLETS AND INJECTION (Rx)**

Tablets: Store at room temperature and protect from high humidity.
Injection: Store premixed flexible containers at room temperature and protect from light. Do not refrigerate because IV solution tends to precipitate. Do not use if particulate matter or discoloration is noted.

▶ **NALBUPHINE HYDROCHLORIDE INJECTION (Rx)**

Store at room temperature and protect from light. Do not use if discolored or contains precipitate.

▶ **NALOXONE HYDROCHLORIDE INJECTION (Rx)**

Store at room temperature and protect from light. Dilute solution before use, and if not used, discard any solution 24 hours after dilution. Do not save partial doses for future use. Do not administer if discoloration, cloudiness, or precipitate are observed. Protect from freezing, and do not use if frozen.

▶ **NEOSPORIN OINTMENT (OTC)**

Store at controlled room temperature.

▶ **NIFEDIPINE CAPSULES, TABLETS, AND INJECTION (Rx)**

Capsules: Store between 15° C and 25° C (59° F and 77° F) and protect from light.
Tablets: Store at room temperature and protect from light.
Injection: Store below 25° C (77° F). Ready-to-use infusion retains potency for only 1 hour in daylight and 6 hours in artificial light. Keep in light-sealed container until absolutely ready to use.

▶ NITROGLYCERIN SUBLINGUAL TABLETS, SPRAY, TOPICAL, AND INJECTION (Rx)

Oral preparations: Keep sublingual tablets in original glass container, tightly capped. Discard cotton once removed. Store at room temperature. Protect from moisture, heat, cold, and humidity. Discard unused sublingual tablets after 6 months. Translingual spray has guaranteed potency for 4 years from the date of manufacture when stored below 50° C (122° F).

Topical ointment: Keep tube tightly closed, and store at room temperature.

Injection: Nitroglycerin solutions (diluted in 5% dextrose or 0.9% sodium chloride solutions in glass containers) are stable for up to 2 days at room temperature and up to 7 days when refrigerated. Extemporaneous solutions of nitroglycerin in concentrations ranging from 0.035 to 1 mg/mL were stable in glass for up to 70 days at room temperature and for 6 months when refrigerated. Brief exposure up to 40° C (104° F) does not adversely affect the potency or stability of the solution. Do not freeze.

▶ NORFLOXACIN TABLETS AND OPHTHALMIC SOLUTION (Rx)

Tablets: Store at room temperature and definitely below 40° C (104° F). Store in tightly closed containers.

Ophthalmic solution: store at room temperature and protect from light.

▶ OFLOXACIN TABLETS, OTIC SOLUTION, AND INJECTION (Rx)

Tablets: Store below 30° C (86° F) in a tightly closed container.

Otic solution: Store at room temperature in airtight container.

Injection: Store single-use vials and premixed bottles at room temperature. Store premixed mini-bags at or below 25° C (77° F). Avoid light, freezing, and excessive heat. Brief exposure to 40° C (104° F) has not been shown to damage product.

▶ PENICILLIN G PROCAINE INJECTION (Rx)

Penicillin should be refrigerated but is stable at room temperatures for 6 months. Higher temperatures increase hydrolysis and decrease potency. May be frozen and retain potency. Solutions prepared for injection are stable at room temperature for at least 1 day and up to 1 week if refrigerated.

▶ PENICILLIN GK INJECTION (Rx)

Penicillin is stable in powder form for 2 to 3 years if stored at no greater than 30° C (86° F). Higher temperatures cause decreased potency. Solutions prepared for injection are stable at room temperature for at least 1 day and up to 1 week if refrigerated.

▶ PHENOBARBITAL INJECTION (S IV)

Store at room temperature and protect from light. Not stable in aqueous solutions. Inspect for precipitate and discoloration before use, and do not administer if present.

▶ PHENYLEPHRINE NASAL (OTC), OPHTHALMIC SOLUTION (Rx), AND INJECTION (Rx)

Do not use nasal, ophthalmic, or parenteral solutions if brown in color or if there is precipitation. Store parenteral solution at room temperature and definitely below 40° C (104° F). Protect all forms from light and freezing.

▶ PHENYTOIN TABLETS AND INJECTION (Rx)

Oral preparations: Store at room temperature. Protect from moisture and light.

Injection: Store at room temperature. Solution is stable if there is no precipitation or haziness. A precipitate may form when refrigerated or frozen but will dissolve when warmed to room temperature. A faint yellow color has no effect on potency. More stable in normal saline than in 5% dextrose. Infuse within 2 hours of mixing the solution, then discard.

▶ POLYSPORIN OINTMENT (Rx)

Store between 15° C and 25° C (59° F and 77° F).

▶ POTASSIUM PERMANGANATE ASTRINGENT SOLUTION (OTC)

Diluted form is used to clean wounds, ulcers, abscesses, and dermatoses. Use 0.1% solution in water to be diluted 1 in 10 before use to provide a 0.01% solution. Undiluted potassium permanganate is composed of dark purple or almost black crystals or granular powder and is soluble in cold and boiling water. It is incompatible with iodides, reducing agents, and most organic substances and may be explosive if it contacts organic or other oxidizable substances.

▶ POVIDONE IODINE SOLUTION (OTC)

Do not heat because iodine concentration may decrease due to interaction with dissolved oxygen or increase due to water evaporation. Store between 37° C and 42° C (99° F and 108° F).

▶ PREDNISONE TABLETS, ORAL SOLUTION, AND SUSPENSION (RX)

Store at room temperature and definitely below 40° C (104° F). Protect from light using airtight container. A suspension prepared using 50 mg of prednisone powder, 100 mg of sodium benzoate, and a sufficient quantity of simple syrup to bring the volume to 100 mL was stable for 12 weeks at room temperature. Shake well before use.

▶ PROCHLORPERAZINE INJECTION, SOLUTION, TABLETS, AND CAPSULES (Rx)

Store at room temperature in airtight, light-resistant containers. Avoid freezing. Discard discolored solution.

▶ PROMETHAZINE INJECTION, TABLETS, SOLUTION, AND SUPPOSITORIES (Rx)

Store oral and parenteral products at room temperature. Refrigerate suppositories between 2° C and 8° C (36° F and 46° F). Protect all forms from light, and avoid freezing.

▶ PSEUDOEPHEDRINE AND PSEUDOEPHEDRINE/ TRIPROLIDINE TABLETS AND CAPSULES (OTC)

Pseudoephedrine tablets and capsules: Store between 15° C and 25° C (59° F and 77° F) in a dry place and protect from light. Do not crush.
Triprolidine tablets and capsules: Store at room temperature and protect from light.

▶ SILDENAFIL TABLETS (Rx)

Store at room temperature.

▶ SIMETHICONE TABLETS, CAPSULES, AND DROPS (OTC)

Store at room temperature in airtight container. Protect from light and freezing.

▶ **SODIUM BICARBONATE INJECTION (Rx)**

Store 50 mL injection ampules at room temperature. Brief exposure to 40° C (104° F) will not compromise efficacy. Do not freeze, and do not use if product has been frozen.

▶ **SODIUM SULFACETAMIDE OPHTHALMIC SOLUTION AND OINTMENT (Rx)**

Ophthalmic solution: Store in a light-resistant container in a cool place, between 8° C and 15° C (46° F and 59° F). Discard if solution darkens to brown.

Ophthalmic ointment: Store at room temperature and do not freeze.

▶ **TEMAZEPAM CAPSULES (S IV)**

Store at room temperature in airtight container. Protect from light.

▶ **TETANUS TOXOID (Rx)**

Injection: Toxoid should be refrigerated; however, it remains stable for months when stored at room temperature. Do not freeze, and do not use if product has been frozen.

▶ **TETRACAINE HYDROCHLORIDE OPHTHALMIC SOLUTION (Rx)**

Protect ampules from light. Refrigerate between 2° C and 8° C (36° F and 46° F) to prevent crystallization and oxidation. Stable for several days at room temperature. If then returned to cool storage, the stability is as labeled by the manufacturer.

▶ **TETRACYCLINE TABLETS, TOPICAL SOLUTION, AND INJECTION (Rx)**

Outdated products may cause renal tubular disease.

Tablets: Store at room temperature. Protect from moisture or light (product will darken).

Topical: Solution prepared with diluent from the manufacturer is stable for 2 months at room temperature.

Injection: Reconstituted solutions are stable at room temperature for 12 hours (6 to 12 hours in 5% dextrose in water).

▶ **TOLNAFTATE TOPICAL ANTIFUNGAL (OTC)**

Store between 2° C and 30° C (36° F and 86° F). Do not freeze. May solidify at low temperatures but liquefies easily when warmed; its potency is not affected. Aerosol products are under pressure. Do not puncture or place in proximity to heat/flame.

▶ TRIAZOLAM TABLETS (S IV)

Store at room temperature, and protect from light.

▶ TRIMETHOPRIM/SULFAMETHOXAZOLE TABLETS, SUSPENSIONS, AND INJECTION (Rx)

Oral preparations: Store tablets and suspensions in a dry place, either between 15° C and 25° C (59° F and 77° F) or at room temperature, depending on the formulation.

Injection: should be used within 4 or 6 hours (depending on dilution in D5W). Injection (16 mg/80 mg per mL) has been shown to maintain greater than 90% stability for more than 60 hours when stored in polypropylene syringes. Discard if cloudy or if precipitate is present. Use within 24 hours if using multiple-use vial for injection. Protect from light. Do not refrigerate or freeze.

▶ VERAPAMIL HYDROCHLORIDE TABLETS AND INJECTION (Rx)

Store at controlled room temperature 15° C to 30° C (59° F to 86° F). Protect from light. Store extended-release tablets at controlled room temperature 20° C to 25° C (68° F to 77° F). Dispense oral forms in tight, light-resistant container. Protect from moisture. Discard any unused amount of parenteral solution.

▶ ZINC SALTS (OTC)

Zinc oxide (e.g., calamine) is practically insoluble in alcohol and water but dissolves in dilute mineral acids. Store zinc acetate in airtight containers and zinc chloride and sulfate in airtight nonmetallic containers. Zinc sulfate ophthalmic solutions should be stored below 40° C (104° F) in tightly closed or airtight containers. Avoid freezing.

▶ ZOLPIDEM TABLETS (S IV)

Store at controlled room temperature in airtight container.

Index

Note: Page numbers followed by b, f, or t refer to boxes, figures, and tables, respectively.